Flexible
Bronchoscopy

Flexible Bronchoscopy

Ko-Pen Wang, MD, FCCP
Director, Interventional Bronchology,
Johns Hopkins Bayview Medical Center
Professor of Medicine,
Chest Diagnostic Center,
Division of Pulmonary Medicine,
Harbor Medical Center,
Baltimore, Maryland

Atul C. Mehta, MB, BS, FACP, FCCP
Head, Section of Bronchology
Staff Physician, Department of Pulmonary and
Critical Care Medicine,
Associate Professor of Medicine,
Cleveland Clinic Foundation,
Health Sciences Center of Ohio State University,
Cleveland, Ohio
Secretary, American Association for Bronchology,
Associate Editor, *Journal of Bronchology*

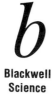

Blackwell Science

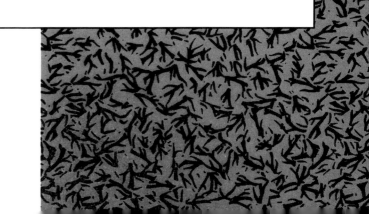

Blackwell Science

Editorial offices:

238 Main Street, Cambridge, Massachusetts
02142, USA

Osney Mead, Oxford OX2 0EL, England

25 John Street, London WC1N 2BL, England

23 Ainslie Place, Edinburgh EH3 6AJ, Scotland

54 University Street, Carlton, Victoria 3053,
Australia

Arnette Blackwell SA, 1 rue de Lille, 75007
Paris, France

Blackwell-Wissenschafts-Verlag GmbH,
Kurfürstendamm 57, 10707 Berlin,
Germany

Feldgasse 13, A-1238 Vienna, Austria

Distributors

North America

Blackwell Science, Inc.

238 Main Street

Cambridge, Massachusetts 02142

(Telephone orders: 800-215-1000 or
617-876-7000)

Australia

Blackwell Science Pty Ltd

54 University Street

Carlton, Victoria 3053

(Telephone orders: 03-347-5552)

Outside North America and Australia

Blackwell Science, Ltd.

c/o Marston Book Services, Ltd.

P.O. Box 87

Oxford OX2 0DT

England

(Telephone orders: 44-865-791155)

Acquisitions: Victoria Reeders
Development: Coleen Traynor
Production: Michelle Choate
Manufacturing: Kathleen Grimes
Typeset by A-R Editions, Madison, WI

Designed by Joyce C. Weston
Printed and bound by Braun-Brumfield, Inc.,
Ann Arbor, MI

© 1995 by Blackwell Science, Inc.

Printed in the United States of America

95 96 97 98 5 4 3 2 1

Notice: The indications and dosages of all drugs in
this book have been recommended in the medical
literature and conform to the practices of the general medical community. The medications
described do not necessarily have specific approval
by the Food and Drug Administration for use in
the diseases and dosages for which they are recommended. The package insert for each drug
should be consulted for use and dosage as
approved by the FDA. Because standards of usage
change, it is advisable to keep abreast of revised
recommendations, particularly those concerning
new drugs.

*Library of Congress Cataloging-in-Publication
Data*

Flexible bronchoscopy [edited by] / Ko-Pen Wang,
Atul Mehta.

    p. cm.

    Includes bibliographical references and
index.

    ISBN 0-86542-289-3

    1. Bronchoscopy.   I. Wang, Ko-Pen.

    II. Mehta, Atul.

RC734.B7F54 1995   95-4235

616.2'307545—dc20   CIP

To my loving wife, Shu-Lian, for all the support you have given to me over the years.

Ko-Pen Wang

To my wife Shuva, whose career has been to support mine.

Atul C. Mehta

Contents

Contributors

Muzaffar Ahmad, MD
Chairman of Medicine
Cleveland Clinic Foundation
Cleveland, Ohio

Alejandro C. Arroliga, MD
Staff Physician
Department of Pulmonary and Critical Care
    Medicine
Cleveland Clinic Foundation
Cleveland, Ohio

Heinrich D. Becker, MD
Assistant Medical Director
Departments of Internal Medicine/Oncology and
    Endoscopy
Hospital for Chest Diseases
Heidelberg, Germany

Glen E. DeBoer, MD
Staff Physician
Department of Anesthesiology
Cleveland Clinic Foundation
Cleveland, Ohio

Philip Eng, MD
Consultant
Department of Medicine III
Singapore General Hospital
Singapore

Elliot K. Fishman, MD
The Russell H. Morgan Department of Radiology
    and Radiological Science
Director, Abdominal Imaging and Body CT
The Johns Hopkins University School of Medicine
Baltimore, Maryland

Randall J. Harris, MD
Senior Fellow
Department of Pulmonary and Critical Care
    Medicine
Cleveland Clinic Foundation
Cleveland, Ohio

Edward M. Harrow, MD, FCCP, FACP
Director, Respiratory Department
Eastern Maine Medical Center
Bangor, Maine

Richard A. Helmers, MD
Chair, Thoracic Diseases and Critical Care
    Medicine
Mayo Clinic Scottsdale
Scottsdale, Arizona

Basil S. Hilaris, MD, FACR
Chief, Department of Radiation Oncology
New York Medical College
Valhalla, New York

Gary W. Hunninghake, MD
Professor and Director
Division of Pulmonary, Critical Care and
    Occupational Medicine
University of Iowa Hospital and Clinic
Iowa City, Iowa

Mani S. Kavuru, MD
Director, Pulmonary Function Laboratory
Department of Pulmonary and Critical Care
    Medicine
Cleveland Clinic Foundation
Cleveland, Ohio

Akira Kawashima, MD
The Russell H. Morgan Department of Radiology
    and Radiological Science
The Johns Hopkins Medical Institutions
Baltimore, Maryland

Janet E. Kuhlman, MD
The Russell M. Morgan Department of Radiology
    and Radiological Science
The Johns Hopkins Medical Institutions
Baltimore, Maryland

Francis Y. W. Lee, MD, MBBS, FCCP
Consultant, Respiratory Medicine
Tan Tock Seng Hospital
Singapore

Mark S. Lingenfelter, MD, FCCP
Director, Intensive Care Unit
Eastern Maine Medical Center
Bangor, Maine

David P. Meeker, MD
Medical Director
Genzyme
Cambridge, Massachusetts

Atul C. Mehta, MB, FCCP, FACP
Head, Section of Bronchology
Department of Pulmonary and Critical Care
  Medicine
Cleveland Clinic Foundation
Cleveland, Ohio

Chitti R. Moorthy, MD
Professor, Department of Radiation Medicine
New York Medical College
Valhalla, New York

Frederick A. Oldenburg, Jr., MD, FCCP
Director, Respiratory Department
St. Joseph Hospital
Bangor, Maine

Anwar R. Padhani, MRCP, FRCR
Department of Radiology
Guy's Hospital
London, England

Sunit R. Patel, MD
Staff Physician
Merced Community Medical Center,
  Merced Hospital, and Merced Pulmonary
  Medical Associates
Merced, California

Michael S. Porrazzo, MD
Department of Radiation Medicine
New York Medical College
Valhalla, New York

Udaya B. S. Prakash, MD, FRCP, FACP, FCCP
Director of Bronchoscopy
Mayo Clinic and Medical Center
Thoracic Diseases and Internal Medicine
Rochester, Minnesota

Navdeep S. Rai, MD
Staff Physician
Kelsey-Bold Clinic
Houston, Texas

Marc S. Rovner, MD
Senior Fellow
Department of Pulmonary and Critical Care
  Medicine
Cleveland Clinic Foundation
Cleveland, Ohio

David A. Schenk, MD, FCCP
San Antonio, Texas

Raul J. Seballos, MD
Senior Fellow
Department of Pulmonary and Critical Care
  Medicine
Cleveland Clinic Foundation
Cleveland, Ohio

A. Marshall Smith, Jr., MD, FCCP
Department of Medicine
Eastern Maine Medical Center
Bangor, Maine

Paul C. Stillwell
Head, Section of Pediatric Pulmonary Medicine
Cleveland Clinic Foundation
Cleveland, Ohio

James K. Stoller, MD
Head, Section of Respiratory Medicine
Staff, Pulmonary and Critical Care Medicine
Cleveland Clinic Foundation
Cleveland, Ohio

James P. Utz, MD
Senior Associate Consultant in Thoracic Diseases
  and Internal Medicine
Mayo Clinic and Medical Center
Rochester, Minnesota

Ko-Pen Wang, MD
Associate Professor of Medicine, Otolaryngology,
  Head and Neck Surgery
Division of Pulmonary Medicine
Johns Hopkins University
Director, Chest Diagnostic Center
Harbor Hospital Center
Baltimore, Maryland

Foreword

We are approaching the centennial anniversary of when physicians first began to insert instruments into the airways for visualization and sampling capabilities. Indeed, it was in 1897 that Killian first reported to his colleagues that a system to inspect the airway lumen was possible, and that he had removed a foreign body. The response of his peers to such a report was far from enthusiastic; they felt that purposeful instrumentation of the airway was far more dangerous than any potential benefit that might be derived. From that meager beginning, we have seen an avalanche of advancing technology in bronchoscopy. Nineteen sixty-six was another landmark year. That was when Shigeto Iketa introduced the flexible bronchoscope for clinical practice. The airways suddenly became much more accessible, and not just because more peripheral branches could be visualized. Rather, the types of physicians who could master the use of a flexible bronchoscope underwent drastic changes, and many more patients, along with their problems, became accessible to this new type of instrument and the skills of the physicians who use flexible bronchoscopes.

This book is written for and is intended to be used by flexible bronchoscopists. It is not about rigid bronchoscopes. That is not to say that the editors and their contributing authors do not recognize that there is still a place for rigid bronchoscopes in the practice and management of airway problems. Instead it is an effort by the editors of this book to place emphasis upon the great utility and widespread application of the flexible bronchoscope in the practice of pulmonary medicine and related disciplines in the 1990s and beyond. Even as this text is being published, we who use flexible bronchoscopes are adapting to another major advance in technology: the video bronchoscope. Newer students of flexible bronchoscopy will learn their skills while watching the image on nearby monitors; those of us who have looked directly through optical fiberoptic bronchoscopes are adapting to this change. The quality of the images is vastly superior with video bronchoscopes, but there are limitations and pitfalls with this new set of instruments, too. Thus, as there is still room and need for rigid bronchoscopes, there is a continuing need for optical and video flexible bronchoscopes as well.

This is also a textbook with a practical intent. That is to say, the editors envision that those who read this book will open it frequently to "brush up" on specific points as they plan an approach to specific problems with the patients they plan to bronchoscope. One chapter contains side-by-side color photographs and diagrams to illustrate the endoscopic anatomy; clockface orientation of the findings is used for description, which is a common way for teacher and student to communicate. There are step-by-step text instructions concerning how and where to insert needles or to use other sampling devices for optimal yield and avoidance of complications. Similar step-by-step instructions are given for aiming lasers or other therapeutic maneuvers with flexible bronchoscopes. Many other practical points also receive detailed attention, from the care and maintenance of delicate and expensive equipment through a broad spectrum of diagnostic and therapeutic applications.

The combined experience of the contributing authors includes well over one thousand articles written and published in referred periodicals, and over one hundred thousand bronchoscopic procedures. From this vast experience, the individual practitioner of flexible bronchoscopy should view this text as a familiar friend and a helping hand in the community application of a procedure for many individual situations.

Paul A. Kvale, MD
Senior Staff Physician, Division of Pulmonary
and Critical Care Medicine,
Henry Ford Hospital, Detroit, Michigan
Professor of Medicine, Case Western Reserve
University School of Medicine, Cleveland, Ohio
Clinical Professor of Medicine,
University of Michigan School of Medicine,
Ann Arbor, Michigan

Preface

Almost a quarter of a century ago, Shigeto Iketa invented the flexible bronchoscope. Today, flexible bronchoscopy has become one of the most frequently performed invasive procedures in pulmonary medicine. Proliferation of diagnostic and therapeutic indications has led to design modifications of the instrument and the emergence of fancy flexible accessories. Furthermore, laser technology has added a new dimension to the field of bronchology. Insuring the welfare of lung transplant recipients would be difficult, if not impossible, without aid from the instrument.

Interest in the field of bronchology has brought pulmonologists of the world together, as evidenced by establishment of various associations, scientific meetings, and peer reviewed publications.

It is obvious that neither flexible bronchoscopy nor the endobronchial tree remain a total curiosity. Several beautiful monographs, atlases, and worthy textbooks have gallantly served the interest of bronchoscopists over the last several years. We, as the editors and contributors of this publication, make an attempt to take a step further toward the horizons of flexible bronchoscopy. We believe that "non-diagnostic bronch" is a failure for any modern day pulmonologist and a deception to the patient, as it creates problems with time, discomfort, and high cost. We emphasize proper selection of the patient and discourage misuse of the procedure. Newer diagnostic and therapeutic procedures have been described in a "cookbook" fashion for practical application. We hope the chapter on applied anatomy will be helpful in reducing complications and increase diagnostic yield, while information on repair and maintenance should help reduce the cost of the procedure.

The field of bronchology is ever growing and no book remains the ultimate. We hope readers will find this book a step closer to the frontiers of bronchology.

Flexible Bronchoscopy

Part 1

Fundamentals of Bronchoscopy

1 | Bronchoscopy: Current Status and Future Prospects

Muzaffar Ahmad

Bronchoscopy was first performed by Killian in 1895 to directly visualize the trachea and bronchi and to remove foreign bodies. The indications gradually expanded and with the advent of fiberoptic bronchoscopy (FOB) in the late 1960s the tracheobronchial tree could be visualized to the level of subsegmental divisions. This ability coupled with significant technical improvements in various biopsy instruments has made FOB the most useful technique for the diagnosis of lung cancer. The maneuverability of the fiberoptic bronchoscope, along with the comfort of the patient, improved diagnostic accuracy, and the documented safety as an outpatient procedure, has enabled the rigid bronchoscope to be replaced by the fiberoptic models. Rigid bronchoscopy is now being used for selective indications such as massive hemoptysis, resectional procedures of central airways (lasers or otherwise), and stent placements. Indications for rigid and fiberoptic bronchoscopy are listed in Tables 1.1 and 1.2.

Fiberoptic bronchoscopy has also achieved an increasing role in staging of lung cancer. This is due to its ability to detect proximal extension of lesions, to evaluate major carina, and to document mediastinal node involvement through various transbronchial and transtracheal needle aspiration techniques (1).

Portions of text have been reproduced or adapted with permission from Ahmad M, Kavuru MS. Flexible bronchoscopy: current status and future directions. J Bronchology 1994;1:89–91.

FOB along with transbronchial biopsy can be performed safely on an outpatient basis, thus avoiding extra costs related to hospitalization (2). These significant advantages, unfortunately, have not changed the dismal survival rate from bronchogenic carcinoma. There is lack of evidence to recommend FOB as a component of a lung cancer screening program (3). This is also true of some newer lung cancer

Table 1.1. Indications for Fiberoptic Bronchoscopy

Abnormal chest x-ray (mass/nodule)
  Suspicion of cancer/infection
Hemoptysis
Respiratory infections (specimen retrieval)
Diffuse lung disease
Chronic cough
Immunocompromised patient (cancer patient, HIV positive)
Therapeutic bronchoscopy (mucous plug, atelectasis, foreign bodies)
Laser procedures
Intubation
Upper airway examination
Research applications (bronchoalveolar lavage, biopsies)

Table 1.2. Indications for Rigid Bronchoscopy

Massive hemoptysis
Central tumors
Laser procedures
Endobronchial resection
Foreign body removal
Stent placement

detection techniques, namely, endobronchial scintillation, photodynamic lasers, and endobronchial sonography.

The role of FOB in lung infections depends on the likely infecting organisms, the clinical setting, and the underlying immune status of the patient. The use of protected specimen brushes does not seem justified in patients who have received prior antibiotics. In pulmonary tuberculosis, FOB contributes to evaluation of patients who are clinically suspected of having tuberculosis but have negative smears for acid-fast bacilli. In this setting segmental lavage in combination with transbronchial biopsy may provide important diagnostic information. This may become even more important with the reemergence of tuberculosis as a major health hazard in the United States. FOB is being increasingly used in immunocompromised hosts and critically ill patients. Bronchoalveolar lavage (BAL) fluid when processed properly has been of immense help in this regard. The diagnostic yield of FOB in combination with BAL in immunocompromised patients with diffuse pulmonary infiltrates varies from 30% to almost 100% (4). These studies have concentrated on patient-specific diagnostic yields. Information in the future should include patient outcomes, namely, survival and performance status.

In diffuse interstitial lung disease, the role of FOB is still evolving. Its usefulness for specific diagnostic yield in sarcoidosis, hypersensitivity pneumonitis, chronic eosinophilic pneumonia, pulmonary histiocytosis X, chronic berylliosis, and pulmonary alveolar proteinosis has been established; however, its role along with BAL in assessment of alveolitis and as a guide to therapy are controversial. Because of conflicting data and variable laboratory standards, it is prudent to be cautious against over-interpretation and use the serial lavage for its research application.

Bronchoscopy has a therapeutic role in several areas. FOB is useful in removal of mucous plugs, treatment of segmental and lobar atelec-

tasis, resection of benign lesions, and extension of laser technology to both malignant and non-malignant lesions. The patient groups for these indications are small and there is potential for misuse of therapeutic bronchoscopy as it relates to the evacuation of secretions and treatment of atelectasis.

In recent years FOB and BAL have become exciting research tools. Great insight has been provided into the mechanism of airway inflammation in bronchial asthma (5) and also lung injury in acute respiratory distress syndrome. BAL studies have also contributed a large amount of information in immune altered states such as sarcoidosis, idiopathic pulmonary fibrosis, hypersensitivity pneumonitis, and chronic berylliosis. Access to molecular biology as a diagnostic aid has also occurred through BAL.

In the era of escalating health care costs, it is important that indications of bronchoscopy be optimized (6). This encompasses a cost-effective approach to bronchoscopy. Bronchoscopic procedures have the great potential for overutilization and need constant reappraisal. The indications that need to be looked at include chronic cough with normal chest x-ray, mild hemoptysis in association with acute bronchitis in a nonsmoker, and pleural effusion without an accompanying pulmonary or hilar lesion. Alternative strategies to the use of bronchoscopy need to be studied in these and other conditions. As an example, empirical therapy may be a better management strategy than early bronchoscopy in patients infected with human immunodeficiency virus (HIV) with presumptive *Pneumocystis carinii* pneumonia. Principles of medical technology assessment must be applied to newer bronchoscopic technologies while emphasizing the complex learning curves of new techniques.

There is indeed a most promising future in the continued application of FOB and its related technology for specimen retrieval to enhance research. The emphasis will continue to be at the molecular level. BAL analysis in asthmatics has provided a considerable fund of new knowledge through study of inflammatory cells and mediators. This knowledge is complemented by bronchial biopsies. BAL analysis has contributed to the information regarding surfactant abnormalities in acute lung injury. Availability of DNA probes to diagnose various bacterial, parasitic, and viral diseases should extend the use of BAL and result in early identification of these infectious agents, thus facilitating early and optimum treatment.

The challenge of the future in bronchoscopy, especially FOB, is to continue to expand its horizon in research at the molecular biology and cellular levels. Additional clinical studies are required to study the impact of this technology on patient outcomes and cost-effective management.

REFERENCES

1. Shure D. Fiberoptic bronchoscopy—diagnostic applications. Clin Chest Med 1987;8:1–13.
2. Ahmad M, Livingston DR, Golish JA, Mehta AL, Wiedemann HP. The safety of outpatient transbronchial biopsy. Chest 1986;90:403–405.
3. Berlin NI, Buncher CF, Fontana RS, et al. The National Cancer Institute Cooperative Early Lung Cancer Detection Program. Am Rev Respir Dis 1984;130:545–549.
4. Broaddus C, Dake MD, Stulbarg MS, et al. Bronchoalveolar lavage and transbronchial biopsy for the diagnosis of pulmonary infections in acquired immunodeficiency syndrome. Ann Intern Med 1985;102:747–752.
5. Smith DL, Deshazo RD. Bronchoalveolar lavage in asthma. An update and perspective. Am Rev Respir Dis 1993;148:523–532.
6. Prakash UBS, Stubbs SE. Optimal bronchoscopy. J Bronchology 1994;1:44–62.

Applied Anatomy of the Airways | 2

Mani S. Kavuru and Atul C. Mehta

The Pharynx and the Larynx

Flexible bronchoscopy is usually performed either via the oral or nasal route. Familiarity with the normal anatomy in this region is important to gain access to the trachea as well as to recognize local pathology. Certainly, bronchoscopy performed for the evaluation of hemoptysis or wheezing should include a careful evaluation of the upper airway. The nose extends from the external nares through the nasal cavity and the nasal pharynx. Each nasal cavity is bounded medially by the nasal septum, laterally by the three bony projections called turbinates or conchae, and inferiorly by the hard palate, which separates the nasal cavity from the mouth. The paranasal sinuses open into an area below each turbinate called a meatus. The blood supply to the nasal mucosa is via branches of the maxillary artery and the facial artery, which anastomose to form the Kisselbach's plexus at the anterior medial wall of the nose, which is a common site of nasal bleeding (1).

The pharynx is 12 to 15 cm long; it communicates anteriorly with the nasal cavity (nasopharynx) and the oral cavity (oropharynx) and extends to the cricoid cartilage inferiorly to encompass the hypopharynx or larynx (1). The pharyngeal muscles, including the cricopharyngeous muscle, act as a sphincter to the proximal esophagus and help to prevent the reflux of esophageal contents. The adenoids or nasopharyngeal tonsils lie on the posterior wall of the nasopharynx. The oropharynx is bounded laterally by the tonsillar pillars, superiorly by the soft palate, anteriorly and inferiorly by the tongue, and posteriorly by the C-2 and C-3 vertebrae. The oropharyngeal cavity is not rigid and is subject to collapse easily. The hypopharynx lies between the epiglottis and the inferior border of the cricoid cartilage. The larynx, which is 5 to 7 cm in length and lies at the level of C-4, C-5, and C-6, is a complex organ composed of cartilages, ligaments, and muscles (1). The endoscopic view of the larynx would demonstrate the epiglottis anteriorly and superiorly, aryepiglottic folds bilaterally with the pyriform sinuses alongside. The glottis is bounded anteriorly and laterally by the vestibular folds (false cords) and vocal folds (true cords) and posteriorly by the arytenoid cartilage (2). During inspiration, the vocal cords are abducted away from the midline and the rima glottidis has a triangular appearance. On expiration, the vocal cords are adducted medially with a very small opening between them. During maximal abduction the distance between the vocal processes is 19 mm in men and 12 mm in women. In adults, unlike children, the glottic chink is the narrowest part of the larynx (2).

The Tracheobronchial Tree

The normal adult trachea begins at the lower margin of the cricoid cartilage and extends 10 to 14 cm until the bifurcation into the left and right main stem bronchi at the level of T-5. One third of the trachea is "extrathoracic," above the level of the suprasternal notch, and two thirds is "intrathoracic" or below the notch. The average tracheal diameter is 2.5 cm and is supported anteriorly by 18 to 24 incomplete C-shaped cartilaginous elements and posteriorly by the membranous trachealis muscle. In the normal adult, the diameter of the entire trachea is well maintained throughout the respiratory cycle by the rigid support of the tracheal elements. In patients with obstructive airways disease or older individuals, the tracheal lumen may be dynamically reduced with coughing or during expiration because of collapse of the posterior membranous wall anteriorly (3). Normally, the aortic arch compresses the mid to distal left lateral wall of the trachea to the right. The adult tracheal width/depth ratio can vary from 0.6 (high-domed variant) to 3.0 (lunate variant). The main carina is normally quite sharp and is mobile during the respiratory cycle (4). The right main stem bronchus normally bifurcates at an angle of 25° to 30° from the midline with a luminal diameter of around 16 mm and an average length of 2 cm before the bifurcation of the right upper lobe bronchus from the right main stem bronchus. The right upper lobe orifice averages 10 mm and it usually branches into the apical, posterior, and anterior segmental bronchi (5). After the bifurcation of the right upper lobe bronchus, the right main stem bronchus continues as the bronchus intermedius. The anterior wall of the intermedius bronchus continues to become the right middle lobe, which divides into the medial and lateral subsegments. By virtue of its anterior location, foreign bodies have a propensity to continue from the trachea and fall into the right middle lobe. The right lower lobe bronchus represents the posterior continuation of the bronchus intermedius, further dividing into five subsegments with frequent variation (6). The superior or apical subsegment usually arises posteriorly opposite to the origin of the middle lobe bronchus. Next, the medial basal subsegment arises on the medial wall and

may subdivide further. The right lower lobe subsequently divides into the anterior, lateral, and posterior basal subsegments. These latter three subsegments are usually stacked one on top of the other proceeding from anterior to posterior configuration (A-L-P-).

The left main stem bifurcates from the trachea at a sharp angle of 45° from the midline. It is narrower and much longer than its counterpart with an average length of 5 cm. The distal left main stem bronchus primarily divides into the left upper and the left lower lobe. The upper divides into the lingular division (which is composed of the superior and inferior lingular subsegments) and the upper lobe division (composed of the apical posterior and anterior subsegments). The lower lobe initially gives rise to the superior or apical subsegment, which is posteriorly located. The left lower lobe subsequently divides into the anterior-medial, lateral, and posterior basal subsegments. There is again considerable variability in the basilar subsegments of the left lower lobe (6,7).

The Relationship of Airways to Lymph Nodes and Vessels

As important as a thorough understanding of the normal endobronchial anatomy and the frequent congenital variations is a thorough familiarity with normal structures that are outside of the airway in intimate juxtaposition to the airway (8). This knowledge is mandatory with the increasing use of endobronchial diagnostic and therapeutic modalities including transbronchial needle aspiration (TBNA), laser therapy, and endobronchial radiation therapy. This anatomic knowledge will help facilitate access to lymph nodes or extraluminal mass lesions that may be important in either diagnosis or staging (9,10). This understanding will hopefully avoid inadvertent access of vascular structures that are intimately associated with the airways in several areas.

The posterior aspect of the trachea is closely

associated with the esophagus. The aortic arch lies anterior and to the left of the distal one third of the trachea and makes an easily recognizable pulsatile imprint on the anterolateral tracheal wall and this area should be avoided for obvious reasons (8). The superior vena cava and the azygos vein lie anteriorly and to the right of the distal third of the trachea. The aortic arch and the inominate artery lie directly anterior to the trachea at the level of the main carina. The right pulmonary artery lies immediately anterior to the right main stem bronchus and the origin of the right upper lobe bronchus. There is significant variability of the relationship of vascular structures to the right middle lobe and lower lobe bronchi. The aortic arch and the left pulmonary artery are in close association to the left main stem bronchus and left upper lobe bronchus.

Lymph nodes lie in close association to the airway. The paratracheal lymph nodes lie on either side of the length of the trachea in a posterolateral distribution. The right paratracheal lymphatic drainage is most easily accessed at one or two tracheal rings above the main carina before the bifurcation on the right posterolateral aspect (Figure 2.1). The subcarinal mediastinal lymph nodes normally lie immediately inferior to the main carina. This chain can be most easily sampled not by direct aspiration of the main carina itself, but by entry with a transbronchial needle 3 to 5 mm below on either side of the main carina with a lateral to inferomedial entry (Figure 2.2). This would minimize having to go through the cartilaginous element itself. Hilar lymph nodes may be sampled at either the secondary carina where the right upper lobe bifurcates from the bronchus intermedius or at the level of the secondary carina where the left upper lobe bifurcates from the left main stem bronchus (Figure 2.3). The right pulmonary artery is in close association with the anterior wall of the right upper lobe bronchus; therefore, TBNA and other procedures are not recommended (Figure 2.4, Figure 2.5) at this site.

The left paratracheal lymth nodes are located at the origin of the left main stem bronchus from the main trachea (Figure 2.6). This chain is particularly difficult to sample, however, aspiration can be performed by using a transbronchial needle anchored to the lateral tracheal wall of the distal trachea at the level of the carina with a subsequent downward or inferior movement of the entire bronchoscope, hence facilitating entry of the needle laterally. Figure 2.7 demonstrates the association of left upper lobe bronchus and the left pulmonary artery. Figure 2.8 demonstrates location of left hilar lymph nodes.

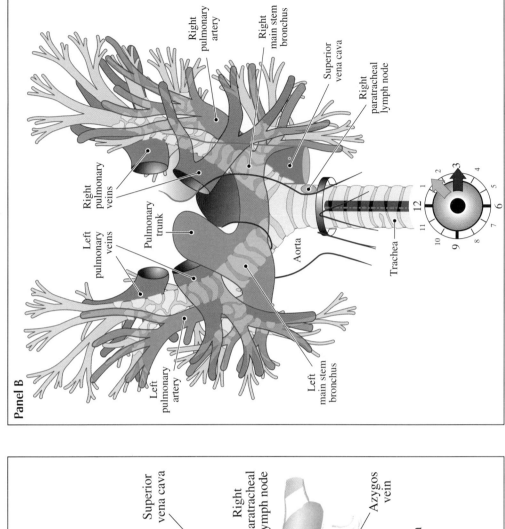

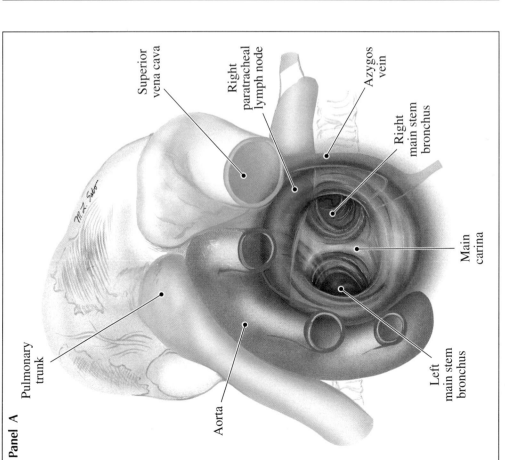

Figure 2.1. Schematic representation of normal anatomic relationships at the level of the distal trachea.
Panel A demonstrates the endoscopic view of the distal trachea, with adjacent vessels and lymph nodes superimposed. The right paratracheal lymph node is between the one and two o'clock position, whereas the azygous vein is located at the three o'clock position.
Panel B shows an endoscopic clock face view, with green arrow indicating proper site for TBNA of right paratracheal lymph node. The red arrow indicates the unsafe location for aspiration (azygous vein).

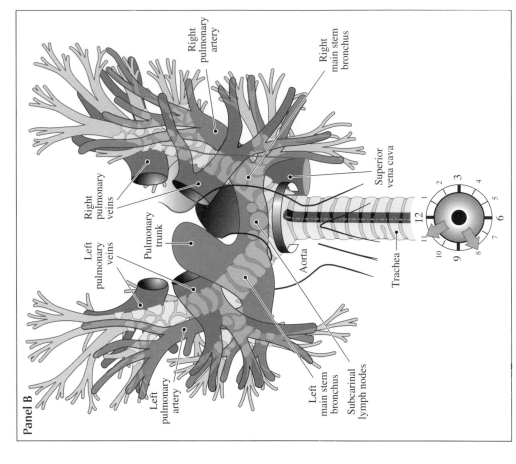

Panel B

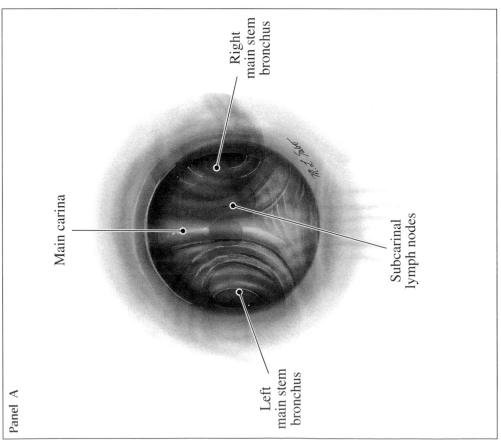

Panel A

Figure 2.2. Schematic representation of normal anatomic relationships at the level of the main carina.
Panel A demonstrates the endoscopic view of the main carina, with surrounding lymph nodes superimposed.
Panel B shows an endoscopic clock face view at the right main stem bronchus orifice. Green arrows at the eight and eleven o'clock positions indicate the proper site for TBNA of subcarinal lymph nodes.

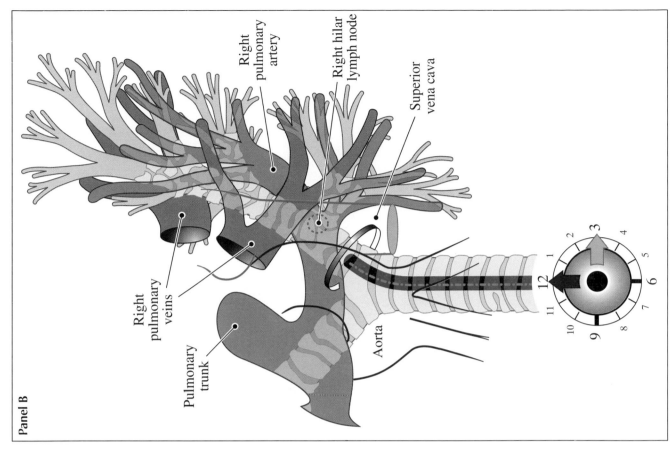

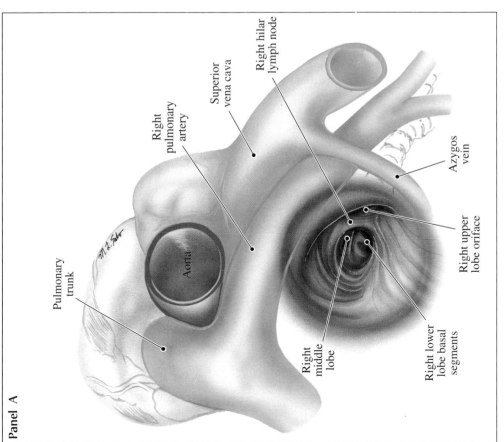

Figure 2.3. Schematic representation of normal anatomic relationships at the level of the proximal bronchus intermedius.
Panel A demonstrates the endoscopic view of the bronchus intermedius, with vessels and lymph nodes superimposed.
Panel B shows an endoscopic clock face view, with green arrow indicating proper site for TBNA of the right hilar lymph node. Red arrow indicates unsafe location for TBNA (right pulmonary artery).

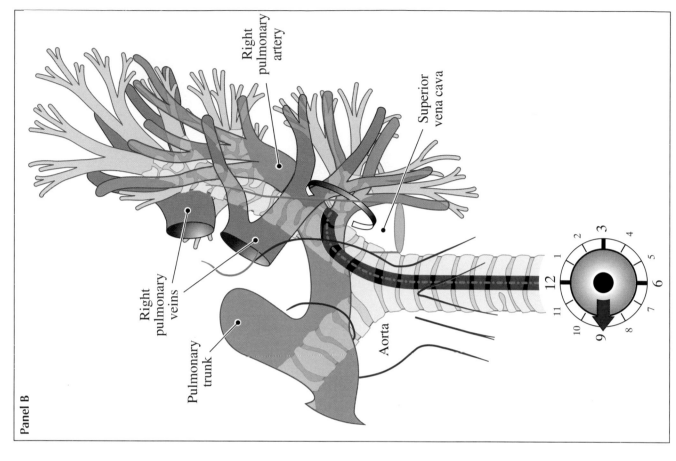

Panel B

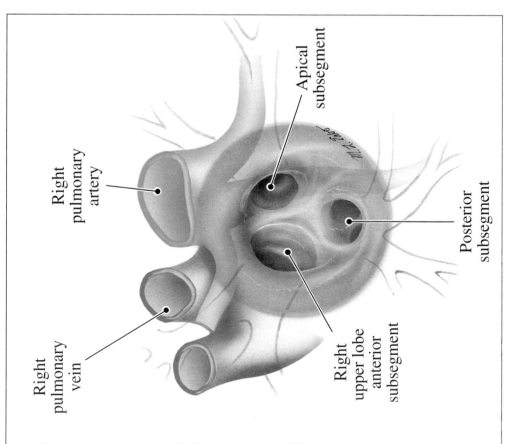

Figure 2.4. Schematic representation of normal anatomic relationships at the level of the right upper lobe orifice.
Panel A demonstrates the endoscopic view of the right upper lobe orifice, with sur–rounding vessels and lymph nodes superimposed.
Panel B shows an endoscopic clock face view, with red arrow indicating location of the right pulmonary artery.

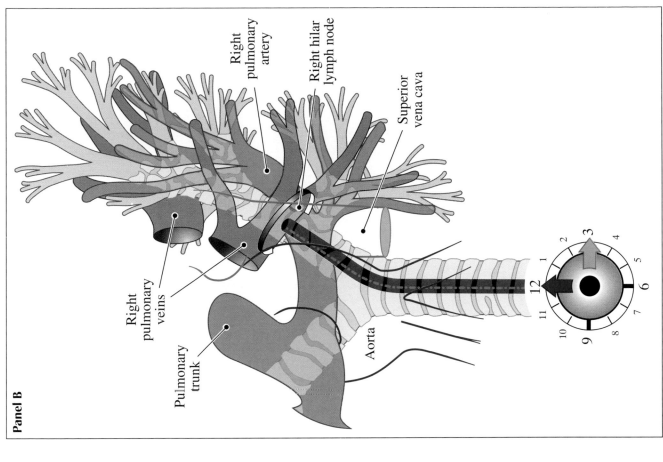

Panel B

Right pulmonary artery

Right hilar lymph node

Superior vena cava

Right pulmonary veins

Pulmonary trunk

Aorta

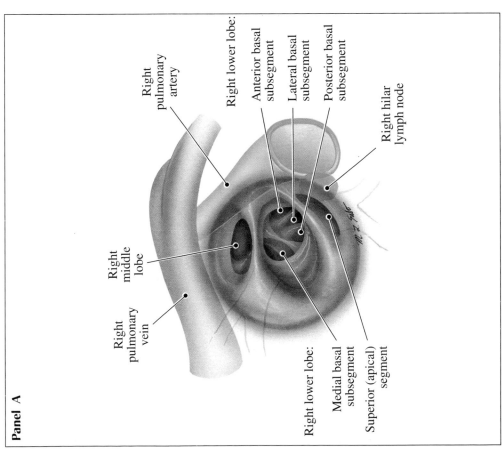

Panel A

Right pulmonary artery

Right middle lobe

Right pulmonary vein

Right lower lobe:

Anterior basal subsegment

Lateral basal subsegment

Posterior basal subsegment

Right hilar lymph node

Right lower lobe:

Medial basal subsegment

Superior (apical) segment

Figure 2.5. Schematic representation of normal anatomic relationships at the level of the distal bronchus intermedius. Note the relationship of the right middle lobe bronchus with surrounding vascular structures.
Panel A demonstrates the endoscopic view of the bronchus intermedius with hilar lymph node superimposed at the three o'clock position.
Panel B shows an endoscopic clock face view with the green arrow indicating the proper site for TBNA of right hilar lymph node. The red arrow indicates unsafe location (right pulmonary vein).

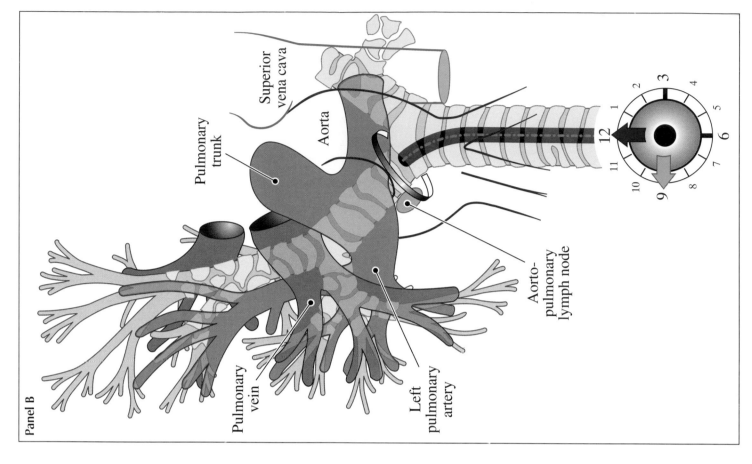

Panel B

Superior vena cava

Aorta

Pulmonary trunk

Aorto-pulmonary lymph node

Pulmonary vein

Left pulmonary artery

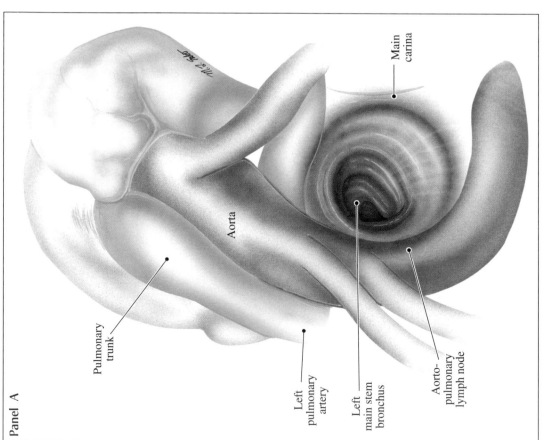

Panel A

Pulmonary trunk

Left pulmonary artery

Left main stem bronchus

Aorto-pulmonary lymph node

Aorta

Main carina

Figure 2.6. Schematic representation of normal anatomic relationships at the level of the left main stem bronchus orifice.

Panel A demonstrates the endoscopic view of the left main stem bronchus, with vessels and the aortopulmonary lymph node superimposed at the nine o'clock position.

Panel B shows an endoscopic clock face view, with green arrow indicating proper site for TBNA of aortopulmonary lymph node below the aortic knob. Red arrow indicates unsafe location (left pulmonary artery).

Panel B

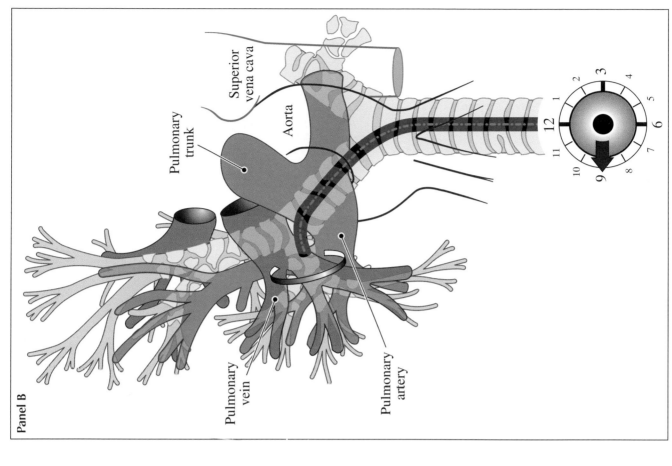

Superior vena cava

Pulmonary trunk

Aorta

Pulmonary vein

Pulmonary artery

Panel A

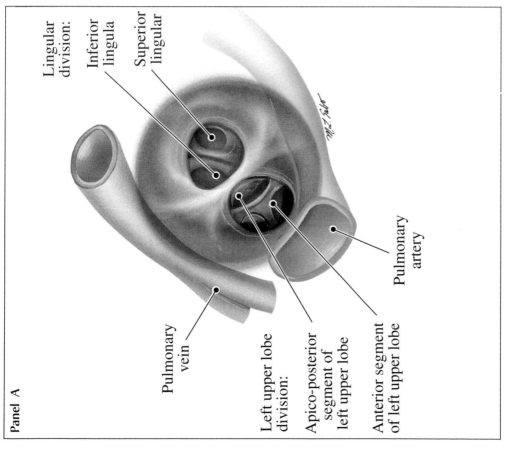

Pulmonary vein

Lingular division:

Inferior lingula

Superior lingular

Left upper lobe division:

Apico-posterior segment of left upper lobe

Anterior segment of left upper lobe

Pulmonary artery

Figure 2.7. Schematic representation of normal anatomic relationships at the level of the left upper lobe orifice.
Panel A demonstrates the endoscopic view of the left upper lobe bronchus, with vessels superimposed.
Panel B shows an endoscopic clock face view, with red arrow at nine o'clock indicating the location of the left pulmonary artery.

Panel B

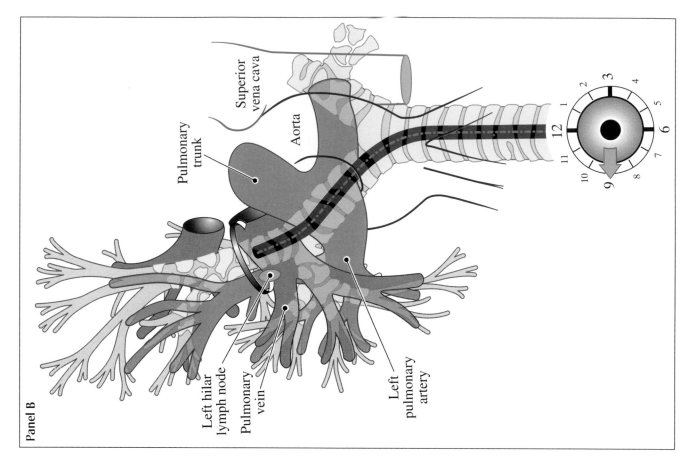

Panel A

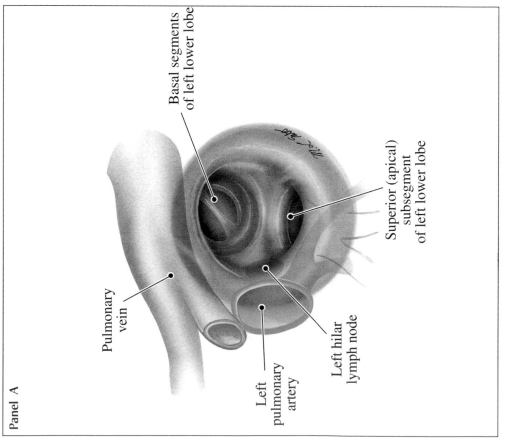

Figure 2.8. Schematic representation of normal anatomic relationships at the level of the left lower lobe orifice.

Panel A demonstrates the endoscopic view of the distal left main stem bronchus, with the left hilar lymph node at the nine o'clock position and vessels superimposed.

Panel B shows an endoscopic clock face view, with green arrow indicating proper site for TBNA of the left hilar lymph node.

REFERENCES

1. Ovassapian A. Anatomy of the airway. In: Ovassapian A, ed. Fiberoptic airway endoscopy in anesthesia and critical care. New York: Raven Press, 1990:15–25.
2. Peter LG, Sasaki CT. Laryngeal anatomy and physiology. In: Heffner JE, ed. Clinics in chest medicine: airway management in the critically ill patient. Philadelphia: WB Saunders, 1991: 415–423.
3. Stradling P. Diagnostic bronchoscopy, 4th ed. Edinburgh: Churchill Livingstone, 1981:34–59.
4. Ikeda S. Atlas of flexible bronchofiberscopy. Baltimore and London: University Park Press, 1974.
5. Zavala DC. Flexible fiberoptic bronchoscopy: a training handbook. Iowa City: Iowa University Press, 1978.
6. Boyden EA. Developmental anomalies of the lung. Am J Surg 1955;89:78–89.
7. Mehta AC, Ahmad M, Golish JA, Buonocore E. Congenital anomalies of the lung in the adult. Cleve Clin Q 1983;50:401–416.
8. Dumon JF, Meric B. Handbook of endobronchial laser surgery. Marseilles, France: Salvator Hospital Publication; 1983:7–22.
9. Mehta AC, Kavuru MS, Meeker DP, Gephardt GN, Nunez C. Transbronchial needle aspiration for histology specimens. Chest 1989;96: 1228–1232.
10. Mountain CF. A new international staging system for lung cancer. Chest 1986;89:225S–233S.

Examination of the Larynx through the Flexible Bronchoscope | 3

David P. Meeker

By definition, bronchoscopy emphasizes examination of the lower airway. However, with the exception of procedures performed via an endotracheal tube or tracheostomy, the procedure also permits a detailed laryngoscopic examination. The bronchoscopist should be well grounded in normal laryngeal anatomy and physiology. Laryngeal findings at the time of bronchoscopy may range from the incidental finding of a benign or malignant lesion to a specific finding that may explain the patient's reason for presenting to the pulmonologist. This chapter contains a brief review of laryngeal anatomy and physiology followed by a review of the more common pathophysiologic changes likely to be seen by the pulmonologist.

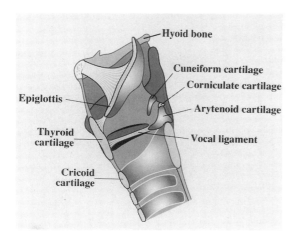

Figure 3.1. Midline cutaway view of the larynx.

Reproduced by permission from Tucker HM. Anatomy of the larynx. In: Tucker HM, ed. The larynx. New York: Thieme Medical Publishers, 1993:1–18.

Anatomy

The support structures of the larynx include the hyoid bone, three paired cartilages, and three unpaired cartilages (Figure 3.1) (1). The hyoid bone is located at the level of C-3 and forms the anterior aspect of the preepiglottic space. The hyoid bone does not articulate with any other cartilage or bony structure and is suspended between the supra- and infrahyoid musculature. The three unpaired cartilages consist of the nonossifying epiglottic cartilage, the thyroid cartilage that articulates with the cricoid cartilage at the inferior cornua bilaterally, and the cricoid cartilage that forms the base of the larynx. The three paired cartilages include the arytenoid cartilages—pyramidal shaped structures whose anteromedial pointed process (vocal process) is the point of attachment of the vocal ligament, small paired cone-shaped corniculate cartilages that form the apex of the arytenoids; and the cuneiform cartilages—rod-shaped structures located within the aryepiglottic folds.

The internal cavity consists of the supraglottic or vestibular area, which is bounded by the epiglottis, aryepiglottic folds, and the lower margin of the false vocal cords (Figure 3.2) (1). The true vocal cords form the glottis and consist of a cartilaginous portion supported by the vocal process of the arytenoid cartilage—and a membranous portion comprising the anterior two thirds of the cords. Reinke's space is a potential space lying just beneath the mucosal layer of the vocal cords. As will be discussed, trauma to the cords frequently results in edema fluid collecting within this space. The glottis separates the supra- from the subglottic space, which extends down to the lower margin of the cricoid cartilage. The pyriform sinuses lie lateral to the aryepiglottic folds (Figure 3.3).

The associated ligaments and muscles of the larynx are defined by their attachments (e.g., thyrohyoid ligament) (1). The extrinsic muscles of the larynx include the suprahyoid muscles, which elevate the larynx, and the infrahyoid muscles, which displace it downward. During swallowing the elevator muscles lift the larynx anteriorly and superiorly, which, combined with posterior downward movement of the tongue, compresses the epiglottis over the laryngeal introitus, preventing aspiration. Subsequent contraction of the cricopharyngeus muscle helps prevent swallowed material from spilling over into the glottis.

The intrinsic muscles are demonstrated in Figure 3.4. The posterior cricoarytenoideus (PCA) muscle is the sole laryngeal abductor, whereas contraction of the remaining muscles adduct the vocal cords and increase vocal cord tension (2). At rest the vocal cords lie in the paramedian position, slightly more adducted due to the greater muscle mass of the adductors. As shown in Figure 3.4B, PCA contraction internally rotates the muscular processes of the arytenoids, swinging the vocal processes and laterally widening the glottis. Conversely, contraction of the interarytenoideus muscles (Figure 3.4A), vocalis and lateral thyroarytenoideus muscles (Figure 3.4C), and cricoarytenoideus muscles (Figure 3.4D) result in adduction and tensing of the vocal cords.

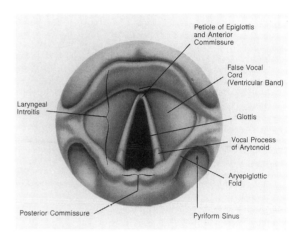

Figure 3.3. *A,* Schematic bronchoscopic view of the larynx.

Reproduced by permission from Tucker HM. Anatomy of the larynx. In: Tucker HM, ed. The larynx. New York: Thieme Medical Publishers, 1993:1–18.

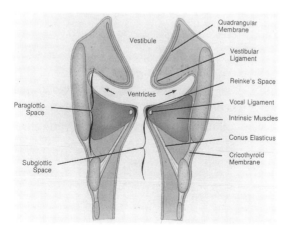

Figure 3.2. Coronal section of larynx (semidiagrammatic).

Reproduced by permission from Tucker HM. Anatomy of the larynx. In: Tucker HM, ed. The larynx. New York: Thieme Medical Publishers, 1993:1–18.

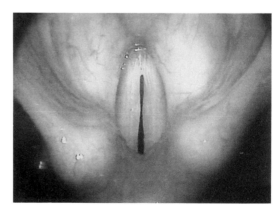

B, The normal larynx on phonation.

Photo courtesy of Eiji Yanagisawa, MD.

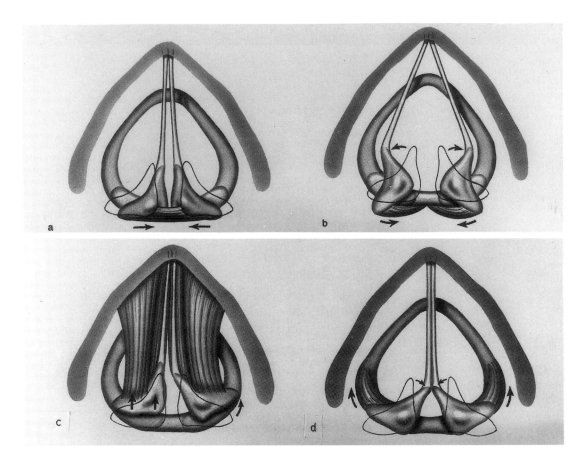

Figure 3.4. *A,* Action of interarytenoideus and oblique arytenoideus muscles to draw the bodies of the arytenoid cartilages together. *B,* contraction of the posterior cricoarytenoid muscles abduct the vocal cords. *C,* The vocalis and lateral thyroarytenoideus muscles serve as both adductors and tensors of the vocal cords depending somewhat on arytenoid position. *D,* The cricoarytenoideus muscles adduct the vocal cords. Complete glottic closure requires simultaneous activity of the interarytenoideus muscles.

Reproduced by permission from Tucker HM. Physiology of the larynx. In: Tucker HM, ed. The larynx. New York: Thieme Medical Publishers, 1993:23–34.

The larynx is innervated by the superior laryngeal nerves (SLNs) and recurrent laryngeal nerves (RLNs), which branch off from the vagus nerve (2). The SLNs carry afferent information from the supraglottic area derived from sensory and proprioceptive nerve endings concentrated on the laryngeal surface of the epiglottis and less so on the vocal cords. The SLNs innervate only the cricothyroideus muscle. The RLNs carry sensory information from the glottic and infraglottic area and innervate the remaining laryngeal musculature. The right RLN travels a shorter path, looping around the subclavian artery before rising in the tracheoesophageal groove, whereas the left RLN loops around the aorta before also rising in the tracheoesophageal groove. Stimulation of the supraglottic mucosa triggers the glottic closure reflex, which may be abolished by topical anesthesia.

Physiology

In addition to the critical functions of airway protection and phonation, the larynx plays a vital dynamic role during respiration. The RLN discharges rhythmically in synchrony with inspiration, leading to PCA muscle contraction just prior to diaphragmatic contraction (3). Downward movement of the larynx and contraction of the PCA muscles during inspiration result in inspiratory vocal cord abduction. Conversely, during expiration the cords adduct slightly due to reversal of the above process, Bernoulli's effect, and relaxation of the PCA muscles. The increase in expiratory laryngeal resistance may play a role in modulating expiratory time.

The relationship between glottic area, lung volume, and a variety of respiratory loads including hypoxemia, hypercarbia, and hyperpnea have been examined in both human beings (4–6) and animal models (3,7). Brancatisano and colleagues (5) observed a change in glottic area from a maximum of 126 ± 8 mm^2 during inspiration to a low of 70 ± 7 mm^2 during expiration in normals performing tidal breathing. Panting minimized swings in glottic diameter, predominantly by widening expiratory glottic width. Conversely, tidal breathing at elevated lung volumes ($75\% \pm 6\%$ total lung capacity) decreased inspiratory glottic width by $19.5\% \pm 8.8\%$ and expiratory width by $24.8\% \pm 12.4\%$, suggesting a coupling between glottic width and lung volume.

With increased ventilatory demand, the glottis widens secondary to a greater downward pull on the larynx and increased activity of the PCA muscles—a factor that also contributes to expiratory widening of the glottis in this state. Exercise, hypoxia, and hypercapnia all attenuate expiratory narrowing of the glottis (6). Interestingly, hypoxia and hypercarbia have differing quantitative effects on expiratory glottic width, with substantially greater expiratory narrowing during isocapnic hypoxia despite a similar increase in ventilation (4).

Obstructive Lung Disease

Obstructive lung disease produces characteristic changes at the level of the glottis. Patients with chronic obstructive pulmonary disease (COPD) and obstructed asthmatic patients exhibit exaggerated expiratory glottic narrowing (8–11). Higgenbottam and Payne (8)

observed glottic narrowing during expiration that increased as a function of airway obstruction. Individuals with a forced expiratory volume at 1 second (FEV_1) greater than 80% predicted had an expiratory glottic width during forced exhalation equal to $97.8\% \pm 20\%$ (SEM) of an inspiratory value, whereas obstructed patients with an FEV_1 less than 80% predicted achieved an expiratory width of only $36.3\% \pm 18.5\%$ (SEM) of the inspiratory value. Unlike nonobstructed individuals, expiratory glottic narrowing persisted with panting. Although the mechanism governing expiratory adduction in this setting is unknown, the authors postulated it may serve to control respiratory time in a similar fashion to pursed-lip breathing. Interestingly, pursed-lip breathing in this setting diminishes expiratory glottic adduction, shifting the level of extrathoracic resistance to the lips (unpublished observations).

Experimentally induced bronchoconstriction with either histamine (9,11) or methacholine (10) produces expiratory glottic narrowing. Collett and coworkers (9) observed a $46\% \pm 12\%$ decrease in midexpiratory width with a histamine-induced $35\% \pm 4\%$ decrease in FEV_1. Inspiratory width remained unchanged although other authors have observed a mild decrease in inspiratory glottic width following bronchoconstriction in some asthmatics (11,12). Expiratory pharyngeal narrowing may accompany the expiratory glottic adduction (9,10). Continuous positive airway pressure temporarily reverses the glottic narrowing, and reversing the bronchoconstriction with a bronchodilator returns the glottic area to baseline values (12).

Vocal Cord Dysfunction

Vocal cord dysfunction (VCD) encompasses a group of related disorders variously labelled factitious asthma (13), functional airway obstruction (14,15), Münchausen's stridor (13,15), laryngeal dyskinesia (16), and emotional wheezing (17). VCD is characterized by inappropriate vocal cord adduction that may occur during inspiration, expiration (17), or both (18). These patients often carry the diagnosis of asthma and have suffered morbidity from long-term steroid therapy. In severe cases, patients have required intubation during an acute attack (14,19). The disorder is more common in young women (20), although it has been reported in men (14,20). The reported ages have ranged from 14 to 74. VCD is believed to represent a form of conversion disorder with most individuals having a history of psychiatric illness or psychologically traumatic experience (20). Although originally termed Münchausen's stridor, most patients do not have volitional control over their vocal cord adduction during an attack and lack evidence of malingering.

Diagnostic clues include the presence of stridor on examination. Although hypoxemia has been described (19), arterial blood gases usually reveal a respiratory alkalosis with a preserved alveolar-arterial gradient (20). Flow volume loops performed during an attack may reveal flattening of the inspiratory and expiratory loops (16,20). Laryngoscopy confirms the presence of inspiratory adduction although the patient's respiratory distress may make the procedure technically difficult. Although sedation may facilitate performance of the procedure, it may also alleviate the VCD, rendering the procedure nondiagnostic (21). Examinations performed between attacks are characteristically normal, although heightened patient anxiety at the time of the examination may reproduce the finding. Christopher and colleagues (20) described a characteristic narrowing of the glottis to a posterior diamond-shaped chink; however, this finding is not universally present. Bronchial provocation using histamine or methacholine between attacks helps determine the presence of associated bronchial hyperreactivity (13,20).

Treatment is centered around therapy for the underlying psychiatric disorder. Video recordings of the larynx during an acute attack may provide important visual feedback to the patient. Speech therapy with emphasis on laryngeal relaxation techniques will benefit some patients. In the acute setting, sedatives have been safely used, although one must be secure in the diagnosis. As an interim measure, panting lowers laryngeal resistance and has successfully aborted attacks (22). Similarly, inhalation of a helium/oxygen mixture may provide symptomatic relief in the acute setting (14).

Gastroesophageal Reflux

Although the relationship between gastroesophageal reflux (GER) and chronic cough has received increasing attention in the pulmonary literature, the etiologic role of GER in other upper airway symptoms and related pathology is less well appreciated (23). Hoarseness, frequent throat clearing, foreign body sensation, chronic sore throat, and nocturnal laryngospasm may all be related to GER (24–29). The history is unreliable because classic symptoms of GER may be absent in 50% or more of patients (25,29–31). Use of 24-hour pH monitoring has significantly improved our ability to diagnose GER. Laryngoscopic findings in the patient with GER are highly variable, which probably reflects the intermittent nature of the irritation. For example, Cherry and colleagues (28) found no laryngeal abnormalities in 12 patients with oropharyngeal or laryngeal complaints, which improved or resolved with antireflux therapy. Conversely, Jacob and associates (24) noted laryngeal findings in 10 of 25 patients with GER-related laryngeal symptoms as compared to normal findings in 15 patients with GER but no laryngeal complaints. In a similar investigation, Wilson and coworkers (32) studied 97 patients with complaints of hoarseness, burning pharyngeal discomfort, or globus sensation. Laryngeal disease was found in association with prolonged acid exposure time in only 17 of 97 (17.5%) of patients studied and 24 patients had laryngeal disease without evidence of reflux by 24-hour monitoring.

The laryngoscopic arytenoid findings associated with GER include erythema and edema and thickening of the intra-arytenoid mucosa (posterior laryngitis). Although these laryngoscopic findings lack both the sensitivity and specificity to qualify as a valid screening test, the finding of posterior laryngitis in the appropriate clinical setting is an important clinical clue. Unfortunately, additional testing may not confirm the presence of GER. Although 24-hour esophageal monitoring is highly specific for the finding of GER, it lacks sensitivity and, therefore, fails as the gold standard examination. Modification of the diet while the pH probe is in place, technical failure of the probe, and the intermittent nature of GER may all contribute to false negative studies. For example, Koufman (29) reported abnormal pH monitoring studies in 113 (62%) of 182 patients with suspected GER-related laryngologic disorders. Fifteen (27%) of 55 patients with normal 24-hour pH monitoring demonstrated free reflux or evidence of esophagitis on barium esophagography. An additional 6 patients (3%) had an abnormal test on a repeat 24-hour pH monitoring study performed when symptoms had worsened, documenting the intermittent nature of the reflux. Finally, 12 patients with normal esophageal studies had evidence of pharyngeal reflux, documented by dual-probe pH monitoring, suggesting that the incidence of false negative esophageal pH monitoring studies in otolaryngologic patients with GER may be as high as 19% to 38%.

Contact ulcers and granulomas represent a more severe form of injury and probably a more complicated pathogenesis (27,33,34). The laryngeal irritation produced by GER leads to continual throat clearing or coughing. Both maneuvers are accompanied by vigorous approximation of the vocal processes of the arytenoids, producing the classic "kissing ulcer" (27). Superimposed bacterial infection may compound the injury (27). Symptoms range from hoarseness to a sharp stabbing unilateral pain that radiates to the ear (33). Control of GER and cessation of maneuvers such as throat clearing that traumatize the vocal processes of the arytenoids facilitate healing.

Gastroesophageal reflux may also play a role in the development of subglottic stenosis and laryngeal cancer. Although prolonged tracheal intubation is the major risk factor for the development of subglottic stenosis, several animal models and case reports implicate GER as a cofactor (35,36). The combination of acid and pepcid appears particularly damaging. Failure to treat GER may lead to recurrent stenosis following surgical revision (35). The role GER plays in carcinogenesis is less clear. Smoking, the major risk factor for squamous cell carcinoma of the larynx, lowers lower esophageal sphincter tone and may exacerbate GER. Alcohol, the other major risk factor, may also worsen GER. Koufman (29) found evidence of GER in 81% of 31 patients with carcinoma of the larynx; 58% of these patients had documented pharyngeal reflux. The group included six lifetime nonsmokers who developed carcinoma of the larynx.

In summary, GER may be responsible for a variety of laryngeal signs and symptoms. GER may be clinically silent in more than 50% of these patients. Use of 24-hour pH monitoring has significantly improved our understanding of the role of GER in these disorders but may have a significant incidence of false negative results. The laryngoscopic examination may provide important clues identifying GER as the cause of the patient's particular complaint or examination finding.

Neurologic Disorders

Neurologic disorders affecting the larynx include both central (CNS) and peripheral nervous system lesions. As previously outlined, neurons from the speech cortex partially decussate at the level of the medulla prior to synapsing in the nucleus ambiguus so each vocal cord receives input from both hemispheres (2). Consequently, unilateral CNS lesions may only produce subtle laryngeal signs and symptoms. However, bilateral hemisphere involvement will produce the classic findings of an upper motor neuron lesion with a flaccid paralysis followed by a spastic paresis of the laryngeal muscles (37).

Sensory information from the supraglottic larynx is carried via the SLN, whereas sensory information from the glottic and subglottic area is carried by the RLN. The patient with unilateral SLN sensory loss may be asymptomatic or present with a foreign body sensation. Laryngoscopy may reveal pooling of secretions in the pyriform sinus on the affected side. The signs and symptoms of both sensory and motor unilateral SLN palsy may be equally subtle because the SLN innervates only the cricothyroid muscle, which increases vocal cord tension. The accompanying dysphonia may be most readily observed in the professional voice user. In addition to pooling of secretions in the ipsilateral pyriform sinus, laryngoscopy may reveal deviation of the posterior commissure to the affected side with rotation of the anterior larynx to the unaffected side. Mild flaccidity of the vocal cord on the affected side may also be noted (38,39). Isolated SLN involvement is most commonly idiopathic although herpes simplex virus reactivation has been implicated (38). Surgical intervention is not required, with most patients improving or developing adequate compensatory mechanisms within one year (38). The glottic closure reflex is mediated by the SLN and modulated by CNS input. Loss of central control may lead to easily triggered and prolonged periods of laryngospasm (37,38).

Involvement of the RLN results in unilateral or bilateral vocal cord paralysis (40,41). Surgical trauma in series up to 1980 remained the primary cause of both single and bilateral vocal cord paralysis. In addition to both sur-

gical and nonsurgical trauma, endotracheal intubation is a rare but well-documented cause of both unilateral and bilateral vocal cord paralysis (42–44). Cadaveric dissection suggests the point of injury lies just below the body of the arytenoid where the anterior branch of the RLN is unprotected, lying in the submucosa between the endotracheal tube and the thyroid lamina (43,44).

Neoplasms of the neck, mediastinum, and lung most commonly cause unilateral vocal cord paralysis (41). Hoarseness may be the presenting symptom. The left RLN is more frequently involved, given its longer course through the mediastinum. Computed tomography (CT) of the neck and thorax helps differentiate malignant causes from the neuropathic and idiopathic categories. Malignancy accounted for 19 of 22 cases of left vocal cord paralysis and 8 of 11 cases of right vocal cord paralysis in one study of 33 patients undergoing CT evaluation for their paralysis (45). Nonmalignant etiologies for the remaining cases included diabetes (2), aortic aneurysm (1), and idiopathic causes (3). Interestingly, idiopathic vocal cord paralysis also occurs more commonly on the left side (46).

On laryngoscopy, the paralyzed cord lies in the paramedian position due to the unopposed action of the cricothyroid muscle (innervated by the SLN) (46). With phonation, the involved cord may tense and move slightly due to bilateral innervation of the transverse arytenoid muscle. In the rare instance of combined unilateral involvement of the SLN and RLN, the flaccid cord lies in the intermediate position. With phonation, the posterior commissure deviates toward the paralyzed side. The patient with unilateral vocal cord paralysis usually presents with hoarseness without associated dyspnea because abduction of the functioning cord maintains an adequate airway (40). With bilateral vocal cord paralysis, both cords lie in the paramedian position sufficiently adducted to vibrate with expiration and produce speech (40,47). However, in contrast to patients with unilateral vocal cord paralysis, patients with bilateral vocal cord paralysis may present with inspiratory stridor despite relatively normal speech. Rarely patients with bilateral vocal cord paralysis may present with respiratory failure (47).

Systemic neurologic diseases that may involve the larynx include (1) a group of closely related disorders—Parkinson's disease, olivopontocerebellar atrophy (OPCA), and Shy-Drager syndrome (SDS), otherwise known as multiple systems atrophy and autonomic dysfunction; (2) amyotrophic lateral sclerosis (ALS); and (3) myasthenia gravis (MG). Although peripheral manifestations of each disease usually clarify the diagnosis, isolated laryngeal involvement may be the presenting feature.

Both the clinical history and the flow volume loop may suggest laryngeal involvement in patients with extrapyramidal disorders (48,49). Vincken and coworkers (48) described upper airway muscle involvement in 27 patients (21 with Parkinson's and 6 with essential tremor). Flow volume loops were abnormal in 24 of 27 (89%) and demonstrated two basic patterns; 18 patients exhibited regular flow oscillations appearing as a saw-tooth pattern with a frequency comparable to their peripheral tremor and 6 patients demonstrated irregular flow oscillations. Laryngoscopy revealed rhythmic changes in glottic area in the first instance and irregular, jerky movements of the glottic and supraglottic structures in the second. Ten patients had physiologic evidence of upper airway obstruction and 4 had clinical symptoms. In patients with extrapyramidal disorders, upper airway obstruction may improve after administration of levodopa (50).

Olivopontocerebellar atrophy is a chronic degenerative neurologic illness that may occur in isolation or in association with signs of Parkinson's disease and autonomic insufficiency (SDS). The laryngeal presentation may be varied, ranging from vocal cord paralysis precipitating respiratory failure (51,52) to a more occult presentation with laryngeal involvement preceding other systemic manifestations of SDS by up to 2.5 years (53,54). Laryngeal involvement may be more common than generally appreciated because vocal cord paresis was found in 11 of 12 patients with SDS undergoing careful laryngeal examination (51).

Amyotrophic lateral sclerosis is characterized by progressive motor neuron loss and a variable presentation dictated by the areas involved. Laryngeal findings are present in approximately 25% or more of patients, often accompanied by complaints of dysarthria and dysphagia (55). Both upper and lower motor neurons may be involved, leading to spastic and atrophic findings. Laryngoscopy most commonly reveals normal vocal cord positioning at rest although spasticity or flaccidity may be present with phonation (55). Patients with MG may present with dyspnea and dysphonia (56,57). Respiratory failure secondary to vocal cord paresis has been reported and improves with anticholinesterase therapy (57,58). Because both patients with ALS and MG more commonly develop respiratory insufficiency due to respiratory muscle involvement, the possibility that vocal cord paresis could be contributing may be overlooked.

Granulomatous Diseases

A variety of granulomatous diseases including infectious and noninfectious diseases may involve the larynx. Because the larynx rarely is the primary site of involvement, a careful search for a systemic disease may clarify the diagnosis.

Tuberculosis

In the preantibiotic era, tuberculosis caused by *Mycobacterium tuberculosis* (MTB) was the most common granulomatous disease to involve the larynx (59). With the development of effective antituberculosis therapy, laryngeal involvement is now rarely seen; laryngeal MTB was noted in 1.5% of 1383 patients with pulmonary MTB (60). Originally, spread to the larynx was presumed to occur via the bronchus with laryngeal findings localized to the posterior larynx. However, cases of laryngeal involvement in the absence of significant chest radiographic findings and with negative sputum smears are well documented (61–63), suggesting involvement occurs due to lymphatic or hematogenous spread (64). The high rate of infection previously associated with laryngeal involvement probably reflected the high incidence of associated cavitary pulmonary disease; laryngeal involvement in the absence of smear positivity is not a highly infectious lesion (61).

Clinically, most patients present with hoarseness; the presence of dysphagia and odynophagia suggest the presence of perichondritis and chondritis (63,65). The laryngoscopy findings may be quite varied with edema, erythema, and granuloma formation of laryngeal structures including the epiglottis (59,64,66). Ulceration with associated fibrosis may be seen with more extensive involvement. Inflammatory and hyperplastic changes respond well to antituberculous therapy, whereas fibrotic change may result in permanent laryngeal compromise (64). MTB may involve the larynx indirectly with mediastinal fibrosis or mediastinal node involvement causing RLN paralysis and unilateral vocal cord paralysis (67).

Virtually any fungal infection may also involve the larynx. Blastomycosis involves the larynx approximately 5% of the time (68). Laryngeal findings range from erythema to an ulcerative lesion covered by a grayish membrane to fibrosis and vocal cord fixation late in the disease. Findings may be difficult to differentiate from laryngeal cancer and multiple biopsies are often required to make the diag-

nosis (69). Coccidioidomycosis uncommonly involves the larynx with 13 reported cases (70). Laryngeal involvement occurs in the setting of disseminated disease. Laryngeal findings reveal erythema and granulomatous lesions, which in some cases have produced respiratory compromise (70). Similarly, disseminated histoplasmosis may involve oropharyngeal and laryngeal sites (71). The characteristic painful ulcerative lesions must also be differentiated from MTB and malignancy (71).

Noninfectious granulomatous diseases that may involve the larynx include Wegener's granulomatosis (WG) and sarcoidosis. WG classically involves the upper and lower respiratory tract and kidneys. At some point, 145 of 158 patients followed at the National Institutes of Health had upper respiratory tract involvement; 25 of 158 (16%) had subglottic stenosis (SGS) (72). The pediatric and adolescent age groups are more likely to present with SGS as compared to the adult age group (11 of 23 [48%] versus 14 of 135 [10%]) (72). For unclear reasons, WG has a clear predilection for the subglottic area as opposed to the glottis or supraglottis (72–75). Endoscopy may reveal circumferential erythematous narrowing of the subglottic area (73) or subglottic mass lesions (75). SGS may cause dyspnea and alterations in the flow volume loop and ultimately may require tracheostomy. Biopsies may be nondiagnostic because granulomatous vasculitis is rarely identified. Antineutrophilic cytoplasmic antibodies (C-ANCA) have improved diagnostic yield, particularly in the unusual case of isolated laryngotracheal involvement (75). A positive C-ANCA is highly specific for the diagnosis of WG (76).

Upper respiratory tract involvement in sarcoidosis is uncommon, with reported incidences of 9% (77) to 16% (78). Laryngeal involvement is present in 6% (77) to 15% (78) of these cases. Hoarseness is the most common presenting symptom although posterior laryngeal involvement may lead to dysphagia.

Nasal mucosal involvement frequently accompanies laryngeal involvement (78). Laryngoscopy classically reveals edematous enlargement of supraglottic structures often described as a turban-like thickening (77,79). Focal reddened granular areas may also be seen. Biopsy reveals the characteristic noncaseating granulomas (77,78). Laryngoscopy has precipitated acute upper airway obstruction requiring tracheostomy (80). Steroids have been effective in cases of severe laryngeal involvement and a compromised airway (77,78,80,81). Unilateral vocal cord paralysis due to mediastinal node enlargement with involvement of the left RLN is uncommon despite the high frequency of mediastinal node involvement (82,83).

Amyloidosis

Amyloidosis has been classified as primary or secondary with subcategories of localized and generalized disease (84). In a literature review of 235 cases of respiratory tract involvement by localized amyloid reported since 1875, the larynx was involved in 177 (75%) of cases (85). Recent biochemical characterization of biopsies from localized laryngeal amyloidosis suggests that abnormal light chains are being produced locally by plasma cells, possibly representing a form of plasma cell dyscrasia (86). On laryngoscopy, the lesion has a waxy, translucent yellow or yellow-gray swelling without ulceration of the underlying mucosa (Plate 1). Congo red staining of the biopsy confirms the diagnosis.

Degenerative Disorders

Vocal cord irritation or trauma leads to characteristic changes that have been variously labeled polypoid degeneration or chronic hypertrophic laryngitis (87). Tucker argues that degenerative change rather than an inflammatory response is the common pathologic denominator (87). Vocal abuse, smoking, alcohol use, chronic sinusitis, and allergies are all common potential irritants that may contribute to the observed laryngeal changes. Reinke's edema represents the earliest pathologic response to irritation and resolves with elimination of the irritant. Reinke's edema is a fairly common, easily recognized laryngeal abnormality accounting for approximately 10% of benign laryngeal lesions (Plate 2) (88). Reinke's space as previously defined is a potential space lying between the lamina propria and vocal ligament filled with loose sheets of connective tissue. Poor lymphatic drainage and well-defined borders retard resolution of the edema. Microsurgical vocal fold stripping prevents recurrence of this entity by eliminating the space, but compromises vocal cord function by altering the complex "flowing" of the mucosa necessary for normal phonatory function. Reinke's edema is not a premalignant lesion with only 1 of 120 patients followed over 8 years developing laryngeal cancer (89). Smoking is a common risk factor for both disorders and probably accounts for the one case in that series.

Sustained laryngeal irritation may lead to polypoid changes. Vocal cord polyps are more common in men and most often associated with chronic vocal abuse (Plate 3). Polyps have been described as gelatinous with a loose edematous stroma seen on histologic examination and as telangiectatic with grossly visible convoluted blood vessels and a tightly filled homogeneous eosinophilic material on histologic examination (90). Large pedunculated polyps may compromise the airway and precipitate acute respiratory failure (91).

Vocal cord nodules are pathologically similar to vocal cord polyps but represent a clinically distinct lesion developing at the junction of the middle and anterior aspect of the vocal cords (Plate 4). This is the point of maximal vibratory amplitude between the two cords during phonation at higher pitch levels. The nodule appears as a whitish elevation if fibrous tissue predominates, pearly gray if edema predominates, and red if blood vessels or hemorrhage predominates (92). The early changes of mucosal hypertrophy, edema, and occasionally hemorrhage are potentially reversible. Repeated hemorrhage and inflammation lead to development of a mature fibrotic nodule. These lesions have been variously termed screamer's nodes or singer's nodes, emphasizing the importance of vocal abuse in their development.

Contact ulcers and granulomas are less common entities that should be considered with lesions attributed to vocal abuse (Plate 5). As previously discussed, GER in combination with habitual throat clearing, and excessive glottic attack—forceful initiation of speech—leads to the development of unilateral or bilateral kissing lesions on the vocal processes of the arytenoids (27,33,34).

Prolonged endotracheal intubation may produce a similar form of injury with ulceration and granuloma formation of the posterior larynx. Large endotracheal tubes and significant movement of the tube while intubated increase the likelihood of injury (93). Benjamin and Croxson (94) have argued ulcers and granulomas are distinct entities developing at similar sites and sharing similar pathophysiology. The specific factors favoring the development of one lesion over the other remain unclear. Denudation of the mucosa overlying the bodies or vocal processes of the arytenoids in combination with bacterial contamination and GER favor granuloma formation. The absence of a submucosa limits the regional blood supply and prolongs healing (87). Postintubation granulomas, unlike those caused by GER and vocal abuse, should resolve following intubation without further therapy (93) although antibiotics, steroids, and speech therapy may be useful (87).

Less common sequelae of endotracheal intubation include the development of laryngeal and subglottic stenosis. Forms of laryngeal involvement range from submucosal intra-arytenoid scarring, to isolated fibrous bands between the vocal cords to more extensive fibrosis in both the glottic and subglottic areas (95). A significant proportion may be managed endoscopically (95,96), whereas some patients will require open reconstructive procedures (95,97).

Benign Neoplasms

Benign neoplasms encompass those benign growths not including the more common laryngeal changes previously described, caused by laryngeal irritants. In a study encompassing the years 1955–1982, and consistent with other published series, papillomas were the predominant tumor (Table 3.1) (98). Historically, papillomas have been divided into juvenile and adult forms although this distinction has been blurred (98). The juvenile type has a female predominance, tends to occur at multiple sites, and is more likely to recur following treatment. Both adult and juvenile types most commonly involve the true vocal cord but may occur on any site in the upper respiratory tract and may extend down into the tracheobronchial tree with occasional parenchymal involvement (99). The lesion is most likely related to the DNA human papillomavirus (100). Malignant degeneration has been reported (100,101). On laryngoscopy, the papilloma has a characteristic cauliflower appearance and may attain suffi-

Table 3.1. Benign Neoplasms of the Larynx	
Papilloma	227
Oncocytic tumor	15
Granular cell tumor	7
Hemangioma	5
Lymphangioma	3
Paraganglioma	2
Neurilemoma	2
Neurofibroma	2
Lipoma	1
Chondroma	1
Pleomorphic adenoma	1
Nodular fascitis	1
Fibrous histiocytoma	1
Fibromatosis	1
Rhabdomyoma	1
Total	270

cient size to produce airway compromise (Plate 6). Treatment options have included surgical excision, radiation, and photodynamic therapy combined with laser ablation (99,102).

Premalignant and Malignant Lesions

A variety of lesions are recognized as having malignant potential (Table 3.2) (103). Although the classification scheme is patterned after that developed for the gynecologic tract, laryngeal lesions do not exhibit the same orderly progression from benign to malignant (103). Leukoplakia is a purely descriptive term describing a whitish plaque and encompassing both the malignant and benign lesions (103). The remaining lesions are pathologically defined. Hyperplasia simply describes thickening of the mucosal layer, whereas keratosis represents a conversion of the normal nonkeratinizing stratified squamous epithelium of the vocal cords to a keratinizing epithelium (103). Hyperplasia and keratosis should reverse if the inciting irritant (most commonly smoking or vocal trauma) is eliminated. Keratosis with atypia and carcinoma in situ describe those lesions with varying degrees of cellular dysplasia (103). Microinvasive carcinoma by definition describes lesions with limited invasion through the basement membrane (103). Plate 7 demonstrates squamous cell carcinoma of the left vocal cord.

Unfortunately, no clinical finding reliably separates benign from premalignant or frankly malignant lesions. Series following patients with leukoplakia suggest the likelihood of developing cancer ranges from 0.13% to 6% (104). Silverman and colleagues (105) observed a 17.5% incidence of cancer in 257 patients with oral leukoplakia followed for a mean period of 8.1 years, suggesting that with longer follow-up the incidence may be higher. Patients at highest risk were nonsmokers with leukoplakia and verrucous papillary hyperkeratotic lesions (105). The presence of erythroplakia (reddish patches of raised epithelium) appears to correlate with greater degrees of cellular atypia and a higher malignant potential (104,105), although not all studies have confirmed this increased malignant potential (106). Management of these lesions requires either a biopsy or close follow-up to ensure resolution of the observed changes.

Table 3.2. Premalignant Lesions

Leukoplakia
Hyperplasia
Keratosis without atypia
Keratosis with atypia
Carcinoma in situ
Microinvasive carcinoma

REFERENCES

1. Tucker HM. Anatomy of the larynx. In: Tucker HM, ed. The larynx, 2nd ed. New York: Thieme Medical Publishers, 1993:1–18.
2. Tucker HM. Physiology of the larynx. In: Tucker HM, ed. The larynx, 2nd ed. New York: Thieme Medical Publishers, 1993: 23–34.
3. Suzuki M, Kirchner JA. The posterior cricoarytenoid as an inspiratory muscle. Ann Otol Rhinol Laryngol 1969;78:849–864.
4. England SJ, Bartlett D, Knuth SL. Comparison of human vocal cord movements during isocapnic hypoxia and hypercapnia. J Appl Physiol Respirat Environ Exercise Physiol 1982;53:81–86.
5. Brancatisano T, Collett PW, Engel LA. Respiratory movements of the vocal cords. J Appl Physiol Respirat Environ Physiol 1983;54:1269–1276.
6. England SJ, Bartlett D. Changes in respiratory movements of the human vocal cords during hyperpnea. J Appl Physiol Respirat Environ Exercise Physiol 1982;52:780–785.
7. Dixon M, Szereda-Przestaszewski M, Widdicombe JG, Wise JCM. Studies on laryngeal calibre during stimulation of peripheral and central chemoreceptors, pneumothorax and increased respiratory loads. J Physiol 1974;239:347–363.

8. Higenbottam T, Payne J. Glottis narrowing in lung disease. Am Rev Respir Dis 1982;125: 746–750.

9. Collett PW, Brancatisano P, Engel LA. Upper airway dimensions and movements in bronchial asthma. Am Rev Respir Dis 1986;133:1143–1149.

10. Brown IG, Zamel N, Hoffstein V. Pharyngeal and glottic changes following methacholine challenge in normal subjects. Bull Eur Physiopathol Respir 1986;22:251–256.

11. Higenbottam T. Narrowing of glottis opening in humans associated with experimentally induced bronchoconstriction. J Appl Physiol 1980;49:403–407.

12. Collett PW, Brancatisano T, Engel LA. Changes in the glottic aperture during bronchial asthma. Am Rev Respir Dis 1983;128:719–723.

13. Downing ET, Braman SS, Fox MJ, Corrao WM. Factitious asthma—Physiological approach to diagnosis. JAMA 1982;248: 2878–2881.

14. Heiser JM, Kahn ML, Schmidt TA. Functional airway obstruction presenting as stridor: a case report and literature review. J Emerg Med 1990;8:285–289.

15. Sim TC, McClean SP, Lee JL, Naranjo MS, Grant JA. Functional laryngeal obstruction: a somatization disorder. Am J Med 1990; 88:293–295.

16. Ramirez J, Leon I, Rivera LM. Episodic laryngeal dyskinesia: clinical and psychiatric characterization. Chest 1986;90:716–721.

17. Rodenstein DO, Francis C, Stanescu DC. Emotional laryngeal wheezing: a new syndrome. Am Rev Respir Dis 1983;127: 354–356.

18. Goldman J, Muers M. Vocal cord dysfunction and wheezing. Thorax 1991;46: 401–404.

19. Appelblatt NH, Baker SR. Functional upper airway obstruction—a new syndrome. Arch Otolaryngol 1981;107:305–306.

20. Christopher KL, Wood RP, Eckert RC, Blager FB, Raney RA, Souhrada JF. Vocal-cord dysfunction presenting as asthma. N Eng J Med 1983;308:1566–1570.

21. Seiner JC, Staudenmayer H, Koepke JW, Harvey R, Christopher K. Vocal cord dysfunction: the importance of psychologic factors and provocation challenge testing. J Allergy Clin Immunol 1987;79:726–733.

22. Pitchenik AE. Functional laryngeal obstruction relieved by panting. Chest 1991;100: 1465–1467.

23. Koufman JA. Aerodigestive manifestations of gastroesophageal reflux: what we don't know yet. Chest 1993;104:1321–1322.

24. Jacob P, Kahrilas PJ, Herzon G. Proximal esophageal pH-metry in patients with reflux laryngitis. Gastroenterology 1992;100:305–31.

25. Weiner GJ, Koufman JA, Wu WC, Cooper JB, Richter JE, Castell DO. Chronic hoarseness secondary to gastroesophageal reflux disease: documentation with 24-H ambulatory pH monitoring. Am J Gastroenterol 1989;84:1503–1508.

26. McNally PR, Maydonovitch CL, Prosek RA, Collette RP, Wong RKH. Evaluation of gastroesophageal reflux as a cause of idiopathic hoarseness. Dig Dis Sci 1989;34:1900–1904.

27. Ward PH, Berci G. Observations on the pathogenesis of chronic non-specific pharyngitis and laryngitis. Laryngoscope 1982;92: 1377–1382.

28. Cherry J, Siegel CI, Margulies SI, Donner M. Pharyngeal localization of symptoms of gastroesophageal reflux. Ann Otol Rhinol Laryngol 1970;79:912–914.

29. Koufman JA. The otolaryngologic manifestations of gastroesophageal reflux disease (GERD): a clinical investigation of 225 patients using ambulatory 24-hour pH monitoring and an experimental investigation of the role of acid and pepsin in the development of laryngeal injury. Laryngoscope 1991;101:1–78.

30. Irwin RS, French CL, Curley FJ, Zawacki JK, Bennett FM. Chronic cough due to gastroesophageal reflux: clinical, diagnostic, and pathogenetic aspects. Chest 1993;104: 1511–1517.

31. Irwin RS, Zawacki JK, Curley FJ, Frence CC, Hoffman PJ. Chronic cough as the sole presenting manifestation of gastroesophageal reflux. Am Rev Respir Dis 1989;140: 1254–1300.

32. Wilson JA, White A, Von Haacke NP, Maran AGD, Heading RC, Pryde A, Piris J. Gastroesophageal reflux and posterior laryngitis. Ann Otol Rhinol Laryngol 1989;98: 405–410.

33. Ward PH, Zwitman D, Hanson D, Berci G. Contact ulcers and granulomas of the larynx: new insights into their etiology as a basis for

more rational treatment. Otolaryngol Head Neck Surg 1980;88:262–269.

34. Cherry J, Margulies SI. Contact ulcer of the larynx. Laryngoscope 1967;78:1937–1940.

35. Little FB, Kohut RI, Koufman JA, Marshall RB. Effect of gastric acid on the pathogenesis of subglottic stenosis. Ann Otol Rhinol Laryngol 1985;94:516–519.

36. Wynne JW, Ramphal R, Hood CI. Tracheal mucosal damage after aspiration: a scanning electron microscope study. Am Rev Respir Dis 1981;124:728–732.

37. Ward PH, Hanson DG, Berci G. Observations on central neurologic etiology for laryngeal dysfunction. Ann Otol 1981;90: 430–441.

38. Adour KK, Schneider GD, Hilsinger RL. Acute superior laryngeal nerve palsy: analysis of 78 cases. Otolaryngol Head Neck Surg 1980;88:418–424.

39. Hartman DE, Daily WW, Morin KN. A case of superior laryngeal nerve paresis and psychogenic dysphonia. J Speech Hearing Disorders 1989;54:526–529.

40. Holinger LD, Holinger PC, Holinger PH. Etiology of bilateral abductor vocal cord paralysis: a review of 389 cases. Ann Otol 1976;85:428–436.

41. Tucker HM. Vocal cord paralysis—1979: etiology and management. Laryngoscope 1980;90:585–590.

42. Holley HS, Gildea JE. Vocal cord paralysis after tracheal intubation. JAMA 1971; 215:281-284

43. Brandwein M, Abramson AL, Shikowitz MJ. Bilateral vocal cord paralysis following endotracheal intubation. Arch Otolaryngol Head Neck Surg 1986;112:877–882.

44. Cavo JW. True vocal cord paralysis following intubation. Laryngoscope 1985;95: 1352–1359.

45. Glazer HS, Aronbert DJ, Lee JKT, Sagel SS. Extralaryngeal causes of vocal cord paralysis: CT evaluation. AJR 1983;141:527–531.

46. Berry H, Blair RL. Isolated vagus nerve palsy and vagal mononeuritis. Arch Otolaryngol 1980;106:333–338.

47. Baumann MH, Heffner JE. Bilateral vocal cord paralysis with respiratory failure: a presenting manifestation of bronchogenic carcinoma. Arch Intern Med 1989;149: 1453–1454.

48. Vincken WG, Gauthier SG, Dollfuss RE, Hanson RE, Darauay CM, Cosio MG. Involvement of upper-airway muscles in extrapyramidal disorders: a cause of airflow limitation. N Engl J Med 1984;311: 438–442.

49. Schiffman PL. A saw-tooth pattern in Parkinson's disease. Chest 1985;87:124–126.

50. Vincken WG, Darauay CM, Cosio MG. Reversibility of upper airway obstruction after levodopa therapy in Parkinson's disease. Chest 1989;96:210–212.

51. Hanson DG, Ludlow CL, Bassich CJ. Vocal fold paresis in Shy-Drager syndrome. Ann Otol Rhinol Laryngol 1983;92:85–90.

52. Drury PME, Williams EGN. Vocal cord paralysis in the Shy-Drager syndrome: a cause of postoperative respiratory obstruction. Anaesthesia 1991;46:466–468.

53. Kew J, Gross M, Chapman P. Shy-Drager syndrome presenting as isolated paralysis of vocal cord abductors. BMJ 1990;300:1441.

54. Martinovits G, Leventon G, Goldhammer Y, Sadeh M. Vocal cord paralysis as a presenting sign in the Shy-Drager syndrome. J Laryngol Otol 1988;102:280–281.

55. Carpenter RJ III, McDonald TJ, Howard FM Jr. The otolaryngologic presentation of amyotrophic lateral sclerosis. Otolaryngology 1978;86:479–484.

56. Friedman S, Goffin FB. Abductor vocal weakness in myasthenia gravis: report of a case. Laryngoscope 1966;76:1520–1523.

57. Schmidt-Nowara WW, Marder EJ, Feil PA. Respiratory failure in myasthenia gravis. Arch Neurol 1984;41:567–568.

58. Colp C, Kriplani L, Nussbaum M. Vocal cord paralysis in myasthenia gravis following anesthesia. Chest 1980;77:218–220.

59. Travis LW, Hybels RL, Newman MH. Tuberculosis of the larynx. Laryngoscope 1976;86:549–558.

60. Brodovsky DM. Laryngeal TB in an age of chemotherapy. Can J Otolaryngol 1975;4: 168–176.

61. Horowitz G, Kaslow R, Friedland G. Infectiousness of laryngeal tuberculosis. Am Rev Respir Dis 1976;114:241–244.

62. Kilgore TL, Jenkins DW. Laryngeal tuberculosis. Chest 1983;83:139–141.

63. Thaller SR, Gross JR, Pilch BZ, Goodman ML. Laryngeal tuberculosis as manifested in the decades 1963–1983. Laryngoscope 1987; 97:848–850.

64. Soda A, Rubio H, Salazar M, Ganem J, Berlanga D, Sanchez A. Tuberculosis of the larynx: clinical aspects in 19 patients. Laryngoscope 1989;99:1147–1149.

65. Riley EC, Amundson DE. Laryngeal tuberculosis revisited. Am Fam Physician 1992;46: 759–762.

66. Rupa V, Mathew J, Bhanu TS, Date A. Paediatric laryngeal tuberculosis presenting with stridor. J Laryngol Otol 1989;103: 787–788.

67. Shah P, Ramakantan R. Hoarseness of the voice due to left recurrent laryngeal nerve palsy in tuberculous mediastinitis. Arch Otolaryngol Head Neck Surg 1990;116: 108.

68. Reder PA, Neel HB. Blastomycosis in otolaryngology: review of a large series. Laryngoscope 1993;103:53–58.

69. Payne J, Koopmann CF. Laryngeal carcinoma—or is it laryngeal blastomycosis? Laryngoscope 1984;94:608–611.

70. Boyle JO, Coulthard W, Mandel RM. Laryngeal involvement in disseminated coccidioidomycosis. Arch Otolaryngol Head Neck Surg 1991;117:433–438.

71. Rajah V, Essa A. Histoplasmosis of the oral cavity, oropharynx and larynx. J Laryngol Otol 1993;107:58–61.

72. Lebovics RS, Hoffman GS, Leavitt RY, et al. The management of subglottic stenosis in patients with Wegener's granulomatosis. Laryngoscope 1992;102:1341–1345.

73. McDonald TJ, Neel HB, DeRemee RA. Wegener's granulomatosis of the subglottis and the upper portion of the trachea. Ann Otol Rhinol Laryngol 1982;91:588–592.

74. Illum P, Thorling K. Wegener's granulomatosis—long term results of treatment. Ann Otol 1981;90:231–235.

75. Hoare TJ, Jayne D, Evans PR, Croft CB, Howard DJ. Wegener's granulomatosis, subglottic stenosis and antineutrophil cytoplasm antibodies. J Laryngol Otol 1989;103: 1187–1191.

76. Gaughan RK, DeSanto LW, McDonald TJ. Use of anticytoplasmic autoantibodies in the diagnosis of Wegener's granulomatosis with subglottic stenosis. Laryngoscope 1990;100: 561–563.

77. Neel HB, McDonald TJ. Laryngeal sarcoidosis: report of 13 patients. Ann Otol Rhinol Laryngol 1982;91:359–362.

78. James DG, Barter S, Jash D, MacKinnon DM, Carstairs LS. Sarcoidosis of the upper respiratory tract (SURT). J Laryngol Otol 1982;96:711–718.

79. Fallivan GJ, Landis JN. Sarcoidosis of the larynx: preserving and restoring airway and professional voice. J Voice 1993;7:81–94.

80. Bower JS, Belen JE, Weg JG, Dantzker DR. Manifestations and treatment of laryngeal sarcoidosis. Am Rev Respir Dis 1980;122: 325–332.

81. Becker GL, Tenholder MF, Hunt KK. Obligate mouth breathing during exercise: nasal and laryngeal sarcoidosis. Chest 1990; 98:756–757.

82. Tobias JK, Santiago SM, Williams AJ. Sarcoidosis as a cause of left recurrent laryngeal nerve palsy. Arch Otolaryngol Head Neck Surg 1990;116:971–972.

83. El-Kassimi FA, Ashous M, Vijayaraghavan R. Sarcoidosis presenting as recurrent left laryngeal nerve palsy. Thorax 1990;45:565–566.

84. Mitrani M, Billner HF. Laryngeal amyloidosis. Laryngoscope 1985;95:1346–1347.

85. McAlpine JC, Fuller AP. Localized laryngeal amyloidosis, a report of a case with a review of the literature. J Laryngol Otol 1964; 78:296–314.

86. Berg AM, Troxler RF, Kane K, Grillone G, Cohen AS, Kasznica J, Skinner M. Localized amyloidosis of the larynx: evidence for light chain composition. Ann Otol Rhinol Laryngol 1993;102:884–889.

87. Tucker HM. Degenerative disorders of the larynx. In: Tucker HM, ed. The larynx, 2nd ed. New York: Thieme Medical Publishers 1993:217–229.

88. Remenar E, Elo J, Frint T. The morphological basis for development of Reinke's oedema. Acta Otolaryngol 1984;97:169–176.

89. Nielsen VM, Hojslet PE, Palvio D. Reinke's oedema: a premalignant condition? J Laryngol Otol 1986;100:1159–1162.

90. Kleinsasser O. Pathogenesis of vocal cord polyps. Ann Otol Rhinol Laryngol 1982; 91:378–381.

91. Yanagisawa E, Hausfeld JN, Pensak ML. Sudden airway obstruction due to pedunculated laryngeal polyps. Ann Otol Rhinol Laryngol 1983;92:340–343.

92. Strong MS, Vaughan CW. Vocal cord nodules and polyps—the role of surgical treatment. Laryngoscope 1971;81:911–923.

93. Feder RJ, Michell MJ. Hyperfunctional hyperacidic and intubation granulomas. Arch Otolaryngol 1984;110:582–584.

94. Benjamin B, Croxson G. Vocal cord granulomas. Ann Otol Rhinol Laryngol 1985;94: 538–541.

95. Hawkins DB, Luxford WM. Laryngeal stenosis from endotracheal intubation: a review of 58 cases. Ann Otol 1980;89:454–457.

96. Mehta AC, Lee FYW, Cordasco EM, Kirby T, Eliachar I, De Boer G. Concentric tracheal and subglottic stenosis. Chest 1993;104: 673–677.

97. McCaffrey TV. Management of subglottic stenosis in the adult. Ann Otol Rhinol Laryngol 1991;100:90–94.

98. Jones SR, Myers EN, Barnes L. Benign neoplasms of the larynx. Otolaryngol Clin North Am 1984:151–178.

99. Basheda SG, Mehta AC, De Boer G, Orlowski JP. Endobronchial and parenchymal juvenile laryngotracheobronchial papillomatosis: effect of photodynamic therapy. Chest 1991;100:1458–1461.

100. Byrne JC, Tsao MS, Fraser RS, Howley PM. Human papillomavirus-11 DNA in a patient with chronic laryngotracheobronchial papillomatosis and metastatic squamous-cell carcinoma of the lung. N Engl J Med 1987; 317:873–878.

101. Bewtra C, Krishnan R, Lee SS. Malignant changes in nonirradiated juvenile laryngotracheal papillomatosis. Arch Otolaryngol 1982;108:114–116.

102. Kavuru MS, Mehta AC, Eliachar I. Effect of photodynamic therapy and external beam radiation therapy on juvenile laryngotracheobronchial papillomatosis. Am Rev Respir Dis 1990;141:509–510.

103. Tucker HM. Malignant neoplasms. In: Tucker HM, ed. The larynx, 2nd ed. New York: Thieme Medical Publishers 1993: 287–323.

104. Mashberg A. Erythroplasia vs leukoplakia in the diagnosis of early asymptomatic oral squamous carcinoma. N Engl J Med 1977;297:109–110.

105. Silverman S, Gorsky M, Lozada F. Oral leukoplakia and malignant transformation: a follow-up study of 257 patients. Cancer 1984;53:563–568.

106. Hellquist H, Olofsson J, Grontoft O. Carcinoma in situ and severe dysplasia of the vocal cords: a clinicopathological and photometric investigation. Acta Otolaryngol 1981;92:543–555.

Indications, Contraindications, and Medications | 4

Navdeep S. Rai and Alejandro C. Arroliga

Since its introduction in 1897 by Killian, the role of the bronchoscope has been expanding (1). Each new technical development has resulted in yet another application. The original rigid bronchoscope was used initially only for visual examination of the trachea and proximal bronchi. Its only therapeutic utility was the removal of foreign bodies (2). With the development of biopsy forceps and other accessories, the rigid bronchoscope's role expanded. The flexible fiberoptic bronchoscope, introduced in 1966 (3), represents a tremendous leap forward in the field of bronchoscopy. With this new instrument, the bronchoscopist could now reach further into the lungs. Additionally, its flexibility allowed better visualization of the upper lobes as well as the distal subsegments of the lower lobes. The continued development of small caliber scopes and new accessory tools has allowed further expansion of the role of the flexible fiberoptic bronchoscope. This chapter reviews the current indications and contraindications of bronchoscopy and discusses the medications used in the patient undergoing flexible bronchoscopy.

Rigid Bronchoscopy

In recent years, the ever-expanding role of the flexible fiberoptic bronchoscope has led to a decline in the use of the rigid bronchoscope. This decline has been so marked that 92% of bronchoscopists never use the rigid scope in their clinical practice (4). The majority of training centers in the United States no longer offer training in rigid bronchoscopy to future pulmonologists. This is an unfortunate trend, because the rigid bronchoscope, in certain circumstances, offers benefits over the flexible fiberoptic bronchoscope. The larger working channel of the rigid bronchoscope allows easier control of massive hemoptysis (5). The larger size is also advantageous in the removal of foreign body and placement of airway stents. Because mechanical ventilation can be provided through the rigid scope, it is ideally suited for patients with tight tracheobronchial stenosis. Although laser therapy is now frequently performed through the flexible fiberoptic bronchoscope, the rigid scope is preferred by some (6). The rigid scope can be used to core the obstructing lesion to expedite removal of the mass. In addition, larger forceps remove bigger pieces with each "bite." The metal of the rigid bronchoscope greatly reduces the risk of endobronchial ignition as compared to the flexible fiberoptic bronchoscope with its rubber housing. Additionally, because the rigid scope can deliver mechanical ventilation, the endotracheal intubation tube is deemed unnecessary, further reducing the risk of an endobronchial ignition. Finally, in case of mishap, the rigid scope is better suited to maintaining a clear airway and controlling hemorrhage.

The major disadvantage of the rigid bronchoscope is the limited access to the distal airway. Furthermore, the rigid bronchoscope requires the use of general anesthesia in most patients. The rigid scope cannot be used in patients with unstable necks, severely ankylosed cervical spines, or restricted temporomandibular joints (6).

Flexible Fiberoptic Bronchoscopy

The flexible fiberoptic bronchoscope, introduced by Ikeda in 1966, has now become the most versatile tool available to the chest physician (3). Available in a range of sizes, the flexible scope can now be used in pediatric and adult populations. Its flexibility allows visualization of a significantly larger portion of the tracheobronchial tree. In addition, it is better tolerated by the patient, obviating the need for general anesthesia. Thus, the procedure can now be routinely performed in the outpatient department. With its accompanying accessories, the flexible fiberoptic bronchoscope is now used for a variety of therapeutic and diagnostic applications (Table 4.1).

Diagnostic Bronchoscopy

Malignancy

Lung cancer is the most common fatal malignancy in the United States. Its prevalence would explain why, in a recent survey of North American bronchoscopists, the presence of a mass on a chest radiograph was the most frequent indication for bronchoscopy (4). From the bronchoscopist's viewpoint, masses can be divided into those centrally and those peripherally located (7). Central masses are endobronchial lesions directly visualized through the bronchoscope or submucosal masses that cause visible airway compression. These lesions may be biopsied using the forceps. Generally, three to four biopsies are considered sufficient for sampling (8,9). The diagnostic yield of forceps biopsy of central lesions ranges from 55% to 85%, depending on the

cell type (7). Flat lesions located on the wall of the bronchus may be better sampled using the

---

Table 4.1. Indications for Diagnostic Bronchoscopy

Malignancy
    Diagnosis of bronchogenic carcinoma
    Staging of bronchogenic carcinoma
    Abnormal sputum cytology
    Follow-up after treatment of carcinoma
    Evaluation of patients with head and neck
        malignancy
    Evaluation of patients with esophageal
        malignancy
    Metastatic carcinoma
Mediastinal mass
Infection
    Recurrent or unresolved pneumonia
    Infiltrate in an immunocompromised patient
    Cavitary lesion
Unexplained lung collapse
Interstitial lung disease
Hemoptysis
Unexplained chronic cough
Localized wheezing
Stridor
Foreign body aspiration
Chest trauma
    Blunt or penetrating
    Chemical
    Thermal
Unexplained pleural effusion
Evaluation of the patient after lung transplantation
Endotracheal intubation
    Confirm tube position
    Evaluate for tube-related injury
    Confirm position of transtracheal oxygen
        catheter
Tracheobronchial stricture and stenosis
Hoarseness or vocal cord paralysis
Superior vena cava syndrome
Fistula
    Bronchopleural
    Tracheo- or bronchoesophageal
    Tracheo- or bronchoaortic
Persistent pneumothorax
Postoperative assessment of tracheal, tracheobronchial, bronchial, or stump anastomosis
Bronchography

spear forceps (7). Cytologic analysis of central lesions can be conducted through the collection of washings and cytology brushes. The yield of bronchial washings for cytologic evaluation ranges from 62% to 79% (10–12). If washings are to be collected, it is generally recommended that the collection be performed after the lesion has been biopsied to increase the number of cells within the washings (10). The reported diagnostic yield of washings ranges from 62% to 79% (10–14). Whether a collection of bronchial washings, in addition to forceps biopsy and bronchial brushings, results in an increased diagnostic yield (10,11,15–18) or does not increase a diagnostic yield (19–23) remains controversial. False positive results are rarely reported with washings. False positive results generally occur in the case of infection, radiation therapy to the chest, air pollution, interstitial lung disease, or tracheostomy (11). Collection of cytology specimens with a cytology brush appears to be effective as well, especially when used in combination with biopsies. Diagnostic yield of brushings ranges from 62% to 78% (10,11,13,20,21,24).

The role of the transbronchial needle aspiration (TBNA) in central lesions remains controversial (4,24,25). TBNA is felt to be useful with submucosal lesions or lesions that cause extrinsic compression of the bronchus (26–29). TBNA is also recommended for use in those lesions that are necrotic or likely to bleed (30,31). The diagnostic yield for TBNA is increased with proper, immediate preparation of the specimen. The most important role of TBNA is in the staging of lung cancer, as discussed below, where it can be used to aspirate hilar or mediastinal lymph nodes (28,32,33).

Peripheral lesions are those that cannot be directly viewed through the bronchoscope. In the setting of lung cancer, the diagnostic yield of the combination of transbronchial biopsies, brushings and washings with guidance of biplanar fluoroscopy varies from 40% to 80% (21,34–37). There is some controversy as to which procedure should be used first to sample

these lesions (38). Although successful transbronchial biopsies have been reported without the use of fluoroscopy, we believe fluoroscopy is essential for localization of these lesions. Additionally, there is a lower incidence of pneumothoraces when a fluoroscope is used (39). The use of biplanar fluoroscopy results in a higher yield as compared to a single-plane fluoroscope, where the yield is 10% to 30% (17,21). If a single-plane fluoroscope is used, turning the patient to the side to confirm localization results in an increased yield (40).

The size of the lesions plays a significant role in the diagnostic yield. Lesions less than 2 cm have a diagnostic yield of 30%, compared with 80% in those over 4 cm (34,36, 37,41,42). If a cytology brush is to be used to sample a peripheral lesion, it should be used before the transbronchial biopsy is performed, so as not to contaminate the airway with blood that may later cover the brush (36). Some have suggested that bronchoalveolar lavage (BAL) with 100 to 200 mL normal saline increases the yield for peripheral lesions as compared to brushings (43,44).

The use of transthoracic needle aspiration as an alternative to fiberoptic bronchoscopy (FOB) in the evaluation of peripheral masses remains controversial. The diagnostic yield of transthoracic needle aspiration is twice that of transbronchial biopsies without regard for the size of the lesions (7,42). However, FOB allows direct examination of the airway where an incidental endobronchial malignancy is found in 3.5% of the cases of lung cancer (42). FOB also offers a significantly lower rate of complications versus that of thoracic needle aspiration (0.01% versus 32% to 36%) (42,44,45).

Some less commonly used techniques for assessing peripheral masses are also used. These include high resolution computer tomography (CT)-guided transbronchial needle biopsies, use of a needle brush, and transbronchial curettage. TBNA biopsy produces a higher yield as compared to a transbronchial biopsy (46,47). The addition of TBNA to transbronchial biopsies, washings, and brushings increases a yield from 48% to 69% (46). However, lack of experience and increased risk of damage to the bronchoscope has resulted in a reluctance among many bronchoscopists to perform peripheral TBNA (4). The needle brush, which combines the advantages of the brush and a needle, has recently been introduced and offers the highest yield of any technique used to sample a lesion (7). Transbronchial curettage is a multiphase procedure whose yields are significantly higher than those of brushings and biopsies (48,49). When single-hinged curettage is used, the diagnostic yield for lesions less than 2 cm in size is 76%, and the yield is 97% for any two-hinged curettage (37,49). This procedure is not sensitive if the lesions are less than 1.1 cm in size, the tumors are pleural based, or in cases of adenocarcinoma, including alveolar cell carcinoma (48). The need to undergo at least two bronchoscopies (first to localize the lesion with a bronchoscopic-guided bronchogram and the second bronchoscopy, approximately 2 weeks later, to obtain the biopsy) make this technique less favorable. Ultrathin FOB has been proposed to increase the yield of transbronchial biopsies. This involves passage of a 1.8- to 2.2-mm scope through a standard bronchoscope, allowing viewing of 10 to 12 generations of bronchi (50,51). Although specimens cannot be collected through the ultrathin bronchoscope, preliminary visualization may result in increased success of biopsy. More experience is necessary to assess the utility of this procedure.

In addition to the diagnosis of bronchogenic carcinoma, the bronchoscopy can be used to stage the patient. If surgical resection of a suspected bronchogenic carcinoma is anticipated, staging should be performed even before the diagnosis is firmly established. This is most important in situations where a parenchymal mass is clinically suspected to be malignant and there is mediastinal or hilar adenopathy. In such situations, transtracheal or transbronchial needle aspiration and transbronchial needle biopsies could be used to sample the enlarged lymph nodes. This should be done before the parenchymal lesion is disturbed because of the risk of contaminating the bronchoscope with malignant cells. If the parenchymal lesion is disturbed, the malignant cells could then be mixed with the specimen from the lymph nodes. The patient would then be considered to have inoperable disease, eliminating the option of potentially curative surgery for the patient. Shure and Fedullo studied the role of TBNA of subcarinal lymph nodes in patients with clinical stage I lung cancer (29). The transbronchial needle aspirate provided the only evidence of nonresectability in 69% of these patients, thus saving the patient a staging surgical procedure (29). Overall, TBNA can preclude the need for staging surgery in one half of the patients whose tumors are unresectable because of mediastinal invasion (52). TBNA has a sensitivity of 50%, with a specificity of 96% and an accuracy of 78% (52). Thus, if transbronchial needle aspirate is negative, a mediastinoscopy or mediastinotomy must still be performed. In such situations, 15% of the patients were found to have positive lymph nodes at mediastinoscopy (53).

Although the role of sputum cytology in large population screening remains controversial, when positive sputum cytology is noted in a patient with normal chest roentgenogram, the process of tumor localization is well defined (54). The stepwise approach starts with a thorough examination of the mouth, pharynx, and larynx. If negative, bronchoscopy is performed. If no endobronchial lesion is noted, a detailed analysis of each segment and subsegmental bronchi is conducted, including collecting separate cytology specimens from each area. Because of the time and detail required, general anesthesia is preferred. The recent introduction of the use of fluorescent light in the detection of occult endobronchial carcinoma also holds significant promise (55). The procedure involves the injection of a photosensitizer (hematoporphyrin), which is retained by malignant cells. The introduction of ultraviolet light results in fluorescence of the tumor cells, which can be detected using a special fluorescence detection endoscopy system. Biopsy of the area for histologic confirmation is required to exclude false results.

In patients undergoing chemotherapy, generally in clinical trials at present, tumor response is best assessed with CT scan of the chest. However, among patients having an endobronchial lesion, prior to initiation of treatment, a bronchoscopy tempers the degree of response as determined by the CT scan. Parrat and colleagues were able to assess tumor response in 86% of patients with a bronchoscope as compared to 99% with CT scan (56). However, the same study noted that in 33 of 88 patients (39%), CT scan either over- or under-evaluated tumor response as compared to direct visualization and biopsy assessment via bronchoscopy. Thus, FOB and CT scan should be viewed as complementary studies in evaluating the response to chemotherapy.

Because of common risk factors, patients with head and neck cancer frequently have multiple synchronous or metachronous tumors of the aerodigestive system (57,58). It is recommended that all patients with head and neck cancer undergo screening endoscopy at the time of diagnosis of the index lesion and at 2 years after diagnosis (59). Screening panendoscopy, including head and neck examination, esophagoscopy, and bronchoscopy, results in a 2.5-fold increase in the diagnosis of synchronous tumors (59).

Esophageal cancer, because of its close proximity, frequently involves the respiratory tract. The degree of involvement has an impact on resectability. In a review of 525 bronchoscopies on patients with esophageal cancer, Choi and associates noted 91 (17.3%) had impingement of the airway, whereas 87 (16.6%) had direct invasion through the respiratory mucosa (60,61). Although the surgical implications of the latter group are obvious, bronchoscopy has its shortcomings in patients found to have a normal airway or simple compression without obvious invasion. Seven percent of the "normal" and 20% of the "compression" patients have frank invasion at the time of surgery (62%).

The lung is frequently involved with metastatic carcinoma. Bronchoscopy plays an important role in the evaluation of these patients. In a report of 111 patients with metastatic disease, Argyros and Torrington noted that 44 patients (39.6%) had abnormal bronchoscopic findings (63). Patients who present with cough, hemoptysis, and chest pain and those with localized wheeze or rhonchi are more likely to have abnormal findings on bronchoscopy (63,64). Additionally, abnormality is more likely to occur if atelectasis is present on chest roentgenogram (63). Malignancies most likely to have endobronchial metastases include renal cell carcinoma, the adenocarcinomas, melanoma, sarcoma, Kaposi's sarcoma, and lymphoma (63).

Mediastinal Mass

In the evaluation of mediastinal masses, bronchoscopy can often spare the patient a more aggressive mediastinoscopy. Because it can be safely performed in the outpatient setting, cost is reduced. In a report of 183 patients with mediastinal lesions, Brynitz and coworkers reported positive transcranial needle biopsies in 37 of 159 patients (23%) with malignant lesions (65). Although the report did not provide the yield of benign diagnoses, a negative needle biopsy result alone should never be an end point and further evaluation must be considered to exclude malignant disease.

Infection

Pneumonia is a frequent disease encountered by the chest physician. Such infections are frequently treated empirically or by microbiologic evaluation of sputum. The rate of radiographic resolution of community-acquired pneumonia depends on the patient's age. Overall, 73% of patients have resolution within 6 weeks (66). However, when pneumonia is recurrent or fails to resolve, bronchoscopy may be necessary. Feinsilver and colleagues, in a review of 35 patients, reported on the role of the flexible fiberoptic bronchoscope in nonresolving pneumonia (67). When a specific diagnosis other than community-acquired pneumonia was present, flexible FOB was able to yield the correct diagnosis in 12 of 14 patients. Of the 23 patients with nondiagnostic bronchoscopy, 21 had no other explanation for their infiltrate except community-acquired pneumonia, suggesting a high negative predictive value of a nondiagnostic bronchoscopy. Bronchoscopy is more likely to yield a specific diagnosis when the infiltrate has been present for more than 30 days and is multilobar rather than lobar or segmental, and when the patient is less than 55 years old (67). Patients who are older or those with impaired immune systems (e.g., those with chronic obstructive pulmonary disease, alcohol abuse, and diabetes) have slower resolution of their pneumonia (67). Thus, bronchoscopy may be delayed in these patients.

Immunocompromised patients are particularly prone to opportunistic pulmonary infection by a variety of organisms. Bronchoscopy with BAL offers a safe and relatively rapid means of sampling the lower respiratory tract. In patients with acquired immunodeficiency syndrome, *Pneumocystis carinii* is a major concern, and obtaining both BAL and transbronchial biopsy provides nearly 100% sensitivity (68). In a study of 100 immunocompromised patients, Martin and associates were able to demonstrate opportunistic infection in 33%, obviating the need for open lung biopsy (69). Through the use of smear, stains, and monoclonal antibody detection methods, the lavage fluid can be rapidly screened. If the preliminary results are negative and an open lung biopsy is deemed necessary, it can be done within a few hours. Thus, even a negative BAL need not cause significant delay in proceeding with the more definitive open lung biopsy.

Cavitary lung lesions represent a special diagnostic challenge for the chest physician. Although many are of an infectious origin, the incidence of associated carcinoma has been reported to be 7.6% to 17% (70). Thus, bronchoscopic examination may be necessary to evaluate the possibility of cancer in patients presenting with cavitary lesions. In evaluating which patients are more likely to have underlying cancer, Sosenka and Glassroth noted that the cavitary lesion is more likely to be benign in patients with higher fevers, greater leukocytosis, and greater prevalence of systemic symptoms and who have risk factors for aspiration (70). In patients with bronchogenic carcinoma, bronchoscopy was diagnostic of cancer in 58% and precipitated additional studies leading to diagnosis in another 16%. In addition to assessing for malignancy, bronchoscopy offers an opportunity to collect specimens for microbiologic studies. There are also reports of successful drainage of abscess via transbronchial catheters (discussed below) (71,72).

Lobar Collapse

Of all of the abnormal radiographic patterns, the diagnostic yield of bronchoscopy is highest when lobar collapse is being evaluated (73). Persistent atelectasis may be a manifestation of an endobronchial lesion with postobstructive consolidation. Such a process requires endoscopic evaluation and appropriate treatment. Of the 54 patients undergoing bronchoscopy for lobar collapse, Su and coworkers noted that 35 (65%) had an endobronchial mass, 8 (15%) had abnormal bronchial mucosa, and 4 (7%) had narrowed, compressed, or stenosed airway (73).

Fiberoptic bronchoscopy has also been used therapeutically in critically ill patients with lobar collapse. In this situation insufflation of air using the bronchoscope with careful monitoring of pressure applied has been advocated (74). However, additional study is required to document benefit over traditional treatment.

Interstitial Lung Disease

Interstitial lung disease encompasses a wide range of diagnoses (75). Similarly the role of bronchoscopy in the evaluation of these diseases is varied. Bronchoscopy can be diagnostic in diseases such as sarcoidosis, lymphangitic carcinomatosis, eosinophilic pneumonia, and pulmonary alveolar proteinosis. BAL, when demonstrating the presence of materials or cells not typically found in the lung, can lead to the diagnosis of diseases such as histiocytosis X, pulmonary alveolar proteinosis, asbestos exposure, and berylliosis (76–79). The cell differential count, although not diagnostic, may provide clues to many diseases. In sarcoidosis, berylliosis, hypersensitivity pneumonitis, tuberculosis, and fungal infections, the T helper/T suppressor ratio is altered (80,81). It should be noted that at present the T helper/T suppressor ratio is not commonly used in the clinical setting. Elevation of polymorphonuclear cells is noted in idiopathic pulmonary fibrosis, collagen vascular diseases, pneumoconiosis, and bronchiolitis obliterans organizing pneumonia (82,83). Eosinophils are increased in chronic eosinophilic pneumonia and Churg-Strauss syndrome (84,85). Lipid-laden macrophages provide clues to amiodarone exposure, whereas the hemorrhagic syndromes produce hemosiderin-laden macrophages (75). It should be noted that although much is written about the use of BAL in interstitial lung disease, no clear role has been established for its use in prognosis or therapy.

Hemoptysis

Hemoptysis is a frequent pulmonary symptom. Its causes range from benign tracheobronchitis to malignancy. Although it is the second most common reason for bronchoscopy (4), not all cases of hemoptysis should undergo bronchoscopy. Distinction between gastrointesti-

nal, pharyngeal, nasal, and pulmonary sources is critical (86). Additionally, hemoptysis resulting from benign, self-limited processes (e.g., tracheobronchitis) need not undergo bronchoscopy. The procedure should be reserved for those having persistent bleeding, bleeding that is brisk or of large volume, or those at increased risk for malignancy. The search for the source of bleeding must be meticulous. Applied appropriately, the bronchoscopy can successfully localize the bleeding site in 75% to 93% of the cases (87). A small-caliber bronchoscope may be needed to conduct a thorough examination of the distal bronchial tree (88). If the initial examination is nondiagnostic, a repeat bronchoscopy following subsequent episodes of hemoptysis may be necessary. Although early bronchoscopy (within 48 hours) has a higher diagnostic yield than late bronchoscopy, its impact on overall patient management has not been shown (89–91). Despite the lack of any formal study, it is our impression that knowledge of cause of hemoptysis and its location is critical in the patient's management, and thus we favor earlier evaluation.

The role of rigid versus flexible bronchoscope in the evaluation of hemoptysis has also been argued, but not studied in a head-to-head comparison. The rigid instrument offers greater suction capacity, better control of the airway, and may afford the ability to tamponade the bleeding site, while the flexible scope offers greater visibility to the smaller airways. Ultimately the choice depends on the bronchoscopist's training and comfort level with the given instrument.

Cough

Cough is another frequent pulmonary complaint and often leads to bronchoscopy. The frequency with which bronchoscopy is performed for cough (4) and its low yield (92) indicate that this is an overutilized procedure. We recommend early bronchoscopy be performed only if the cough is associated with localizing lesion on chest roentgenogram, hemoptysis, or localized wheezing. If the cough has been persistent for at least 6 months (without smoking) and is not associated with any of the above conditions, a methacholine provocation challenge test, esophageal pH monitoring (or barium swallow), and otorhinolaryngologic examination should be performed prior to bronchoscopy (93).

Wheezing

Although wheezing is frequently associated with asthma, the differential diagnosis is varied and large (94). The evaluation of the wheezing in the nonasthmatic patient requires a thorough history and examination and ancillary studies, including a bronchoscopy. A chest roentgenogram and pulmonary function testing with flow volume loops can provide important diagnostic clues (95). However, if diagnosis remains elusive, FOB offers direct airway examination in search of an obstructing airway lesion. Additionally, bronchoscopy may be an important therapeutic tool for removing the offending lesion. Along with localized wheezing, an obstructing lesion may produce evidence of air trapping on roentgenogram, the evaluation of which may require bronchoscopy.

Stridor

Stridor is an important sign of life-threatening upper airway obstruction. The etiology must be rapidly elucidated. The causes are varied and can be grouped by age of presentation (96). In children the differential diagnosis should include epiglottis, croup, laryngomalacia, laryngeal papillomas, and tracheal foreign bodies (6). In adults the diagnostic considerations include acute bilateral vocal cord paralysis, rapidly growing tracheal lesions, and extrinsic compression of the trachea by mediastinal or esophageal lesions (6). The radiographic studies should include evaluation of the neck as well as the chest. Soft tissue roentgenograms of the neck may be diagnostic

of epiglottis or retropharyngeal abscess. Correct visualization of the upper airway can be diagnostic and occasionally therapeutic if the offending lesion or foreign body can be removed. Prior to starting the endoscopy, the bronchoscopist should ensure that equipment and the expertise to perform endobronchial intubation or emergent tracheostomy are immediately available.

Foreign Body Aspiration

Aspiration of a foreign body served as the impetus for the first bronchoscopy (1). The bronchoscope continues to play a major role in this entity, avoiding the need for major surgical procedures. Older children and adults can often provide a reliable history of foreign body aspiration. However, in younger children, and occasionally in adults, a clear history of aspiration may not be available. Pasaoglu and colleagues noted that 48% of 822 children gave a clear statement of aspiration (97). Although radiopaque objects can be detected by roentgenologic examination, radiolucent objects present with normal chest roentgenogram or with focal hyperinflation, infiltrate, or atelectasis (97). Traditionally, the rigid bronchoscope has been preferred, with successful removal in 85% of the cases (98). However, similar success has been reported with the FOB with lower morbidity and mortality (99,100). If sufficient time has passed since the aspiration, the foreign body may be completely surrounded by granulation tissue. The granuloma should be removed and dissected carefully to find the foreign body.

Trauma

The chest is frequently subjected to various types of trauma. Physical trauma injuries may be due to either blunt or penetrating insult. Bronchoscopy is frequently necessary following major thoracic trauma, both blunt and penetrating, to assess for airway damage. Hara and Prakash, in a retrospective review, noted bronchoscopy was of diagnostic value in

28 (53%) of 53 patients admitted with trauma (101). Although they did not discuss the decision process in selecting patients for bronchoscopy, others have suggested that all cases of major thoracic trauma be evaluated by bronchoscopy (102,103). In addition to the initial evaluation of the trauma victim, bronchoscopy may also be necessary to diagnose and manage posttrauma complications including aspiration and mucous plugging. Those with severe neck injury may require flexible bronchoscopy to perform oral intubation, although in case of emergent intubation, or intubation outside of the hospital setting, nasal intubation can be performed without direct visualization of the pharynx.

Thermal inhalation injury to the lungs can be devastating, with a mortality rate of 82% when patients have combined cutaneous burns and inhalation injury (104,105). Reliance on clinical criteria, such as facial or oral pharyngeal burns, production of carbonaceous sputum, wheezing, hoarseness, or singed nasal hairs, also fails to diagnose a number of patients with burn injury (106,107). Early radiographic diagnosis is also difficult (106,108). Moylan and associates evaluated 25 consecutive patients with thermal injury, who were admitted into a burn unit (108). Sixty percent were noted to have inhalation injury. These patients had an average burn size of 38% of the total body surface area, with a range of as little as 1% up to 80%. The presence of airway injury was associated with higher rates of pulmonary complications and overall mortality (108). Acute injury may produce severe airway edema, erythema, and mucosal sloughing. Subacute injury may cause mucosal necrosis and hemorrhagic tracheobronchitis, whereas chronic injury leads to scarring and stenosis, bronchiectasis, and formation of granulation tissue. Transbronchial biopsy in the chronic phase may demonstrate bronchiolitis obliterans (6). The use of the bronchoscope early in the evaluation of airway injury allows earlier diagnosis, with resul-

tant rapid institution of treatment, including corticosteroids, humidified air, antibiotics, and assistance in clearing airway plugs (107).

Chemicals released during industrial accidents and during war also pose a substantial risk of injury to the lungs. Freitag and colleagues reported their experience in managing 21 Iranian soldiers who suffered lung injury following inhalation of mustard gas (dichlorodiethyl sulfide) and other poisonous gases during the Iran–Iraq War in the 1980s (109). In the acute stage of injury bronchoscopy is used to assess the extent of damage and remove charred, necrotic debris from the airways. These patients produced large amounts of purulent thick mucus that could not be expectorated by the patients in their weakened state. Later sequelae, including tracheobronchial stenosis and granulation tissue, may necessitate the use of the bronchoscope in a more aggressive therapeutic role, as discussed below (109).

Pleural Effusions

Pleural effusions are generally evaluated by thoracentesis and closed pleural biopsy. The majority of effusions that remain undiagnosed have a high incidence of malignancy (110). In such situations, FOB may play a role, particularly in the presence of cough or hemoptysis or if the chest roentgenogram shows a concurrent pulmonary lesion. Chang and Perng performed thoracentesis, closed pleural biopsy, and bronchoscopy on 140 patients with pleural effusions (111). The combination of these procedures resulted in a diagnosis in 100 (71%) of the patients. Sixty-eight patients were diagnosed by thoracentesis or pleural biopsy or both. Bronchoscopy provided diagnosis in an additional 32 patients. Bronchoscopy was more likely to be positive if the patient had hemoptysis or if the chest roentgenogram demonstrated a parenchymal lesion in addition to the pleural effusion. In fact in the latter case, bronchoscopy was diagnostic more often than the pleural examination (111). Others have suggested that the presence of cough also increases the yield of bronchoscopy (112). The recent widespread use of thoracoscopically guided pleural biopsies may serve as an alternative to bronchoscopy in the search for the elusive causes of perplexing pleural effusions.

Lung Transplantation

With improved operative survival of patients undergoing lung transplant, the postoperative management of such patients presents a special challenge to the chest physician. The transplant patient is susceptible to complications related to the bronchial anastomosis, rejection, infection, and bronchiolitis obliterans. Bronchoscopy is of critical importance in the evaluation and management of airway complications and in the differentiation of rejection versus infection. Although recent surgical advances have decreased the incidence of anastomotic dehiscence, bronchoscopy should be performed in patients with persistent chest tube air leak to assess the anastomotic site. The lung transplant patient may also develop suture granuloma with compromise of the airway. Bronchoscopy is used to evaluate these patients and may also serve a therapeutic role (e.g., stent placement or laser resection of the granulomas and offending suture material) (113).

In the lung transplant patient, infection and rejection can present with similar clinical and radiographic findings. Because the treatment for either is different, bronchoscopy with transbronchial biopsy must be performed to differentiate between the two entities (114). The development of bronchiolitis obliterans remains a major obstacle to long-term survival of the lung transplant patient. Its manifestation includes the presence of new or increasing airway obstruction or restriction on pulmonary function testing. However, histologic confirmation requires tissue sampling via transbronchial biopsy (115).

Endotracheal Intubation

Traditionally, the laryngoscope is used to visualize the glottis for correct intubation of the airway. However, in difficult cases a fiberoptic bronchoscope offers an excellent alternative. Situations where the need for flexible bronchoscopy may be anticipated include patients with either fixed or unstable cervical spines, ankylosis of the temporal mandibular joint, and patients with large oral pharyngeal tumors (116). Additionally, the fiberoptic bronchoscope may be emergently needed when the glottis is unexpectedly difficult to visualize. Another role of the fiberoptic bronchoscope in the management of airways is confirmation of correct endotracheal tube position. Although a portable chest roentgenogram is frequently adequate to confirm position, a few settings are better suited for the bronchoscope. These include the obese patient where radiographic penetration of the mediastinum is insufficient and in unstable patients where a delay is anticipated in obtaining a chest x-ray. Some have also advocated the use of the bronchoscope to check endotracheal tube position in the pediatric patient to decrease the radiation dose from routine chest roentgenogram (117).

Endobronchial intubation and tracheostomy are potential sources for iatrogenic airway injury (118). Direct trauma to the vocal cords during passage of the endotracheal tube can lead to scarring of the anterior commissure. The pressure at the various contact points along the path of the endotracheal tube results in ischemic ulceration (119). Frequently, these injuries heal properly. However, with prolonged injury, cricoarytenoid joint fixation and scarring of the posterior commissure can occur (120,121). Overinflation of the cuff leads to circumferential ischemic necrosis of the trachea. The result may be loss of cartilagineous support and tracheomalacia or formation of fibrous stenosis during the repair process (122). The transmission of cuff pressure through the tracheal wall may injure the recurrent laryngeal nerve, with a resultant vocal cord paresis (119). Although tracheostomy eliminates the risk of glottic and subglottic injury, the stoma site is subject to stenosis by granulation, scarring, and contraction (119). Bronchoscopy and laryngoscopy allow full anatomic assessment of these injuries and the institution of proper therapeutic maneuvers. Both the flexible and rigid scope can be used to assess the airway proximal to the narrow airway. However, in situations of tight stricture, examination distal to the lesion may not be possible with the flexible scope. In these situations a rigid bronchoscope, which is capable of delivering mechanical ventilation, may be used to complete the airway examination. The bronchoscopist should be aware that any manipulation of a critically narrowed stenosis may precipitate complete obstruction by increasing secretions, hemorrhage, or edema. Thus, one should be prepared to perform immediate dilation.

Bronchoscopy may be used to assess the proper length and placement of transtracheal oxygen catheters. Patients receiving transtracheal oxygen therapy may have a catheter that has retroflexed through the vocal cord or is too long, thus producing irritation and traumatizing the carina or bronchi. Although these conditions may be assessed by chest roentgenogram, direct visualization with the bronchoscope may be needed. Irritation from the transtracheal oxygen catheter may also lead to granulation tissue formation along the cutaneotracheal tract, requiring bronchoscopic visualization and treatment. The transtracheal catheter also serves as a nidus for large mucous plug formation, which may require bronchoscopic evaluation and removal (123).

Vocal Cord Paralysis

Most patients with hoarseness and vocal cord paralysis tend to present to otolaryngologists rather than chest physicians. The etiologies of vocal cord paralysis are many (124) and the offending lesion may be located in the chest,

necessitating a referral to the chest physician. In a review of 20 years of literature on the etiologies of vocal cord paralysis, Terris and associates noted that 36% were the result of a neoplastic process (125). Of these, 55% were due to lung cancer. When history, physical examination, and imaging are nondiagnostic, endoscopy should be used because it can provide diagnosis in 20% of the patients (125). The left recurrent laryngeal nerve, because of its circuitous path into the chest, can be involved with diseases in the area of the left hilum. Lesions in this area can be biopsied via transbronchial needles. The right laryngeal nerve is involved only if the lesion extends into the right side of the neck.

Superior Vena Cava Syndrome

Mediastinal lesions can compromise venous return, producing the superior vena cava syndrome. The bronchoscope may be used to perform transtracheal or transbronchial needle aspiration and biopsy on masses or enlarged lymph nodes in these areas. Knowledge of the location of the great vessels is of critical importance when sampling these areas. When patients with superior vena cava syndrome are being evaluated, vascular anomalies should be excluded prior to any invasive procedure. Superior vena cava syndrome in the era of antibiotic therapy is predominantly related to malignancy (126). However, benign causes must also be kept in mind. Pathologic confirmation of the cause is needed before definitive treatment can be initiated. Bronchoscopic biopsy can establish the diagnosis in 60% to 70% of the cases (127,128). This is particularly important in avoiding unnecessary thoracotomy under general anesthesia, which may be associated with prolonged intubation in patients with large mediastinal masses (129).

Fistula

Fistulas are known to occur between the airway and its surrounding structure. Bronchopleural fistulas are the most common and generally occur after surgery. Bronchopleural fistulas are also associated with tuberculosis, pneumonia, empyema, and lung abscess (130,131). Proximally located fistulas may be directly visualized. However, localization of fistulas distal to the reach of the flexible bronchoscope are more challenging. In such situations an occluding balloon is systematically passed into each bronchial segment and inflated. When the correct segment is located, inflation of the balloon will result in a reduction in the air leak (130,132). Once localized, the bronchoscope can also be used therapeutically to seal the leak with a variety of tissue sealants (130).

Tracheoesophageal fistulas may be the result of a congenital defect, or more commonly in the adult, related to a malignancy of the aerodigestive system and its treatment. The most frequent symptom indicating the presence of a fistula is cough, especially triggered by swallowing or being in the decubitus position (133). The overall yield of bronchoscopic detection of a tracheal esophageal fistula is 83% (133). In addition to this diagnostic role, bronchoscopy performed in conjunction with esophagoscopy allows preoperative analysis and planning for surgical correction.

Aortobronchial fistula represents an uncommon but often lethal problem. The most common setting of aortobronchial fistula is prior surgical repair of the aorta (134). Other causes include syphilitic and atherosclerotic aneurysms and tuberculous involvement of the aortic wall (134). Aortograms frequently fail to demonstrate the fistula. Graeber and coworkers reported only one of five aortograms to be positive (134). Bronchoscopy is diagnostic in 50% of cases (7 of 14 cases) (135).

The bronchoscopist must understand the inherent danger of performing bronchoscopy in the presence of an aortobronchial fistula. Manipulation of the fistula or its overlying clot, may precipitate massive hemorrhage (134). Thus, one must be prepared to quickly isolate the hemorrhaging lung and proceed to immediate surgical repair.

Postoperative Assessment of Anastomosis

Patients undergoing lung resection or lung transplantation have the potential of developing a variety of problems at the surgical site. The stump or the anastomotic site is subject to dehiscence, recurrence of cancer, and suture granuloma. Bronchoscopy allows direct visualization and often can also be used therapeutically as discussed below.

Bronchography

Prior to the advent of the bronchoscope and CT, bronchography was frequently used to define the airway anatomy. Although it is used infrequently in the United States, bronchography continues to play a role in the detection of radiographically occult lung cancer, particularly in Europe and Japan (49,136). Ono and associates described mapping of the location of the peripheral lung lesion by selective peripheral bronchograms, performed through the flexible bronchoscope (49). Combining this mapping technique with a double-hinged curet, Ono was able to establish diagnosis of peripheral lesions in 41 of 46 patients (89%) on the first bronchoscopy and 45 of 46 patients (98%) within two bronchoscopies (49).

Therapeutic Bronchoscopy

Although frequently used in a diagnostic role, the bronchoscope was originally used as a therapeutic tool to remove a chicken bone (1). Since that time, both the therapeutic and diagnostic role of the bronchoscope have expanded greatly. The therapeutic applications of the bronchoscope are listed in Table 4.2. Frequently, the diagnostic and therapeutic applications of the bronchoscope occur simultaneously. Many of the indications listed in Table 4.2 have previously been discussed in the preceding section on diagnostic

Table 4.2. Indications for Therapeutic Bronchoscopy

Pulmonary toilet
Removal of foreign bodies
Removal of obstructive endobronchial tissue
    Malignant
        Brachytherapy
        Laser
        Photodynamic therapy
        Cryotherapy
        Electrosurgery
    Nonmalignant
Stent placement
Bronchoalveolar lavage
Aspiration of cysts
    Mediastinal
    Bronchogenic cysts
Drainage of abscesses
Pneumothorax
Lobar collapse
Intralesional injection
Thoracic trauma
Intubation
Airway maintenance (tamponade for bleeding)

bronchoscopy and discussion will not be repeated in this section.

Pulmonary Toilet

Pulmonary toilet is probably the most common therapeutic application of the bronchoscope. This is commonly required in patients who have an impaired cough mechanism from a variety of causes. Generally the scope with the largest working channel is preferred to enhance removal of the secretions.

Foreign Body Removal

Although the rigid bronchoscope traditionally is the preferred instrument for the removal of foreign bodies (98), the flexible scope, used with a variety of forceps and baskets, has also been proved to be safe and effective (99,100). As training of new pulmonologists offers increasingly less experience in the use of the rigid scope, the flexible scope will be used more and more to remove foreign bodies. The flexible scope offers the advantage of greater access to the periphery. It can also be used in patients with an unstable neck or those on mechanical ventilation.

Removal of Obstructive Endobronchial Tissue (Malignant)

Brachytherapy

The presence of an endobronchial obstruction, whether due to malignant cancer, benign tumor, or other benign lesion, often requires urgent medical attention. Bronchoscopy offers a unique means of delivering local treatment for these lesions. Large malignant endobronchial tumors can be treated by a variety of methods depending on the characteristics of the tumor and previous treatment. Because the endobronchial tumor represents only "the tip of the iceberg" with substantial submucosal and parenchymal tumor load, external beam radiation is a preferred modality to attack the entire tumor burden. When external beam radiation cannot be provided because of the danger of exposure to adjacent structures, brachytherapy offers an alternative mode of radiation delivery. Paradelo and coworkers, using a bronchoscopically positioned catheter to deliver radioactive seeds to the area of obstruction caused by tumor, noted symptomatic improvement in 30 of 34 patients (88%) (137). Radiographic improvement or stability was noted in 22 of 24 patients (92%) (137). Complications of brachytherapy include necrotic cavitation, fistula formation, and hemorrhage (138). A recent development of an implantable cylindrical capsule may allow a more homogenous delivery of the radiation dose and perhaps decrease the complication rate (139). This technique requires further study before widespread use.

Laser Photoresection

Tumor that has eroded through the mucosal wall into the lumen of the bronchus is amenable to laser photoresection. The application of laser to an obstructive lesion allows rapid reestablishment of airway patency, which in turn allows ventilation of the distal lung and drainage of postobstructive pneumonia. Coagulative effects of the laser energy can be used to palliate patients with hemorrhagic endobronchial tumors. Several reports have demonstrated improved airway patency in 79% to 92% of patients (140–142). Laser light can only be applied to the visible endobronchial part of the lesion and a significant amount of extraluminal tumor may be left behind. This extraluminal tumor may be amenable to adjuvant radiotherapy, either via external beam or bronchoscopically administered brachytherapy. Once a lumen has been reestablished, stent placement may delay reocclusion. Laser treatments may be used multiple times as the tumor grows back into the lumen. The complications of laser include hypoxemia, hemorrhage, perforation into adjacent structures, and endobronchial ignition of equipment (143). Despite its increasing popularity, laser bronchoscopy has not been demonstrated to increase survival in patients with malignant disease. In these patients it is only a palliative instrument.

The therapeutic role of laser is more apparent in the less commonly occurring benign airway obstructions. Its use in benign endobronchial tumor has been well described and can obviate the need for more aggressive surgical resection (140,141). Other causes of benign airway obstruction treatable by laser photoresection include tracheal granulomas (e.g., suture granuloma), tracheal stenosis (e.g., postintubation injury), endobronchial amyloidosis, syphilis gumma, and osteoplastic tracheopathy (140,141,144).

Photodynamic Therapy

The application of photodynamic therapy in the lung is the subject of ongoing research. The process requires the injection of a hematoporphyrin derivative, which serves as a photosensitizer. The subsequent delivery of laser light through the bronchoscope activates a hematoporphyrin derivative, resulting in tissue necrosis. The indications for photodynamic therapy are not yet fully defined. Imanmura and colleagues have reported its application in roentgenographically occult lung cancer, in which 25 of 39 patients (64%) had complete response (145). Another 10 had complete response with adjuvant radiotherapy (145). Balchum and McCoughan have reported a palliative role in patients with unresectable endobronchial tumor (146,147). Abramson has noted a reduction in the growth rate of endobronchial polyps in patients with juvenile laryngotracheobronchial papillomatosis (148). Preliminary analysis of a recent prospective trial of photodynamic therapy in patients with juvenile laryngotracheobronchial papillomatosis indicates that 50% have been disease free for at least one year (149).

Cryosurgery

Although bronchoscopic cryosurgery has been available since the 1970s (150), its use has been rather limited. Its utility in comparison with laser and brachytherapy is a matter of some debate. Proponents argue that cryotherapy is safer because of the lack of risk of bronchial wall perforation and endobronchial ignition (151,152). Additionally, there is no danger to the operator's eyes, no limitation of supplemental oxygen that may be used during the procedure, and a lower startup cost (151,152). The pros are balanced by those who note that the cryotherapy requires the use of a rigid scope and several follow-up bronchoscopies to remove tissue slough (153). Additionally, there is a delay between application of the treatment and the establishment of maximal airway patency (153).

Electrosurgery

In addition to serving as a vehicle for the delivery of laser light and radiation catheters, the bronchoscope can also be used to deliver electricity to perform electrocautery. The method is similar to that used to remove colonic polyps via a colonoscope. A snare is used to lasso the lesion and then electric current is passed to cut the mass. The mass is then removed as any other foreign body. In comparison with laser photoresection, electrosurgery offers the advantage of lower startup cost and shorter procedure time (154). However, unlike the colonoscope, the bronchoscope is not an electrically grounded instrument. This poses a significant danger of electrocution to the bronchoscopist should the snare contact the tip of the bronchoscope while electricity is turned on.

Removal of Obstructive Endobronchial Tissue (Nonmalignant)

Many of the techniques used for the removal of malignant tumors can also be used to remove benign tumors and nontumorous obstructive lesions. Laser is the most common technique used to remove nontumorous tissue. However, cryotherapy and balloon dilation have also been used (151,155). The most commonly encountered lesion requiring intervention is suture granuloma following thoracic surgery (156). Granulomas may also arise as a consequence of infection (e.g., tuberculosis), mechanical trauma (e.g., intubation), and inflammatory processes (e.g., sarcoidosis and Wegener's granulomatosis). A recent new application has been the photoablation of a granuloma that had formed at the stoma of a transtracheal catheter (157).

Tracheal stenosis presents a particularly difficult therapeutic dilemma for the chest physician. Treatment options include open surgical resection and reanastomosis, or nonsurgical/endoscopic procedures. The latter has included attempts at mechanical dilatation, electrocautery, cryosurgery, and laser ablation (151,155,158). The former three methods produce a significant amount of trauma to the tracheal mucosa, with a resultant increased risk of restenosis. A less traumatic technique, using radial laser incision of the scar tissue, followed by gentle dilation, was introduced by Shapsay, and produces good results in appropriately selected patients (158,159).

Stents

Most of the above methods of removing airway obstruction are limited in their application to only endobronchial lesions. In situations where the airway is compromised by extrinsic compression or by loss of tracheal cartilaginous rings, placement of a prosthetic stent may be able to provide patency. Stents have also been used in patients with anastomotic stenosis following sleeve resection or lung transplant (113,160,161). Stent placement usually requires the use of the rigid scope (162). However, placement using a flexible scope has also been described (163).

Bronchoalveolar Lavage

Bronchoalveolar lavage has several known diagnostic applications. Additionally, in patients with pulmonary alveolar proteinosis, the lavage plays a unique diagnostic and therapeutic role. The diagnosis by analysis of the lavage fluid can obviate the need for an open lung biopsy. Therapeutically, the lavage allows mechanical removal of intra-alveolar phospholipids (164,165). Multiple lavages are often necessary in patients with pulmonary alveolar proteinosis (165).

Aspiration of Cysts

Bronchogenic cysts present a diagnostic and therapeutic dilemma, often in otherwise healthy asymptomatic patients. Often surgery is required for histologic confirmation or to relieve compression on adjacent structures. However, there are several reports of successful diagnosis and decompression of cysts using transbronchial needle aspiration (166,167).

Drainage of Lung Abscesses

Lung abscesses are treated with antibiotics and adequate drainage. Drainage is usually attempted with chest physiotherapy and postural drainage. Surgical intervention is generally considered to be the next step in patients who do not respond to these drainage maneuvers (168,169). However, the bronchoscope can be used not only to obtain culture material, but also to effectively drain the cavity (71,170). Bronchoscopic placement of an indwelling drainage catheter has been attempted in a small number of patients with good results (72). This technique not only allows avoidance of surgery, but also circumvents the problem of inadequate drainage that may occur when the catheter is removed at the end of the bronchoscopic session. The indwelling catheter not only maintains a patent route for drainage, but can also be used to irrigate the cavity when spontaneous drainage ceases (72). Care must be exercised in using this technique to avoid spillage of the abscess fluid in the airway.

Contraindications

Bronchoscopy has been shown to be a safe procedure since its early beginning (171,172). The American Thoracic Society guidelines give only four contraindications to bronchoscopy (173). Of these, three (absence of informed consent, inexperienced operator, and inadequate facilities) are applicable to any medical intervention. The fourth contraindication is the inability to adequately oxygenate the patient for the procedure. Additionally, when considering rigid bronchoscopy, the patient must not have an unstable neck, severely ankylosed cervical spine, or restricted temporomandibular joint (6). For patients on mechanical ventilation, flexible FOB is preferred to rigid bronchoscopy (173).

Although generally a safe procedure, the risk of complications of bronchoscopy are increased in the presence of several conditions (Table 4.3). The risk is especially increased in the presence of malignant cardiac arrhythmia,

Table 4.3. Contraindications to Bronchoscopy

Contraindications
Inadequate oxygenation during the procedure
For rigid bronchoscopy
  Unstable neck
  Severely ankylosed cervical spine
  Restricted temporomandibular joint

Relative contraindications
Malignant arrhythmia
Unstable cardiac status
Refractory hypoxemia
Bleeding diathesis (if biopsy is anticipated)

Factors associated with increased risk of complications
Uncooperative patient
Recent or unstable angina
Unstable asthma
Moderate to severe hypoxemia
Hypercarbia
Uremia
Pulmonary hypertension
Lung abscess
Immunosuppression
Superior vena cava obstruction
Debility, advanced age, or malnutrition

Data derived from Sokolowski JW. Guidelines for fiberoptic bronchoscopy in adults. Am Rev Respir Dis 1987;136:1066.

severe refractory hypoxemia, or severe bleeding diathesis (if biopsy is anticipated) (173,174).

The importance of bleeding diathesis depends on the bronchoscopic procedure. Airway examination and BAL can generally be performed safely. To decrease the risk of nasal hemorrhage, oral rather than nasal intubation is preferred. If biopsy or resection is anticipated, the coagulopathy should be corrected. Uncorrected thrombocytopenia (less than 50,000/dL) or platelet dysfunction in the setting of uremia, are considered to be relative contraindications to bronchoscopy (25,172). However, when absolutely necessary, transbronchial biopsy can be successfully obtained with lower platelet counts. We have performed a number of transbronchial biopsies on immunocompromised bone marrow transplant recipients with platelet counts of less than 20,000/dL who were not candidates for open lung biopsy. All patients received platelet transfusion during the procedure and the flexible bronchoscope was firmly wedged into a segment before the biopsy was obtained. After the biopsy, suction was turned off and the scope was left in the wedged position to tamponade any bleeding for at least 5 minutes. Three to four biopsies were obtained from each patient without complication.

Medications

The need for sedation during bronchoscopy is a matter of some debate in the literature (175,176). However, surveys of practicing pulmonologists demonstrate that a majority prefer to use a sedative during the procedure. The use of sedative agents can facilitate the completion of the bronchoscopic examination in an efficient and comfortable manner. A survey of bronchoscopic practices in the United Kingdom showed 94% of physicians used a sedative, whereas in North America 77% routinely obtained intravenous access for sedation (4,39). In the same surveys, 12% to 16% of physicians used general anesthesia, although most flexible bronchoscopies can be performed with intravenous sedation and topical anesthesia (25). In addition to its well-known medical risks, general anesthesia has been demonstrated to decrease BAL fluid recovery and to elevate airway neutrophil counts as compared with awake, spontaneously breathing patients (177). General anesthesia is usually required only for rigid bronchoscopy and laser photoresection because of the duration of the procedure.

Those who favor no routine use of sedation argue that the risk of complications, especially respiratory depression, is a major contributor of up to one half of all bronchoscopic complications (176,178). However, with a thorough understanding of the pharmacology of agents used and their judicious use, the risk can be minimized. Immediate access to resuscitative equipment is critical to minimize the adverse effects of any untoward effects that may occur. The careful use of sedatives has been proven to be safe, even in the elderly (179,180). The proper use of sedation can decrease patient anxiety, discomfort, and unwanted negative physiologic responses. Although a variety of agents are used (4) the combination of an opiate and benzodiazepine is preferred (178). While providing sedation, the opiates offer analgesic and antitussive properties, and the benzodiazepines offer anxiolytic effects and antegrade amnesia.

Benzodiazepines

Midazolam is the most commonly used benzodiazepine (4). It offers rapid onset of action, short duration, and better amnesia, as compared to diazepam (181–184). Additionally, diazepam may be associated with pain and thrombophlebitis at the site of intravenous injection (181). Men tend to require a slightly higher dose as compared to women (178). Effects are also more pronounced in patients with cirrhotic livers (185). As with other benzodiazepines, midazolam can cause respiratory depression and even apnea if injected rapidly. Although the effect on the cardiovascular system is minimal, when combined with narcotics, both respiratory and cardiovascular depression is more pronounced (186).

Opiates

The opiates provide excellent sedation, cough suppression, and analgesia. Of the group, meperidine is the most commonly used (4). Onset of action is within 15 minutes and peaks within 2 hours. Meperidine has little effect on cough (187). Codeine, morphine, and fentanyl provide good cough control (175). Fentanyl, a synthetic opioid, has the fastest onset of action and shortest duration. It is 80 times as potent as morphine, necessitating extreme caution against overdose (187). At high doses fentanyl can cause muscular rigidity. Impaired liver and renal function may delay clearance of the opioids (175).

Other Agents

Propofol, a phenol derivative, provides excellent sedation with rapid onset and extremely short duration. It has been demonstrated to be as effective as midazolam in providing sedation (188). However, its potential to cause hypotension and myocardial and respiratory depression makes this a less than ideal agent for bronchoscopy.

Hydroxyzine, a piperazine antihistamine, has sedative and anxiolytic properties. It also has some analgesic effect. It potentiates the effect of opiates, allowing a reduction in the dose of the latter. Its anticholinergic effects may decrease respiratory secretions, facilitating the airway examination.

Droperidol, a butyrophenone, is a potent dissociative neuroleptic and an antiemetic. It is available in a premixed formula with fentanyl, allowing one to attain neuroleptic analgesia (186). It can cause extrapyramidal muscle movement. Its prolonged duration of action (up to 6 hours) makes this a less desirable agent (186).

Antagonists

Flumazenil is a benzodiazepine antagonist. Although it effectively reverses benzodiazepine-induced sedation, its effect on respiratory depression is less reliable (189).

Naloxone is a potent opiate antagonist. At low dose, it will reverse the opiate-induced ventilatory depression, without affecting analgesia (190). Its short half-life may necessitate redosing to maintain effect for the duration of the narcotic agent's effect.

Topical Anesthesia

Although nerve blocks can be used to provide excellent analgesia to the airway, most physicians rely on topical administration of local anesthetics to provide adequate analgesia. For the transnasal approach, a cotton-tipped applicator is used to deliver the medication. The pharynx can be anesthetized by gargling a solution of a topical anesthetic agent, by applying the anesthetic with an atomizer, or by inhaling a nebulized anesthetic solution. The approach should be individualized to the patient's skills and capacity.

Lidocaine

Although a variety of agents may be used for local anesthesia, lidocaine is the most widely used. It offers the widest margin of safety. It has a rapid onset of action and sufficient duration to allow completion of most bronchoscopic procedures. It is absorbed from the mucosa, and therefore poses some risk of systemic toxicity, particularly when levels exceed 5 μg/mL (191). Generally, up to 300 mg may be administered safely in small aliquots into the tracheobronchial tree. The dosage should be reduced in patients with hepatic dysfunction (192). Although inhaled lidocaine has been shown to induce bronchoconstriction in patients with asthma, its clinical implications are not clear because most would avoid performing bronchoscopy on patients with moderate to severe asthma (192,193). When a specimen is being collected for microbiologic culture, one must avoid use of preservative-containing solutions so as not to impede growth of organisms in the laboratory.

Cocaine

Cocaine, a naturally occurring alkaloid, produces both topical anesthesia and vasoconstriction. Its vasoconstrictive effects may be helpful in shrinking the nasal mucosa to ease passage of the bronchoscope. The same vasoconstrictive effects can cause myocardial and cerebral vascular infarction. Its side effects, addictive potential, and possibility of abuse should all favor the discontinuation of its use in bronchoscopy.

Antisialagogue

Several agents are available to help limit secretions to facilitate airway examination and also increase effectiveness of topical anesthesia. Atropine, a tertiary amine antimuscarinic agent, is the most commonly used agent (4). In addition to decreasing secretions, it is a potent bronchodilator. Glycopyrrolate, a quaternary ammonium antimuscarinic agent, does not cross the blood–brain barrier, and thus does not have a sedating effect (194). It is a better antisialagogue and also produces less tachycardia, a useful characteristic in patients with coronary artery disease (194).

REFERENCES

1. Nakhosten J. History of bronchoscopy: removal of tracheobronchial foreign body, Gustav Killian. J Bronchology 1994;1:76.
2. Jackson C. Bronchoscopy; past, present and future. N Engl J Med 1928;199:759–763.
3. Ikeda S, Yawai N, Ishikawa S. Flexible bronchofiberscope. Keio J Med 1968;17:1–133.
4. Prakash UBS, Stubbs SE. Bronchoscopy in North America: The ACCP survey. Chest 1991;100:1660–1675.
5. Wedzicha JA, Pearson MC. Management of massive hemoptysis. Respir Med 1990;84: 9–12.
6. Prakash UBS. Bronchoscopy. In: Bone RC, ed. Pulmonary and critical care medicine. St. Louis: Mosby-Yearbook, 1993;F(5):1–18.
7. Arroliga AC, Matthay RA. The role of bronchoscopy in lung cancer. Clin Chest Med 1993;14:87–98.
8. Popovich J Jr, Kvale PA, Eichenhorn, et al. Diagnostic accuracy of multiple biopsies from flexible fiberoptic bronchoscopy: a comparison of central versus peripheral carcinoma. Am Rev Respir Dis 1982;125:521–523.
9. Shure D, Astarita RW. Bronchoscopic carcinoma presenting as an endobronchial mass: optimal number of biopsy specimens for diagnosis. Chest 1983;83:865–867.
10. Chaudhary BA, Yoneda K, Burki NK. Fiberoptic bronchoscopy: comparison of procedures used in the diagnosis of lung cancer. J Thorac Cardiovasc Surg 1978;76:33–37.
11. Jay SJ, Wehr K, Nicholason DP, et al. Diagnostic sensitivity and specificity of pulmonary cytology: comparison of techniques used in conjunction with flexible fiberoptic bronchoscopy. Acta Cytol 1980;24:304–312.
12. Payne CR, Hadfield JW, Stovin PG, et al. Diagnostic accuracy of cytology and biopsy in primary bronchial carcinoma. J Clin Pathol 1981;34:773–778.
13. Bedrossian CWM, Rybka DL. Bronchial brushing during fiberoptic bronchoscopy for the cytodiagnosis of lung cancer: comparison with sputum and bronchial washings. Acta Cytol 1976;20:446–453.
14. Castella J, del la Heras P, Puzo C, et al. Cytology of post bronchoscopically collected sputum samples and its diagnostic value. Respiration 1981;42:116–121.
15. Buccheri G, Barberis P, Delfino MS. Diagnostic, morphologic and histopathologic correlates in bronchogenic carcinoma: a review of 1,045 bronchoscopic examinations. Chest 1991;99:809–814.
16. Cummings CLM, Brooks IO, Stinson JM. Increases in diagnostic yield of fiberoptic bronchoscopy by fluoroscopy. J Natl Med Assoc 1982;74:239–241.
17. Mak VHF, Johnston IDA, Hetzel MR, et al. Value of washings and brushings at fiberoptic bronchoscopy in the diagnosis of lung cancer. Thorax 1990;45:373–376.
18. Skitarelic K, von Haam E. Bronchial brushings and washings: a diagnostically rewarding procedure? Acta Cytol 1974;18:321–326.
19. Chopra SK, Genovesi MG, Simmons DH, et al. Fiberoptic bronchoscopy in the diagnosis of lung cancer: comparison of pre- and post-bronchoscopy sputa, washings, brushings, and biopsies. Acta Cytol 1977; 21:524–527.
20. Funahashi A, Browne TK, Houser WC, et al. Diagnostic value of bronchial aspirate and post bronchoscopic sputum in fiberoptic bronchoscopy. Chest 1979;76:514–517.
21. Kvale PA, Bode FR, Kini S. Diagnostic accuracy in lung cancer: comparison of techniques used in association with flexible fiberoptic bronchoscopy. Chest 1976;69:752–757.
22. Solomon DA, Solliday NH, Gracey DR. Cytology in fiberoptic bronchoscopy: comparison of bronchial brushing, washing, and post-bronchoscopy sputum. Chest 1974;65: 616–619.

23. Struve-Christensen E, Michaelsen M, Mossing N. The diagnostic value of bronchial washing in lung cancer. J Thorac Cardiovasc Surg 1974;68:313–317.

24. Matsuda N, Horai T, Nakamura S, et al. Bronchial brushing and bronchial biopsy: comparison of diagnostic accuracy and cell typing reliability in lung cancer. Thorax 1986;41:475–478.

25. Prakash UBS, Stubbs SE. The bronchoscopy survey: some reflections. Chest 1991;100: 1660–1667.

26. Gay PC, Bruntinel WM. Transbronchial needle aspiration in the practice of bronchoscopy. Mayo Clin Proc 1989;64:158–162.

27. Horsley JR, Miller RE, Amy RWM, et al. Bronchial submucosal needle aspiration performed through the fiberoptic bronchoscope. Acta Cytol 1984;28:211–217.

28. Shure D. Transbronchial needle aspiration—current status. Mayo Clin Proc 1989;64: 251–254. Editorial.

29. Shure D, Fedullo PF. The role of transcarinal needle aspiration in the staging of bronchogenic carcinoma. Chest 1984;86:693–696.

30. Schenk DA, Bryan CL, Bower JH, et al. Transbronchial needle aspiration in the diagnosis of bronchogenic carcinoma. Chest 1987;92:83–85.

31. Shure D. Is transbronchial needle aspiration worthwhile? Pulmonary Perspectives 1991; 8:1–13.

32. Harrow E, Halbert M, Hardy S, et al. Bronchoscopic and roentgenographic correlates of a positive transbronchial needle aspiration in the staging of lung cancer. Chest 1991;100:1592–1596.

33. Wang KP, Gupta PK, Haponik EF, et al. Flexible transbronchial needle aspiration: technical considered. Ann Otol Rhinol Laryngol 1984;93:233–236.

34. Cortese DA, McDougall JC. Biopsy and brushing of peripheral lung cancer with fluoroscopic guidance. Chest 1979;75:141–145.

35. Kovnat DM, Rath GS, Anderson WM, et al. Bronchial brushing through the flexible fiberoptic bronchoscope in the diagnosis of peripheral pulmonary lesions. Chest 1975; 67:179–184.

36. Radke JR, Conway WA, Eyler WR, et al. Diagnostic accuracy in peripheral lung lesions. Chest 1979;76:176–179.

37. Zavala DC. Diagnostic fiberoptic bronchoscopy: techniques and results of biopsy in 600 patients. Chest 1975;68:12–19.

38. Cummings SR, Lillington GA, Richard RJ. Managing solitary pulmonary nodules: the choice of strategy is a close call. Am Rev Respir Dis 1986;134:453–460.

39. Simpson FG, Arnold AG, Purvis A, et al. Postal survey of bronchoscopic practices by physicians in the United Kingdom. Thorax 1986;41:311–317.

40. Ellis JH. Transbronchial lung biopsy via the fiberoptic bronchoscope. Chest 1975;68: 524–532.

41. Stringfield JT, Markowitz DJ, Bentz RR, et al. The effect of tumor size and location on diagnosis by fiberoptic bronchoscopy. Chest 1977;72:474–476.

42. Wallace JM, Deutsch AL. Flexible fiberoptic bronchoscopy and percutaneous needle lung aspiration for evaluating the solitary pulmonary nodule. Chest 1982;81:665–671.

43. Pirozynski M. Bronchoalveolar lavage in the diagnosis of peripheral, primary lung cancer. Chest 1992;102:372–374.

44. Shiner RJ, Rosenman J, Katz I, et al. Bronchoscopic evaluation of peripheral lung tumors. Thorax 1988;43:887–889.

45. Swinburn CR, Veale D, Peel ET, et al. A prospective randomized comparison of fine needle aspiration biopsy and fiberoptic bronchoscopy in the investigation of peripheral pulmonary opacities. Respir Med 1989;83: 493–495.

46. Shure D, Fedullo PF. Transbronchial needle aspiration of peripheral masses. Am Rev Respir Dis 1983;128:1090–1092.

47. Wang KP, Haponik EF, Britt EJB, et al. Transbronchial needle aspiration of peripheral pulmonary nodules. Chest 1984;86: 819–823.

48. Mori K, Yanasc N, Kaneko M, et al. Diagnosis of peripheral lung cancer in cases of tumors 2 cm or less in size. Chest 1989; 95:304–308.

49. Ono R, Loke J, Ikeda S. Bronchofiberscopy with curette biopsy bronchography in the evaluation of peripheral lung lesions. Chest 1981;79:162–166.

50. Ovchinikov A, Narizhny A. Value of ultrathin bronchofibroscope in the diagnostics of peripheral cancer. Chest 1991;100:89S. Abstract.

51. Tanaka M, Kohda E, Satoh M, et al. Diagnosis of peripheral lung cancer using a new type of endoscope. Chest 1990;97: 1231–1234.

52. Schenk DA, Bower JH, Bryan CL, et al. Transbronchial needle aspiration staging of bronchogenic carcinoma. Am Rev Respir Dis 1986;134:146–148.

53. Wang KP. Needle biopsy for the diagnosis of intrathoracic lesions: transbronchial needle biopsy. In: Keetle, ed. Current controversy in thoracic surgery. Philadelphia: WB Saunders, 1986.

54. Martini N, Melamed MR. Occult carcinomas of the lung. Ann Thorac Surg 1980;30: 215–223.

55. Kato M, Cortese DA. Early detection of lung cancer by means of hematoporphyrin derivative fluorescence and laser photoradiation. Clin Chest Med 1985;6:237–253.

56. Parrat E, Pujol JL, Gautier V, Michel FB, Godard P. Chest tumor response during lung cancer chemotherapy: computed tomography vs fiberoptic bronchoscopy. Chest 1993;103: 1495–1501.

57. Abemayor E, Moore DM, Hanson DG. Identification of synchronous esophageal tumors in patients with head and neck cancer. J Surg Oncol 1988;38:94–96.

58. Leipzig B, Zellmer JE, Klug D. The role of endoscopy in evaluating patients with head and neck cancer: a multi-institutional prospective study. Arch Otolaryngol 1985; 111:589–594.

59. Haughey BH, Gates GA, Arfken CL, Harvey J. Meta-analysis of second malignant tumors in head and neck cancer: the case for an endoscopic screening protocol. Ann Otol Rhinol Laryngol 1992;101:105–112.

60. Choi TK, Siu KF, Lam KH, Wong J. Bronchoscopy and carcinoma of the esophagus I: findings of bronchoscopy in carcinoma of the esophagus. Am J Surg 1984;147: 757–759.

61. Choi TK, Siu KF, Lam KH, Wong J. Bronchoscopy and carcinoma of the esophagus II: carcinoma of the esophagus with tracheobronchial involvement. Am J Surg 1984;147:760–762.

62. Giuli R, Sancho-Garnier H. Diagnostic, therapeutic, and prognostic features of cancers of the esophagus: results of the international prospective study conducted by the OESO group (790 patients). Surgery 1986;99: 614–622.

63. Argyros GJ, Torrington KG. Fiberoptic bronchoscopy in the evaluation of carcinoma metastatic to the lung. Chest 1994; 105:454–457.

64. Poe RH, Ortiz C, Isreal RH, et al. Sensitivity, specificity, and predictive values of bronchoscopy in neoplasm metastatic to lung. Chest 1985;88:84–88.

65. Brynitz S, Struve-Christensen E, Borgeskov S, Bertelsen S. Transcarinal mediastinal needle biopsy compared with mediastinoscopy. J Thorac Cardiovasc Surg 1985;90:21–25.

66. Mittle RL Jr, Schwab RJ, Duchin JS, et al. Radiographic resolution of community acquired pneumonia. Am J Respir Crit Care Med 1994;149:630–635.

67. Feinsilver SH, Fein AM, Niederman MS, et al. Utility of fiberoptic bronchoscopy in nonresolving pneumonia. Chest 1990;98: 1322–1326.

68. Gal AA, Klatt EC, Koss MN, et al. The effectiveness of bronchoscopy in the diagnosis of Pneumocystis carinii and cytomegalovirus pulmonary infections in acquired immunodeficiency syndrome. Arch Pathol Lab Med 1987;111:238–241.

69. Martin WJ II, Smith TF, Sanderson DR, et al. Role of bronchoalveolar lavage in the assessment of opportunistic pulmonary infections: utility and complications. Mayo Clin Proc 1987;62:549–557.

70. Sosenko A, Glassroth J. Fiberoptic bronchoscopy in the evaluation of lung abscesses. Chest 1985;87:489–494.

71. Jeong MP, Kim WS, Han SK, et al. Transbronchial catheter drainage via fiberoptic bronchoscope in intractable lung abscess. Korean J Int Med 1989;4:54–58.

72. Schmitt GS, Ohar JM, Kanter KR, Naunheim KS. Indwelling transbronchial catheter drainage of pulmonary abscess. Ann Thorac Surg 1988;45:43–47.

73. Su WJ, Lee PY, Perng RP. Chest roentgenographic guidelines in the selection of patients for fiberoptic bronchoscopy. Chest 1993;103: 1198–1201.

74. Tsao TCY, Tsai YH, Lan RS, Shieh WB, Lee CH. Treatment for collapsed lung in critically ill patients: selective intrabronchial air

insufflation using the fiberoptic broncho-scope. Chest 1990;97:435–438.

75. Depaso WJ, Winterbauer RH. Interstitial lung disease. Dis Mon 1991;37:61–133.

76. Chollet S, Soler P, Dournovo P, et al. The diagnosis of pulmonary histiocytosis X by immunodetection of Langerhan's cell in BALF. Am J Pathol 1984;115:225–232.

77. Martin RJ, Coalsen JJ, Rogers RM, et al. Pulmonary alveolar proteinosis: the diagnosis by segmental lavage. Am Rev Respir Dis 1980;121:819–825.

78. Helmers RA, Hunninghake GW. Broncho-alveolar lavage in the non-immunocompro-mised patient. Chest 1989;96:1184–1190.

79. Rossman MD, Kern JA, Elias JA, et al. Proliferative response of bronchoalveolar lymphocytes to beryllium, a test for chronic beryllium disease. Ann Intern Med 1988;108:687–693.

80. Hunninghake GW, Crystal RG. Pulmonary sarcoidosis: a disorder mediated by excess helper T-lymphocyte activity at sites of dis-ease activity. N Engl J Med 1981;305:429–434.

81. Semenzato G. Current concepts on bron-choalveolar lavage cells in extrinsic allergic alveolitis. Respiration 1988;54:59–65.

82. Studdy PR, Rudd RM, Gellert AR, et al. Bronchoalveolar lavage in the diagnosis of diffuse pulmonary shadowing. Br J Dis Chest 1984;78:46–54.

83. Hunninghake GW, Kawanami O, Ferrans VJ, et al. Characterization of inflammatory and immune effector cells in the lung parenchyma of patients with interstitial lung disease. Am Rev Respir Dis 1981;123:407.

84. Aguayo SM, Niccole SA, Martin RJ, et al. Is BAL eosinophilia clinically useful in the dif-ferential diagnosis of unexplained pulmonary infiltrates? Am Rev Respir Dis 1989;139:385. Abstract.

85. Pesci A, Bertorelli G, Manganelli P, et al. Bronchoalveolar lavage in chronic eosin-ophilic pneumonia: analysis of six cases in comparison with other interstitial lung dis-eases. Respiration 1988;54:16–22.

86. Lyons HA. Differential diagnosis of hemoptysis and its treatment. Basics of RD 1976;5:26–30.

87. Smiddy JF, Elliot RC. The evaluation of hemoptysis with fiberoptic bronchoscopy. Chest 1973;92:77–82.

88. Prakash UBS. The use of the pediatric fiberoptic bronchoscope in adults. Am Rev Respir Dis 1985;132:715–717.

89. Pursel SE, Lindskog GE. Hemoptysis: a clin-ical evaluation of 105 patients examined con-secutively on a thoracic surgical service. Am Rev Respir Dis 1961;84:329–336.

90. Gong H Jr, Salvatierra C. Clinical efficacy of early and delayed fiberoptic bronchoscopy in patients with hemoptysis. Am Rev Respir Dis 1981;124:221–225.

91. Stoller JK. Diagnosis and management of massive hemoptysis: a review. Respir Care 1992;37:6:564–581.

92. Poe RH, Israel RH, Utell MJ, Hall WJ. Chronic cough: bronchoscopy or pulmonary function testing? Am Rev Respir Dis 1982;126:160–162.

93. Irwin RS, Curley FJ, French CL. Chronic cough: the spectrum and frequency of causes, key components of the diagnostic evaluation, and outcome of specific therapy. Am Rev Respir Dis 1990;141:640–647.

94. Holden DA, Mehta AC. Evaluation of wheez-ing in the non-asthmatic patient. Cleve Clin J Med 1990;57:345–352.

95. Kryger M, Bode F, Antic R, Anthonisen N. Diagnosis of obstruction of the upper and central airways. Am J Med 1976;61:85–93.

96. O'Hollaren MT, Everts EC. Evaluating the patient with stridor. Ann Allergy 1991;67:301–305.

97. Pasoglu I, Dogan R, Demircin M, et al. Bronchoscopic removal of foreign bodies in children: retrospective analysis of 822 cases. Thorac Cardiovasc Surg 1991;39:95–98.

98. Weissberg D, Schwartz I. Foreign bodies in the tracheobronchial tree. Chest 1987;91:730–773.

99. Cunanan OS. The flexible fiberoptic bron-choscope in foreign body removal: experience in 300 cases. Chest 1978;73:725–726.

100. Lan RS, Lee CH, Chaing YC, Wang WJ. Use of fiberoptic bronchoscopy to retrieve bronchial foreign bodies in adults. Am Rev Respir Dis 1989;140:1734–1737.

101. Hara KS, Prakash UBS. Fiberoptic bron-choscopy in the evaluation of acute chest and upper airway trauma. Chest 1989;96:627–630.

102. Payne WS, DeRemee RA. Injuries of the

trachea and major bronchi. Postgrad Med 1971;49:152–158.

103. Travis SPL, Layer GT. Traumatic transection of the thoracic trachea. Ann R Coll Surg Engl 1983;65:240–241.

104. Bartlett RH, Niccole M, Travis MJ, et al. Acute management of the upper airway in facial burns and smoke inhalation. Arch Surg 1976;111:744.

105. Schneider W, Berger A, Mailander P, Tempka A. Diagnostic and therapeutic possibilities for fiberoptic bronchoscopy in inhalation injury. Burns 1988;14:1:53–57.

106. Hunt JL, Agee RN, Pruitt BA. Fiberoptic bronchoscopy in acute inhalation injury. J Trauma 1975;15:641.

107. Moylan JA. Smoke inhalation and burn injury. Surg Clin North Am 1980;60:1533–1540.

108. Moylan JA, Adib K, Birnbaum M. Fiberoptic bronchoscopy following thermal injury. Surg Gynecol Obstet 1975;140:541–543.

109. Freitag L, Firusian N, Stamatis G, Greschuchuna D. Bronchoscopy: the role of bronchoscopy in pulmonary complications due to mustard gas inhalation. Chest 1991;100:1436–1441.

110. Gunnels JJ. Perplexing pleural effusion. Chest 1978;74:390–393.

111. Chang SC, Perng RP. The role of fiberoptic bronchoscopy in evaluating the causes of pleural effusions. Arch Intern Med 1989;149:855–857.

112. Upham JW, Mitchell CA, Armstrong JG, Kelly WT. Investigation of pleural effusion: the role of bronchoscopy. Aust N Z J Med 1992;22:41–43.

113. Seballos RJ, Mehta AC, McCarthy PM, Kirby TJ. The management of airway complications following lung transplantation. Am Rev Resp Dis 1993;147:A602. Abstract.

114. Sibley RK, Berry GJ, Tazelaar HD, et al. The role of transbronchial biopsies in the management of lung transplant recipients. J Heart Lung Transplant 1993;12:308–324.

115. Paradis I, Yousem S, Griffith B. Airway obstruction and bronchiolitis obliterans after lung transplantation. Clin Chest Med 1993;14:751–763.

116. Edens ET, Sia RL. Flexible fiberoptic endoscopy in difficult intubations. Ann Otol 1981;90:307–309.

117. Dietrich KA, Strauss RH, Cabalka AK, et al. Use of flexible fiberoptic endoscopy for determination of endotracheal tube position in the pediatric patient. Crit Care Med 1988;16:884–887.

118. Streitz JM, Shapshay SM. Airway injury after tracheotomy and endotracheal intubation. Surg Clin North Am 1991;71:1211–1231.

119. Bishop MJ. Mechanisms of laryngotracheal injury following prolonged tracheal intubation. Chest 1989;96:185–186.

120. Colice GL, Stukel TA, Dain B. Laryngeal complications of prolonged intubation. Chest 1989;96:877–884.

121. Whited RE. A prospective study of laryngotracheal sequelae on long term intubation. Laryngoscope 1984;94:376–377.

122. Kastanos N, Estopa Miro R, Marin Perez A, et al. Laryngotracheal injury due to endotracheal intubation: incidence, evolution, and predisposing factors. A prospective long-term study. Crit Care Med 1983;11:362–367.

123. Rai NS, Mehta AC, Meeker DP, Stoller JK. Transtracheal oxygen therapy—does practice make perfect? J Bronchology 1994;1:205–212.

124. Parnell FW, Brandenburg JH. Vocal cord paralysis: a review of 100 cases. Laryngoscope 1970;80:1036–1045.

125. Terris DJ, Arnstein DP, Nguyen HH. Contemporary evaluation of unilateral vocal cord paralysis. Otolaryngol Head Neck Surg 1992;107:84–90.

126. Abner A. Approach to the patient who presents with superior vena cava obstruction. Chest 1993;103:394S–397S.

127. Armstrong BA, Perez CA, Simpson JR, et al. Role of irradiation in the management of superior vena cava syndrome. Int J Radiat Oncol Biol Phys 1987;13:531–539.

128. Chen JC, Bongard F, Klein SR. A contemporary perspective on superior vena cava syndrome. Am J Surg 1990;160:207–211.

129. Ferrari LR, Bedford RF. General anesthesia prior to treatment of anterior mediastinal masses in pediatric cancer patients. Anesthesiology 1990;72:991–995.

130. Baumann MH, Sahn SA. Medical management and therapy of bronchopleural fistulas in the mechanically ventilated patient. Chest 1990;97:721–728.

131. Steiger Z, Wilson RF. Management of bronchopleural fistulas. Surgery 1984;158:267–271.

132. Regal G, Sturm A, Neumann C, et al. Occlusion of bronchopleural fistula after lung injury: a new treatment by bronchoscopy. J Trauma 1989;29:223–226.

133. Campion JP, Bourdelat D, Launois B. Surgical treatment of malignant esophagotracheal fistulas. Am J Surg 1983;148:641–646.

134. Graeber GM, Farrell BG, Neville JF Jr, Parker FB Jr. Successful diagnosis and management of fistulas between the aorta and the tracheobronchial tree. Ann Thorac Surg 1980; 29:555–561.

135. Ishizaki Y, Tada Y, Takagi A, et al. Aortobronchial fistula after an aortic operation. Ann Thorac Surg 1990;50:975–977.

136. Brown SD, Foster WL. Localization of occult bronchogenic carcinoma by bronchography. Chest 1991;100:1160–1162.

137. Paradelo JC, Waxman MJ, Throne BJ, et al. Endobronchial irradiation with ^{192}Ir in the treatment of malignant endobronchial obstruction. Chest 1992;102:1072–1074.

138. Khanavkar B, Stern P, Alberti W, Nakhosteen JA. Complications associated with brachytherapy alone or with laser in lung cancer. Chest 1991;99:1062–1065.

139. Marsh BR, Colvin DP, Zinreich ES, et al. Clinical experience with an endobronchial implant. Radiology 1993;189:147–150.

140. Brutinel WM, Cortese DA, McDougall JC, et al. A two-year experience with the neodymium-YAG laser in endobronchial obstruction. Chest 1987;91:159–165.

141. Cavaliere S, Foccoli P, Farina PL. Nd:YAG laser bronchoscopy: a five-year experience with 1,396 applications in 1,000 patients. Chest 1988;94:15–21.

142. Unger M. Bronchoscopic utilization of the Nd:YAG laser for obstructing lesions of the trachea and bronchi. Surg Clin North Am 1984;64:931–938.

143. Unger M. Lasers and their role in pulmonary medicine: present and future. In: Fishman AP, ed. Update: pulmonary diseases and disorders. New York: McGraw Hill, 1992: 419–432.

144. Mehta AC. Laser applications in respiratory care. In: Kacmarek RM, Stoller JK, eds. Current respiratory care. Toronto: Mosby-Year Book, 1988:100–106.

145. Imamura S, Kusunoki Y, Takifuji N, et al. Photodynamic therapy and/or external beam radiation therapy for roentgenological occult lung cancer. Cancer 1994;73: 1608–1614.

146. Balchum O, Doiron DR. Photoradiation therapy of endobronchial lung cancer. Clin Chest Med 1985;6:255–275.

147. McCaughan JS. Overview of experience with photodynamic therapy for malignancies in 192 patients. Photochem Photobiol 1987; 46:903–909.

148. Abramson AL, Shikowitz MJ, Mullooly VM, et al. Clinical effects of photodynamic therapy on recurrent laryngeal papillomas. Ann Otol Head Neck Surg 1992;118:25–29.

149. Patel SR, DeBoer G, Mehta AC. Role of photodynamic therapy in juvenile laryngotracheobronchial papillomatosis. Chest 1993; 104:161S. Abstract.

150. Carpenter RJ, Neel HB, Sanderson DR. Cryosurgery of bronchopulmonary structures. Chest 1977;72:279–284.

151. Marasso A, Gallo E, Massaglia GM, et al. Cryosurgery in bronchoscopic treatment of tracheobronchial stenosis: indications, limits, personal experience. Chest 1993;103:472–474.

152. Walsh DA, Maiwand MO, Nath AR, et al. Bronchoscopic cryotherapy for advanced bronchial carcinoma. Thorax 1990;45: 509–513.

153. George PJM, Rudd RM. Bronchoscopic cryotherapy for advanced bronchial carcinoma. Thorax 1990;150.

154. Gerasin VA, Shafrovsky BB. Endobronchial electrosurgery. Chest 1988;93:270–274.

155. Cohen MD, Weber TR, Rao CC. Balloon dilatation of tracheal and bronchial stenosis. Am J Radiol 1984;142:477–478.

156. Dumon JF, Rebound E, Grabe L, et al. Treatment of tracheobronchial lesions by laser photoresection. Chest 1982;81:278–284.

157. Punzal PA, Myers R, Ries AL, Harrell JH. Laser resection of granulation tissue secondary to transtracheal oxygen catheter. Chest 1992;101:269–271.

158. Shapshay SM, Beamis JF, Hybels RL, Bohigian RK. Endoscopic treatment of subglottic and tracheal stenosis by radial laser incision and dilation. Ann Otol Rhinol Laryngol 1987;96:661–664.

159. Mehta AC, Lee FYW, Cordasco EM, et al. Concentric tracheal and subglottic stenosis; management using the Nd-YAG laser for mucosal sparing followed by gentle dilatation. Chest 1993;104:673–677.

160. Colt HG, Janssen JP, Dumon JF, Noirclerc MJ. Endoscopic management of bronchial stenosis after double lung transplantation. Chest 1992;102:10–16.

161. Tsang V, Goldstraw P. Endobronchial stenting for anastomotic stenosis after sleeve resection. Ann Thorac Surg 1989;48:568–571.

162. Dumon JF. A dedicated tracheobronchial stent. Chest 1990;97:328–332.

163. deCastro FR, Lopez L, Varela A, et al. Tracheobronchial stents and fiberoptic bronchoscopy. Chest 1991;99:792. Letter.

164. Goldstein RA, Rohatgi PK, Bergofsky EH, Block ER. Clinical role of bronchoalveolar lavage in adults with pulmonary disease. Am Rev Respir Dis 1990;142:481–486.

165. Prakash UBS, Barham S, Carpenter HA, et al. Pulmonary alveolar phospholipoproteinosis: experience with 34 cases and a review. Mayo Clin Proc 1987;62:499–518.

166. Schwartz DB, Beals TF, Wimbish KJ, Hammersley JR. Transbronchial fine needle aspiration of bronchogenic cysts. Chest 1985;88:573–575.

167. Schwartz AR, Fishman EK, Wang KP. Diagnosis and treatment of a bronchogenic cyst using transbronchial needle aspiration. Thorax 1986;41:326–327.

168. Delarue NC, Pearson FG, Nelems JM, Cooper JD. Lung abscess: surgical implications. Can J Surg 1980;23:297–302.

169. Estrera AS, Platt MR, Mills LJ, Shaw RR. Primary lung abscess. J Thorac Cardiovasc Surg 1980;79:275–282.

170. Connors JP, Roper CL, Ferguson TB. Transbronchial catheterization of pulmonary abscesses. Ann Thorac Surg 1975; 19:254.

171. Pereira W Jr, Kovnat DM, Snider GL. A prospective cooperative study of complications following flexible fiberoptic bronchoscopy. Chest 1978;73:813–816.

172. Suratt PM, Smiddy JF, Gruber B. Deaths and complications associated with fiberoptic bronchoscopy. Chest 1976;69:747–751.

173. Burgher LW, Jones FL, Patterson JR, Selecky PA. Guidelines for fiberoptic bronchoscopy in adults. Am Rev Respir Dis 1987;136: 1066.

174. Katz AS, Michelson EL, Stawicki J, Holford FD. Cardiac arrhythmias: frequency during fiberoptic bronchoscopy and correlation with hypoxemia. Arch Intern Med 1981;141: 603–606.

175. Kvale PA. Is sedation necessary for brochoscopy? Pro Sedation. J Bronchology 1994; 1:246–249.

176. Colt HG. Is sedation necessary for bronchoscopy? Con Sedation. J Bronchology 1994;1:250–253.

177. deBlasio F, Daughton DM, Thompson AB. General vs. local anesthesia; effect on bronchoalveolar lavage findings. Chest 1993; 104:1032–1037.

178. Shelly MP, Wilson P, Norman J. Sedation for fiberoptic bronchoscopy. Thorax 1989;44: 769–775.

179. O'Hickey S, Hilton AM. Fiberoptic bronchoscopy in the elderly. Age Ageing 1987; 16:229–233.

180. Knox AJ, Mascie-Taylor BH, Page RL. Fiberoptic bronchoscopy in the elderly: 4 years' experience. Br J Dis Chest 1988; 82:290–293.

181. Whitwam JG, Al-khudhairi D, McCloy RF. Comparison of midazolam and diazepam in doses of comparable potency during gastroscopy. Br J Anaesth 1983;55:773–776.

182. Al-khudhairi D, Whitwam JG, McCloy RF. Midazolam and diazepam for gastroscopy Anaesthesia 1982;37:1002–1006.

183. Dundee JW, Wilson DB. Amnesic action of midazolam. Anaesthesia 1980;35:459–461.

184. Sanders LD, Davies-Evans J, Rosen M, Robinson JO. Comparison of diazepam with midazolam as I.V. sedation for outpatient gastroscopy. Br J Anaesth 1989;63:726–731.

185. Macgilchrist AJ, Brinie GG, Cook A, et al. Pharmacokinetics and pharmacodynamics of intravenous midazolam in patients with severe alcoholic cirrhosis. Gut 1986;27: 190–195.

186. Marshall BE, Longnecker DE. General anesthetics. In: Gilman AG, ed. The pharmacological basis of therapeutics, 8th ed. New York: Pergamon Press, 1990:285–310.

187. Jaffe JH, Martin WR. Opioid analgesics and antagonists. In: Gilman AG, ed. The pharmacological basis of therapeutics, 8th ed. New York: Pergamon Press, 1990:485–521.

188. Clarkson K, Camillus PK, O'Connell F, et al. A comparative evaluation of propofol and midazolam as sedative agents in fiberoptic bronchoscopy. Chest 1993;104:1029–1031.

189. Klotz U, Ziegler G, Ludwig L, Reimann IW. Pharmacodynamic interaction between midazolam and a specific benzodiazepine antagonist in humans. J Clin Pharmacol 1985; 25:400–406.

190. Evans JM, Hogg MIJ, Lunn JN, Rosen M. Degree and duration of reversal by naloxone of effects of morphine in conscious subjects. Br Med J 1974;2:589.

191. Bigger JT, Hoffam BF. Antiarrhythmic agents. In: Gilman AG, ed. The pharmacological basis of therapeutics, 8th ed. New York: Pergamon Press, 1990:840–873.

192. Kirkpatrick MB. Lidocaine topical anesthesia for flexible bronchoscopy. Chest 1989;96: 965–966.

193. McAlpine LG, Thomson NC. Lidocaine-induced bronchoconstriction in asthmatic patients: relation to histamine airway responsiveness and effect of preservative. Chest 1989;96:1012–1015.

194. Kennedy SK, Longnecker DE. History and principles of anesthesiology. In: Gilman AG, ed. The pharmacological basis of therapeutics, 8th ed. New York: Pergamon Press, 1990:269–284.

When Routine Flexible Bronchoscopy Is Not Indicated | 5

Randall J. Harris, Marc S. Rovner, Muzaffar Ahmad, and Atul C. Mehta

Flexible fiberoptic bronchoscopy (FOB) was introduced in the late 1960s as a relatively noninvasive procedure to assess and treat a wide variety of bronchopulmonary diseases. It is invaluable for diagnosing opportunistic infections and for identifying tumors. It is safe, versatile, and convenient. These same qualities, however, may result in overuse. Certain clinical situations do not benefit from bronchoscopy. Given these concerns and the increasing emphasis on cost effectiveness (1), it is imperative to better define patient selection for bronchoscopy. This review focuses on the clinical situations in which bronchoscopy has been shown to have limited value (Table 5.1).

Atelectasis

Pulmonary atelectasis is the most common respiratory complication occurring in the postoperative period after thoracic or abdominal surgery. The incidence of atelectasis varies with the nature of the surgery, ranging from 20% to 60% (2). Secretions and atelectasis also occur frequently in patients in general medical and medical intensive care units. Atelectasis can predispose to pneumonia, impair gas exchange, and prolong hospital stay. Although therapeutic FOB has been widely implemented, it has not been shown through controlled studies to improve the outcome or rate of resolution of clinically stable atelectasis.

Marini and colleagues (3) reported data on 31 patients in a prospective, randomized, controlled study comparing therapeutic bronchoscopy with a standard, conservative treatment regimen for hospital-acquired lobar atelectasis. Patients were randomized to receive either initial bronchoscopy or a repeated regimen of nebulized aerosols, chest physiotherapy with percussion and postural drainage, coughing (if not intubated), and suctioning. Delayed bronchoscopy was undertaken if this conservative regimen failed. Arterial blood gases and chest roentgenograms were obtained after the initial intervention, at 24 hours, and at 48 hours. There were no significant differences in objective data between the two treatment groups at any time. Although it was a small study, the authors concluded that FOB was not superior to respiratory therapy maneuvers. Importantly, the presence of an air bronchogram on the chest roentgenogram predicted delayed resolution of collapse regardless

Table 5.1. Clinical Conditions in Which Routine Bronchoscopy Has Limited Value

Atelectasis
Solitary pulmonary nodule
Isolated pleural effusion
Chronic cough with negative chest roentgenogram
Hemoptysis with negative chest roentgenogram
Lower respiratory bacterial infection
Acute stridor in children
Foreign body removal in children

which form of treatment was used. The air bronchogram may represent regional compliance changes, infection, or microatelectasis. Olopade and Prakash (4) reported on 90 therapeutic FOB procedures undertaken in the intensive care setting. Clinical improvement in atelectasis was noted in only 19% as evidenced by oxygenation and radiologic data. These authors also reviewed several published series and concluded that therapeutic bronchoscopy in the intensive care setting is safe, with no deaths reported in over 1150 procedures. Nevertheless, FOB can cause transient hypoxemia and intense bronchospasm and should not be considered risk free (5–7).

The development of atelectasis is particularly hazardous in patients undergoing lobectomy for lung carcinoma. In a recent study (8), 20 patients who underwent lobectomy were randomized to either a standard postoperative regimen of respiratory maneuvers that included chest physiotherapy and aerosols every 4 hours or to immediate postoperative FOB in addition to the standard regimen. No significant differences were noted in forced vital capacity, arterial blood gas values, sputum quantity, degree of postoperative atelectasis, or lengths of intensive care or hospital stay.

Firm guidelines for the treatment of atelectasis do not exist. Bronchoscopy has not been found superior to conservative therapy. Clinically stable patients with limited atelectasis or intubated patients who can receive adequate tracheobronchial care may be effectively treated by less aggressive measures (9). However, each patient's status must be meticulously assessed and therapeutic bronchoscopy not be denied for those patients uncooperative with respiratory maneuvers, requiring immediate intervention, or failing conservative regimens.

Solitary Pulmonary Nodule

By definition, a solitary pulmonary nodule (SPN) is a discrete nodule less than 3 cm in diameter that is completely surrounded by lung and not associated with parenchymal disease or adenopathy (10). Approximately 150,000 new SPNs are detected each year in the United States (11). Over 80 different etiologies have been reported (10). Approximately 40% to 50% of all SPNs are malignant (12). The risk of malignancy depends on nodule size, growth rate, patient age, patient smoking exposure, and certain radiographic findings (11,13).

Options for managing an SPN include observation, histologic investigation through either percutaneous transthoracic needle aspiration (TTNA) or bronchoscopy, and surgical intervention. TTNA is reported to have a diagnostic sensitivity ranging from 43% to 97% for malignant lesions, but is less effective in yielding a definitive benign diagnosis (14). However, TTNA has a pneumothorax complication rate of 15% (15–17). It has a false positive rate of 1.5% to 3%; the false negative rate in the presence of malignancy ranges from 3% to 11% (15,16). Bronchoscopy is useful for large central lesions but has low diagnostic yield (approximately 10% to 20%) for the smaller peripheral lesions (18,19).

A prospective study (20) clearly showed that the diagnostic yield of FOB for SPN depends on the size of the nodule. The yield for periperal lung lesions was higher for lesions greater than 2 cm (64%) than for smaller lesions (28%). The same investigators observed a lower yield for nodules less than 2 cm located in the peripheral third of the lung field compared to more proximal lesions. A retrospective study (21) involving 143 bronchoscopic procedures in 137 patients with SPN reported a 19% overall yield. Again, yield significantly increased with the size of the nodule. FOB had less than 20% yield for lesions less than 3 cm. The presence of a "bronchus sign" on computed tomography scan has been shown to improve patient selection for bronchoscopy with regard to peripheral lesions (22,23).

Despite the low diagnostic yield for peripheral lesions, many patients with SPN scheduled to undergo curative surgery continue to be screened for malignancy with FOB. Three potential reasons to perform FOB preoperatively are to obtain a benign tissue diagnosis of the lesion, to exclude synchronous primary bronchogenic or metastatic malignant neoplasms in the airway, and to evaluate tracheobronchial anatomy to assist surgical management. However, the benefit of preoperative inspection of the lower respiratory tract with FOB in patients with suspected clinical stage I disease has not yet been proven. Torrington and Kern (24) retrospectively reviewed all records of patients who underwent a preoperative FOB for SPN evaluation over a 4-year period. Patients with mediastinal or pleural abnormalities were excluded. Seventy-nine (87%) of 91 patients in this study were subsequently diagnosed with bronchogenic carcinoma at thoracotomy. Sixteen patients (18%) had malignancy identified preoperatively by FOB. Five of these patients had endobronchial tumors. The preoperative FOB revealed only one unsuspected vocal cord carcinoma and no occult synchronous primary carcinomas. The FOB findings did not obviate the need for surgery nor alter the stage of the lung cancer. A preoperative diagnosis of malignancy did not affect the operative time, the operative procedure, or patient survival. In another study (12) undertaken to assess the value of staging FOB for the asymptomatic SPN, endobronchial examination failed to detect a single lesion that precluded surgery. Importantly, all 33 patients in this study reported no symptoms of weight loss, chest pain, hemoptysis, localized wheeze, or hoarseness. The authors concluded that when the history, physical examination, radiographic assessment, and laboratory evaluations fail to document contraindications to surgery or to suggest metastatic disease, routine airway inspection is of limited value.

Thus, bronchoscopy is not routinely indicated in the diagnostic evaluation or staging of an SPN—especially if the lesion is less than 2 cm, a bronchus sign is absent on imaging studies, and the patient is asymptomatic. Routine preoperative FOB in an asymptomatic patient does not measurably benefit the patient who is suspected of having stage I bronchogenic carcinoma. If malignancy is highly suspected or a definitive benign diagnosis has not been proven by other minimally invasive techniques, the SPN should be resected by thoracoscopy or open thoracotomy.

Isolated Pleural Effusion

Many patients presenting with a pleural effusion undergo FOB to exclude an associated bronchogenic carcinoma. The pleural effusion is first evaluated by direct sampling to assess for both benign and malignant disease. The relative ease of access to the pleural space allows for the immediate study of pleural fluid and tissue for diagnostic evaluation. Conventional sampling includes thoracentesis and closed pleural biopsy. Cytologic analysis of pleural fluid by thoracentesis is positive in 45% to 80% of malignant pleural effusions but is positive in as few as 20% of patients with mesothelioma (25–28). Repeat cytologic analysis can increase the yield for a malignant diagnosis by an additional 17% to 22% (25,29). Some advocate the addition of a closed pleural biopsy to further increase the diagnostic yield (29). Closed pleural biopsy is reported to be successful in diagnosing pleural malignancy in approximately 50% of cases (30,31). However, Prakash (31) reported that only 20 (7%) of 281 patients with malignant pleural effusions had a closed pleural biopsy that revealed malignant disease when the fluid cytology was negative.

The role of bronchoscopy is limited in the investigation of unexplained isolated pleural effusion. Many studies have shown that bronchoscopy is unlikely to aid in the diagnosis of an isolated pleural effusion in the absence of concurrent radiographic evidence of atelectasis, mass, adenopathy, or without accompanying clinical signs and symptoms of endobronchial disease (32–36). In a study of 245 patients with pleural effusion, only 13 of 46 patients who had bronchoscopy had a positive yield (32). Symptomatic cough was present in 12 of these 13 patients. Five of the 13 patients had a second plural aspirate that was equally diagnostic. In another study of 115 patients undergoing FOB for unilateral effusion, FOB diagnosed bronchogenic carcinoma in only 33 patients (37). Importantly, the diagnostic yield was highest for those patients presenting with hemoptysis or who had other chest roentgenogram abnormalities. Patients with just an isolated small- or moderate-sized effusion overwhelmingly had a nondiagnostic FOB (47 of 48). On the other hand, patients with a massive effusion (defined as greater than three-fourths the hemothorax) were more likely to have bronchogenic carcinoma identified (7 of 18). One publication did conclude that bronchoscopic examination is of significant value in the evaluation of patients with undiagnosed isolated effusions without other roentgenographic abnormalities (38). In this small retrospective study of 28 patients, 4 patients had a diagnosis established by bronchoscopy (3 carcinoma, one tuberculosis). In agreement with others (37,39), we do not believe routine bronchoscopy is indicated for the evaluation of isolated pleural effusion if airway symptoms are absent, and chest roentgenogram is otherwise normal.

Chronic Cough with a Negative Chest Roentgenogram

In the absence of any abnormality on the chest roentgenogram, routine bronchoscopy is unrewarding for the evaluation of chronic cough (40–42). FOB should be undertaken only after multiple directed empirical therapies have failed and cough persists despite smoking cessation. The etiology of cough in a patient who is a nonsmoker, who is not taking an angiotensin-converting enzyme inhibitor, and who has a normal chest roentgenogram can be elucidated in nearly all cases by applying a systematic algorithm approach that does not include early bronchoscopy (40). There are reports of endobronchial obstruction with negative chest roentgenograms, but this is a rare entity (43). Cough with associated recurrent hemoptysis, localized wheeze, or an abnormal chest roentgenogram provides more compelling indication for bronchoscopy than chronic cough alone (39).

Hemoptysis with a Negative or Nonlocalizing Chest Roentgenogram

Hemoptysis is responsible for approximately 15% of all pulmonary consultations (44). Although there is agreement that patients with focal chest roentgenogram abnormalities benefit from bronchoscopy (45), the indication for FOB in cases in which the chest roentgenogram is normal or shows only nonspecific, nonlocalizing findings is controversial. Earlier studies by Zavala (46), Gong and Salvarierra (47), and Richardson and colleagues (48) found bronchogenic carcinoma in 22%, 7%, and 13%, respectively. More recently, Peters and coauthors (49), Weaver and coworkers (45), and Heimer and associates (50) failed to identify bronchogenic carcinoma in a total of 86 patients with hemoptysis and a normal roentgenogram. Jackson and colleagues (51) identified bronchogenic carcinoma in 4.2%, and their literature review noted 3% of patients with hemoptysis and a normal chest roentgenogram had carcinoma. Differences in the above studies have been attributed to errors secondary to small sample size, differences in the patient population being studied, smoking history, and differences between patients with normal and nonlocalizing chest roentgenograms (44,49). O'Neill and Lazarus (44) reviewed 119 bronchoscopies performed for hemoptysis in patients with a normal (n = 75) or nonlocalizing (n = 44) chest roentgenogram and attempted to identify predictors of malignancy. A neoplasm was identified in 5% and bronchogenic carcinoma was identified in 2.5%. They reported the risk factors of male gender, age greater than 40 years, and a more than 40 pack-year smoking history appeared to identify patients in whom the yield of FOB is higher. Poe and colleagues (52) reviewed 196 procedures and identified bronchogenic carcinoma in 6% and another specific cause (including bronchitis) of hemoptysis in 17%. Univariate and multivariate analyses showed that the three factors of age greater than 50 years, male gender, and a more than 40 pack-year smoking history were significant risk factors for malignancy. The presence of two of the three factors or bleeding in excess of 30 mL daily identified 100% of the patients with bronchogenic carcinoma and 82% of all the diagnostic FOB procedures. They concluded that limiting FOB to the patients with two or more risk factors would have reduced the number of FOB procedures by 28%. Thus it seems reasonable to reserve FOB for those select patients with persistent and significant hemoptysis, those who develop focal chest abnormalities, or for those at high risk for malignancy as characterized above. Routinely performing bronchoscopy in all patients presenting with acute, new-onset hemoptysis and a negative chest roentgenogram will eventually result in the earlier diagnosis (weeks, months) of a few occult bronchogenic carcinomas. Whether this approach is cost effective or truly improves patient outcome is not clear (53).

The clinical outcome is favorable if FOB is performed, is nondiagnostic, and the patient has a normal or nonlocalizing chest roentgenogram. Adelman and colleagues (54) reported that 90% of their 67 patients with "cryptogenic hemoptysis" had resolution by 6 months and only 5 (7.5%) patients had intermittent episodes of bleeding for more than one year. Only one patient developed bronchogenic carcinoma during follow-up, 20 months after the FOB and resolution of his symptoms. These data indicate that the negative predictive value of a nondiagnostic FOB in the setting of an unremarkable chest roentgenogram is high.

Lower Respiratory Bacterial Infection

Community-acquired pneumonia in an immunocompetent patient can be successfully managed by empirical therapy directed toward the common pathogens. Sputum Gram stain and culture can help direct therapy (55,56). Bronchoscopy is typically reserved for atypical infection, possible postobstructive pneumonia, lack of response to broad-spectrum antibiotics, and as a more aggressive approach to the patient ill enough to require intensive care unit management.

Bronchoalveolar lavage (BAL) has been used extensively to evaluate pulmonary infiltrates in both immunocompetent and immunosuppressed patients. The reported diagnostic sensitivity of BAL for lower respiratory infection ranges from 39% to 100% (55–61). The wide range in sensitivities reflects differences in patient population, the prevalence of specific pathogens, prior use of antibiotics, laboratory technique, and diagnostic criteria (55–61). BAL is most often used for evaluating for opportunistic organisms in the immunosuppressed host. There is considerable controversy as to its necessity and usefulness in diagnosing community-acquired pneumonia, especially for bacterial pneumonia and for patients already receiving antibiotics.

Antibiotic exposure can affect both the sensitivity and specificity of the microbial studies (55,56,58,61). Ortqvist and colleagues (62) studied 24 patients admitted to the hospital with community-acquired pneumonia who underwent FOB with protected specimen brush (PSB) sampling. The diagnostic sensitivity of PSB culture was much higher in the patients who had bronchoscopy before antibiotic therapy (80% to 12%). In Chastre's series of ventilated patients with pneumonia (58), PSB specificity was 87% in patients not taking antibiotics as compared to 42% in patients receiving antibiotics. Antibiotics can result in higher incidence of both false negative and false positive results (61,62). BAL for bacteria is most accurate in patients not receiving antibiotics, antibiotic duration less than 72 hours, or BAL within 5 days of presentation (55,56,58,61).

Pneumocystis carinii pneumonia (PCP) is the defining diagnosis in the majority of patients with the acquired immunodeficiency syndrome (AIDS) and occurs in up to 80% of all patients with AIDS at some time in their disease (63). Induced sputum samples may be diagnostic, but the reported sensitivities vary widely due to differences in the ability to collect good specimens and laboratory experience (63,64). Some experts have advocated bronchoscopic confirmation of the diagnosis in all cases, whereas others have stated that empirical therapy can safely be used for the classic presentation of PCP (with FOB reserved for those who fail empirical therapy) (65). The arguments against empirical therapy include the delay in diagnosing pathogens other than PCP, anti-PCP therapy is potentially toxic, and patients may deteriorate to the point that they cannot undergo delayed bronchoscopy without significant increased risk. The outcomes of the two strategies, early bronchoscopy versus empirical therapy, were recently compared using a decision analysis model (65). This was not a clinical trial. The proposed population included patients who did not have a history of PCP but fulfilled the Centers for Disease Control and Prevention case definition for presumptive PCP (dyspnea, nonproductive cough, hypoxemia, and bilateral infiltrates). The expected one-month survival rate was the primary outcome. This survival rate was found to be essentially the same for the two strategies (85% for each) using mean base-

line probabilities derived from published literature and expert opinion (surveys). The results of this analysis have to be interpreted with caution because of the use of multiple assumptions and must only apply to those patients not receiving prophylaxis. The results of this analysis, however, are consistent with several clinical studies that have reported equivalent efficacies and survival rates between the two strategies (66–68). Empirical therapy for PCP is now an option, but large prospective, randomized trials are needed to confirm its role.

Acute Stridor in Children

Chronic stridor is one of the most common indications for endoscopy of the airways of infants and young children (69). Acute stridor is usually the manifestation of infectious croup, epiglottitis, or laryngeal foreign body (70). It is sometimes difficult to make the important distinction between stridor caused by croup from epiglottitis and there is a great temptation to visualize the airway. The primary reason not to perform bronchoscopy or laryngoscopy in this setting is the high likelihood of making children with acute stridor worse by causing total upper airway obstruction. Because the clinical information needed can be obtained safely in other ways, routine endoscopy for acute stridor is contraindicated.

Epiglottitis is an acute febrile illness, almost exclusively caused by the bacteria *Haemophilus influenzae* type b, that results in inflammation of the supraglottic structures. Infectious croup (laryngotracheobronchitis) is of viral etiology and is rarely associated with any life-threatening complication (71). Although specific data are lacking with regard to the risk of complete obstruction or death secondary to airway manipulation in patients with epiglottitis, most authors agree that both can be provoked by any disturbance of the hypopharynx or larynx and should be avoided

(71–73). In cases of suspected epiglottitis, direct visualization of the upper airway, either by tongue blade or endoscopy, should only be done in the operating room with the expectation for emergent airway management. This is generally accomplished by a team of physicians ("epiglottitis code team") including an anesthesiologist, pediatric intensivist, and surgeon. The patient is intubated or, rarely, has a tracheostomy placed at the time of the first manipulation of the airway. Bronchoscopy is not done. In children with epiglottitis who undergo controlled, elective intubation at the time of the first airway manipulation, survival is excellent (73).

Foreign Body Removal from the Pediatric Airway

Although the *diagnosis* of a foreign body in the airway of a child is an appropriate indication for FOB, *removal* of foreign body should be done via the rigid bronchoscope rather than the flexible instrument (69). In one series of 29 patients in whom the history, physical examination, or chest roentgenogram suggested a high likelihood for the presence of a foreign body, 27 (93%) patients actually had a foreign body at the time of bronchoscopy. Therefore, in cases of high clinical suspicion, rigid bronchoscopy should be done for both diagnosis and removal, without the initial flexible procedure (74).

In less obvious cases, foreign bodies are found in only 19% to 25% of cases and multiple foreign bodies have been reported to occur in 5% to 26% of suspected cases (69,74). Therefore, FOB has the most utility in equivocal cases, in that rigid bronchoscopy can be avoided in 75% of these cases. FOB is also useful for identifying the location of multiple foreign body fragments and for postrigid bronchoscopy follow-up.

The vast majority (85%) of children who have a foreign body in the airway are less than 5 years old (75). The instruments used for foreign body removal cannot fit through the bronchoscopes that these children can tolerate. Although successful removal of foreign bodies in children via the flexible instrument has been reported, the rigid bronchoscope remains the instrument of choice for the removal of foreign bodies in children (76–78). Only in situations where the rigid bronchoscope has failed should removal via the flexible instrument be attempted (79).

Summary

Bronchoscopy has proved a productive diagnostic and therapeutic modality for many bronchopulmonary conditions. It does, however, have limitations. Proper indications are evolving as practical experience is reported through appropriate studies. Acknowledging limitations is paramount to preventing its overuse. We encourage bronchoscopists to continually reevaluate the clinical situations that are not benefited by flexible FOB.

REFERENCES

1. Diamond GA, Denton TA. Alternative perspective on the biased foundations of medical technology assessment. Ann Intern Med 1993;118:455–464.
2. Mahajan VK, Catron PW, Huber GL. The value of fiberoptic bronchoscopy in the management of pulmonary collapse. Chest 1978;73:817–820.
3. Marini JJ, Pierson DJ, Hudson LD. Acute lobar atelectasis: a prospective comparison of fiberoptic bronchoscopy and respiratory therapy. Am Rev Respir Dis 1979;119:971–978.
4. Olopade CO, Prakash UB. Bronchoscopy in the critical-care unit. Mayo Clinic Proc 1989;64:1255–1263.
5. Credle WF, Smiddy JF, Elliot RC. Complications of fiberoptic bronchoscopy. Am Rev Respir Dis 1974;109:67–72.
6. Wiedemann HP. Bronchoscopy in severe chronic obstructive pulmonary disease. J Bronchology 1994;1:177–178. Editorial.

7. Matsushima Y, Jones RL, King EG, Moysa G, Alton JDM. Alterations in pulmonary mechanics and gas exchange during routine fiberoptic bronchoscopy. Chest 1984;86:184–188.

8. Jaworski A, Goldberg SK, Walkenstein MD, Wilson B, Lippmann ML. Utility of immediate postlobectomy fiberoptic bronchoscopy in preventing atelectasis. Chest 1994;1:38–43.

9. Meyrs DJ. Can fiberoptic bronchoscopy reverse acute lobar atelectasis? Indiana Med 1986;595–605.

10. Viggiano RW, Swensen SJ, Rosenow EC. Evaluation and management of solitary and multiple pulmonary nodules. Clin Chest Med 1992;13:83–95.

11. Lillington GA. Management of solitary pulmonary nodules. Dis Mon 1991;37:271–318.

12. Goldberg SK, Walkenstein MD, Steinbach A, Aranson R. The role of staging bronchoscopy in the preoperative assessment of a solitary pulmonary nodule. Chest 1993;104:94–97.

13. Cummings SR, Lillington GA, Richard RJ. Estimating the probability of malignancy in solitary pulmonary nodules. Am Rev Respir Dis 1986;134:449–452.

14. Mack MJ, Hazelrigg SR, Landreneau RJ, Acuff TE. Thoracoscopy for the diagnosis of the indeterminate solitary nodule. Ann Thorac Surg 1993;56:825–832.

15. Westcott JL. Direct percutaneous needle aspiration of localized pulmonary lesions: results in 422 patients. Radiology 1980;137:31–35.

16. Westcott JL. Percutaneous transthoracic needle biopsy. Radiology 1988;169:593–601.

17. Khouri NF, Stitik FP, Erozan YS. Transthoracic needle aspiration biopsy of benign and malignant lung lesions. Am J Roentgenol 1985;144:281–288.

18. Richardson RH, Zavala DC, Mukerjee PK, Bedell GN. The use of fiberoptic bronchoscopy and brush biopsy in the diagnosis of suspected pulmonary malignancy. Am Rev Respir Dis 1974;109:63–66.

19. Fletcher EC, Levin DC. Flexible fiberoptic bronchoscopy and fluoroscopically-guided transbronchial biopsy in the management of solitary pulmonary nodules. West J Med 1982;136:477–483.

20. Radke JR, Conway WA, Eyler WR, Kvale PA. Diagnostic accuracy in periperal lung lesions: factors predicting success with flexible fiberoptic bronchoscopy. Chest 1979;76:176–179.

21. Stringfield JT III, Markowitz DJ, Bentz RR, Welch MH, Weg JG. The effect of tumor size and location on diagnosis by fiberoptic bronchoscopy. Chest 1977;72:474–476.

22. Gaeta M. Bronchus sign on CT in peripheral carcinoma of the lung: value in predicting results of transbronchial biopsy. Am J Roentgenol 1991;157:1181–1185.

23. Naidich DP, Sussman R, Kutcher WL, et al. Solitary pulmonary nodules and CT-bronchoscopic correlation. Chest 1988;93:595–598.

24. Torrington KG, Kern JD. The utility of fiberoptic bronchoscopy in the evaluation of the solitary pulmonary nodule. Chest 1993;104:1021–1024.

25. Menzies R, Charbonneau M. Thoracoscopy for the diagnosis of pleural disease. Ann Intern Med 1991;114:271–276.

26. Boutin C, Viallat JR, Cargnino P, Farisse P. Thoracoscopy in malignant pleural effusions. Am Rev Respir Dis 1981;124:588–592.

27. Edmondstone WM. Investigation of pleural effusions: comparison between fiberoptic thoracoscopy, needle biopsy, and cytology. Respir Med 1990;84:23–26.

28. Boutin C, Cargnino P, Viallat JR. Thoracoscopy in the early diagnosis of malignant pleural effusion. Endoscopy 1980;12:155–160.

29. Sayler WR, Eggleston JC, Erozan YS. Efficacy of pleural needle biopsy and pleural fluid cytopathology in the diagnosis of malignant neoplasms invading the pleura. Chest 1975;67:536–539.

30. Loddenkemper R, Grosser H, Gable A, Mai J, Preussler II, Brandt HJ. Prospective evaluation of biopsy methods in the diagnosis of malignant pleural effusions. Intrapatient comparison between pleural fluid cytology, blind needle biopsy, and thoracoscopy. Am Rev Respir Dis 1983;127(suppl 4):114.

31. Prakash U. Comparison of needle biopsy with cytologic analysis for evaluation of pleural effusions: analysis of 414 cases. Mayo Clin Proc 1985;60:158–164.

32. Upham JW, Mitchell CA, Armstrong JG, Kelly WT. Investigation of pleural effusion: the role of bronchoscopy. Aust N Z J Med 1992;22:41–43.

33. Kelly P, Fallouh M, O'Brien A, Clancy L. Fiberoptic bronchoscopy in the management of lone plural effusion: a negative study. Eur Resp J 1990;3:397–398.

34. Heaton RW, Roberts CM. The role of fiberoptic bronchoscopy in the investigation of pleural effusion. Postgrad Med J 1988;64:581–582.

35. Chang SC, Perng RP. The role of fiberoptic bronchoscopy in evaluating the causes of pleural effusions. Arch Intern Med 1989;149: 855–857.

36. Feinsilver SH, Barrows AA, Braman SS. Fiberoptic bronchoscopy and pleural effusion of unknown origin. Chest 1986;90:516–519.

37. Poe RH, Levy PC, Israel RH, Ortiz CR, Kallay MC. Use of fiberoptic bronchoscopy in the diagnosis of bronchogenic carcinoma. Chest 1994;105:1663–1667.

38. Williams T, Thomas P. The diagnosis of pleural effusions by fiberoptic bronchoscopy and pleuroscopy. Chest 1981;80:566–569.

39. Utz JP, Prakash UBS. Indications for and contraindications to bronchoscopy. In: Prakash UBS, ed. Bronchoscopy. New York: Raven Press, 1994.

40. Irwin RS, Curley FJ, French CL. Chronic cough. The spectrum and frequency of causes, key components of the diagnostic evaluation, and outcome of specific therapy. Am Rev Respir Dis 1990;141:640–647.

41. Poe RH, Israel RH, Utell MJ, Hall WJ. Chronic cough: bronchoscopy or pulmonary function testing. Am Rev Respir Dis 1982;126: 160–162.

42. Irwin RS, Curley FJ. Is the anatomic, diagnostic work-up of chronic cough not all that it is hacked up to be? Chest 1989;95:711–713. Editorial.

43. Shure D. Radiologically-occult endobronchial obstruction in bronchogenic carcinoma. Am J Med 1991;91:19–22.

44. O'Neill KM, Lazarus AA. Hemoptysis: indications for bronchoscopy. Arch Intern Med 1991;151:171–174.

45. Weaver LG, Solliday N, Cugell DW. Selection of patients with hemoptysis for fiberoptic bronchoscopy. Chest 1979;76:7–10.

46. Zavala DC. Diagnostic fiberoptic bronchoscopy: techniques and results of biopsy in 600 patients. Chest 1975;68:12–19.

47. Gong H, Salvatierra C. Clinical efficacy of early and delayed fiberoptic bronchoscopy in patients with hemoptysis. Am Rev Respir Dis 1981;124:221–225.

48. Richardson RH, Zavala DC, Mukerjee PK, Bedell GN. The use of fiberoptic bronchoscopy and brush biopsy in the diagnosis of suspected pulmonary malignancy. Am Rev Respir Dis 1974;109:63–66.

49. Peters J, McClung H, Teague R. Evaluation of hemoptysis in patients with a normal chest roentgenogram. West J Med 1984;141: 624–626.

50. Heimer D, Bar-Ziv J, Scharf SM. Fiberoptic bronchoscopy in patients with hemoptysis and nonlocalizing chest roentgenograms. Arch Intern Med 1985;145:1427–1428.

51. Jackson C, Savage P, Quinn D. Role of fiberoptic bronchoscopy in patients with hemoptysis and a normal chest roentgenogram. Chest 1985;87:142–144.

52. Poe RH, Israel RH, Marin MG, et al. Utility of fiberoptic bronchoscopy in patients with hemoptysis and a nonlocalizing chest roentgenogram. Chest 1988;92:70–75.

53. Berger R, Rehm SR. Bronchoscopy for hemoptysis. Chest 1991;99:1553. Letter.

54. Adelman J, Haponik EF, Bleecker ER, Britt EJ. Cryptogenic hemoptysis. Ann Intern Med 1985;102:829–834.

55. Cook DJ, Fitzgerald JM, Guyatt GH, Walter S. Evaluation of the PSB and BAL in the diagnosis of nosocomial pneumonia. J Intensive Care Med 1991;6:196–205.

56. Thorpe JE, Baughman RP, Frame PT, Wesseler TA, Staneck JL. Bronchoalveolar lavage for diagnosing acute bacterial pneumonia. J Infect Dis 1987;155:855–861.

57. Kahn FW, Jones JM. Diagnosing bacterial respiratory infection by bronchoalveolar lavage. J Infect Dis 1987;155:862–869.

58. Chastre J, Viau F, Brun P, et al. Prospective evaluation of the protected specimen brush for the diagnosis of pulmonary infections in ventilated patients. Am Rev Respir Dis 1984; 130:924–929.

59. Guerra LF, Baughman RP. Use of bronchoalveolar lavage to diagnose bacterial pneumonia in mechanically ventilated patients. Crit Care Med 1990;18:169–173.

60. Pisani RJ, Wright AJ. Clinical utility of bronchoalveolar lavage in immunocompromised hosts. Mayo Clin Proc 1992;67:221–227.

61. Meduri GU, Baselski V. The role of bronchoalveolar lavage in diagnosing nonopportunistic bacterial pneumonia. Chest 1992; 100:179–190.

62. Ortqvist A, Kalin M, Lefdeborn L, Lundberg B. Diagnostic fiberoptic bronchoscopy and protected brush culture in patients with community-acquired pneumonia. Chest 1990;97:1208–1219.

63. Kirsch CM, Azzi RL, Yenokida GG, Jensen WA. Analysis of induced sputum in the diagnosis of *Pneumocystis carinii* pneumonia. Am J Med Sci 1990;299:386–390.

64. Kirsch CM, Jensen WA, Kagawa FT, Azzi RL. Analysis of induced sputum for the diagnosis of recurrent *Pneumocystis carinii* pneumonia. Chest 1992;102:1152–1154.

65. Tu JV, Biem HJ, Detsky AS. Bronchoscopy versus empirical therapy in HIV-infected patients with presumptive *Pneumocystis carinii* pneumonia. A decision analysis. Am Rev Respir Dis 1993;148:370–377.

66. Pozniak AL, Tung KT, Swinburn CR, Stovey S, Semple SJG, Johnson NM. Clinical and bronchoscopic diagnosis of suspected pneumonia related to AIDS. Br Med J 1986;293:797–799.

67. Miller RF, Jillar AB, Weller IVD, Sempel SJG. Empirical treatment without bronchoscopy for *Pneumocystis carinii* pneumonia in the acquired immunodeficiency syndrome. Thorax 1989;44:559–564.

68. Marino WD. Is fiberoptic bronchoscopy in AIDS cost- and risk-effective? Chest 1991;41S. Abstract.

69. Wood RE. Spelunking in the pediatric airways: explorations with the flexible fiberoptic bronchoscope. Pediatr Clin North Am 1984; 31:785–799.

70. Wood RE. Bronchoscopy. In: Laughlin GM, Eigen H, eds. Respiratory diseases in children: diagnosis and management. Baltimore: Williams & Wilkins, 1994:123.

71. Levine DS, Springer MA. Croup and epiglottitis. In: Hilman B, ed. Pediatric respiratory disease: diagnosis and treatment. Philadelphia: WB Saunders, 1993:238–240.

72. Vernon DD, Sarnaik AP. Acute epiglottitis in children: a conservative approach to diagnosis and management. Crit Care Med 1986; 14:23–25.

73. Sivan Y, Newth CJL. Acute upper airway obstruction. In: Laughlin GM, Eigen H, eds. Respiratory diseases in children: diagnosis and management. Baltimore: Williams & Wilkins, 1994:319–333.

74. Wood RE, Gauderer WL. Flexible fiberoptic bronchoscopy in the management of tracheobronchial foreign bodies in children: the value of a combined approach with open tube bronchoscopy. J Pediatr Surg 1984;19:693–698.

75. Cohen SR, Lewis GB, Herbert WI, Geller KA. Foreign bodies in the airway: five-year retrospective study with special reference to management. Ann Otol 1980;89:437–442.

76. Cunanan OS. The flexible fiberoptic bronchoscope in foreign body removal. Experience in 300 cases. Chest 1979;73:725–726.

77. Rayet I, Navez M, Freycon MT, Prades JM. Endoscopic extraction of a foreign body from the distal bronchus in the middle lobe, inaccessible by usual techniques, in a 3-year-old child. Pediatrics 1992;47:589–591.

78. Castro M, Midthun DE, Edell ES, Stelck MJ, Prakash UBS. Flexible bronchoscopic removal of foreign bodies from pediatric airways. J Bronchology 1994;1:92–98.

79. Wood RE. Flexible bronchoscopy to remove foreign bodies in children—Yes, maybe—But... J Bronchology 1994;1:87.

ACKNOWLEDGMENT: We are indebted to Dr. Paul Stillwell for his review of this manuscript.

Accessories for the Flexible Bronchoscope | 6

Atul C. Mehta and Philip Eng

The flexible fiberoptic bronchoscope has dramatically changed the practice of pulmonary medicine since its introduction into clinical practice by Shigeto Ikeda at the National Cancer Center Hospital in Tokyo in 1966. Invasive evaluation of radiographic chest abnormalities is now possible with relatively low morbidity and mortality even in critically ill patients. Aside from direct visualization of the airway, the availability of a number of flexible accessories has extended the diagnostic and therapeutic capabilities of the flexible fiberoptic bronchoscope. This chapter describes many of these accessories and their applications in the clinical arena (Table 6.1).

Conventional Instruments

Biopsy Forceps

A variety of biopsy forceps are available for the retrieval of pieces of bronchial mucosa, endobronchial lesion, and lung parenchyma for histopathologic studies. Forceps design vary in relation to size of the cups and with the presence or absence of alligator teeth, fenestration, mechanisms to rotate the cups (rotating forceps), and centrally placed needle assembly. Cup forceps provide tissue specimens by cutting it between its edges, whereas alligator forceps do so by shearing the tissue during its withdraw. Despite the difference, there are no reports of significant difference in bleeding following the use of

Table 6.1

Conventional instruments
Biopsy forceps
3-mm cytology brush
Protected specimen brush
Balloon catheters
Dormia basket
3-prong snare
Flexible scissors
Magnet extractor
Mouth guard
Endotracheal tube adaptor

Newer instruments
7-mm cytology brush
Flexible biopsy scraper
Transbronchial aspiration needle
Bronchoscope through bronchoscope
Protected bronchoalveolar lavage catheter
Bipolar cautery
Polypectomy snare
Flexible cryoprobe
Endobronchial suture scissors

either type of forceps. Transbronchial biopsy (TBB) is usually performed using alligator forceps. Fenestration of the cups of the forceps may allow retrieval of a larger volume of the tissue. Forceps with the needle assembly are particularly useful in sampling mucosal lesions of the trachea and main bronchi as they allow the bronchoscopist to "spear" the lesion, hence fixing the forceps before taking a specimen (Figure 6.1). "Rotating forceps" allows proper positioning of the cups after its insertion through the working channel without manipulation of the flexible bronchoscope.

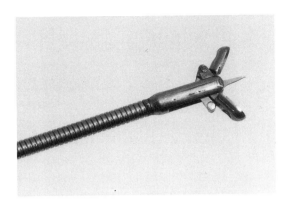

Figure 6.1. Alligator forceps with needle assembly used for sessile mucosal lesions.

In recent years, several manufacturers have introduced disposable forceps in an attempt to avoid the theoretical concern of transmission of communicable diseases. The overall cost of the reusable forceps is about five times that of the disposable model and to date, we are not aware of any instances of cross contamination of specimens or transmission of infection due to the reusable forceps. The most popular agent used for cleansing and sterilizing of the biopsy forceps and the flexible bronchoscope is the alkaline glutaraldehyde (Cidex®) (1,2). Forceps can also be gas sterilized or cleansed using ultrasound devices.

Biopsy forceps have many uses, including the sampling of endobronchial/submucosal lesions under direct visualization and abnormal lung parenchyma under fluoroscopic guidance. Small foreign bodies including sutured material from prior thoracic surgery can also be easily retrieved with the biopsy forceps.

Even though statistically insignificant, it appears that biopsy forceps may be somewhat superior to cytology brushes in the definitive diagnosis of endobronchial lesions. In a study of 600 patients, Zavala (3) was able to establish a diagnosis of bronchogenic carcinoma in 182 of 193 patients (94%) with a visible endoscopic lesion. In 97% of these patients, the diagnosis was rendered with biopsy forceps, whereas the brush yielded the diagnosis in 93%. Another similar study showed a significant difference between these two modalities; 80% with biopsy versus 46% with brushings and a combined yield of 88% (4). Thus, the forceps may provide a superiority over the brush for the diagnosis of endobronchially visible lesions.

3-mm Cytology Brush

A conventional 3-mm cytology brush contains short nylon bristles of total length of 3 mm with a retractable sheath. Circular, spiral, and loop style brushes are available from different manufacturers. Some manufacturers incorporate a blunt, rounded end at the tip of the brush to minimize airway trauma, whereas other designs lack this feature. No one design has proven to produce better cytologic yield in the definitive diagnosis of endobronchial or parenchymal lesions (5–7).

Because of the stiff nature of the bristles, these brushes produce significant mucosal trauma and may not be suitable in patients with extremely vascular lesions or coagulopathies. Under such circumstances, sampling of lesions may be better performed with the use of small cutting cup forceps, transbronchial needle aspiration (TBNA) (8,9), or by a less traumatic 7-mm cytology brush (Figure 6.2).

Peripheral lung lesions can be accurately

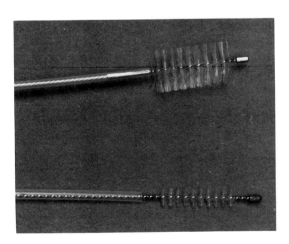

Figure 6.2. 7-mm and 3-mm cytology brushes.

localized using either single- or double-image fluoroscopy, and brushings can be performed. Diagnostic yield on specimens thus obtained approaches that of the TBB. Zavala (3) reported a 69% and 70% diagnostic yield by the forceps and the "brush biopsy" of parenchymal masses performed under fluoroscopy, respectively, in patients with lung cancer. Whether the brush technique can be used to obviate the need for TBB in the evaluation of chest malignancy would require further studies. Our practice is to obtain as many types of specimens as felt necessary (i.e., biopsy, brush, TBB, TBNA, etc.) to maximize diagnostic yield (10). Bronchoscopy is an expensive, time consuming, and uncomfortable procedure for the patient and we make every effort to limit the need for further diagnostic procedures.

Protected Specimen Brush

The protected specimen brush (PSB) is designed to obtain microbiologic specimen from deep within the lung parenchyma without contamination by upper airway organisms. This brush was first introduced by Wimberley, Faling, and Bartlett (11) in 1979 (so-called BFW brush) after studying several catheter designs to obviate the problem of upper airway contamination while the flexible bronchoscope traverses through the airways to reach the site of interest within the lung. This telescoping brush is contained inside a pair of plastic catheters. A paraffin plug placed at the distal end of the outer catheter prevents contamination of the brush during its passage through the working channel. Once this telescopic catheter is advanced into the bronchopulmonary segment of interest, the "plug" is expelled by advancing the inner catheter and the sterile brush is then advanced into the area of interest to obtain a specimen. Specimen retrieval can be performed blindly or under fluoroscopic guidance (Figure 6.3).

The PSB technique is simple and well tolerated and has a relatively high diagnostic yield depending on the cut-off value of colony

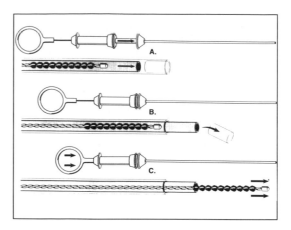

Figure 6.3. Schematic diagram of use of protected specimen brush.

counts used to define infection and if used before antibiotics are given to the patient. The PSB has been most frequently studied in the setting of nosocomial pneumonia. Among the larger studies appearing in the literature, Fagon and colleagues (12) were able to demonstrate positive brush cultures (greater than 10^3 cfu/mL) in 45 of 174 mechanically ventilated patients suspected of having nosocomial pneumonia. Pneumonia was subsequently confirmed either by autopsy or on clinical grounds in 34 of these 45 patients and false positive results were noted in only 4 of the 45 patients. One hundred and two patients with less than 10^3 cfu/mL for the PSB did not develop pneumonia clinically and recovered without specific antibiotic therapy. Other studies have reported a diagnostic yield using this technique varying from 50% to 96% with the majority in the range of 70% to 90% (13–22).

Balloon Catheters

Inflatable angioplasty balloon catheters are used in conjunction with the flexible bronchoscope in three main instances: 1) to palliate endobronchial obstruction, 2) to tamponade the airway during excessive bleeding, and 3) to assist in the removal of endobronchial foreign bodies. A size 4 to 7 F Fogarty catheter can be passed through the working channel of the

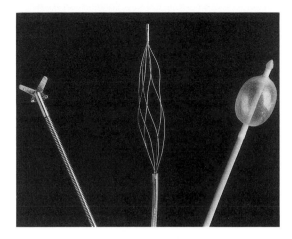

Figure 6.4. Flexible scissors, Dormia basket, and Fogarty balloon catheter.

bronchoscope and into the bronchial segment of interest (Figure 6.4). A 3-cc syringe is used to inflate the balloon to the desired size (1 to 3 cc) with air while traction is placed at the proximal portion of the catheter. Once the catheter is pulled through the obstructed bronchus, the balloon is deflated allowing withdrawal through the flexible bronchoscope (23). This method is often used in association with neodymium:yttrium-aluminum-garnet (Nd:YAG) laser photoresection of airway lesions either to identify and dilate the lumen of the bronchus or to pull tumor tissue into more

proximal airways (i.e., from lobar to main bronchi) for safer targeting of laser energy.

Fogarty catheters have also been used in a similar fashion to dislodge impacted foreign bodies prior to removal with more conventional instruments (i.e., forceps and snares) (24,25).

The balloon catheter can also be used to tamponade a bleeding airway in uncontrollable hemorrhage. A special 200-cm long balloon catheter inflatable to different dimensions can provide more long-term tamponade because the bronchoscope can be removed over the catheter from the airway with the inflated balloon left in place (Figure 6.5). A proximal portion of the catheter protruding from the patient's airway is clamped and cut, thus freeing the flexible bronchoscope. Although not providing definitive control of bleeding, this device may serve as a temporary measure until a more definitive procedure can be performed.

Dormia Basket

A modified version of the Dormia basket (used by gastroenterologists and urologists to retrieve calculi from the common bile duct and the bladder, respectively) is now available. It can be passed through the working channel of the flexible bronchoscope to retrieve foreign

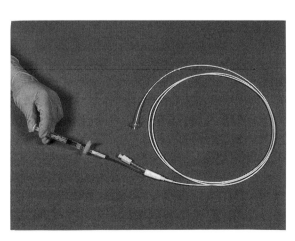

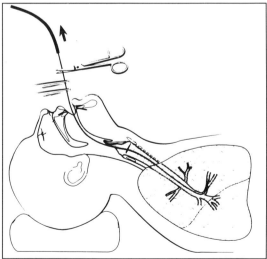

Figure 6.5. 200-cm balloon tamponade catheter and schematic diagram depicting its use.

bodies lodged in the distal bronchi. The wings of the basket are normally retracted within a 1.6-mm diameter Teflon catheter and by manipulating the proximal end these wings can be made to open up, hence ensnaring the foreign bodies. In our experience, the Dormia basket is especially useful for retrieving hard objects such as peanuts or dislodged teeth (24–26).

Three-Prong Snare

Three-prong snares, similar to the Dormia basket, can also be used to remove foreign bodies (25). When the handle of the snare is squeezed, the three prongs of the distal end come together on the foreign body and, once secured, the object, the snare, and the flexible bronchoscope are simultaneously withdrawn from the airway (Figure 6.6). With this open ended snare, larger objects such as coins can be easily removed from the endobronchial tree.

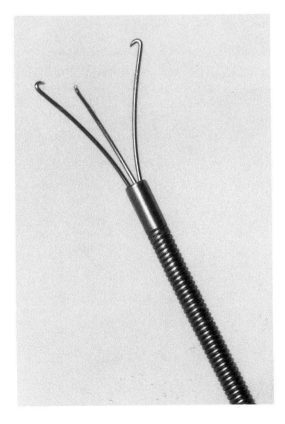

Figure 6.6. Three-prong snare used for foreign body removal.

Flexible Scissors

Flexible scissors are useful for base excision of a large pedunculated airway lesion, which, once freed, can be extracted using forceps. The stainless steel device has 5-mm blades and is limited in flexibility and maneuverability; hence, its use is confined mainly to the larger airways. The blades are sharp enough to cut the tumor tissue, yet it is blunted at the tip to avoid damage to the tracheobronchial tree. We use this instrument often for the excision of the lesion following laser coagulation. Use of this instrument is discussed in detail in successive chapters.

Magnet Extractor

A magnetic cylinder forms the tip of a flexible probe (Olympus 1E-2P) and this is passed through the working channel of the flexible bronchoscope and is useful for retrieving metallic foreign bodies lodged in major airways. Cases have been reported of forceps and cytology brushes breaking during their use, possibly due to metal fatigue (27–29). Saito (27) first described its use on a patient in whom an alligator forceps that broke during the procedure was subsequently removed with the magnetic extractor.

Mouth Guard

Historically, when the Japanese first introduced the flexible fiberoptic bronchoscope, it was inserted transorally. In the United States today, most would favor the transnasal approach except in instances where the patient has a deviated nasal septum, nasal polyps, or bleeding diatheses or when removal of a foreign body is planned. When choosing the transoral route, most would insert the flexible bronchoscope through a mouth guard to prevent the anxious patient from damaging the scope by biting on it. The mouth guard is made of hard plastic and it would be prudent to secure it by taping it to the sides of the mouth before introducing the bronchoscope (Figure 6.7).

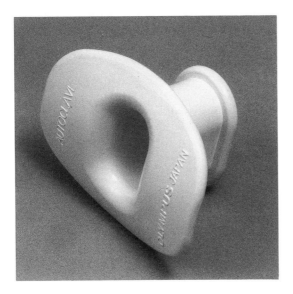

Figure 6.7. Mouth guard.

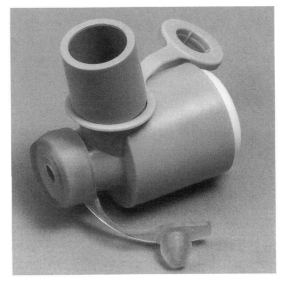

Figure 6.8. Endotracheal tube adaptor.

Endotracheal Tube Adaptor

The endotracheal tube adaptor (Portex®, Keene, NH 03431, USA) is essential while performing bronchoscopy in an intubated patient (e.g., during laser bronchoscopy) to prevent air leak at the point where the scope is inserted through the endotracheal tube. This T-shaped gadget allows for uninterrupted mechanical ventilation during the procedure (Figure 6.8).

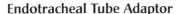

Newer Instruments

7-mm Brush

The 7-mm brush is unsheathed and has much longer Teflon-coated bristles (total length 7 mm) than the conventional 3-mm cytology brush. Aside from producing less airway mucosal trauma, the developer claims it provides a superior yield of sample for cytologic analysis compared to standard brushes. One study at the Cleveland Clinic Foundation comparing the 7-mm brush with the conventional brush on 13 patients with proven endobronchial carcinoma showed no significant diagnostic improvement with the use of a larger brush although, according to the cytologist, the cellular yield was somewhat higher with the larger brush (7). A possible disadvantage with the 7-mm brush arises from its large size, which will not allow its withdrawal through the working channel of the scope. After retrieving the sample, the scope and the brush must be removed simultaneously from the airway, mandating reinsertion of the scope if further examination is required.

Flexible Biopsy Scraper

This instrument originally developed by Zavala (3) was modified by Kato and colleagues (30) and reintroduced into clinical practice in 1985. The scraper has a smooth blunt tip and sharp blade, which is housed within a polyethylene sheath. The device is introduced via the working channel of the bronchoscope and is pushed out of the sheath at the target site. Its blade is then extended and specimens are obtained by scraping action. Kato and coworkers used the instrument in 20 patients with peripheral lung lesions and established the diagnosis in 11. The major advantages of the device are purportedly a lower pneumothorax rate given the blunt end and minimal bleeding.

Transbronchial Aspiration Needles

Transbronchial needle aspiration (TBNA) extends the diagnostic capabilities of the flexible fiberoptic bronchoscope by allowing the retrieval of specimens beyond the confines of the tracheobronchial mucosa. Previously, paratracheal masses or lymph nodes required mediastinoscopy or thoracotomy under general anesthesia to fully ascertain their nature. In 1983, Wang introduced flexible needles that could be inserted through the flexible scope to obtain extrabronchial specimens (8). Since its initial introduction, this instrument has undergone several design modifications. Depending on the size of the metal needle used to obtain specimens, there are two main versions: 1) cytology needle and 2) histology needle.

The cytology needle consists of a 22 G 13-mm long beveled needle that is retracted into a polyethylene flexible tube at the time of its passage through the working channel. At the intended site of aspiration, the beveled needle is advanced out of the polyethylene tube under direct vision via a rigid stylet that provides stiffness to the entire system. The stylet can be withdrawn proximally to add flexibility to the catheter while sampling peripheral lesions. The specimen is obtained by applying suction using a 60-mL plastic syringe containing 2 to 3 mL sterile saline. The material obtained in this fashion is then flushed out for cytologic examination. Usually two to three passes at the site of interest are made with the same needle. A number of companies have produced different versions of this needle incorporating spring-loaded versus fixed needles, metal versus plastic needles, 20 G versus 22 G, and 10 mm versus 13 mm length, without any documented benefits.

The histology needle (31) consists of a main 19 G retractable needle 15 mm in length with a beveled tip connected to a 120-cm long thin hollow spring that controls the needle movement. A 21 G beveled retractable needle 5 mm long is housed within the 19 G needle and is attached to a guidewire. The entire assembly is placed inside a 120-cm long flexible plastic catheter that can be easily advanced through the working channel. Once the biopsy site is localized both needles are extended and locked into position. The 21 G needle is advanced into the tracheobronchial wall and suction is applied at the proximal end using a 60-mL syringe containing 3 mL normal saline to ascertain that the needle has not entered a vessel. Once this is confirmed, suction is released and the 19 G needle is advanced by a few millimeters through the tracheobronchial wall, following which the 21 G needle is withdrawn. A core of tissue is obtained by advancing the 19 G needle to its fullest extent and by applying suction.

Both techniques require experience to enhance their usefulness. Its safe use necessitates an intimate knowledge of the anatomic relationships of the tracheobronchial tree. Use of both needles is discussed in detail elsewhere in this book.

Bronchoscope through Bronchoscope

Use of a new bronchoscope (BF-1.8T) measuring 1.8 mm in external diameter and 1120 mm in total length and providing a visual angle of 75° was reported by Tanaka and coworkers (32) in 1984. This instrument can be passed through the 2.6-mm working channel of the standard flexible fiberoptic bronchoscope and can be extended in a straightforward manner along the bronchioles of a luminal size down to 1.8 mm (corresponding to the eighth order branches of the air tracts). The smaller scope has neither controls nor a working channel and thus can only be used for visualization and photographic documentation of peripheral, small airway lesions. The utility of this scope may lie with its ability to guide biopsies of suspicious areas or to localize lesions or mucosal abnormalities for photodynamic therapy.

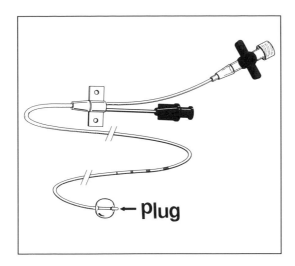

Figure 6.9. Schematic of protected BAL catheter.

Protected Bronchoalveolar Lavage Catheter

This catheter was developed by Meduri and colleagues (33) to reduce upper airway contamination of bronchoalveolar lavage (BAL) fluid, yet maintain the greater alveolar sampling compared to the PSB. The catheter is similar to the Swan-Ganz catheter with an inflatable high-compliance, low-pressure latex balloon that when fully inflated with 1.5 to 2 mL of air reaches a diameter of about 10 mm, enabling occlusion of the third generation bronchi (Figure 6.9). The catheter, measuring about 120 cm in length, has a second lumen about one mm in diameter used for injecting the BAL fluid and has a polyethylene glycol diaphragm at the distal tip to prevent contamination. This diaphragm is pushed out by flushing the catheter with 2 mL sterile saline after the balloon is inflated before performing the BAL in the usual fashion. In our experience, the main drawback of this technique is poor return of BAL fluid through the small lumen of the catheter. Design modifications by increasing the diameter of the lumen for fluid injection might possibly correct this. Overall, its superiority compared to the PSB remains to be proven. The role of this accessory is discussed in detail in successive chapters.

Bipolar Cautery

This instrument was first used by gastroenterologists for the control of upper gastrointestinal hemorrhage. Marsh (34) reported its endobronchial use in 1987. The device is a 1.6-mm multipolar probe with equally spaced electrodes along its 6-mm active distal element and grounded at its proximal end (Figure 6.10). An important feature of this instrument is that the localized electric field passes through a narrow arc between its electrodes, minimizing the risk of transmural injury and without requiring grounding. It should be noted that unlike flexible gastroscopes, bronchoscopes are not grounded instruments. The passage of current from probe to tissue generates heat. The amount of current, the type of current, and the area of contact between the probe and tissue determines the heat generated. The results of the current can range from simple drying to complete vaporization of the tissue at the point of contact (35). The distal tip of the flexible scope is made of metal and because the instrument is not grounded, electrical polypectomy snares should not be used

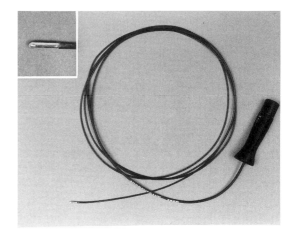

Figure 6.10. Bipolar cautery (*inset:* distal tip).

A

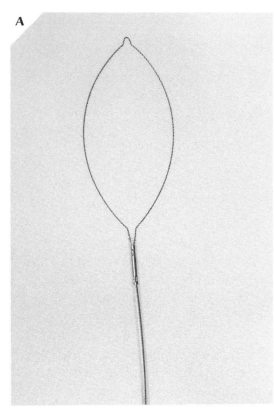

B

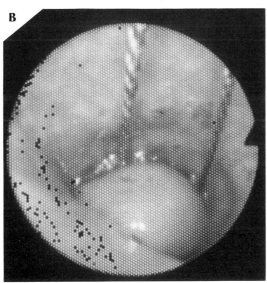

Figure 6.11. *A*, Polypectomy wire loop snare and its (*B*) application in removal of a polypoid endobronchial lesion.

through the bronchoscope; inadvertent contact between the wire loop and the distal tip can cause endobronchial ignition and damage to the scope may result (36,37). Electrosurgery

through the flexible fiberoptic bronchoscope is still considered experimental.

Polypectomy Snare

Wire loop snares of various different sizes, capable of removing colonic polyps through a colonoscope, can be used to snare off selected exophytic and polypoid endobronchial lesions (Figure 6.11). We mainly use this instrument in conjunction with Nd:YAG laser photoresection. Opening and closing the wire loop can be easily carried out using the proximal handle.

Flexible Cryoprobe

Cryotherapy was first used as early as 1907 in dermatology and was first applied in the endobronchial tree in the mid 1970s. The effect of cold temperature on tissues results in necrosis through crystallization and thrombosis. The endobronchial lesion can be frozen by applying a cryoprobe tip inserted through a rigid bronchoscope and cooled to a minimum of −70°C with circulating nitrous oxide. The probe is allowed to thaw and then the lesion is refrozen (38). Homasson (39) used a prototype flexible cryoprobe through the flexible bronchoscope. The main drawback to this technique was that it was not possible to produce complete clearance of an obstructing bronchial lesion with a single application of cryotherapy. As such, the use of flexible cryoprobes is still experimental and further studies are required prior to its widespread application. Detailed discussion of this modality is dealt with in successive chapters.

Endobronchial Suture Scissors

Shure and coworkers (42) described use of endobronchial suture scissors (Olympus) through a flexible bronchoscope to remove suture material involving the endobronchial tree. Unlike the flexible scissors described above, the blades of this instrument are shaped like a hook, which makes grabbing the suture material easier. Of the two blades, one is fixed while the movement of the other can be controlled with a proximal handle. We usually use Nd:YAG laser to remove granulomas related to nonmetallic suture material. Metal wire can also be melted with laser energy.

In summary, many accessory instruments can be used with the flexible fiberoptic bronchoscope to increase its utility for diagnostic and therapeutic purposes. The conventional instruments have undergone clinical studies that verify their diagnostic capabilities and their safety record in various clinical situations. The newer instruments have not been studied in an equally rigorous manner clinically, although experience indicates that they can be useful in special circumstances. Yet newer instruments await description and clinical trials by innovative bronchoscopists.

REFERENCES

1. Elford B. Care and cleansing of the fiberoptic bronchoscope. Chest 1978;73:761–763.
2. Mehta AC, Curtis PC, Scalzitti ML, Meeker DP. The high price of bronchoscopy. Chest 1990;98:448–454.
3. Zavala DC. Diagnostic fiberoptic bronchoscopy; techniques and results of biopsies in 600 patients. Chest 1975;68:12–19.
4. Saltzein SL, Harrell JH, Cameron T. Brushings, washings, or biopsy. Chest 1977;71:630–632.
5. Kinnear WJM, Wilkinson, MJ, James PD, Johnston ID. Comparison of the diagnostic yields of disposable and reusable cytology brushes in fiberoptic bronchoscopy. Thorax 1991;46:667–668.
6. Hamson FN, Wesselius LJ. Effect of bronchial brush size on cell recovery. Am Rev Respir Dis 1987;136:1450–1452.
7. Mehta AC, Ahmad M, Nunez C, Golish JA. Newer procedures using the fiberoptic bronchoscope in the diagnosis of lung cancer. Cleve Clin J Med 1987;54:195–203.
8. Wang KP, Terry PB. Transbronchial needle aspiration in the diagnosis and staging of bronchogenic carcinoma. Am Rev Respir Dis 1983;127:344–347.
9. Harrow EM, Odlenburg FH, Smith AH. Transbronchial needle aspiration in clinical practice. Thorax 1985;40:756–759.
10. Schenk DA, Bryan CL, Bower JH, Myers DL. Transbronchial needle aspiration in the diagnosis of bronchogenic carcinoma. Chest 1987;92:83–85.
11. Wimberley N, Faling LJ, Bartlett JG. A fiberoptic bronchoscopy technique to obtain uncontaminated lower airway secretions for bacterial culture. Am Rev Respir Dis 1979;119:337–343.
12. Fagon JY, Chastre J, Hance AJ, et al. Detection of nosocomial lung infection in ventilated patients; use of a protected specimen brush in quantitative culture techniques in 147 patients. Am Rev Respir Dis 1988;138:110–116.
13. Matthay RA, Moritz ED. Invasive procedures for diagnosing pulmonary infections. Clin Chest Med 1981;2:3–18.
14. Fletcher EC, Mohr JA, Levin DC, Flourney DJ. Bronchoscopic diagnosis of pulmonary infections. West J Med 1983;138:364–370.
15. Lennette EH, Ballows A, Hausler WJ Jr, Shadomy EJHJ, eds. Manual of clinical microbiology. Washington, DC: American Society of Microbiology, 1985.
16. Glanville AR, Marlin GE, Hartnett BJJ, Yap JM, Bradbury R. The use of fiberoptic bronchoscopy with sterile catheter in the diagnosis of pneumonia. Aust N Z J Med 1985;15:309–319.
17. Bordelon JY, Le Grand P, Gervin WC, Sanders CV. The telescoping plug catheter in suspected anaerobic infections. Am Rev Respir Dis 1983;128:465–468.
18. Teague RB, Wallace RB, Wallace RJ, Awe JR. The use of quantitative sterile brush culture in Gram stain analysis in the diagnosis of lower respiratory tract infection. Chest 1981;79:157–161.
19. Chastre CJ, Dian F, Brun P, et al. Prospective evaluation of the protected brush for the diagnosis of pulmonary infections in ventilated patients. Am Rev Respir Dis 1984;130:924–929.
20. Villers D, Derrienic M, Raffi F, et al. Reliability of the bronchoscopic protected catheter brush in intubation ventilated patients. Chest 1985;88:527–530.
21. Higuchi JH, Coalson JJ, Johanson YWG. Bacteriological diagnosis of nosocomial pneumonia in primates. Am Rev Respir Dis 1982;125:53–57.
22. Torres A. Protected specimen brush versus transtracheal aspiration. A comparative study

in bacterial pneumonia. Am Rev Respir Dis 1982;125:368–369.

23. Carlin BW, Harrel JH, Moser KM. The treatment of endobronchial stenosis using balloon catheter dilation. Chest 1988;93:1148–1151.

24. Fieselmann JF, Zavala DC, Kein LW. Removal of foreign bodies (two teeth) by fiberoptic bronchoscopy. Chest 1972;72:241–243.

25. Zavala DC, Rhodes ML. Foreign body removal: a new role for the fiberoptic bronchoscope. Ann Otol 1975;84:650–656.

26. Hiller C, Lerner S, Varnum R, et al. Foreign body removal with the flexible fiberoptic bronchoscope. Endoscopy 1977;9:216–222.

27. Saito H, Saka H, Sakai S, Shimokata K. Removal of broken fragment of biopsy forceps with magnetic extractor. Chest 1989; 95:700–701.

28. Sanders DM. Needle in a haystack. Chest 1983;83:935–936.

29. Olesen LL, Thorshauge H, Nielsen BA. Breakage of the wire cytology brush during fiberoptic bronchoscopy. Chest 1987;92:188.

30. Kato H, Goto H, Leke R, et al. A new, fully protected biopsy scrapper for transbronchial lung biopsy. Chest 1985;1:143. Communication to the editor.

31. Wang KP. Flexible transbronchial needle aspiration biopsy for histologic specimens. Chest 1985;88:860–863.

32. Tanaka M, Satoh M, Kawanami O, Aihara K. A new bronchofiberscope for the study of diseases of very peripheral airways. Chest 1984;85:590–594.

33. Meduri GY, Beals DH, Maijul AG, Baselski V. Protected bronchoalveolar lavage. Am Rev Respir Dis 1991;143:855–864.

34. Marsh BR. Bipolar cautery for the fiberoptic bronchoscope. Ann Otol Rhinol Laryngol 1987;96:120–121.

35. Hooer RB, Jackson FN. Endobronchial electrosurgery. Chest 1985;87:712–714.

36. Wallace JM. Electrosurgery via the fiberoptic bronchoscope: a useful therapeutic technique. Chest 1985;87:705–706.

37. Hooper RB, Jackson FN. Endobronchial electrocautery. Chest 1988;94:595–598.

38. Walsh DA, Maiwand MO, Nath AR, Lockwood P, Lloyd MH, Saab M. Bronchoscopic cryotherapy for advanced bronchial carcinoma. Thorax 1991;45:509–513.

39. Homasson JP, Renault P, Angebault M, Bonniot JP, Bell NJ. Bronchoscopic cryotherapy for airway strictures caused by tumors. Chest 1986;90:159–164.

40. Homasson JP. Endoscopic palliation of tracheobronchial malignancies. Thorax 1991; 46:861.

41. Angebault M, Bonniot JP, Baud D, Farlet D, Homasson JP. Cryotherapy in the treatment of tracheobronchial obstruction of tumor origin. Revu De Pneumologie Clinique 1987; 43:13–18.

42. Shure D. Endobronchial suture, a foreign body causing chronic cough. Chest 1991; 100:1193–1196.

7 | The Care and Maintenance of the Flexible Bronchoscope

Raul J. Seballos and Atul C. Mehta

Shiget Ikeda first reported the development of the flexible bronchoscope in 1968 (1). Over the last 25 years, the flexible bronchoscope has revolutionized the practice of pulmonary medicine. It has become the field's most utilized medical instrument. Its growing spectrum of diagnostic, therapeutic, and palliative indications range from direct visual airway examination, thermal laser resection of endobronchial tumors, brachytherapy, and photodynamic therapy (2–4). Modifications in design and availability of a wide range of accessories have kept pace with the growing use of the flexible bronchoscope. Correspondingly, the price of the instrument has also risen. The average cost of a new flexible bronchoscope, not including accessories and light source, ranges from $10,000 to $12,000.

This chapter deals with the routine care and prevention of damage of the instrument and includes discussions on cleaning, disinfection, sterilization, storage, and transportation. Because a growing number of immunocompromised patients are undergoing both diagnostic and therapeutic flexible fiberoptic bronchoscopy (FOB) and transmission of infection via contaminated bronchoscopes has been reported (5), the disinfection and sterilization of the bronchoscope are emphasized. Secondly, key areas in the prevention of damage to the instrument are addressed. Lastly, the financial impact of damage and the cost of repair are discussed.

Routine Care

Cleaning

The manufacturer's instruction manual is a valuable resource for routine care instructions. Its cleaning guidelines should be followed closely. Most flexible bronchoscopes available today are fully submersible instruments. In cases of nonsubmersible ones, submersing the proximal control unit, eyepiece, and light connector in the cleaning solution should be avoided.

After each FOB procedure, the exterior surface is wiped with a moist gauze. Approximately 500 mL clean water or saline solution is suctioned (in about 10 seconds) through the working channel. After the suction channel valve pieces are removed, the entire scope is submersed in tap water or cleaning solution. At this stage, a "leak test" is recommended for early detection of damage to the external sheath or working channel of the scope. At our institution, this is done after every transbronchial needle aspiration (TBNA) and endobronchial neodymium: yttrium-aluminum-garnet (Nd:YAG) laser photoresection. Proper methods for the "leak test" are described in the accompanying operator's manual of each bronchoscope. An air leak at either end of the working channel indicates a perforation of the inner channel of the scope, usually resulting from improper handling of the TBNA needle, excessive flexing of the scope, or use of damaged accessories (6). The cost to repair this type of damage is approximately $3500. If an air leak is detected from the external surface of the scope (Figure 7.1), damage to the polyurethane covering on the proximal flexible portion or rubber sheath located on the distal end has occurred. Damage to the external surface usually results from routine wear and tear or abrading the exterior surface against a sharp object. The cost of repair for this type of damage is approximately $400. Once a leak test is identified, immediate repair is indicated.

After a negative "leak test," the bronchoscope is submersed in a cleaning solution. A cleaning brush is passed through the working channel several times until the brush extends beyond the distal end of the scope. After all channel ports and suction connector are brushed, the scope is rinsed with tap water. Tap water is again suctioned through the working channel for approximately 10 seconds, followed by air suction for 30 seconds to air dry the working channel. The bronchoscope is now ready for disinfection or sterilization.

Disinfection

Because of the growing number of immunocompromised patients undergoing endoscopy and the threat of transmission of pathogens between patients due to inadequately processed endoscopes, there has been a heightened awareness of the potential for infection in both public and medical communities. Cross contamination among patients undergoing endoscopic procedures has been reported. In the comprehensive review by Spach and colleagues (5), 96 infections were transmitted by the bronchoscope. Tuberculous and nontuberculous mycobacteria and *Pseudomonas* species were the most commonly reported agents. Outbreaks of endoscopic-related infections can be attributed to improper cleaning and processing procedures, and because of their complex internal structure, the inability to decontaminate endoscopic valves and chan-

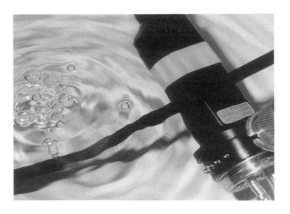

Figure 7.1. Air bubbles from the exterior surface of the flexible bronchoscope or "positive leak test."

Reproduced by permission from Stelck MJ, Kulas MJ, Mehta AC. Maintenance of the bronchoscope and bronchoscopy equipment. In: Prakash UBS, ed. Bronchoscopy. New York: Raven Press, 1994; 382.

nels. More recently, reports of contamination by automated washers have been described (7,8). Fraser and associates (9) reported persistent endoscopic contamination in 11 of 60 endoscopes (18%) despite a three-state decontamination procedure in their study comparing manual and automated endoscope procedures.

Spaulding (10) defined three categories of medical instruments each requiring different levels of microbial cleanliness: noncritical items (those coming in contact with intact skin) requiring low-level disinfection; semicritical items (those coming in direct contact with mucous membranes or nonintact skin without penetration) requiring high-level disinfection; and critical items (those introduced beneath the surface of the body, penetrating either skin or mucous membranes) requiring sterilization. The flexible bronchoscope can therefore be classified as a semicritical item or critical item.

High-level disinfection, defined as a procedure that inactivates all fungi, viruses, and vegetative microorganisms, but not necessarily all bacterial spores (10), can be achieved with 2% glutaraldehyde. Immersion for 10 minutes in 2% glutaraldehyde will destroy bacteria, viruses, and 99.8% of mycobacterial organ-

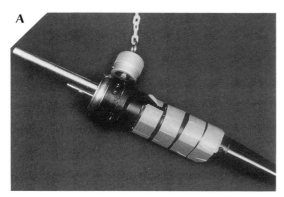

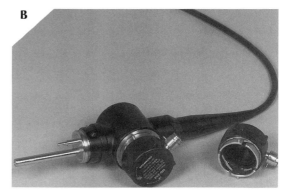

Figure 7.2. Properly placed ETO venting cap on an Olympus fiberoptic bronchoscope (*A*) and on a new Olympus videobronchoscope (*B*). An additional ETO venting cap is shown.

isms. Immersion for 45 minutes at 25°C will eradicate all mycobacterial organisms. We recommend minimal immersion of 20 minutes to achieve high-level disinfection following routine cases. A large pan containing the disinfectant should be used to avoid excessive coiling of the bronchoscope. Repeated excessive coiling of the scope can lead to development of curved-fixed angulation ("memory curve") of the distal portion or kinking of the working channel at its proximal most flexible portion. Following submersion in the disinfectant solution, the bronchoscope exterior is rinsed with tap water and the working channel with sterile water. The working channel is then dried by air suction.

The disadvantages of disinfection by 2% glutaraldehyde include skin and eye irritation, need for adequate ventilation, disposal considerations (certain states prohibit disposal of glutaraldehyde into the sinks because of environmental considerations and its relative toxicity to fish), and lack of means to monitor the necessary conditions (time, temperature, and concentration). Other disinfectants such as phenol and isopropyl alcohol are less toxic, but their sporicidal actions are inferior compared to glutaraldehyde. In addition, the flexible bronchoscope should never be boiled or autoclaved (11).

Sterilization

As stated previously, sterilization is required for critical items; that is, instruments intro-

duced beneath the surface of the body, penetrating either the skin or mucous membranes, as in the case of TBNA. Under this circumstance, the bronchoscope, its accessories, and biopsy forceps require sterilization.

Ethylene oxide (ETO) gas sterilization is highly effective against all types of microorganisms. It is readily available, noncorrosive, and able to penetrate all portions of the bronchoscope. High pressures are not necessary. However, an ETO venting cap must be placed at the proximal end of the umbilical cable, which equalizes the pressure between the exterior and interior of the scope. Failure to use the ETO venting cap will rupture the outer polyurethane sheath (Figures 7.2 and 7.3). The

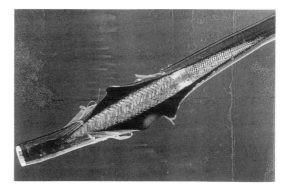

Figure 7.3. Rupture of the external sheath of the bronchoscope resulting from gas sterilization without the ETO venting cap.

Reproduced by permission from Mehta AC, Curtis PS, Scalzitti M, Meeker DP. The high price of bronchoscopy: maintenance and repair of the flexible fiberoptic bronchoscope. Chest 1990;98:448–454.

scope should be secured in a large, hard-walled sterilization pan. ETO gas sterilization guidelines regarding pressure, temperature, humidity, and duration should be followed as stated in the operator's manual.

The disadvantage of ETO sterilization is the lengthy turnover time. ETO sterilization requires approximately 4 hours followed by 12 to 24 hours of degassing time. At our institution, ETO sterilization is done in our central processing department with a turnover time of 3 days. This lengthy turnaround time makes ETO sterilization impractical. In addition, Vesley and coworkers (12) have shown that even after ETO sterilization, viable spores may be present in some scopes, suggesting that ETO processing does not necessarily guarantee sterility. The authors also point out concerns of high ETO residue levels even after 12.5 hours of degassing time.

An attractive alternative to ETO sterilization is the STERIS SYSTEM™. This liquid chemical process is performed, controlled, and monitored in a processor using a sterilant concentrate—peracetic acid (PAA)—as the active biocidal agent. The processor is a tabletop, automated microprocessor-controlled device connected to a potable water supply, drain, and electricity (Figure 7.4). Sterile water is made by the processor via a sterilizing grade

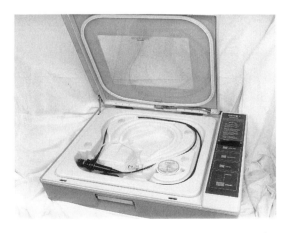

Figure 7.4. The STERIS SYSTEM 1™ processor with a properly placed flexible bronchoscope before sterilization.

filter located upstream in the fluid pathway. The sterilant is automatically mixed with sterile water made by the processor to form a solution that flows into the chamber and comes in contact with all accessible external and internal surfaces of the instrument. The sterilant solution is also distributed throughout the fluid pathway including the downside of the sterilizing grade filter. The processor has simple push button operations and an internal self-diagnostic and monitoring system that produces a printed document confirming that all sterilization parameters have been met during each cycle (13). The total time to process and sterilize the bronchoscope is about 25 minutes.

To assess and confirm that the processor met all sterilization parameters during each cycle, *Bacillus stearothermophilis* spore strips were used to biologically monitor the process. In addition, chemical indicators sensitive to the presence of PAA were used to confirm that the sterilization concentration of PAA was delivered. A detailed description of the sterilization process has been previously described (14).

We prospectively studied the effectiveness of this system in 20 consecutive patients suspected to have a lower respiratory tract infection who underwent an FOB procedure with bronchoalveolar lavage (BAL) and protected specimen brush (PSB) specimen collections. Sterile normal saline was aseptically suctioned and collected through the bronchoscope's suction channel after the procedure (preprocessing fluid). The scope was then cleaned and processed in the liquid chemical sterilization system. After processing, normal saline was again suctioned and collected (postprocessing fluid) in a similar fashion. Cultures of the BAL, PSB, preprocessing, and postprocessing fluids were compared. In addition to the 20 patients studied, deliberate inoculations of the bronchoscope with *Mycobacterium avium* complex (MAC) organisms were done. Cultures of the inoculated, preprocessing, and postprocessing fluids were compared. BAL and PSB cultures predominantly revealed bacterial growth. *Pneumocystis carinii* was noted in 3 patients. Positive viral cultures included cytomegalovirus and herpes simplex virus. All postprocessing fluid cultures were negative except in 2 patients where the rare number of organisms (coagulase-negative staphylococci and diphtheroids) isolated was felt to represent contaminated collection or processing procedures in the laboratory. All postprocessing fluids of the inoculated bronchoscopes revealed no growth for MAC organisms. Our results indicated that our department's cleaning and sterilization protocol was effective in eradicating bacterial, mycobacterial, and viral organisms. This liquid chemical sterilization system using PAA as the active biocidal agent provided an effective and safe sterilization process with a relatively quick turnover time (15).

At our tertiary care center, more than 1100 FOB procedures are done annually. To date, our institution has not reported any infection transported by bronchoscopy. However, infections related to endoscopy can be difficult to document and remain unrecognized because of inadequate surveillance and because some patients may have asymptomatic infections or have prolonged incubation periods before symptoms arise. In addition, since our department has adopted the liquid chemical sterilization system, over 2000 sterilization cycles have been done. We have had no mechanical or sterilization failures. No bronchoscopes have required repairs as a result of damage caused by the sterilant. On two occasions, however, a bronchoscope was damaged by inadvertently closing the lid at the distal end of the insertion tube.

Despite the availability of written policies and recommendations for high-level disinfection (16,17), practices for cleaning and disinfection remain highly variable. Kaczmarek and coworkers (18) reported a 23.9% contamination rate of gastrointestinal endoscopes in a multistate investigation. Many of the facilities did not test the concentration of the disinfecting agent or appropriately sterilize biopsy forceps. Considerable interhospital and intrahospital variability in reprocessing practices of endoscopes and semicritical items have also been reported (19,20). We recommend that each institution follow the current disinfection and sterilization guidelines from the Association for Practitioners in Infection Control (17) as well as those of their respective professional societies (e.g., Society of Gastroenterology Nurses and Associates, American Society for Gastrointestinal Endoscopy, etc.). In addition, we suggest that each institution have periodic evaluations of their disinfection and sterilization protocols.

Storage

Following disinfection and sterilization, the flexible bronchoscope should be dried with close attention to electrical contacts and ocular and objective lenses. The control lock should be released. The scope should be stored in a neutral and vertical position. The storage cabinet should be well ventilated, dry, away from direct sunlight, high humidity, extreme temperatures, and radiation. Excessive radiation exposure may cause yellow discoloration to the lens and darken the fiber bundles. The storage cabinet should also be tall enough to prevent bending of the insertion tube and to avoid development of the "memory curve." For the same reason, the bronchoscope should never be stored in the carrying case. In addition, the carrying case is usually colonized with microorganisms and should only be used for transportation. Storage of the bronchoscope with the ETO venting cap may allow evaporation of moisture that develops over time from leak test.

Transportation

The original carrying case should be used for long distance transportation. The scope should be properly placed in its protective recessed molding before the lid is closed. Closing the lid on the insertion tube can cause damage similar to that caused by a patient biting on the scope (see below). The ETO venting cap should always be placed and secured before high-altitude flights to equalize pressures within the bronchoscope.

Prevention of Damage

The bronchoscopist is responsible for the prevention of damage to the bronchoscope during the procedure. The areas of potential damage include improper handling, TBNA, Nd:YAG photoresection, electrosurgery, inadequate lubrication of the scope, and an uncooperative patient (Table 7.1).

Improper Handling

The objective lens and the delicate quartz filaments are especially vulnerable to trauma. Proper handling requires not allowing the distal end of the scope to strike a hard surface. Excessive angulation of the proximal end of the insertion tube (Figure 7.5A) or twisting the distal half (Figure 7.5B) can damage the quartz fiber bundles. Damaged quartz filaments appear as black spots on the ocular lens (Figure 7.6). Adequate distance between the bronchoscopist and the patient's head can avoid excessive angulation of the insertion tube. The rotation of the scope should be done by flexing or extending the wrist to minimize the scope's torque.

Table 7.1. Areas of Potential Damage to the Flexible Fiberoptic Bronchoscope

Improper handling
Procedural
    Transbronchial needle aspiration
    Nd:YAG photoresection
    Electrosurgery
    Radiation
    Use of lubricants
Patient related
Cleaning and maintenance
    Ethylene oxide gas sterilization

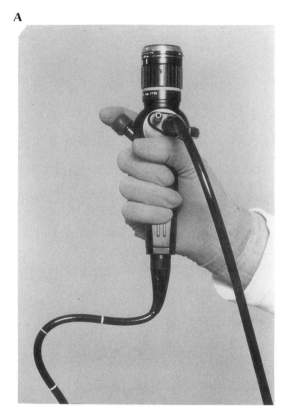

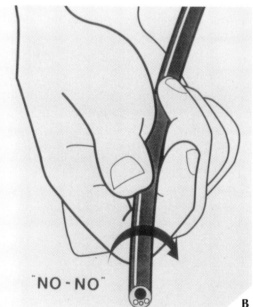

"NO-NO"

Figure 7.5. Excessive angulation of the proximal end of the insertion tube (*A*) and twisting of the distal end of the bronchoscope (*B*) can damage the quartz filaments.

Reproduced by permission from Mehta AC, Curtis PS, Scalzitti M, Meeker DP. The high price of bronchoscopy: maintenance and repair of the flexible fiberoptic bronchoscope. Chest 1990;98:448–454.

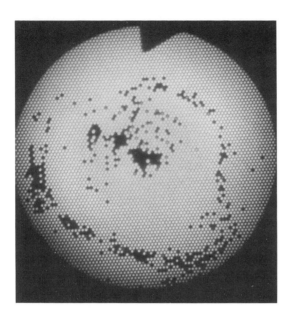

Figure 7.6. Multiple damaged quartz fiber bundles appearing as black spots on the ocular lens.

Procedural

The working channel of the bronchoscope is lined by a delicate plastic tubing. Newer scopes become more flexible with thinner inner plastic tubing, thus making them more vulnerable to perforation, laceration, or fracture. Submersing the scope with a damaged inner plastic channel will allow cleaning solution into the flexible quartz bundles, fogging the ocular lens.

The most proximal portion of the insertion tube is the most vulnerable area of damage because flexible instruments impact on this portion of the tubing while negotiating the angulation. The proximal portion should be kept as straight as possible during insertion of any instrument into the working channel to prevent damage.

The diameter of the working channel should be noted. This can usually be estimated by the size of the green spot found on the proximal unit of most Olympus bronchoscopes. The diameter of flexible instruments such as transbronchial aspiration needles, biopsy forceps, or cleaning brushes should not be larger than the working channel diameter.

In addition, damaged endoscopic accessories should not be used and should be replaced to prevent potential damage to the bronchoscope.

Transbronchial Needle Aspiration

Cytology and histology specimens obtained from TBNA have increased the diagnostic yield of FOB (21,22). The transbronchial needle, if not properly used, is the single most common cause of damage to the inner lining of the working channel (6). The beveled end of the retractable needle must be withdrawn completely within the metal hub that caps the distal end of the plastic catheter. The needle should also not be retracted too far beyond the metal hub or well within the plastic catheter. Advancing the needle in this situation can penetrate the inner plastic and damage the inner lining of the working channel (Figures 7.7 and 7.8).

As previously mentioned, the most proximal portion of the insertion tube should be kept as straight as possible during insertion of any instrument into the working channel, especially when negotiating the angulation. The distal end should be kept in a neutral forward viewing position. The needle must not be extended until its plastic catheter casing is well visualized beyond the tip of the bronchoscope in the endobronchial tree. After the specimens are collected, the scope should be straightened for smooth withdrawal of the needle. The plastic catheter with the exposed needle is withdrawn in one swift motion back through the working channel. We recommend that a "leak test" be performed after TBNA procedures to identify any damage to the working channel of the bronchoscope. This will assist in identifying flaws in one's technique and prevent future damage to the scope.

Nd:YAG Photoresection

The Nd:YAG laser is now widely used for the ablation of malignant or benign unresectable endobronchial lesions (2,23–25). This modality

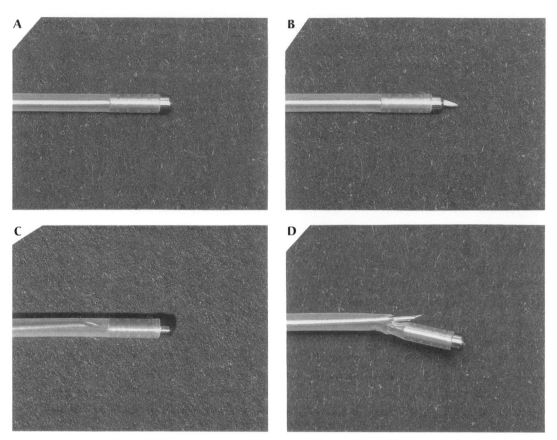

Figure 7.7. *A,* Correct position of the metal needle prior to TBNA: the entire beveled end is placed inside the metal hub. *B,* Incorrect position of the metal needle: the sharp end of the needle is extending beyond the metal hub, which can potentially lacerate the working channel of the bronchoscope. *C* and *D,* Incorrect position of the metal needle: the needle is placed too proximal to the metal hub and can perforate its own plastic catheter during forward thrust and potentially damage the working channel of the bronchoscope.

Reproduced by permission from Stelck MJ, Kulas MJ, Mehta AC. Maintenance of the bronchoscope and bronchoscopy equipment. In: Prakash UBS, ed. Bronchoscopy. New York: Raven Press, 1994;386.

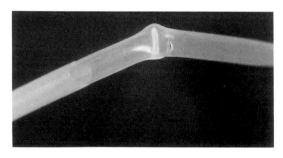

Figure 7.8. Perforation (*arrow*) of the inner plastic channel of the bronchoscope during TBNA. Note kinking of the plastic channel, which occurred at the most proximal flexible portion of the flexible bronchoscope as a result of repetitive excessive bending.

Reproduced by permission from Mehta AC, Curtis PS, Scalzitti M, Meeker DP. The high price of bronchoscopy: maintenance and repair of the flexible fiberoptic broncho-scope. Chest 1990;98:448–454.

can be administered through either a rigid or a flexible bronchoscope and can penetrate to depths of 5 mm, providing good hemostasis is maintained through photocoagulation of vessels. The potential risks of Nd:YAG photoresection include endobronchial ignition due to the use of a combustible polyvinyl chloride endotracheal tube (ETT) and combustible materials that make up the bronchoscope. We propose the "Rule of Fours" to minimize the risk of endobronchial ignition. The fraction of inspired oxygen (FIO_2) should be less than 0.40. The distal end of the ETT should be more than 4 cm from the lesion. The tip of the laser fiber should extend at least 4 mm from the scope and be 4 mm from the lesion. We recommend using single-pulse mode with a pulse duration of 0.4 seconds, under 40 watts, and pausing every 40 pulses to clean the fiber (see Table 7.2 for complete listing). Alcohol or alcohol-based solutions should not be used to clean the laser fiber tip to avoid the possibility of combustion. In addition, the tip of the laser fiber and bronchoscope should be free of any carbon particles because these absorb a higher degree of energy than surrounding tissue and may potentially start an ignition. Finally, a coaxial flow of air or saline solution should be continuously maintained to keep the laser tip cool. An overheated metal tip of the noncontact laser fiber can damage the inner channel of the scope on withdrawal (Figure 7.9).

Table 7.2. "Rule of Fours" to Prevent Laser-Induced Damage to the Flexible Bronchoscope

Distance	
Endotracheal tube to lesion	> 4 cm
Fibertip to lesion	4 mm
Flexible bronchoscope to fibertip	4 mm
FIO_2	< 0.40
Power (watts)	
Noncontact	40 W
Contact	4 W
Pulse duration	0.4 s
Number of pulses between cleaning	40
Operating room time	< 4
Laser team (bronchoscopist, assistant, anesthesiologist, bronchoscopy nurse)	4

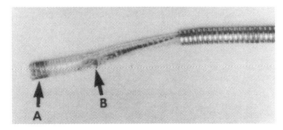

Figure 7.9. Damaged distal end of the working channel of the flexible bronchoscope. The charring (A) and perforation (B) were caused by heated metal casing of the noncontact laser fiber when the coaxial gas flow was accidentally shut off.

Reproduced by permission from Mehta AC, Curtis PS, Scalzitti M, Meeker DP. The high price of bronchoscopy: maintenance and repair of the flexible fiberoptic bronchoscope. Chest 1990;98:448–454.

Electrosurgery

The use of endobronchial cautery in treating endotracheobronchial lesion has been described (26–28). An electrocautery unit consists of two electrodes connected to terminals on a high-frequency AC generator. One electrode acts as the active instrument with a small surface area and high current density. The opposite electrode is a large surface area grounding plate with a low current density that is attached to the patient's back. Heat is generated with electrical resistance causing interaction ranging from drying to vaporization depending on the type and amount of current and the contact area between tissue and probe (29).

Electrocauterization via the flexible gastrointestinal scopes has been used to treat gastrointestinal bleeding. However, unlike the gastrointestinal endoscope, the bronchoscope is not grounded. Therefore, if a wire loop snare or cautery probe inadvertently touches the distal metal tip of the bronchoscope, it can cause an endotracheal ignition, especially in the setting of high oxygen concentration, and damage the scope. Though not yet approved and considered experimental, bipolar cautery, because of its unique design, has been advocated as safer than wire loop cautery (30).

Lubrication

A water-soluble lubricant should be used to lubricate the bronchoscope. Petroleum-based products should be avoided because they may cause premature wear and stretching of the external, distal rubber sheath of the scope. The use of a lubricant is especially important in performing FOB in an intubated patient. An adult bronchoscope requires a minimum size 8.0 ETT. In addition, a pediatric bronchoscope may be necessary in cases where the FOB procedure is done through a tracheostomy tube (Figure 7.10).

Patient-Related Damages

A cooperative patient with adequate sedation is important in performing FOB. We

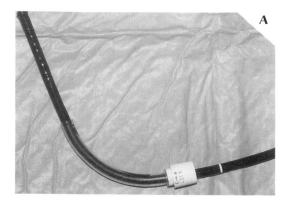 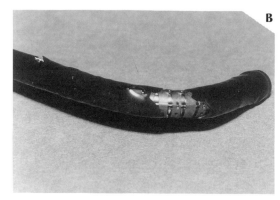

Figure 7.10. *A,* An improperly selected size bronchoscope "stuck" in a tracheostomy tube led to patient distress, requiring immediate removal of both. *B,* Removing the tracheostomy tube damaged the external sheath.

A reproduced by permission from Stelck MJ, Kulas MJ, Mehta AC. Maintenance of the bronchoscope and bronchoscopy equipment. In: Prakash UBS, ed. Bronchoscopy. New York: Raven Press, 1994;387.

recommend patients to be in supine positions for greater comfort and the less likelihood of a vasovagal attack. A transnasal approach is also recommended for greater stability and to avoid the problem of patient biting on the scope. If FOB is performed via ETT or transoral approach, a bite guard, well fastened to the patient's face, must be used to protect the bronchoscope from being bitten (Figure 7.11).

Videobronchoscope

Some centers now use a videobronchoscope system. Our pulmonary department is now using the EVIS video system manufactured by Olympus Corporation (Lake Success, New York); however, our experience with this equipment is limited. This system consists of a videobronchoscope, a light source, a video system center, and a video monitor. Ancillary equipment that can be used includes a videotape recorder, video printer, and a compact video trolley. Special care and handling are essential. The care and maintenance of this new system are fully described in the accompanying manuals.

Financial Impact

The flexible bronchoscope is an expensive medical instrument. The cost of repair and maintenance can be substantial unless proper care and maintenance, as previously articulated, are undertaken. In addition, the life span of the bronchoscope can also be extended when following these guidelines.

The manufacturer's instruction manual is one of the most important sources of information in the care and maintenance of the bronchoscope. A survey conducted by Mehta and colleagues (6) related to pulmonologists in the local community, pulmonary fellows, and other personnel involved in handling the bronchoscope revealed that only 11% have actually read the accompanying manufacturer's instruction manual. The authors conclude that the manual is significantly underused and should be readily available to all personnel involved.

We have reviewed our institution's cost of repair of damaged flexible bronchoscopes between 1985 and 1989 (6). The frequency and average cost of preventable and nonpreventable repairs were especially looked at. More than 1000 FOB procedures are now done annually at our institution. In comparing the time period of the original survey of 1985–1989 to the period of 1990–1993, the number of FOB procedures increased (922/y versus 1056/y, respectively). However, the number of repairs per year (10.3/y versus

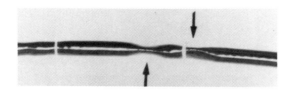

Figure 7.11. External damage (*arrows*) to the flexible insertion tube of the bronchoscope was caused by the patient biting during the procedure.

Reproduced by permission from Mehta AC, Curtis PS, Scalzitti M, Meeker DP. The high price of bronchoscopy: maintenance and repair of the flexible fiberoptic bronchoscope. Chest 1990;98:448–454.

10.5/y, respectively) and repair cost per procedure per year ($25.36/procedure/y versus $27.23/procedure/y) have not significantly changed, despite our department's emphasis on the care and maintenance of the scope. The lack of significant improvement in the number of repairs and the cost per repair per year may in part be due to the increased number of procedures done per year, the increase in the number of pulmonary fellow trainees, or the increase in the number of pulmonary attendings at our institution doing FOB and related diagnostic procedures such as TBNA.

Conclusion

In conclusion, all personnel involved in FOB procedures should be aware of all areas of potential damage to the bronchoscope. Proper handling and manipulation of the scope, its accessories, and particularly close attention to cleaning, disinfection, sterilization, storage, and shipping are all important aspects in the care and maintenance of the bronchoscope. Patient cooperation, adequate sedation, and proper positioning of both the patient and bronchoscopist are other key important issues to a successful bronchoscopy procedure. Constant vigilance in these areas is highly recommended.

REFERENCES

1. Ikeda S. Flexible bronchofiberscope. Ann Otol Rhinol Laryngol 1970;79:916–917.
2. Unger M. Neodymium:YAG laser therapy for malignant and benign endobronchial obstruction. Clin Chest Med 1985;6: 277–290.
3. Schray MF, McDougall JC, Martinez A, Cortese DA, Brutinel NW. Management of malignant airway compromise with laser and low dose rate brachytherapy: Mayo Clinic experience. Chest 1988;93:26–69.
4. Edell E, Cortese DA. Bronchoscopic phototherapy with hemalto-porphyrin derivative for treatment of localized bronchogenic carcinoma: a 5-year experience. Mayo Clin Proc 1987;62:8–14.
5. Spach DH, Silverstein FE, Stamm WE. Transmission of infection by gastrointestinal endoscopy and bronchoscopy. Ann Intern Med 1983;118:117–128.
6. Mehta AC, Curtis PS, Scalzitti M, Meeker DP. The high price of bronchoscopy: maintenance and repair of the flexible fiberoptic bronchoscope. Chest 1990;98:448–454.
7. Alvarado CJ, Stolz SM, Maki DM. Nosocomial infections from contaminated endoscopes: a flawed automated endoscope washer, an investigation using molecular epidemiology. Am J Med 1991;91(suppl 3B): 272–280.
8. Alvarado CJ, Stolz SM, Maki DM, et al. Nosocomial infections and pseudoinfections from contaminated endoscopes and bronchoscopes, Wisconsin and Missouri. MMWR 1991;40:675–678.
9. Fraser V, Zuckeman G, Clouse RE, et al. A prospective randomized trial comparing manual and automated endoscope disinfection methods. Infect Control Hosp Epidemiol 1993;14:383–389.
10. Spaulding EH. Chemical disinfection of medical and surgical materials. In: Lawrence CA, Block SS, eds. Disinfection, sterilization, and preservation. Philadelphia: Lee and Febiger, 1968.
11. Elford B. Care and cleansing of the fiberoptic bronchoscope. Chest 1978;73:761–763.
12. Vesley D, Norlien KG, Nelson B, Ott B, Streifel AJ. Significant factors in the disinfection and sterilization of flexible endoscopes. Am J Infect Control 1992;20:291–300.

13. STERIS Operator Manual for the Olympus Scope Processing Instructions. STERIS CORPORATION, Mentor: Publication I.D. #1008.20115, 1992.

14. Malchesky PS. Peracetic acid and its application to medical instrument sterilization. Artif Organs 1993;17:147–152.

15. Seballos RJ, Walsh A, Mehta AC. Clinical evaluation of a liquid chemical sterilization system for the flexible bronchoscope. J Bronchology 1995 (in press).

16. Centers for Disease Control. Guidelines for the prevention of human immunodeficiency virus and hepatitis B virus to health care and public safety workers. MMWR 1989;38: 1–37.

17. Rutala WA. APIC guidelines for selection and use of disinfectants. Am J Infect Control 1990;18:99–117.

18. Kaczmarek RG, Moore RM Jr, McCrohan J, et al. Multi-state investigation of the actual disinfection/sterilization of endoscopes in health care facilities. Am J Med 1992; 92:257–261.

19. Reynolds CD, Rhinehart E, Dreyer P, Goldmann DA. Variability in reprocessing policies and procedures for flexible fiberoptic endoscopes in Massachusetts hospitals. Am J Infect Control 1992;20:283–290.

20. Rutala WA, Clontz EP, Weber DJ, Hoffman KK. Disinfection practices for endoscopes and semicritical items. Infect Control Hosp Epidemiol 1991;12:282–288.

21. Wang KP. Flexible transbronchial needle aspiration for histological specimens. Chest 1985;86:860–863.

22. Kelly SJ, Wang KP. Transbronchial needle aspiration. J Thorac Imaging 1987;2:33–44.

23. Personne C, Colchan A, Leroy M, et al. Indications and techniques for endoscopic laser resections in bronchology: a critical analysis based on 2,284 resections. J Thorac Cardiovasc Surg 1986;91:710–715.

24. Cavaliere S, Foccoli P, Farina PL. Nd:YAG laser bronchoscopy: a five-year experience with 1,396 applications in 1,000 patients. Chest 1988;94:15–21.

25. Desai SJ, Mehta AC, Medendorp SV, et al. Survival experience following Nd:YAG laser photoresection from primary bronchogenic carcinoma. Chest 1988;94:939–944.

26. Hooper RG, Jackson FN. Endobronchial electrocautery. Chest 1985;87:712–714.

27. Gerasin VA, Shafirovsky BB. Endobronchial electrosurgery. Chest 1988;93:270–274.

28. Hooper RG, Jackson FN. Endobronchial electrocautery. Chest 1988;94:595–598.

29. Barlow DE. Endoscopic applications of electrocautery: a review of basic principles. Gastrointest Endosc 1982;28:73–76.

30. Marsh BR. Bipolar cautery for the fiberoptic bronchoscope. Ann Otol Rhinol Laryngol 1987;96:120–121.

31. Stelck MJ, Kulas MJ, Mehta AC. Maintenance of the bronchoscope and bronchoscopy equipment. In: Prakash UBS, ed. Bronchoscopy. New York: Raven Press, 1994.

Part 2

Diagnostic Bronchoscopy

8 | Basic Techniques in Flexible Bronchoscopy

Francis Y. W. Lee and Atul C. Mehta

Endobronchial examination dates back to 1897 when Killian (1) used a translaryngeal approach to perform the first bronchoscopy. The first indication for bronchoscopy was the location and recovery of a foreign body. In 1917, Jackson reported the first peroral bronchoscopic resection of an endobronchial tumor (2). He subsequently proposed the use of bronchoscopy to drain retained secretions (3). Over the next two decades, the role of bronchoscopy shifted from removing foreign bodies to the diagnosis of lung cancer. This coincided with the rising popularity of cigarette smoking and lung cancer during this period. The next major advancement was Shigeto Ikeda's development of flexible fiberoptic bronchoscopy (FOB) reported in 1968 (4). Up to this point only the rigid scope was used, and the introduction of a flexible bronchoscope widened the application of this procedure even further. Although the role of rigid bronchoscopy is widely recognized, we will emphasize the role of flexible FOB in routine practice. We will direct our discussion at the novice bronchoscopist who will be taken through basic diagnostic and therapeutic techniques step by step in a "cookbook" fashion. We hope that in this way, the rite of passage will be an easier one for the reader. Each section will close with a brief review of the literature as well as the authors' own recommendations for achieving the best results.

The diagnostic techniques described are:

- Bronchial washings (BW)
- Bronchoalveolar lavage (BAL)
- Protected catheter lavage
- Cytology brushing
- Lung mapping
- Protected catheter brush
- Endobronchial forceps biopsy

Transbronchial biopsy and needle aspiration are advanced techniques and will be discussed in Chapters 9, 12, 13,14, 15, and 16.

Therapeutic techniques discussed include:

- Mechanical debulking of obstructive endobronchial tumor with biopsy forceps
- Balloon catheter dilatation of endobronchial stenosis
- Endobronchial electrocautery
- Endobronchial cryosurgery
- Bronchial toilet

Laser photoresection, brachytherapy, and removal of foreign bodies—advanced therapeutic techniques—are described in Chapters 18 through 20 of this book. We close the chapter with a practical "bedside" discussion on managing hypoxemia and hemorrhage, the most common complications seen in the bronchoscopy suite. Our recommendations for flexible FOB in mechanically ventilated patients are also included.

Diagnostic Procedures

Bronchial Washings

Bronchial washings are usually obtained for cytologic diagnosis. They are a useful by-product of FOB; however, the advent of BAL has superseded their role in identifying infective agents. At our institution, we routinely send BW for cytology and appropriate staining for fungi and mycobacteria. The utility in most of our cases, however, is largely for the diagnosis of primary or metastatic lung carcinoma. BW should be taken in combination with endobronchial forceps biopsy and cytology brushings (5,6). FOB is an uncomfortable, expensive, and time-consuming procedure. Efforts should be made to use all techniques available to establish the diagnosis at one sitting. Besides, obtaining a greater variety of specimens increases the diagnostic yield. If the tumor is *endoscopically visible*, proceed with BW over the surface of the lesion. If it is a submucosal infiltrative process, the likelihood for success is higher if the integrity of the bronchial mucosa is lost. Otherwise BW are taken from both bronchial trees and pooled together for analysis. BW should be performed before forceps biopsy and cytology brushings to avoid contamination of the specimen with blood (5). Wedging of the segmental bronchus is not required for BW. Place a specimen trap in series with the suction catheter. The trap should be oriented vertically during the procedure to ensure proper collection and prevent inadvertent loss of BW. Two percent lidocaine and normal saline instilled through the working channel of the bronchoscope as part of the usual procedure of FOB is collected in the trap. Only 15 mL of BW is required for acid-fast bacilli, fungi, and cytology if no lavage is obtained. Disconnect the trap before biopsy and brushings are performed to prevent contamination from any bleeding resulting from the latter procedures. If different sites are sampled, use individual traps to distinguish the segment or a lobe with pathology. Routine BW are seldom performed in isolation; the discussion will be carried in the section on endobronchial biopsy.

Bronchoalveolar Lavage

The focus of our discussion will be on the technique of performing BAL for infectious as well as noninfectious diseases (7,8) and the possible complications and their prevention. Although it is not within the scope of this chapter to discuss indications for BAL, we have included Tables 8.1 and 8.2, which provide the reader with a sense of perspective of both the capabilities and limitations of BAL and apply this technique in the appropriate setting.

Technique of Bronchoalveolar Lavage

LAVAGE FOR INFECTIOUS DISEASES: The technique for BAL is not standardized. As such, we will present the method performed at our institution, which is consistent with the American Thoracic Society guidelines (7).

Impact of ongoing antibiotic therapy: Antibiotics should be avoided as far as possible before the BAL. The chances of obtaining a true positive culture was found to rise by 47% for each additional day off antibiotics (9). Where possible, stop antibiotics for at least 48 hours before proceeding with the FOB. Antibiotic prophylaxis for bacterial endocarditis is not required for FOB (10) and thus will not interfere with the BAL culture results.

Premedication: Premedication is given in the usual manner. Atropine in particular should be used to minimize oropharyngeal secretions and improve visibility through the bronchoscope as well as to prevent vasovagal attack.

Local anesthesia: Local anesthesia should be induced using sterile, methylparaben-free 2% lidocaine because this preservative has bacteriostatic properties (11). At our institution the lidocaine is freshly prepared by our pharmacy and stored in the refrigerator to prevent dete-

Table 8.1. Infectious Diseases

Infective organisms that can be identified from BAL
Pneumocystis carinii
Toxoplasma gondii
Strongyloides
Legionella
Histoplasma
Mycobacterium tuberculosis
Mycoplasma
Influenza
Respiratory syncytial virus

Infections that are not confirmed from BAL but may aid diagnosis and management
Herpes simplex
Cytomegalovirus
Bacteria
Aspergillus
Candida
Cryptococcus
Atypical mycobacteria

Modified from Goldstein RA, Rohatgi PK, Bergofsky FH, et al. Clinical role of bronchoalveolar lavage in adults with pulmonary disease (ATS statement). Am Rev Respir Dis 1990;142:481–486.

Table 8.2. Noninfectious Diseases

Noninfectious diseases that are diagnostic from BAL
Alveolar proteinosis
Eosinophilic granuloma (electron microscopy required)
Malignancy including lymphoma

Noninfectious diseases that are nondiagnostic from BAL but may aid diagnosis
Pulmonary hemorrhage
Eosinophilic pneumonia
Berylliosis
Hypersensitivity pneumonitis
Asbestosis
Silicosis
Sarcoidosis

Noninfectious diseases that are nondiagnostic from BAL but may aid management
Idiopathic pulmonary fibrosis
Collagen vascular disease
Sarcoidosis

Modified from Goldstein RA, Rohatgi PK, Bergofsky EH, et al. Clinical role of bronchoalveolar lavage in adults with pulmonary disease (ATS statement). Am Rev Respir Dis1990;142:481–486.

rioration. Previous workers have preferred nebulized lidocaine (12,13); we favor having our patients gargle to induce local anesthesia. We believe that the degree of oropharyngeal contamination is no worse with our technique. Gargling is much less time consuming compared to inhaled lidocaine. The key practical point is to avoid injecting lidocaine into the suction channel before the lavage is completed to avoid contamination of the endobronchial tree with oropharyngeal secretions (12). The bronchoscope is then passed through the nostril in the usual fashion.

Suction: While performing FOB for the purpose of diagnosing infectious diseases, suction should not be used until BAL sampling (and protected catheter brushing) have been completed through the working channel (13).

Selection of a bronchial segment for lavage: For focal infiltrates on the chest film, the seg-

mental bronchus chosen for BAL should be the one in the area of new or progressive radiologic abnormality. In patients with more than one radiologic opacity, the segmental bronchus with the most purulent secretions should be chosen under direct visualization. If the infiltrates are diffuse, the superolateral segment of the right middle lobe or the superior segment of the lingula are recommended to maximize percentage of fluid recovery by the less dependent anatomy of these lobes (14,15). Lavage performed in the right middle lobe can yield up to 20% more fluid returned when compared to the lower lobes (14).

Technique of wedging the bronchoscope in a segmental bronchus: Ensure that the nonsuction channel port (Olympus Corp., Medical Instrument Division, 4 Nevada Drive, Lake Success, NY 11042-1179; non-suction syringe valve #MB163) is placed at the proximal end of the working channel. The bronchoscope is introduced into the endobronchial tree in the usual fashion without the use of suction or introduction of lidocaine into the working channel. The scope is then advanced to a segmental bronchus and wedged in place to completely occlude the lumen. Proper wedging prevents seepage of the lavage fluid proximally, which causes irritation and cough. Preventing cough is important because this can cause trauma, contamination with blood or mucus, and loss of instillate. If the wedge is incomplete, air will be seen bubbling into the syringe with a diminished return on aspiration with the syringe. An excessively tight wedge can lead to a poorer return and unnecessary trauma to the bronchial mucosa.

Bronchoalveolar lavage: Insert the syringe and three-way valve (Figure 8.1) into the nonsuction channel port. BAL is then performed with sterile pyrogen-free saline in 20–50-mL aliquots until a return of 40 mL or more is obtained as required by our microbiology laboratory (Table 8.3). We use the smallest aliquots (20 mL) for BAL in our lung transplant patients and limit the total volume instilled to 200 mL per lavage (16) in all patients. Slow, deep inhalation during instillation and prolonged controlled exhalation during aspiration of lavage fluid increases the return (8,17). Gentle, steady suction should be applied to the syringe plunger. Uncontrolled suction can result in less fluid recovery because the segmental bronchial wall may collapse from the excessive negative pressure applied. In our experience, it may also traumatize the bronchial mucosa and contaminate the effluent with blood. Each aliquot is immediately aspirated following instillation to minimize dwell time of lavage fluid in the lungs.

A description of the protocol we use for collection, transport, storage, and processing of lavage fluid at our institution is detailed in Table 8.3.

LAVAGE FOR NONINFECTIOUS CONDITIONS: The technique is essentially the same as above, only made easier by the fact that suction and a standard nonrefrigerated lidocaine preparation containing methylparaben can be used. Table 8.2 describes conditions in which BAL can be diagnostic, helpful in diagnosis, or aid in management.

Safety and Complications of Lavage

Bronchoalveolar lavage has been associated with transient declines in arterial oxygen saturation (PaO_2), forced expiratory volume in one second (FEV_1), vital capacity (VC), total lung capacity (TLC), forced expiratory flow (FEF_{25-75}), residual volume (RV), and airway resistance (R_{AW}). These disturbances in lung function have been attributed to bronchoscopic technique, volume instilled, temperature of fluid, lavage site, and number of segments/lobes lavaged.

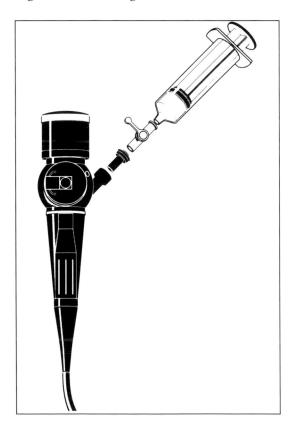

Figure 8.1. Use of syringe, three-way valve, and a special nonsuction adapter for BAL.

Table 8.3. Infectious Bronchoalveolar Lavage Protocol

1. Specimen collection
   a. 40 mL of BAL fluid is collected in a leak-proof screw-capped plastic container.
   b. Record lobe or segment BAL fluid is taken from.

2. Transport and storage
   a. BAL specimens should be transported as soon as possible.
   b. If a delay is expected to exceed 1 h, refrigerate the specimen.

3. Microbiology processing procedures

   General
   a. If < 10 mL fluid is received, inoculate fluid directly onto media.
   b. Refrigerate any excess fluid for 48 h.
   c. If volume is inadequate, contact the physician to prioritize the tests.

   Microscopic examination
   a. Prepare 6 cytospin slides:
      i. One for Gram stain
      ii. Two for acid-fast bacilli and nocardia stain
      iii. Three for Legionella direct fluorescent antibody
   b. Cytocentrifugation is the preferred method of slide preparation.
   c. One organism per immersion field (X1000) in the Gram-stained smear is considered a positive result.
   d. Positive results are phoned to the clinical services routinely.

   Bacteriology culture
   a. Use a calibrated 0.001-mL urine loop to inoculate uncentrifuged BAL onto a
      i. Blood agar plate (O_2)
      ii. Chocolate agar plate (CO_2)
      iii. McConkey's agar chocolate plate (O_2)
   b. Streak inoculum as per routine urine specimen.
   c. More than 100,000 bacteria/mL represent a positive culture.

   Virology culture
   a. Add 2-5 mL BAL fluid to 1.5 mL viral transport media (VTM) with antibiotics. Swirl to distribute contents and refrigerate until inoculation.
   b. Viruses routinely cultured include adenovirus, cytomegalovirus, and herpes.

   Legionella, mycobacteria, nocardia, and fungus cultures
   a. 10-20 mL BAL fluid will be divided equally between 2 isolator tubes.
   b. Tube 1 sediment—used for acid-fast bacilli stains, mycobacterial and nocardial culture.
   c. Tube 2 sediment—used for fungus culture, KOH preparation, and legionella culture.
   d. If less than 10 mL of BAL fluid is available, inoculate media directly. Always acid treat fluid for legionella culture and digest fluid for mycobacterial culture.

Adapted from Dr. John A Washington's (Head, Microbiology Department, Cleveland Clinic Foundation) infectious BAL protocol.

Hypoxemia is well documented in BAL-related literature. Pirozynski and colleagues (16) found that the degree of desaturation was related to the volume instilled. Lavage fluid of 100 mL produced desaturation up to 7%, whereas 200 mL produced desaturation up to 15% from baseline. Most patients in this study had returned to normal levels of oxygen saturation 10 minutes after bronchoscopy. However, those who had the most profound falls in saturation needed up to 30 minutes to return to baseline. Gibson and coworkers (18) compared the effect of BAL with and without supplemental oxygen using 300-mL volumes per lavage. In this study, the PaO_2 in 76% of patients breathing room air fell below 60 mm Hg, whereas only 25% of those on supplemental oxygen had a similar decline. The percentage return from the lavage was similar in both cohorts and did not affect the degree of hypoxemia. However, it took both groups about an hour to return to the baseline PaO_2 levels. Burns and associates (19) also compared the effect of BAL with and without supplemental oxygen in 19 healthy nonsmokers using one-liter lobar lavages. All volunteers on room air experienced PaO_2 values of less than 80 mm Hg. Although supplemental oxygen did not always eliminate hypoxemia, it did reduce the magnitude of desaturation to a large extent. They also noted that *both* the time of the procedure and the *volume* of lavage fluid were important factors because volunteers who had falls in PaO_2 below 60 mm Hg experienced it *late* in the lavage. Baseline saturations were again reached only after an hour postlavage. Our recommendations for preventing arterial hypoxemia in BAL are:

1. Measure baseline arterial blood gases before BAL, especially for patients with underlying lung disease, or low baseline Pao_2.
2. Use supplemental oxygen during and for at least one hour after the procedure.
3. Keep the duration of lavage procedure as short as possible.
4. Use judicious volumes of lavage fluid, although volumes of up to one liter have been used in lobar BAL (19).
5. Monitor arterial oxygen saturation and the electrocardiogram continuously during BAL and for at least an hour afterward. The peak incidence of cardiac arrhythmias is related to the nadir of oxygen desaturation (20).

The changes in spirometry appear related to the temperature of the lavage fluid (19). Subjects lavaged with saline at room temperature had falls in VC, TLC, and FEF_{25-75}. There was also an increase in RV and a slight but insignificant elevation of R_{AW}. Saline lavage at body temperature did not produce significant change in any of these parameters except a rise in RV when compared to prelavage values. Dhillon and colleagues (21) examined the effect of BAL on peak expiratory flow (PEF), but found the decline in PEF to be related more to the procedure of bronchoscopy itself rather than BAL. Kirby and coworkers (22) studied the effect of BAL on methacholine challenge sensitivity as measured by PC20 (provocation concentration required to cause a 20% fall in FEV_1). They found no

alteration in airway reactivity after BAL. Kelly and associates (23), however, demonstrated increased responsiveness to methacholine in asthmatics and recommended that although BAL was safe for most asthmatics, special attention should be given to asthmatics with heightened bronchial reactivity. Bronchospasm itself, however, appears to be uncommon in patients who are not reactive to methacholine challenge. Strumpf and colleagues (24) reported an incidence of only 0.7% in their series of 281 BALs in 119 patients with interstitial lung disease. Caution, however, should continue to be exercised in hyperreactive patients (25,26). Wardlaw and coworkers (26) found that asthmatics with a PC20 less than 4 mg/mL to methacholine would wheeze after BAL, whereas those with a PC20 more than 4 mg/mL did not. They reported mild but persistent wheezing for up to 2 weeks following BAL, requiring control with inhaled β_2-agonist therapy. In addition to our recommendations for hypoxemia, we advise the following for all patients with hyperreactive airways:

1. Before BAL, obtain spirometry; perform elective lavage only if FEV_1 is greater than 60% predicted. Otherwise optimize therapy before lavage.
2. Avoid bronchoscopy if the patient has acute bronchospasm. If possible avoid BAL in an asthmatic with a history of status asthmaticus or multiple admissions requiring mechanical ventilation.
3. Pretreat with bronchodilators and steroids especially if PC20 is less than 0.2 mg/mL (26).
4. Have nebulized β_2-agonists on standby especially in patients with PC20 less than 4 mg/mL.
5. Use lavage fluid warmed to body temperature.

Both inspiratory and expiratory crackles can be heard in the dependent/lavaged segments in the initial 24 hours after BAL. This side effect is seen in both normal and asthmatic patients (25) and is felt to be related to the volume of BAL fluid used.

Bronchoalveolar lavage has had an excellent safety record and is not associated with an increased risk of complications over that seen with regular bronchoscopy. The reported overall rate of complications of BAL (0% to 3%) is less than half that of transbronchial biopsy (7%). No mortalities have been reported from BAL. In contrast, transbronchial biopsy has a mortality rate of 0.2% (8). Although rare, pneumothorax has been documented in relation to therapeutic BAL for pulmonary alveolar proteinosis (27) in one patient and in another patient with acquired immunodeficiency syndrome (AIDS) and *Pneumocystis carinii* pneumonia (28). The latter is of particular interest as patients with human immunodeficiency virus (HIV) with *P. carinii* pneumonia have been observed to be at higher risk of developing spontaneous pneumothoraces (29,30).

If the patient has a platelet count of greater than 75,000/mL, a normal coagulation profile, and normal hepatorenal function, the risk of a significant bleed is minimal from FOB (31). For BAL specifically, Strumpf and coworkers (24) reported a bleeding complication rate of only 0.7% not requiring interventional therapy.

Reported rates of fever (greater than 1°C) and chills vary widely from 2.5% to 50% (14,19,21,24,32). Pingleton (14) had the highest incidence and attributed this to the total number of segments/lobes lavaged as opposed to the total lavage volume. Fever and chills were transient (under 24 hours) and did not require antibiotic therapy. Similar experiences have been documented by other workers (19,21,24,32).

Our recommendations are:

1. To avoid a high incidence of fevers/chills, lavage less than four different segments/lobes at each sitting.
2. Unless there is definite clinical or radiologic evidence of infection and the fever does not resolve within 24 hours, antibiotic treatment is not necessary.

The incidence of alveolar infiltrates following BAL varies between 0.4% to 50% (14,24, 32). They usually appear in the dependent lavaged segments and resolve within 24 hours (14). Pingleton again recorded the highest incidence of this complication and observed that all those with fever and chills had subsegmental opacities consistent with atelectasis. This appears to be related to the volume of saline used and the number of segments/lobes lavaged (14). The association between fever/chills and infiltrates has also been reported by Cole and colleagues (32).

Protected Bronchoalveolar Lavage

The role of BAL in opportunistic bacterial pneumonias is well documented but its role in the diagnosis of nonopportunistic bacterial pneumonias is still controversial. Kahn and Jones (33) found that greater than 1% squamous epithelial cells (SEC) in BAL returns was indicative of heavy contamination by oropharyngeal flora. Semiquantitative cultures (more than 10^5 cfu/mL) can no longer identify bacteria accurately once contamination exceeds this breakpoint. Nevertheless, 16 of 18 patients with pneumonias were accurately diagnosed when less than 1% SEC were identified in the effluent. The corollary was also true—no patients with under 1% SEC and no clinical manifestations of bacterial pneumonia had greater than 10^5 cfu/mL on semiquantitative culture. Thorpe and colleagues (34) achieved similar results in 13 of 15 patients using the same breakpoint of significant bacterial growth (more than 10^5 cfu/mL). Technical issues abound, however, on the successful results that these two groups have attained (35). Reproducibility of the less than 1% SEC contamination rate by other laboratories is an unknown factor. Different BAL volumes were used by Kahn (240 mL) and Thorpe (150 mL). The volume of fluid used will affect the dilution of the semiquantitative cultures. The optimal volume to instill has not been determined. Should the first aliquot be discarded? The first aliquot is regarded by some authors as being heavily contaminated by bronchial rather than alveolar organisms (36,37). Studies of nosocomial bacterial pneumonias in mechanically ventilated patients have also revealed inconsistent results. Torres and coworkers (38) compared BAL cultures with protected catheter brush (PCB) cultures using the same breakpoint for both techniques (10^3 cfu/mL). BAL and PCB agreed in 88.5% of the organisms cultured. However, Chastre and colleagues (36) found that quantitative cultures of BAL fluid were of little value compared to PCB using a 10^5 cfu/mL cutoff. In his series of 21 mechanically ventilated patients, 40% with pneumonia and 15% without would have been incorrectly diagnosed. As such, current recommendations (35) for semiquantitative BAL cultures are to adhere closely to the techniques described by Kahn and Jones (33) and Thorpe and coworkers (34). The technique of protected bronchoalveolar lavage (pBAL) was developed by Meduri and associates (39) in an effort to reduce the incidence of false positives stemming from oropharyngeal contaminants found in the working channel of the bronchoscope.

Technique of Protected Bronchoalveolar Lavage

CATHETER CONSTRUCTION: The pBAL catheter is of a polyurethane construction, which is radiopaque. The outer diameter is 2.3 mm, which fits in standard 2.6-mm diameter suction channels (Figure 8.2). It has two lumina. A large 1-mm diameter open-ended irrigation lumen extends the length of the catheter, and a red female Luer-lok is attached proximally for instilling and aspirating BAL effluent. A small lumen communicates with a recessed, high-compliance, low-resistance latex balloon at the distal tip of the catheter and a blue one-way stopcock proximally. The balloon is 12 mm in length and when inflated with 1.5 to 2 mL of air reaches an external diameter of 10 to 12 mm.

This enables occlusion at the level of third generation bronchi. Black stripes have been placed around the catheter at the proximal end of the balloon to guide the bronchoscopist in visually placing the balloon in the correct site. They are also placed at 72 cm from the catheter tip (representing the length of the working channel) and three other points 2 cm apart from this marking. These latter markings help in assessing the length of catheter extending beyond the distal end of the bronchoscope. A thin polyurethane glycol diaphragm is applied at the tip of the larger lumen to prevent contamination. This diaphragm is pushed out by flushing the pBAL catheter with 2 mL sterile saline and will readily dissolve at body temperature.

TECHNIQUE: The earlier considerations we discussed for a BAL for infectious diseases apply equally to pBAL. We will confine the present discourse to the technique of pBAL itself. Select a large-channel bronchoscope because the pBAL catheter itself has an outer diameter of 2.3 mm. Attach a syringe with 2 mL of air to the stopcock and inflate the balloon to verify its patency and integrity. Deflate the balloon after verification. Introduce the bronchoscope in the usual fashion. It is worth repeating at this point that the use of suction and the instillation of lidocaine should be avoided. Do *not* attempt to assess patency of the irrigation channel because this will disrupt the polyethylene glycol diaphragm prematurely.

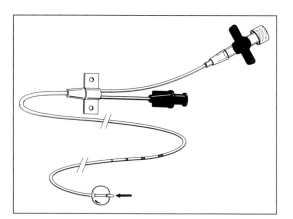

Figure 8.2. A schematic diagram of the protected bronchoalveolar lavage catheter with polyethylene-glycol diaphragm at the tip (*arrow*).

Select the segmental bronchus under direct vision but do not wedge the bronchoscope as done with regular BAL. Insert the pBAL catheter into the working channel of the bronchoscope and advance it until the first black marking on the proximal end of the catheter is flush with the suction channel's proximal orifice. Flush the polyethylene glycol diaphragm out with 2 mL sterile nonpyrogenic saline with a Luer-lok syringe attached to the female Luer-lok. Guide the pBAL catheter into the subsegmental bronchus until the black strip at the proximal end of the balloon is in line with the subsegmental bronchus orifice. Attach a 3-mL Luer-lok syringe to the stopcock. Turn the stopcock handle so that its orientation is in the axis of the body of the stopcock. Inflate the balloon with 2 mL of air, which will occlude the lumen of the subsegmental bronchus. Turn the stopcock handle to a position perpendicular to the stopcock body to prevent air from leaking out of the balloon. Pull on the proximal end of the catheter gently to confirm a good seal. Lavage is performed in the usual fashion. Meduri and colleagues (39) advocate discarding the first aliquot before specimen collection. After the lavage fluid has been collected, deflate the balloon and aspirate the air out with the syringe at hand. The catheter is then removed from the bronchoscope. In our limited experience with 10 cases, we have experienced difficulty in aspirating BAL fluid back through the narrow suction lumen of the pBAL catheter.

Diagnostic Yield

Using a breakpoint of more than 10^4 cfu/mL of a single bacteria as his diagnostic threshold for pBAL and greater than 10^3 cfu/mL for PCB, Meduri's initial experience noted correlation of bacterial growth in 10 of 11 cases when pBAL was compared to PCB. The contamination rate of pBAL specimens was excellent with 91% having under 1% SEC. In this study, pBAL was found to have 96% diagnostic efficacy, 97% sensitivity, and 92% specificity (39). We

also note with interest that in this study time off the antibiotic therapy did not affect pBAL results, whereas PCB cultures were significantly altered for each day off treatment. The chances of a true positive PCB culture increase by 47% ($P < 0.06$) each day off therapy. Injecting lidocaine through the working channel of the bronchoscope led to a higher contamination rate for *both* pBAL and PCB. In this study, PCB sampling before pBAL had less false positives than sampling in the opposite sequence. Our own view is that brushing before lavage may induce bleeding, which will contaminate the BAL cytology specimen. The advantage of pBAL or BAL over PCB is that a greater area of lung parenchyma can be sampled (estimated coverage of one million alveoli). On the other hand, PCB samples a very small portion of the distal airways, retrieving only 0.01 to 0.001 mL of material each time. In conclusion, we feel the technique of pBAL is an innovation with a potential to be at least as efficacious as PCB. However, modification of the design to increase the returns on BAL would increase the acceptance of the technique.

Bronchial Brush Biopsy

Before the advent of FOB, brushings for cytology were performed under fluoroscopic guidance *without* the use of a bronchoscope. Premolded nonmobile catheters were first used by Fennessy (40,41) and Fry (42). Zavala and colleagues (43) described the use of a controlled-tip catheter that made the procedure safer, faster, and more accurate. In their series of 75 patients, they were able to obtain a positive cytology in 82% of cases with lung carcinoma. Brush biopsies through the FOB were subsequently analyzed for the first time in 1973 by Zavala and coworkers (44). He was able to attain a positive or highly suspicious cytology in 89% of cases with lung cancer. Where the lesion was visible endobronchially, direct brushing of the tumor surface yielded a 94% success rate. Despite fluoroscopic control, brushings of peripheral lesions yielded a success rate of only 78%. We will describe both brushing of endobronchially visible tumors and peripheral lung lesions using the regular 3-mm cytology brush and the 7-mm brush only for endobronchial lesions. Brushes with diameters less than 3 mm have the same yield as the 3-mm brush and will not be described further (45).

Technique of Bronchial Brush Biopsy

REGULAR 3-MM CYTOLOGY BRUSH: We use the disposable Mill-Rose Bronchial Cytology Brush (Product code 149R) at our institution. After opening the package, retract the brush into the Teflon catheter until the tip of the brush is flush with the distal end of the catheter. The protective metal tip now prevents the brush from contaminants in the working channel.

Advance the catheter with the brush in place to the segmental bronchus of choice. The brush is then extended out of the catheter under direct vision. By advancing the upper handle, the maximum distance the brush will extend out is 5 cm from the distal end of the catheter.

Visible endobronchial tumor: Brush directly over the surface of the tumor in a back and forth motion 5 to 10 times. Also rotate the upper handle while doing this to maximize the brush contact with the tumor. Pull the brush back into the catheter *before* withdrawing the unit through the working channel. This will prevent contamination and limit cell loss as the catheter is withdrawn. At our institution, the brush is advanced from the catheter and smeared onto two glass slides (per brushing) that are then *immediately* placed in a screw-cap vial containing Carnoy's solution. If the slides are allowed to dry, the cells will become unreadable to the cytologist. We suggest a delay of no more than 10 seconds. Two passes are made with a single brush to obtain specimens from the area of interest. We advise

performing bronchial washings first, followed by endobronchial biopsies before brushings are taken (5). In our experience brushing first may on occasion cause enough bleeding or clot formation over the tumor surface to obscure vision or create false negatives.

Peripheral infiltrate/nodule: When a lesion is not visible endobronchially, brushings can still be performed under single-plane fluoroscopic guidance. The anatomic location is assessed on the chest radiograph in both the posteroanterior view and lateral view. The segmental bronchus is identified under direct vision. The brush is then prepared in the manner similar to that described before and advanced into the selected bronchus. Once it is in place, attention is directed to the fluoroscope and the remainder of the procedure is viewed from there. The catheter is then fluoroscopically guided to the lesion before the brush is extruded in the usual manner. Attempt to "move" the lesion by pushing the tip of the catheter against it. If both the catheter and lesion move in synchrony then the correct segment has been cannulated. Again, following the same sequence described above, the brush is advanced into the infiltrate/nodule under fluoroscopy and samples are taken.

Diagnostic yield of 3-mm brush: Zavala and colleagues (44,46) reported a 94% success rate for endoscopically visible lesions. Peripheral lesions, however, enjoyed a success rate of only 78% (14 of 18). In the latter group, the remaining 4 were falsely negative primarily because of difficulty in positioning the brush on the lesion. Solomon and coworkers (47) were able to diagnose 10 of 11 patients with central tumors and 23 of 25 (92%) with peripheral lesions under fluoroscopic guidance. Without fluoroscopy, the diagnosis of peripheral tumors by brush specimens was made in only 7 of 11 patients. Kvale and colleagues (48) assessed various techniques in diagnosing pulmonary malignancies and found bronchial brushing to be as effective as bronchial biopsy in diagnosing lung cancer (65). When his group analyzed brushings of visible tumors, they were able to make a positive diagnosis in 77% (54 of 70). In fact they were only able to make the diagnosis in 20% of the patients with peripheral tumors despite biplane fluoroscopy. In the section on endobronchial biopsy, we will discuss that it is the combination of procedures that provides the maximal yield in FOB.

THE 7-MM CYTOLOGY BRUSH: This brush is only indicated for central, endobronchially visible lesions. This brush is different from the regular 3-mm brush in several ways. Apart from the diameter, the bristles are Teflon-coated and the brush itself is not sheathed (Figure 8.3). Mehta and associates (49) first described the use of this brush in 20 patients with suspected endobronchial disease. Bronchial brushings were taken with both 7-mm and 3-mm brushes. In 13 patients the diagnosis of bronchogenic carcinoma was made by both brushes in all cases. In the remaining 7 patients, both brushes established true negative cytologies on microscopy. Cell return was greater with the 7-mm brush but did not affect the yield. In terms of bleeding following brushing, both brushes were found equally safe. A key difference in the technique with the 7-mm brush is that it cannot be retracted back into the working channel after obtaining the specimen. Therefore, both the brush and the scope have to be withdrawn simultaneously. To avoid having to reinsert the bronchoscope, we recommend doing this procedure last. A key disadvantage of the 7-mm brush is that it takes away the opportunity to reexamine the upper airway anatomy at the end of the procedure because the brush obstructs the view of the airway as it is being withdrawn. Plate four glass slides with the 7-mm brush and place the slides in Carnoy's solution immediately. A single pass with the 7-mm brush provides an adequate specimen for satisfactory examination. Cut off the tip of the brush with wire cutters into a test tube and add saline to cover the brush. Send all samples to the cytologist immediately.

Lung Mapping

Occult carcinomas of the lung are described in individuals with a normal chest radiograph and positive sputum cytology. This is an uncommon presentation and represents under 0.5% of all lung tumors. Laryngeal carcinomas and other tumors of the upper airway have a higher incidence in lung carcinoma patients (50). In fact, Martini and Melamed (51) found that one third of patients who fit into this criteria will eventually be diagnosed as having tumors originating from the head and neck. Marsh and coworkers (52) noted in their series of 33 patients with positive cytology for squamous cell carcinoma and normal chest radiographs that 4 patients actually had tumors of the upper airways (three laryngeal and one nasopharyngeal). Hence a full clinical examination and a thorough ear, nose, and throat evaluation is essential before the diagnosis of occult lung carcinoma is made. Lung mapping is a technique used to localize the cancer in the hope of diagnosing early disease and performing curative surgical resection (49–52).

Technique

Flexible FOB is performed under general anesthesia because the procedure is a laborious

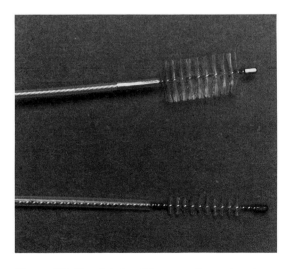

Figure 8.3. The details of 7-mm vs 3-mm brushes.

process taking up to 2 hours to complete. A complete airway examination is performed to confirm the absence of an endobronchial lesion. If the tumor is visible, washings, brushings, and biopsies are taken in the usual fashion. Otherwise systematic washings and brushings are taken from each subsegment of each lung and individually collected and analyzed. Correct labeling and meticulous technique to prevent cross contamination of specimens is required. A maximum of 500 mL saline should be used in each patient (8). Martini and Melamed (51) took up to 45 samples per patient in their series of 21 patients. If the initial cytology was positive, FOB was repeated with washings and brushings taken from the suspected subsegments. Only when cytology was positive from the same subsegment on both occasions, localization was considered accurate. These patients would then be staged and sent for appropriate surgery or other modalities of therapy.

Diagnostic Yield

Martini and Melamed (51) were able to diagnose 14 (67%) of 21 patients using this technique as having stage 1 disease treatable by resection. At time of diagnosis, 28% were in advanced stages of disease despite apparently normal chest radiographs. However, with the advent of photodynamic diagnostic techniques (53,54) and the failure of the national lung cancer detection program, this has not become a popular method for diagnosing occult lung cancer.

Protected Catheter Brush

PCB was first described in 1979 by Bartlett, Faling, and Wimberley (12). They established PCB as a safe and accurate diagnostic tool in 65 patients with suspected pneumonia using quantitative aerobic and anaerobic cultures (55). In our practice, we perform both BAL and PCB for all patients with clinical signs and pulmonary infiltrates suggestive of pneumonia to maximize the yield of FOB. The

indications for PCB (Figure 8.4) specimens are given in Table 8.4. The same considerations for antibiotics, premedication, local anesthesia, suction, and selection of segmental bronchus discussed in the BAL section apply equally for PCB.

Technique

The technique of PCB has been well documented by previous authors (12,13). Advance the bronchoscope to the segmental bronchus of choice without using suction or injecting lidocaine into the working channel. Do *not* wedge the scope. Advance the PCB until the distal end is visible. Then advance the inner cannula, which pushes the polyethylene glycol plug out. Perform this maneuver in the airway just proximal to the selected segmental bronchus to prevent the plug from being pushed into the sampling area. Extend the brush 3 to 4 cm for the inner cannula under direct vision to collect bronchial secretions. Pull the brush back into the inner cannula before removing the catheter from the working channel.

Table 8.4. Indications for Protected Catheter Brush

1. Immunocompromised, diabetic, alcoholic, or institutionalized patients who are at risk for unusual pneumonias
2. Radiographic patterns that do not differentiate between infective and noninfective etiologies
3. Radiographic patterns that suggest coexisting infective and noninfective disease (cytology brushing and forceps biopsy should be added to PCB in this setting)
4. Necrotizing or extensive radiographic infiltrates
5. Recurrent pneumonias
6. Progressive pneumonias despite antibiotics (e.g., bronchiectatic patients)
7. Pulmonary infiltrates in a mechanically ventilated patient

---

Adapted from Broughton WA, Bass JB, Kirkpatrick MB. The technique of protected brush catheter bronchoscopy. J Crit Illness 1987;2:63–70

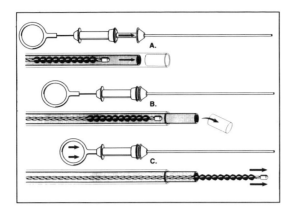

Figure 8.4. Bartlett-Faling-Wimberly brush. *A,* Inner/outer catheter. *B,* Use of remote plungers for plug. *C,* brush.

Processing the Specimen

As with BAL and pBAL, PCB specimens have to be handled in an aseptic manner to avoid contamination for it to remain a useful test for the patient. Considerable microbiologic expertise is required to perform quantitative cultures and interpret the results. Hence, every effort has to be made to ensure the collection and processing of PCB samples is up to mark.

After removing the catheter from the bronchoscope, the inner cannula is cleaned with a sterile swab soaked with 70% alcohol and then wiped dry (12). Cut off the section of inner cannula distal to the brush. This is to prevent potential contamination of the brush as it is advanced. Place a screw-cap vial containing one mL sterile lactated Ringer's below the brush. Then cut the brush from its retracting wire with a pair of sterile scissors, allowing it to fall into the Ringer's solution. Seal the receptacle and send it to the microbiology laboratory within 30 minutes.

Diagnostic Yield

Quantitative cultures are required to separate contaminants from true pathogens. Wimberley and colleagues (12,55) were the first to ascertain that the volume of PCB specimens was between 0.01 to 0.001 mL. They calculated from this that the number of colony-forming units per milliliter (cfu/mL) needed to distinguish true pathogens from contaminants was greater than 10^3 cfu/mL. This breakpoint was confirmed in studies by Chastre and associates (36,56), Torres and colleagues (38), and Fagon and coworkers (57). Wimberley and coworkers (55) studied 65 patients with suspected pneumonia and were able to diagnose 41 with certainty and 23 of the 24 others with probable organisms who all improved with specific antibiotic treatment. Chastre and colleagues (36,56), Fagon and coworkers (57), Villers and associates (58), and Torres and colleagues (38) have also demonstrated the value of PCB in mechanically ventilated patients. PCB quantitative cultures of greater than 10^3 cfu/mL correctly diagnosed all cases in Chastre's series. All patients without pneumonia had cultures of less than 10^3 cfu/mL. Chastre's earlier series (56), however, reported a false positive rate of 31% (8 of 26 patients). Fagon had positive cultures of greater than 10^3 cfu/mL in 45 patients. Of these, 34 of 45 were confirmed on follow-up and only 4 of these 45 were false positives. No patients in his series with less than 10^3 cfu/mL had pneumonias. Torres reported a similar experience with a specificity of 86% for PCB as compared to 71% for BAL. We feel comfortable with the breakpoint of greater than 10^3 cfu/mL but would like to emphasize meticulous technique for those performing this procedure.

Endobronchial Forceps Biopsy

The forceps has become an essential tool in the diagnosis of endobronchial neoplasms. It is used for lesions that can be directly visualized and lesions that can only be seen with fluoroscopic guidance. The latter technique of transbronchial forceps biopsy will be described in another chapter. We will focus on biopsy of lesions within the visual range of flexible FOB. In his series of 600 patients, Zavala was able to visualize endobronchial primary bronchogenic

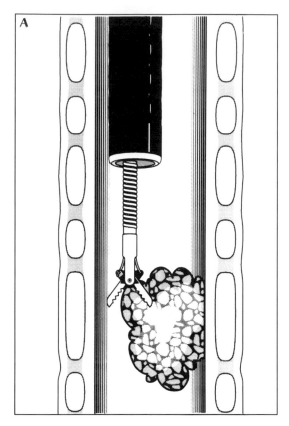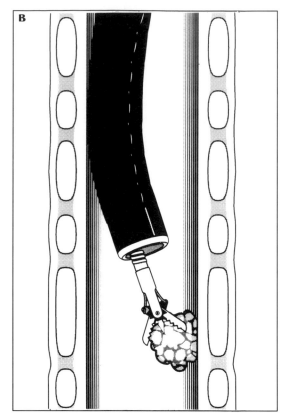

Figure 8.5. *A,* Endobronchial alligator forceps biopsy with tumor seen end-on. *B,* Endobronchial alligator forceps biopsy with tumor on the side wall of bronchus/trachea.

carcinoma in 193 cases (59). Of these, he obtained forceps biopsies from 60 patients with positive cytology in 58 (97%). From the same patient group of 133, brushing was successful in 93% of cases, giving a combined success rate of 94%.

Technique of Endobronchial Forceps Biopsy

We recommend the use of nondisposable "alligator" forceps (7 F gauge) for these biopsies (Figure 8.5). Fenestrated versions do not improve the quality of specimens significantly. Some authors suggest small alligator forceps (5 F gauge) for endobronchial lesions in the upper lobe. We prefer to first extend the large alligator forceps just beyond the distal end of the scope before negotiating the right upper lobe bronchus. This way we are able to take full advantage of the larger forceps and are able to avoid having to pass the forceps beyond the acute curvature of the working channel when the scope is already in the upper

lobe. Where possible, the distal end of the scope should be wedged in a segmental bronchus before a biopsy is taken. This will limit any bleeding to that particular segment. Technical problems are seldom encountered when the lesion is in the bronchial lumen and in the longitudinal axis of the forceps as it emerges from the distal end of the working channel (see Figure 8.5A). The forceps is opened and applied directly with gentle but firm pressure to the tumor surface under direct vision. As much tissue is engaged as possible before the forceps is closed around the specimen. A "tugging" sensation can be felt by the operator as the closed forceps is withdrawn into the working channel and removed from the bronchoscope. The tumor will also be seen being drawn toward the distal end of the scope under direct vision. Each biopsy specimen is teased off the forceps onto a piece of filter paper and placed in Hollande's solution for permanent sections.

When the lesion is on the wall of the trachea or main stem bronchi, it is occasionally difficult to angle the scope to obtain a good biopsy (see Figure 8.5B). In this situation the needle biopsy forceps will enable the operator to fix the forceps in place over the lesion before taking a specimen.

Even when an adequate tissue specimen is obtained, the surface of slow-growing tumors may be necrotic, especially if it has a pallid appearance. Histologic diagnosis may be difficult and false negative reports may result from that. We suggest that in these cases further biopsies should be taken until the core of the lesion is reached and viable tissue obtained as indicated by some degree of surface bleeding. As an alternative, a transbronchial needle aspiration (TBNA) should be performed to obtain specimens from the core of the lesion. TBNA is also useful for hemorrhagic lesions because it produces less trauma than a forceps biopsy.

Diagnostic Yield

How many endobronchial forceps biopsy specimens should be collected to achieve the optimal yield? Shure and Astarita (60) performed five biopsies on each of 18 consecutive tumors. Ten of 90 biopsy specimens were negative. All tumors were diagnosed with the first three biopsies. Further biopsies did not add any further information. There was no evidence to suggest any dependence of successive biopsies. They estimated the probability of obtaining a diagnosis to be 0.889 after one biopsy, 0.9877 after two biopsies and 0.9986 after three biopsies. Other authors (61,62) have suggested the need for more biopsies, but our own experience concurs with Shure and Astarita's findings.

Mark and colleagues (5) studied the yield of FOB with biopsy, brushings, and washings. In the group with endoscopically visible tumors, biopsy alone was positive in 76%. Cytology brushings alone yielded a 52% success rate and washings in 49.6%. A combination of biopsy and washings produced a yield of 94.5%. With biopsy and brushing the yield was 97.2%, comparable to Saita and coworkers (63), who achieved a combined success rate of 94.3%. Shure and Fedullo (64) reviewed the use of all three procedures plus TBNA and found the success rate increased even for submucosal and peribronchial lesions. A combination of all three procedures will maximize the diagnostic yield for visible tumors. Lam and colleagues (65) in a study on a larger series of patients had similar results and also recommended the use of brushings and washings to increase the yield of endobronchial biopsies. At our institution, we routinely perform all three procedures at the same sitting unless contraindicated.

Therapeutic Procedures

Biopsy Excision in the Palliative Management of Endobronchial Obstruction

In the 1920s, Jackson (66,67) used the rigid scope to excise both benign and malignant tumors. More recently, the use of the rigid bronchoscope to relieve malignant airway obstruction has been described by various authors (68–70). Mehta and Livingston (71) were the first to describe forceps biopsy excision through flexible FOB successfully in six symptomatic patients with unresectable lung cancer. All patients had a normal platelet count, coagulation profile, and renal function. The decision to perform a biopsy excision was made on initial evaluation when bleeding from the first biopsy was felt to be readily controllable. Immediate symptomatic relief was attained in all patients. Hence in place of neodymium:yttrium-aluminum-garnet (Nd:YAG) laser photoresection, this modality of treatment is safe, effective, and relatively inexpensive to perform in selected cases.

Balloon Catheter Dilatation of Endobronchial Stenosis

Acquired tracheobronchial stenoses (ATBS) have been attributed to a variety of causes. Medical etiologies include tuberculosis,

Wegener's granulomatosis, sarcoidosis, and carcinoma. Tracheobronchial surgery like sleeve resections or lung transplantation, which involve end-to-end airway anastomosis, can also lead to stenotic lesions. Current therapeutic options include Nd:YAG photoresection, cryotherapy, and surgery. We are aware of five reported cases of ATBS treated with balloon catheter dilatation (BCD) (72–75). All of these cases were treated with the use of angio/valvuloplasty balloon catheters through a rigid bronchoscope or guided into position with the aid of fluoroscopy without bronchoscopy. We have performed BCD through the fiberoptic bronchoscope on a number of occasions (unpublished data) using the Fogarty's arterial embolectomy catheter (American Edwards Laboratories, Anasco, Puerto Rico, size 5–7 F). We have found it useful in dilating stenotic lesions due to sarcoidosis and bronchogenic carcinoma. It is also a useful adjunct in establishing a distal lumen prior to Nd:YAG photoresection. Our technique involves placing the balloon at the stenosed portion of the airway and inflating the balloon with a small amount of air, starting with 1 to 1.5 mL in a 3-mL Luer-lok syringe. We introduce a small amount of air initially to minimize the risk of bleeding from mucosal tears. Withdraw the bronchoscope a reasonable distance so that the balloon is not ruptured as it is drawn back through the stenosis against the distal tip of the scope. If the initial BCD is successful, then gradually increase the amount of air from 2 to 3 mL and repeat the dilatation by drawing the balloon through the stenosis until satisfactory results are obtained.

Endobronchial Electrocautery

Electrosurgery involves using electricity to cut and coagulate tumor tissue (76). Endobronchial electrocautery (EEC) has been used effectively for many years in gastrointestinal surgery. Its use in flexible FOB has only been popularized since 1981. The application of EEC to tracheobronchial lesions has been demonstrated more recently by several authors (77–79). To date there have been 40 reported cases of treatment of obstructive airway lesions with EEC. An electrocautery unit comprises two electrodes connected to terminals on a high-frequency AC generator (2500 to 4000 mA, usually less than 200 V). At these settings, AC can be passed through the body with no effects other than heat production. One electrode acts as the active instrument with a small surface area and high current density. The other dispersive electrode is a large surface area grounding plate with a low current density that is attached to the patient's back. Heat is generated within living tissue with electrical resistance producing interaction ranging from drying to vaporization depending on the type and amount of current and the contact area between tissue and probe. Tissue resistance varies in direct proportion to water content and vascularity. Also, as the tissue dries, the resistance increases accordingly (80). The procedure can be carried out safely under local anesthesia and with flexible FOB. EEC seems best suited for removal of polypoid lesions with a narrow stalk or base using a wire snare (77). The key practical point is to cut with the current rather than the wire itself. The snare is closed around the stalk of the lesion with gentle pressure and the appropriate current applied. Experience is required to apply the right amount of pressure on the snare and in setting the appropriate level of current. Too high a current will lead to cutting without coagulation and excessive bleeding. Too low a current will lead to drying without cutting and hardening of the tissue. The ideal "blending" current setting should allow the operator to coagulate while cutting, hence providing hemostasis and a clear surgical field. Technically it involves mixing vacuum tube (cutting) and spark gap (coagulating) currents (76). The use of EEC for tumor debulking is less successful. EEC leads to tissue destruction with far less vaporization than Nd:YAG laser does. Hence treatment results in burnt tissue, producing lots of smoke and a large amount of debris to clear. Bleeding or a wet surface also interferes with the cautery action by diffusing the contact surface area and diminishes the efficacy of the probe. We also find the Nd:YAG laser far better at achieving hemostasis through photocoagulation than the superficial charring caused by EEC. Compli-cations reported with EEC using a wire loop snare or cautery probe included limited endobronchial bleeding and tracheal fire (81). Since then, the use of bipolar cautery has been advocated as being safer but still requires adequate precautions such as limiting inspired oxygen concentration to less than 30% and keeping the endotracheal tube a good distance away from the snare/probe (82). Potential complications include perforation of an airway or pneumothorax. A unique complication with EEC that is not shared by Nd:YAG laser is electric shock to the bronchoscopist. Bronchoscopes, unlike gastrointestinal endoscopes, are not electrically grounded. Contact between the probe and the distal tip of the bronchoscope can provide an alternate route for the current instead of the grounding plate, giving the bronchoscopist a nasty jolt! As electrocautery equipment generates radio frequencies, electrocardiograph machines should be situated elsewhere to minimize interference. Although EEC is more widely available and costs less than Nd:YAG laser equipment, we favor the latter modality of treatment, especially for vaporization and debulking of tumor and achieving good hemostasis.

Cryosurgery

Cryosurgery involves the application of subfreezing temperatures for the destruction of tissue by coagulation necrosis. Sanderson and colleagues (83,84) performed the first animal experiments using a rigid cryoprobe and standard liquid nitrogen cryosurgical equipment. The sudden transfer of gas from a higher to a lower pressure leads to a drop in temperature. The temperature of the iceball that forms at the tip of the cryoprobe ranges from -80° to -160°C. They then extended this mode of therapy through the rigid bronchoscope to six patients with successful palliation of their endobronchial tumors. Homasson and coworkers (85) extended the use of cryosurgery to more peripheral lesions with the development of a prototype flexible probe that could be used in flexible FOB. They were successful in treating 13 of 21 patients with malignant tumors and 5 patients with benign granulomas. The cryoprobe was passed through the bronchoscope and the iceball appearing on the tip of the probe was applied directly to the surface of the lesion. Up to three cycles of cooling and thawing were applied over one minute. This process of repeated rapid freezing (to between -30° and -60°C at the tissue level) and slow spontaneous thawing has been shown to produce tissue necrosis by intra- and extracellular crystallization (84). Bronchoscopy was repeated 4 to 6 days after the procedure to remove the necrotic debris that forms after cryotherapy. The key drawbacks of cryosurgery are delayed reaction, tumor swelling, a lack of control over cryonecrosis, and vessel perforation (86). Few complications have been reported with cryotherapy. Two episodes of mild fever and three episodes of arrhythmias were documented by Homasson and coworkers (85) in 27 cases. Although the cost of a cryoprobe is less than a Nd:YAG laser system, the effects of cryosurgery are not immediate and would not be indicated in acute respiratory emergencies due to obstructive lesions. However, in appropriate cases cryosurgery has been a simple and efficacious method of treating benign and malignant airway tumors. Presently, application of cryotherapy through FOB remains limited due to a lack of availability of flexible cryoprobes.

Bronchial Toilet

Pulmonary atelectasis is a common complication after surgery. The incidence following thoracic or abdominal surgery is as high as 70% in the postoperative period (87). The role of FOB, however, has remained controversial with authors taking opposing views as to its therapeutic value. Mahajan and colleagues (88) performed 19 FOB procedures on 10 patients for acute collapse of either one or more lobes or an entire lung. Thick and occasionally purulent mucous plugs were aspirated from the main stem bronchi of the involved lung in all but one case. Lavage with physiologic saline was found useful in addition to bronchial toilet in some patients. Improvement was based on radiologic reexpansion of the collapsed lung or lobe and changes in the arterial blood gases. Marini and coworkers (89), however, randomized patients treated with respiratory therapy for acute atelectasis preceded by, without, or followed by bronchial toilet. They found that FOB with bronchial toilet did not improve on the results of respiratory therapy in cases of acute lobar atelectasis. Interestingly, they also observed that the presence of an air bronchogram on chest x-ray often meant that neither respiratory therapy nor bronchial toilet with FOB would be effective. The presence of an air bronchogram often indicated a patent proximal bronchus clear of secretions and was a negative predictor for successful therapy in acute atelectasis. This study has been criticized by Myers for several flaws, the most significant of which was the patients under study were not comparable because most patients in one group were intubated while the majority in the other group were not (90). We have often seen the immediate benefits of bronchial toilet in patients with acute atelectasis from retained secretions in our own practice. We therefore advocate that while hemodynamically stable patients with minor degrees of atelectasis or intubated patients who respond to regular tracheal suctioning do not require FOB and bronchial toilet, acutely hypoxic patients who cannot cooperate or who do not respond to respira-

tory therapy should not be denied this simple and effective modality of treatment.

Management of Hypoxia During Bronchoscopy

Karetzky and colleagues have documented significant falls in arterial oxygen tension as a result of flexible FOB performed on room air, especially when the scope is inserted past the carina and during occlusion of a bronchus of a lobe with radiologic changes of pneumonia (91). Almost all patients showed recovery to pre-FOB levels immediately after removal of the bronchoscope. Two, however, did not recover until 24 hours after FOB. Albertini and associates (92,93) have found mean decreases of 20 mm Hg in arterial PaO_2 due to FOB alone in a group of 18 patients. Although most of their patients recovered baseline PaO_2 values 2 hours after FOB, some required up to 4 hours before full recovery was documented. Albertini and others (94) have recommended supplemental oxygen for all patients with pre-FOB PaO_2 values of less than 70 mm Hg. These authors (93,94) have also suggested FOB through a Venturi mask with 28% to 40% supplemental oxygen flow to prevent hypoxemia during regular FOB. Hypoxia related to BAL has already been described and will not be discussed further in this section. Bronchography using flexible FOB has, however, been shown to produce significant falls in arterial oxygen saturation (SaO_2) by Goldman and coworkers (95). They injected 10 to 20 mL of aqueous propyliodone (Dionosil, Glaxo) through the working channel of the bronchoscope and measured the SaO_2 during the procedure. They demonstrated a mean fall in SaO_2 of 20.5% after bilateral injection of contrast. Recovery to 50% of the total desaturation was rapid in most cases (1 to 10 minutes), but full recovery in half the patients took more than 3 hours. Unilateral injection produced mean desaturation of 12.5%. Both atrial and ventricular arrhythmias have been shown to occur most frequently at the nadir of hypoxemia (20). Because hypoxemia can persist for up to 4 hours after FOB and cardiac arrhythmias can be life-threatening, we recommend the use of supplemental oxygen in all patients during the procedure and for 4 hours afterward. We also recommend judicious use of premedication with narcotic or sedative agents, especially in patients with compromised lung function. Supplemental oxygen would also be recommended for BAL and bronchography. We routinely use intranasal cannulas to deliver oxygen during FOB, but switch to or start off with a Venturi mask if patients have low initial SaO_2 or PaO_2. We monitor SaO_2 continuously during the procedure and advance oxygen requirements accordingly. During hypoxic episodes, we stop applying suction through the working channel to limit "suction steal" of tidal volume. Morgan (96) has noted that suction at 12.5 cm H_2O of vacuum through the working channel may reduce a tidal volume of 700 mL by 40%. If suction at 21 cm H_2O of vacuum is used, the same tidal volume can fall by 75%. If laryngospasm occurs, we advise holding the scope in place or removing it entirely and instituting bronchodilator therapy.

Management of Significant Bleeding following Bronchoscopy

Flexible FOB is a common procedure that is well tolerated with few side effects. Pereira and colleagues (97), in a prospective review of 908 patients, documented the following complications: fever, vasovagal reaction, cardiac arrhythmias, nausea and vomiting, bleeding, pneumonia, and pneumothorax. Bleeding, however, is a difficult management problem for many bronchoscopists. In our own experience (31) with FOB-induced bleeding, all bleeding stops in the bronchoscopy suite if the patient has a normal coagulation profile, platelet count, and hepatorenal function. We do not perform FOB routinely if the patient is

unstable hemodynamically, has unstable arrhythmias, raised intracranial pressure, severe hypoxemia, hypercapnia, thrombocytopenia, or coagulopathies. Pulmonary hypertension alone is not a contraindication for FOB. Platelet count should be above 50,000/mL for FOB and above 75,000/mL for transbronchial biopsy. We found in our series of 6969 FOB and 3096 biopsies that transbronchial biopsy was more often accompanied by bleeding than endobronchial biopsy. Immunosuppressed patients and patients with chest malignancy seemed to bleed more frequently in our series and that of others (98,99). We feel, however, that this high incidence of bleeding is due to the greater number of patients with these conditions who require FOB in our practice. Compromise of the airway as a direct result of bleeding, which required specific emergency intervention or hospitalization, has not been experienced in our practice but has been documented by others (98,100). Sixty two percent of FOB-related bleeding (36 of 58 episodes) in our series stopped spontaneously and required no intervention. Those with profuse bleeds were stopped by wedging the bronchoscope to tamponade the bleed in the offending segmental bronchus. We also instill 2 to 4 mL of 1:10000 epinephrine routinely in these situations and stop suctioning to allow a clot to form over the bleeding point. Other modalities include Fogarty's balloon catheter, 200-cm long balloon

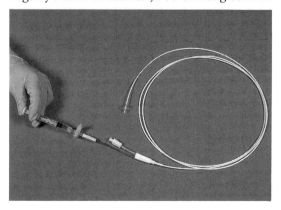

Figure 8.6. A 200–cm balloon tamponade catheter.

tamponade catheter (Figure 8.6) or a rigid bronchoscope to tamponade the bleed, bronchial artery embolization, and open lung surgery as a final resort. In cases where the bleeding point is visible, Nd:YAG laser photocoagulation works well in achieving hemostasis. Maneuvers during FOB to protect the uninvolved lung include turning the patient so that the hemorrhaging lung is in the dependent position and selectively intubating the uninvolved lung with a Carlin's endotracheal tube.

Flexible Fiberoptic Bronchoscopy during Mechanical Ventilation

The indications for flexible FOB during mechanical ventilation are largely the same as those without. However, we recommend some practical considerations during such procedures. Use a polyvinyl-chloride endotracheal tube (ETT) as opposed to a red rubber tube because the latter tends to kink during FOB and has a relatively narrow lumen for a comparable size (101). The adult bronchoscope will have no difficulty in negotiating an ETT of greater than size 8 (32 F). If the ETT is smaller than size 8, use the pediatric bronchoscope (Olympus P10). Shorten the ETT as much as possible by cutting it proximal to the cuff channel. Use a mouth guard to prevent the patient from biting the scope. Take the patient off positive end-expiratory pressure or pressure support where possible because peak airway pressures can increase by as much as 25 cm H_2O during FOB (101). Increase the fraction of inspired oxygen (FIO_2) to 1.0 during FOB and for a short period afterward until SaO_2 is above 90% again. If a pressure-limited ventilator is used, increase the peak pressure setting to compensate for the increased resistance and consequent loss of volume. Use an adapter for the ETT (Portex Fibreoptic Bronchoscope adapter La-090, #625109) so that there is no air leak at the point of insertion of the scope. Finally, transbronchial biopsy done in the intensive care unit setting is usually done without fluoroscopy due to a lack of this piece of equipment in these settings.

REFERENCES

1. Killian G. Direct endoscopy of upper air passages and esophagus: its diagnostic and therapeutic value in search for and removal of foreign body. J Laryngol 1902;18:461–468.
2. Jackson C. Endothelioma of the right bronchus removed by peroral bronchoscopy. Am J Med Sci 1917;153:371–375.
3. Jackson C. Bronchoscopy: past, present and future. N Engl J Med 1928;199:759–763.
4. Ikeda S, Yanai N, Ishikawa S. Flexible bronchofiberscope. Keio J Med 1968;17:16–18.
5. Mak VHF, Johnston IDA, Hetzel MR, Grubb C. Value of washings and brushings at fibreoptic bronchoscopy in the diagnosis of lung cancer. Thorax 1990;45:373–376.
6. Martini N, McCormick PM. Assessment of endoscopically visible bronchial carcinomas. Chest 1978;73:718–720.
7. Goldstein RA, Rohatgi PK, Bergofsky EH, et al. Clinical role of bronchoalveolar lavage in adults with pulmonary disease (ATS statement). Am Rev Respir Dis 1990;142: 481–486.
8. European Pneumology Task Group, Technical recommendation and guidelines for bronchoalveolar lavage. Eur Respir J 1989; 2:561–585.
9. Meduri GU, Beals DH, Maijub AG, Baselski V. Protected bronchoalveolar lavage. Am Rev Respir Dis 1991;143:855–864.
10. Dajani AS, et al. Prevention of bacterial endocarditis. JAMA 1990;264:2919–2922.
11. Wimberley N, Willey S, Sullivan N, Bartlett JG. Antibacterial properties of lidocaine. Chest 1979;76:37–40.
12. Wimberley N, Faling LJ, Bartlett JG. A fibreoptic bronchoscopy technique to obtain uncontaminated lower airway secretions for bacterial culture. Am Rev Respir Dis 1979;119:337–343.
13. Broughton WA, Bass JB, Kirkpatrick MB. The technique of protected brush catheter bronchoscopy. J Crit Illness 1987;2:63–70.
14. Pingleton SK, Harrison GF, Stechschulte DJ, Wesselius LJ, Kerby GR, Ruth WE. Effect of location, pH, and temperature of instillate in

bronchoalveolar lavage in normal volunteers. Am Rev Respir Dis 1983;128:1035–1037.

15. Klech H, Haslam P, Turner-Warwick M, et al. World wide clinical survey on bronchoalveolar lavage in sarcoidosis. Experience in 62 centers in 19 countries. Sarcoidosis 1986; 3:113–122.

16. Pirozynski M, Sliwinski P, Zielinski J. Effect of different volumes of BAL fluid on arterial oxygen saturation. Eur Respir J 1988; 1:943–947.

17. Goldstein RA, et al. Summary and recommendations of a workshop on the investigative use of fiberoptic bronchoscopy and bronchoalveolar lavage in asthmatics. Am Rev Respir Dis 1985;132:180–182.

18. Gibson PG, Breit SN, Bryant DH. Hypoxia during bronchoalveolar lavage. Aust N Z J Med 1990;20:39–43.

19. Burns DM, Shure D, Francoz R, et al. The physiological consequences of saline lobar lavage in healthy human adults. Am Rev Respir Dis 1983;127:695–701.

20. Katz A, Michelson EL, Stawicki J, Holford FD. Cardiac arrhythmias: frequency during fibreoptic bronchoscopy and correlation with hypoxaemia. Arch Intern Med 1981; 141:603–606.

21. Dhillon DP, Haslam PL, Townsend PJ, Primett Z, Collins JV, Turner-Warwick M. Bronchoalveolar lavage in patients with interstitial lung diseases: side effects and factors affecting fluid recovery. Eur J Respir Dis 1986;68:342–350.

22. Kirby JG, O'Byrne PM, Hargreave FE. Bronchoalveolar lavage does not alter airway responsiveness in asthmatic subjects. Am Rev Respir Dis 1987;135:554–556.

23. Kelly C, Hendrick D, Walters H. The effect of bronchoalveolar lavage on bronchial responsiveness in patients with airflow obstruction. Chest 1988;93:325–328.

24. Strumpf IJ, Feld MK, Cornelius MJ, Keogh BA, Crystal RG. Safety of fiberoptic bronchoalveolar lavage in evaluation of interstitial lung disease. Chest 1981;80:268–271.

25. Rankin JA, Snyder PE, Schachter EN, Matthay RA. Bronchoalveolar lavage: its safety in subjects with mild asthma. Chest 1984;85:723–728.

26. Wardlaw AJ, Collins JV, Kay AB. Mechanisms in asthma using the technique of bronchoalveolar lavage. Int Arch Allergy Immunol 1987;82:518–525.

27. Prakash UB, Barham SS, Dines DE, Marsh HM. Pulmonary alveolar phospholipoproteinosis: experience with 34 cases and a review. Mayo Clin Proc 1987;62:499–518.

28. Krueger JJ, Sayre VA, Karetzky MS. Bronchoalveolar lavage-induced pneumothorax. Chest 1988;94:440–441.

29. McClellan MD, Miller SB, Parson DE, Cohn DL. Pneumothorax with *Pneumocystis carinii* pneumonia in AIDS. Chest 1991;100: 1224–1228.

30. Beers FB, Sohn M, Swartz M. Recurrent pneumothorax in AIDS patients with pneumocystis pneumonia. Chest 1990; 98:266–270.

31. Cordasco EM, Mehta AC, Ahmad M. Bronchoscopically induced bleeding. A summary of nine years' Cleveland Clinic experience and review of the literature. Chest 1991;100:1141–1147.

32. Cole P, Turton C, Lanyon H, Collins J. Bronchoalveolar lavage for the preparation of free lung cells: technique and complications. Br J Dis Chest 1980;74:273–278.

33. Kahn FW, Jones JM. Diagnosing bacterial respiratory infection by bronchoalveolar lavage. J Infect Dis 1987;155:862–869.

34. Thorpe JE, Baughman RP, Frame PT, Wesseler TA, Staneck JL. Bronchoalveolar lavage for diagnosing acute bacterial pneumonia. J Infect Dis 1987;155:855–861.

35. Rankin JA. Editorial: getting the bugs out of BAL. Chest 1991;100:1–2.

36. Chastre J, Fagon JY, Soler P, et al. Diagnosis of nosocomial bacterial pneumonia in intubated patients undergoing ventilation: comparison of the usefulness of BAL and the protected specimen brush. Am J Med 1988;85:499–506.

37. Crystal RG, Reynolds HY, Kalica AR. Bronchoalveolar lavage—the report of an international conference. Chest 1986; 90:122–131.

38. Torres A, Bellacasa JP, Xaubet A, et al. Diagnostic value of quantitative cultures of BAL and telescoping plugged catheters in mechanically ventilated patients with bacterial pneumonia. Am Rev Respir Dis 1989; 140:306–310.

39. Meduri GU, Beals DH, Maijul AG, Baselski V. Protected bronchoalveolar lavage. Am Rev Respir Dis 1991;143:855–864.

40. Fennessy JJ. Bronchial brushing in the diagnosis of peripheral lung lesions. Am J

Roentgenol Radium Ther Nucl Med 1966; 98:474–481.

41. Fennessy JJ. Bronchial brushing. Ann Otol Rhinol Laryngol 1970;79:924–931.

42. Fry WA, Manallo-Estrella P. The technical details of bronchial brushing. J Thorac Cardiovasc Surgery 1970;60:636–640.

43. Zavala DC, Rossi NP, Bedell GN. Bronchial brush biopsy. Ann Thorac Surg 1972;13: 519–528.

44. Zavala DC, Richardson RH, Mukerjee PK, Rossi NP, Bedell GN. Use of the bronchofiberscope for bronchial brush biopsy. Chest 1973;63:889–892.

45. Hanson FN, Wesselius LJ. Effect of bronchial brush size on cell recovery. Am Rev Respir Dis 1987;136:1450–1452.

46. Richardson RH, Zavala DC, Mukerjee PK, Bedell GN. The use of fibreoptic bronchoscopy and brush biopsy in the diagnosis of suspected pulmonary malignancy. Am Rev Respir Dis 1974;109:63–66.

47. Solomon DA, Solliday NH, Gracey DR. Cytology in fibreoptic bronchoscopy. Chest 1974;65:616–619.

48. Kvale PA, Bode FR, Kini S. Diagnostic accuracy in lung cancer. Comparison of techniques used in association with flexible fibreoptic bronchoscopy. Chest 1976; 69:752–757.

49. Mehta AC, Ahmad M, Nunez C, Golish JA. Newer procedures using the fiberoptic bronchoscope in the diagnosis of lung cancer. Cleve Clin J Med 1987;54:195–203.

50. Sanderson DR, Fontana RS, Woolner LB, Bernatz PE, Payne WS. Bronchoscopic localization of radiographically occult lung cancer. Chest 1974;65:608–612.

51. Martini N, Melamed MR. Occult carcinomas of the lung. Ann Thorac Surgery 1980; 30:215–223.

52. Marsh BR, Frost JK, Erozan YS, Carter D. Diagnosis of early bronchogenic carcinoma. Chest 1978;73:716–717.

53. Cortese DA, Kinsey JH, Woolner LB, Payne WS, Sanderson DR, Fontana RS. Clinical application of a new endoscopic technique for the detection of in-situ bronchial carcinoma. Mayo Clin Proc 1979;54:635–641.

54. Hayata Y, Kato H, Konaka C, et al. Fibreoptic bronchoscopic laser photoradiation for tumor localisation in lung cancer. Chest 1982;82:10–14.

55. Wimberley NW, Bass JB, Boyd BW, Kirkpatrick MB, Serio RA, Pollock HM. Use of a bronchoscopic protected catheter brush for the diagnosis of pulmonary infections. Chest 1982;81:556–562.

56. Chastre J, Viau F, Brun P, et al. Prospective evaluation of the protected speicmen brush for the diagnosis of pulmonary infections in ventilated patients. Am Rev Respir Dis 1984;130:924–929.

57. Fagon JY, Chastre J, Hance AJ, et al. Detection of nosocomial lung infection in ventilated patients. Use of a protected specimen brush and quantitative culture techniques in 147 patients. Am Rev Respir Dis 1988;138:110–116.

58. Villers D, Demennic M, Raffi F, et al. Reliability of the bronchoscopic protected catheter brush in intubated and ventilated patients. Chest 1985;88:527–530.

59. Zavala DC. Diagnostic fibreoptic bronchoscopy. Techniques and results of biopsy in 600 patients. Chest 1975;68:12–19.

60. Shure D, Astarita RW. Bronchogenic carcinoma presenting as an endobronchial mass. Optimal number of biopsy specimens for diagnosis. Chest 1983;83:865–867.

61. Gellert AR, Rudd RM, Sinha G, Geddes DM. Fibreoptic bronchoscopy: effect of multiple bronchial biopsies on diagnostic yield in bronchial carcinoma. Thorax 1982;37: 684–687.

62. Popovich J Jr, Kvale PA, Eichenhorn MS, Radke JR, Ohorodnik JM, Fine G. Diagnostic accuracy of multiple biopsies from flexible fibreoptic bronchoscopy. A comparison of central versus peripheral carcinoma. Am Rev Respir Dis 1982;125:521–523.

63. Saita S, Tanzillo A, Riscica C, Maresca A, Potenza E, D'Arrigo M. Bronchial brushing and biopsy: a comparative evaluation in diagnosing visible bronchial lesions. Eur J Cardiothorac Surg 1990;4:270–272.

64. Shure D, Fedullo PF. Transbronchial needle aspiration in the diagnosis of submucosal and peribronchial bronchogenic carcinoma. Chest 1985;88:49–51.

65. Lam WK, So SY, Hsu C, Yu DYC. Fibreoptic bronchoscopy in the diagnosis of bronchial cancer: comparison of washings, brushings and biopsies in central and peripheral tumors. Clin Oncol 1983;9:35–42.

66. Jackson C. Bronchoscopy and esophagoscopy: a manual of peroral endoscopy and laryngeal surgery. Philadelphia: WB Saunders, 1922.

67. Jackson C. Bronchoscopy and esophagoscopy: a manual of peroral endoscopy and laryngeal surgery, 2nd ed. Philadelphia: WB Saunders, 1927.

68. Houston HE, Payne WS, Harrison EG Jr, Olsen AM. Primary cancers of the trachea. Arch Surg 1969;99:132–140.

69. Nakratzas G, Wagenaar JPM, Reintjes M, Scheffer E, Swierenga J. Repeated partial endoscopic resections as treatment for 2 patients with inoperable tracheal tumors. Thorax 1974;29:125–131.

70. Mathisen DJ, Grillo HC. Endoscopic relief of malignant airway obstruction. Ann Thorac Surg 1989;48:469–475.

71. Mehta AC, Livingston DR. Biopsy excision through a fibreoptic bronchoscope in the palliative management of airway obstruction. Chest 1987;91:774–775.

72. Cohen MD, Weber TR, Rao CC. Balloon dilatation of tracheal and bronchial stenosis. Am J Roentgenol 1984;142:477–478.

73. Groff DB, Allen JK. Gruentzig balloon catheter dilatation for acquired bronchial stenosis in an infant. Ann Thorac Surg 1985;39:379–381.

74. Fowler CL, Aaland MO, Harris FL. Dilatation of bronchial stenosis with Gruentzig balloon. J Thorac Cardiovasc Surg 1987;93:308–315.

75. Carlin BW, Harrell JH, Moser KM. The treatment of endobronchial stenosis using balloon catheter dilatation. Chest 1988;93:1148–1151.

76. Jackson R. Basic principles of electrosurgery: a review. Can J Surg 1970;13:354–361.

77. Hooper RG, Jackson FN. Endobronchial electrocautery. Chest 1985;87:712–714.

78. Gerasin VA, Shafirovsky BB. Endobronchial electrosurgery. Chest 1988;93:270–274.

79. Hooper RG, Jackson FN. Endobronchial electrocautery. Chest 1988;94:595–598.

80. Barlow DE. Endoscopic applications of electrosurgery: a review of basic principles. Gastrointest Endosc 1982;28:73–76.

81. Hooper RG, Jackson FN. Endobronchial electrocautery. Chest 1985;87:712–714.

82. Marsh BR. Bipolar cautery for the fibreoptic bronchoscope. Ann Otol Rhinol Laryngol 1987;96:120–121.

83. Gorenstein A, Neel HB III, Sanderson DR. Transbronchoscopic cryosurgery of respiratory strictures: experimental and clinical studies. Ann Otol 1976;85:670–678.

84. Carpenter RJ III, Neel HB III, Sanderson DR. Cryosurgery of bronchopulmonary strictures. An approach to lesions inaccessible to the rigid bronchoscope. Chest 1977;72:279–284.

85. Homasson JP, Renault P, Angebault M, Bonniot JP, Bell NJ. Bronchoscopic cryotherapy for airway strictures caused by tumors. Chest 1986;90:159–164.

86. Sanderson DR, Neel HB III, Fontana RS. Bronchoscopic cryotherapy. Ann Otol 1981;90:354–358.

87. Lewis FR. Management of atelectasis and pneumonia. Surg Clin North Am 1980;60:1391–1401.

88. Mahajan VK, Catron PW, Huber GL. The value of fibreoptic bronchoscopy in the management of pulmonary collapse. Chest 1978;73:817–820.

89. Marini JJ, Pearson DJ, Hudson LD. Acute lobar atelectasis: a prospective comparison of fibreoptic bronchoscopy and respiratory therapy. Am Rev Respir Dis 1979;119:971–977.

90. Myers DJ. Can fibreoptic bronchoscopy reverse acute lobar atelectasis? Indiana Medicine 1986;(July):593–595.

91. Karetzky MS, Garvey JW, Brandstetter RD. Effect of fibreoptic bronchoscopy on arterial oxygen tension. NY State J Med 1974;74:62–63.

92. Albertini R, Harrell JH, Moser KM. Hypoxemia during fibreoptic bronchoscopy. Chest 1974;65:117.

93. Albertini R, Harrell JH, Moser KM. Management of arterial hypoxemia induced by fibreoptic bronchoscopy. Chest 1975;67:134–136.

94. Dubrawsky C, Awe RJ, Jenkins DE. The effect of bronchofiberscopic examination on oxygenation status. Chest 1975;67:137–140.

95. Goldman JM, Currie DC, Morgan AD, Collins JV. Arterial oxygen saturation during bronchography via fibreoptic bronchoscope. Thorax 1987;42:694–695.

96. Morgan MDL. Physiological aspects of bronchoscopy. In: du Bois RM, Clarke SW. Fibreoptic bronchoscopy in diagnosis and management. London/New York: Harcourt Brace Jovanovich, Gowers Medical Publishing, 1987;5:5.3.

97. Pereira W Jr, Kovnat DM, Snider GL. A prospective cooperative study of complications following flexible fibreoptic bronchoscopy. Chest 1978;73:813–816.

98. Zavala DC. Pulmonary hemorrhage in fibre-optic transbronchial biopsy. Chest 1976; 70:584–588.

99. Suratt DM, Smiddy JF, Bruber B. Deaths and complications associated with fibreoptic bronchoscopy. Chest 1976;69:747–751.

100. Ackart RS, Foreman DR, Klayton RJ, Doulan CJ, Munzel TL, Schuler MA. Fibreoptic bronchoscopy in outpatient facilities, 1982. Arch Intern Med 1983;143:30–31.

101. Shinnick JP, Johnston RF, Oslick T. Bronchoscopy during mechanical ventilation using the fiberscope. Chest 1974;65: 613–615.

9 | Bronchoscopic Lung Biopsy
Udaya B. S. Prakash and James P. Utz

Bronchoscopic lung biopsy (BLB), also referred to as transbronchoscopic or transbronchial lung biopsy, is the technique by which biopsy of lung parenchyma can be obtained by using either the rigid or the flexible bronchoscope. Before BLB was described, lung biopsies were usually obtained by thoracotomy. Percutaneous needle biopsy using cutting needles and high-speed drills were developed, but these techniques have largely been abandoned because of significant mortality and morbidity (1–6). In 1965, Andersen and colleagues at the Mayo Clinic described the technique and results of BLB in 13 patients (7). BLB was obtained by using the rigid bronchoscope in these and other patients subsequently reported in the literature (8–11). Among the first 450 cases of BLB performed via the rigid bronchoscope, lung tissue was obtained in 84% (8). The introduction of the flexible bronchoscope in the late 1960s increased the popularity of the technique and demonstrated that BLB with the flexible instrument could be obtained with minimal mortality and morbidity (12–14). The initial reports observed positive biopsies in 82% of cases (12). BLB subsequently took the place of thoracotomy lung biopsy in many instances. Presently, BLB is a standard technique used by almost all bronchoscopists, and the flexible bronchoscope is used almost exclusively.

With several newer bronchoscopic techniques now available, there has been some confusion in the nomenclature used to describe various bronchoscopic procedures. The descriptive term BLB should be used to describe the procedure used to obtain specimens from abnormal lung parenchyma. Many bronchoscopists apply this term indiscriminately to describe bronchoscopic brushing and biopsy of peripheral nodules, masses, cavities, and other nonparenchymal lesions. We find that the prefix "trans" in transbronchoscopic lung biopsy does not add much to the description and therefore we prefer the shorter term, *bronchoscopic lung biopsy*. We believe that the word "transbronchial" should be reserved for bronchoscopic needle aspiration of paratracheal, subcarinal, or perihilar lesions.

Indications

As a result of more recent development and application of newer nonbronchoscopic diagnostic tests and techniques, the indications for BLB have diminished. Theoretically, the roentgenologic presence of any diffuse lung disease without an obvious etiology is an indication for BLB. We believe, however, that clinical correlation and evaluation of other less invasive diagnostic tests should be undertaken before performing BLB. These may include studies of respiratory secretions, pleural effusions, blood, and other body fluids or tissues, as well as various imaging procedures. The increasing clinical application of high-resolution computed tomography (HRCT) of the chest has contributed to the decreasing number of BLBs performed in diffuse lung disease. Even though typical HRCT findings in the presence of characteristic clinical features may be highly indicative of the diagnosis of disease entities such as pulmonary eosinophilic granuloma (histiocytosis X), lymphangioleiomyomatosis, idiopathic pulmonary fibrosis, and lymphangitic pulmonary metastases, bronchoalveolar lavage (BAL) and BLB may be needed in many of these to definitely establish the diagnoses. The wide availability of BAL has decreased the need for BLB (and thoracotomy) in many patients with opportunistic infections, particularly those caused by *Pneumocystis carinii,* mycobacteria, and certain mycoses (15–17). The role of BAL in the diagnosis of noninfectious diffuse diseases such as sarcoidosis, idiopathic pulmonary fibrosis, hypersensitivity pneumonitis, pneumoconioses, and others remains limited to the research sphere. The clinical application of BAL to diagnose or monitor these diseases is not recommended. BAL does provide diagnostic information in certain noninfectious diffuse lung diseases such as pulmonary eosinophilic granuloma, pulmonary alveolar proteinosis, and lymphangitic pulmonary metastasis. BLB, however, provides a higher diagnostic yield in all these pathologic entities (18–24). BAL and BLB may be complementary and increase the overall diagnostic yield under these circumstances. More recently, video-assisted thoracoscopy has contributed to the decreased utilization of BLB and is useful to secure larger lung biopsies in patients with diffuse as well as focal lung diseases. Nevertheless, BLB continues to be a valuable diagnostic tool in a variety of situations (Table 9.1).

Contraindications

Even though there are very few absolute contraindications to routine bronchoscopy, there are several contraindications to BLB. BLB is absolutely contraindicated if a patient is unable to cooperate with the procedure or unable to undergo general anesthesia to obtain BLB (25). Other absolute contraindications include an unstable cardiovascular status, status asthmaticus, severe hypoxemia that is likely to worsen during bronchoscopy and BLB, an inadequately trained bronchoscopist or bronchoscopy team, and inadequate instruments to properly perform the procedure. Relative contraindications include cough that is uncontrollable during the procedure, untreated hemorrhagic diatheses, renal failure, pulmonary artery hypertension, significant hypoxemia in a patient with a single lung, extensive bullous changes in areas to be biopsied, and roentgenographic suggestion of vascular malformations adjacent to areas to be biopsied.

Prerequisites

Once the indication for BLB is established, an informed consent should be obtained from the patient after details of the procedure, goals, and risks involved with bronchoscopy and BLB are explained. Table 9.2 indicates certain steps that are essential before bronchoscopy. It is essential that the patient undergo a thorough history and physical examination with particular emphasis on conditions that might pose problems during or after bronchoscopy. In an otherwise healthy individual scheduled to undergo bronchoscopy with or without BLB, it is not essential to perform a complete blood

Table 9.1. Pulmonary Diseases in Which BLB Provides a Higher Diagnostic Yield

Sarcoidosis
Pulmonary eosinophilic granuloma
   (histiocytosis X)
Pneumonia caused by *Pneumocystis carinii*
Diffuse lung infections caused by mycobacteria
   and mycoses
Lymphangitic pulmonary carcinomatosis
Pulmonary alveolar proteinosis
Diffuse alveolar cell carcinoma
Diffuse pulmonary lymphoma
Lymphangioleiomyomatosis
Silicosis

count, blood chemistry, or urinalysis (26,27). It is particularly important to ask the patient about the presence of familial or acquired hemorrhagic diathesis. In the absence of a history of bleeding diathesis, it is not necessary to routinely perform coagulation studies before BLB. Furthermore, no single test designed to examine the integrity of the coagulation system can predict bleeding during surgery (28,29). Therefore, estimation of prothrombin time, activated partial thromboplastin time, bleeding time, platelet count, and other parameters of coagulation is not warranted on a routine basis. If a test is to be obtained, measurement of serum creatinine is probably the most important because platelet dysfunction caused by renal failure is associated with a clinically significant hemorrhagic tendency that can be quite severe (30). Zavala reported a 45% incidence of significant hemorrhage following BLB in uremic patients (31) and remarked that "any biopsy procedure is avoided, if at all possible, on a uremic patient because of hemorrhage" (32). A serum creatinine level of 3 mg/dL or greater or a serum urea level of 30 mg/dL or greater is considered a relative contraindication to BLB (26). Preparation of patients with coagulation disorders who are scheduled to undergo BLB is discussed below.

Most patients with diffuse lung disease who are referred for BLB have significant pulmonary dysfunction and are often hypoxemic. These abnormalities often lead to a decision to perform BLB and their presence should not in general preclude the performance of BLB. Therefore, routine pulmonary function testing and arterial blood gas analysis before BLB are unnecessary. If pulmonary function testing is otherwise planned, it should be performed before bronchoscopy because bronchoscopy can induce mucosal edema and spuriously alter lung function tests (33–35).

Special imaging procedures such as HRCT may occasionally be helpful in identifying the abnormal areas to be biopsied. The identification of a particular roentgenologic pattern and its location by tomography or HRCT may optimize the application and diagnostic yield of BLB. Additionally, these imaging procedures may demonstrate areas that should be avoided by the biopsy forceps, namely, bullous lesions, vascular abnormalities, and pleural based lesions. Some bronchoscopists perform bronchography before brushing and biopsy of peripheral lesions to identify the bronchus leading to the localized lesion (36). We believe

Table 9.2. Prebronchoscopy Checklist*

1. Is there an appropriate indication for bronchoscopy?

2. Has there been a previous bronchoscopy?

3. If the answer to the above question is "yes," were there any problems or complications?

4. Does the patient (and close relative/s if patient is unable to communicate) fully understand the goals, risks, and complications of bronchoscopy?

5. Does the patient's past medical history (allergy to medication and topical anesthesia) and present clinical condition pose special problems or predispose to complications?

6. Are all the appropriate tests completed and the results available?

7. Are the premedications appropriate and the dosages correct?

8. Does the patient require special consideration before (e.g., corticosteroid for asthma, insulin for diabetes mellitus, or prophylaxis against bacterial endocarditis) or during (supplemental oxygen, extra sedation) bronchoscopy?

9. Are the plans for postbronchoscopy care appropriate?

10. Are all the appropriate instruments and personnel available to assist during the procedure and to handle the potential complications?

*Table reproduced with permission from Prakash UBS, Cortese DA, Stubbs SE. Technical solutions to common problems in bronchoscopy. In: Prakash UBS, ed. Bronchoscopy. New York: Raven Press, 1994:111–133.

this is unnecessary and adds time and expense to the procedure as well as adding to the patient's overall discomfort.

Technique

The preparation of the patient for BLB is similar to that for routine bronchoscopy and premedications and sedatives used are likewise identical. Most adult patients can undergo BLB under topical anesthesia. General anesthesia is indicated in patients who cannot cooperate under topical anesthesia. Cough suppression is especially important during BLB and administration of optimal sedation during BLB or preoperative cough suppressive therapy may be necessary. Excessive sedation may inhibit the patient's ability to voluntarily withhold cough when instructed to do so by the bronchoscopist. Before the administration of a sedative, the patient should be instructed to indicate by hand gestures if pain is experienced during the procedure. If fluoroscopic guidance is used, metallic pads and wires to be placed on the patient's thoracic cage for electrocardiographic or other monitoring should be placed in such a way that they do not interfere with the fluoroscopic image of the lesion to be biopsied.

Bronchoscopic examination is performed in the usual manner and both bronchial trees are thoroughly examined prior to BLB. If other procedures such as BAL, transbronchial needle aspiration, endobronchial brushings and biopsies, or bronchial washings are required, they should be obtained before BLB. Performing BLB as the last procedure minimizes cough after BLB by avoiding subsequent instrumentation that frequently results in cough, thereby reducing the risk of pneumothorax resulting from cough-induced barotrauma. After positioning the fluoroscope to obtain the image of the area to be biopsied, the bronchoscope is advanced as far distally as possible, with repeated application of topical anesthetic as needed to suppress cough. The bronchoscope is then maintained in this wedged position while the biopsy forceps is inserted into the working channel of the instrument. Once the distal end of the biopsy forceps exits the distal end of the bronchoscope, the forceps is further advanced distally until its tip is beyond bronchoscopic visualization. At this point, the fluoroscopic image is projected on the monitor and used to monitor the progress of the forceps to the lesion. If the lesion is localized, biplane fluoroscopy is essential to ensure proper placement of the forceps (Figure 9.1). The exact point of biopsy is identified on the fluoroscope monitor. The biopsy forceps is opened 5 to 6 mm proximal to the area to be biopsied. At this juncture, the patient is instructed to inhale deeply (this maneuver may not increase the size of the biopsy specimen but may permit more distal movement of the forceps) and the open forceps is advanced until gentle resistance is encountered, making sure, by fluoroscopic monitoring, that the forceps stays at least 5 mm proximal to visceral pleura. The patient is then instructed to exhale fully and the forceps is closed at the end of exhalation. At this point, the patient is asked if any pain is experienced. If the patient indicates pain (by hand signals previously decided on), the forceps is opened and withdrawn proximally without obtaining biopsy. The biopsy is then attempted in another area. If there is no indication of pain, the biopsy forceps is maintained in closed position for 6 to 8 seconds and gently but firmly withdrawn. During the withdrawal of the forceps, the bronchoscope is actually advanced distally, if possible, so that its tip can be maintained in the wedged position (31). The advantage of this "wedge" technique is twofold: it maintains the tip of the bronchoscope in the optimal position so that more biopsies can be obtained without having to withdraw the bronchoscope to clean the objective lens; and if post-BLB bleeding occurs, the wedged position of the bronchoscope limits the bleeding to the biopsied segment or subsegment of the lung. It is not necessary to apply prolonged

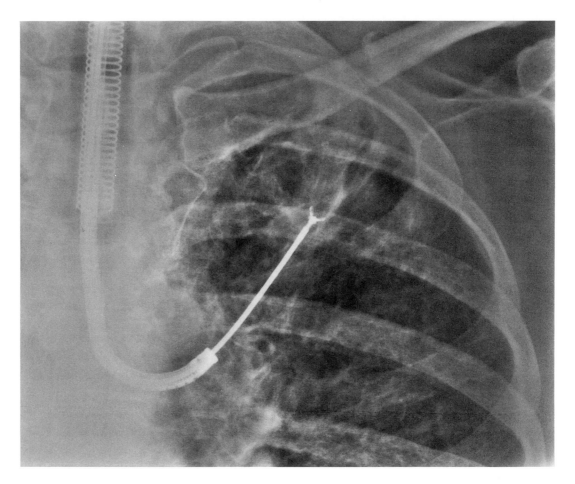

Figure 9.1. Fluoroscopic guidance used to obtain BLB from a localized parenchymal lesion in the left upper lobe. The use of biplane fluoroscopy enables the bronchoscopist to obtain lung specimens from selected areas.

suction to check for serious hemorrhage after each biopsy. If a brief suctioning does not indicate serious hemorrhage, then the bronchoscopist can proceed to obtain more biopsies. Obtaining BLB from peripheral lung zones (very close to pleura) may prevent or minimize hemorrhage because bronchial arteries are smaller in the distal airways (37).

If significant hemorrhage (more than 50 mL) as measured by bronchoscopic suction is encountered immediately after BLB, the wedged position of the bronchoscope is maintained and continuous suction is applied. If bleeding persists or fails to diminish, the bronchoscopist can perform several maneuvers to minimize and control the hemorrhage. First, continuous or prolonged intermittent suction

can be maintained by retaining the tip of the bronchoscope in the wedged position. In the majority of patients, this method alone is sufficient as long as the blood is prevented from escaping around the bronchoscope and flowing into other bronchi. Second, the suction is interrupted while 10 to 15 mL of iced saline is gently instilled through the bronchoscope into the bleeding area. During the slow instillation of iced saline, the bronchoscopist should be able to visualize the distal bronchial tree through the saline. This "saline flooding" of the distal bronchus should be maintained for several seconds after completing the instillation of iced saline. A stream of blood coming from the distal bronchus and mixing with the just instilled saline usually indicates that bleeding from the biopsied area is persistent. Iced saline also produces vasoconstriction and thus thwarts excessive bleeding. If the bleeding persists, the instilled saline should be aspirated by bronchoscopic suction and another aliquot of fresh iced saline instilled as described above. This technique can be repeated several times until bleeding stops. In almost all patients, this technique will diminish and eventually stop the bleeding caused by BLB. Some advocate bronchoscopic instillation of epinephrine to effect vasoconstriction. This technique has no therapeutic value when the bleeding is coming from distal areas because the small aliquot of epinephrine injected through the bronchoscope is pushed back proximally by the blood. We have occasionally added 1.0 mL epinephrine (1:1000) to an aliquot of 15 mL iced saline before injecting the iced saline as described above. This method is more likely to carry epinephrine to the bleeding area.

Other techniques described to control BLB-induced hemorrhage include balloon tamponade, fibrin glue application, rigid bronchoscopic aspiration of blood and endobronchial packing of bleeding bronchus, isolation of bronchial trees by inserting double-lumen endotracheal tubes, and lastly surgical resection of the bleeding segment (38). Some of these techniques are described in other chapters in this volume. In our experience, however, these measures are seldom required to treat BLB-induced hemorrhage.

After the BLB is completed and the lack of bleeding is confirmed, the bronchoscope is withdrawn proximally and the patient is instructed to cough gently to see if this induces further bleeding. If no further bleeding is observed, the bronchoscope is fully withdrawn from the airways to terminate the procedure. Routine chest roentgenography is unnecessary after BLB (39–41). We usually perform an end-expiratory fluoroscopic screening of pleural surfaces to exclude a pneumothorax. Chest roentgenography should be reserved for patients who cough excessively during BLB, repeatedly complain of pain during BLB, or in patients who develop other pulmonary symptoms (dyspnea, chest tightness, or chest pain) after BLB. Routine hospitalization following BLB, as practiced by 12% of North American bronchoscopists (42), is unnecessary (26). Clinical suspicion of post-BLB pneumothorax, presence of pneumothorax following BLB, serious hemorrhage following BLB, and development of unexplained dyspnea or other significant cardiorespiratory symptoms are indications for hospitalization. The patient should be instructed to contact the physician or report to the emergency room if new symptoms develop later.

Processing of the lung specimen obtained by BLB is an important part of the procedure. Crush artifacts should be avoided by careful handling of specimen with pickup forceps. Appropriate preservatives and culture media should be selected before BLB. If touch preparations are required for identification of *P. carinii,* the lung specimen should be gently touched to the surface of a glass slide by carefully holding the lung specimen with a pickup forceps. Crush artifact should be avoided so that histologic analysis of the tissue is not impaired. Communication with the pathologist regarding the clinical features and provisional diagnosis is also essential.

Other Considerations

Coagulation Disorders

The limitation of the tests of coagulation to predict bleeding in BLB is discussed above. As noted, coagulation disorders are relative contraindications to BLB. A low platelet count is perhaps the most common disorder of coagulation encountered by the bronchoscopist. In one report, 25 BLBs were performed in 24 patients with a mean platelet count of 30,000/mm^3 (7000 to 60,000/mm^3); self-limited hemorrhage was noted in three patients and one patient developed fatal bleeding (this patient had a platelet count of 23,000/mm³) (43). Because of this increased risk of hemorrhage, thrombocytopenia is a relative contraindication to BLB. Immunocompromised patients with bone marrow failure frequently require both fresh frozen plasma and platelet transfusions. Despite these measures, a hemorrhage-associated fatality has been reported in a thrombocytopenic patient who underwent these supplementations (43). Failure of the platelet count to increase significantly one hour past platelet infusion indicates the presence of platelet antibodies (44). BLB should be avoided in these patients although BAL can be safely performed (38). In thrombocytopenic (platelet count less than 50,000/mm³) patients, 6 to 10 packs of platelets should be transfused 30 to 40 minutes before BLB (31,32,45).

Platelet dysfunction (despite normal platelet count) in patients with renal failure is associated with increased risk of hemorrhage and may be manifested by prolonged bleeding time. If BLB is an absolute necessity in the presence of platelet dysfunction, the clotting mechanism should be normalized by the administration of deamino-8D-arginine-vasopressin (DDAVP) (46–48). Iatrogenically induced (heparin or coumarin) abnormalities of coagulation should be corrected with discontinuation of the drug and monitoring of appropriate laboratory tests. BLB should be undertaken only after the bleeding tendency is reversed. The incidence of significant blood loss from routine BLB is so low that grouping and crossmatching of blood type before BLB is unnecessary (27).

Fluoroscopy

Fluoroscopic guidance is invaluable in obtaining optimal lung specimens. The main reason for using fluoroscopic guidance is to prevent pneumothorax secondary to BLB. Other important reasons for using fluoroscopic guid-ance include the ability to obtain biopsy specimens from a localized infiltrate as noted by chest roentgenogram and the capability to monitor and guide the distal end of the flexible bronchoscope toward the lesion on the fluoroscopy monitor. The 1989 survey of about 1800 North American bronchoscopists disclosed that more than 75% of the participants routinely used fluoroscopy for BLB (42). Some bronchoscopists, however, believe that fluoroscopy is not necessary to obtain BLB (49–51). Indeed, BLB can be performed without fluoroscopic guidance in the following situations: if the pulmonary parenchymal process involves an entire lung, if the infiltrate is localized to a lung apex, or if the infiltrate is roentgenographically well defined and involves an entire segment of any lobe (52). Using tactile sensation (without fluoroscopy), a study analyzed the complications of BLB in 68 patients, undergoing at least three BLBs; a single pneumothorax was reported and no significant hemorrhage ensued (50). However, a more recent study suggests that the risk of pneumothorax following BLB is higher when fluoroscopy is not used. A mail survey of 231 British bronchoscopists reported that the incidence of pneumothorax following BLB was 1.8% when fluoroscopy was used and the incidence increased to 2.9% when fluoroscopy was not used (53). For this reason, we recommend fluoroscopic guidance when performing BLBs.

The cost of fluoroscopy equipment or the administrative control of the fluoroscopy equipment (usually by the roentgenologist) are the main impediments to the optimal utilization of fluoroscopy (28). If fluoroscopy equipment is readily available, the bronchoscopist should use it to obtain maximal diagnostic yield. Fluoroscopy also provides the advantage of post-BLB assessment of the thoracic cage to exclude pneumothorax and thus preclude routine post-BLB roentgenography (52). The bronchoscopist should be trained in the appropriate use of fluoroscopic equipment or should have a trained person available during the procedure. Every attempt should be made to minimize the exposure of the patient and bronchoscopy personnel to fluoroscopy-associated radiation.

Localized Peripheral Lesions

These lesions include pulmonary parenchymal nodules, localized (segmental, subsegmental, or subsubsegmental) infiltrates, and bronchoscopically invisible endobronchial lesions. The last mentioned include distal carcinoma, carcinoid, hamartoma, or other lesions originating in the mucosa or wall of distal bronchi or bronchioles. The term BLB is a misnomer to describe biopsy of such lesions because the lung parenchyma is not biopsied. The lesions originating in the bronchoscopically invisible bronchi and very dense alveolar infiltrates (such as alveolar cell carcinoma and alveolar lymphoma) are less likely to result in pneumothorax following bronchoscopic biopsy because the biopsied area is either endobronchial or airless.

Rigid Bronchoscopy

Although the first BLBs were obtained via the rigid bronchoscope and with rigid bronchoscopy forceps (1,7,8), currently it is unlikely that many bronchoscopists use the rigid bronchoscope for this purpose. Nevertheless, BLB can be safely obtained using rigid bronchoscopic techniques. The technique is similar to that used with the flexible bronchoscope. The rigid bronchoscopic biopsy forceps indeed provides better tactile feedback when the lung parenchyma is approached and the biopsy forceps is withdrawn after obtaining a biopsy. Fluoroscopic guidance should be used to obtain BLB via the rigid bronchoscope. A disadvantage is the relative difficulty is introducing the rigid bronchoscope and biopsy forceps into upper lobe bronchi. We have used a rigid bronchoscope, through which flexible bronchoscopic biopsy forceps is introduced, to obtain BLB in pediatric patients (see below).

Biopsy Forceps

No special biopsy forceps are designed solely for the purpose of BLB. The forceps used to biopsy endobronchial lesions are usually used to obtain BLB. Among these, the two main types are the cup (without teeth) and alligator (toothed) forceps. Although during the early years of BLB, toothed biopsy forceps were purported to induce more hemorrhage because of a "tearing" action, no data support this notion. We believe that either type of forceps can be used to obtain BLB. Another somewhat traditional technique, as discussed above, is to instruct the patient to inhale deeply, advance the open forceps as far distally as possible during this maneuver, and close the forceps at the end of full exhalation. This technique is purported to increase the amount of lung tissue. It is unclear if this concept is correct.

The small size (usually measures 5 to 20 mm^2) of the tissue obtained by BLB may be inadequate to establish a histopathologic diagnosis (54). The size of the specimen depends on the size of the cups in the biopsy forceps. Rigid bronchoscopic forceps are much larger compared to the flexible biopsy forceps and our earlier experience (unpublished data) suggested that the biopsy specimens obtained with rigid forceps were larger. Some publications observed that larger tissue pieces obtained by BLB do not provide additional diagnostic yield (55,56). However, a recent publication reported that larger flexible biopsy forceps (cup size $3X \times 2 \times 0.9$ mm) obtained significantly more tissue in 74% of 27 patients in contrast to small biopsy forceps (cup size $2 \times 1.5 \times 0.6$ mm), which obtained more tissue in only 19% of 27 patients (57). Large forceps also obtained more alveolar tissue in 73%, whereas small forceps obtained more alveolar tissue in only 27%. There was no difference in the post-BLB bleeding with either forceps. The results of this study may be of clinical significance because another study demonstrated that the presence of a greater number of alveoli per individual tissue piece resulted in a statistically significant increase in the ability to make a diagnosis of infection (58). Potential problems with the use of larger forceps include the inability to pass the forceps through the working channel of smaller adult flexible bronchoscopes and difficulty in getting the jaws to open in small peripheral airways (57). To assess the adequacy of the biopsy specimens as soon as the biopsy is obtained, many bronchoscopists use the "float sign" (59). The biopsied lung tissue, if part of it contains aerated alveoli, may float when put into the liquid fixative. This sign is not completely reliable because dense nonaerated lesions may not float.

Number of Biopsies

In addition to the size of the biopsy forceps, the number of biopsies also determines the diagnostic yield. However, it is intuitively obvious that the risk of pneumothorax is proportional to the number of BLBs obtained. Therefore, the least number of BLBs to establish the diagnosis is the optimal number. The optimal number of BLBs required, however, depends on the underlying pulmonary process and several other factors. The availability of frozen section technique to immediately analyze the biopsy specimen also determines the number of biopsies obtained. For instance, if the first biopsy specimen is subjected to frozen section examination and if it reveals a definitive diagnosis (e.g., lymphangitic carcinomatosis, noncaseous granulomas, or caseous granulomas), an additional biopsy for permanent section may be all that is required. Nonspecific findings on frozen section analysis may require a larger number of biopsies. BLB in peribronchial or peribronchiolar disease processes (such as lymphangitic malignancy, sarcoidosis, or disseminated infections) is more likely to provide higher diagnostic yield (60).

In patients with stage II or stage III sarcoidosis, the diagnostic sensitivity of at least four BLBs is in excess of 95% (50,61–66). In patients with stage I sarcoidosis, as many as 10 BLBs may be needed to obtain the similar diagnostic yield (67). The overall diagnostic accuracy of BLB in all stages of sarcoidosis is 73% to 80% but is improved to 85% when both BLB and bronchial mucosal biopsy are combined (68). In patients with acquired immunodeficiency syndrome (AIDS) complicated by *P. carinii* pneumonia, a minimum of two biopsies is required if the chest roentgenograph exhibits severe abnormalities and at least four biopsies if the chest roentgenograph is normal, to obtain a diagnostic rate of 97% (69). The size of the biopsy specimens may also influence the diagnostic utility of BLB. A study of 116 patients who underwent BLB observed that this relationship was applicable for the diagnosis of infection and not malignancy (58).

Diagnostic Accuracy

By definition, BLB denotes biopsy of lung or pathologic process occurring within the pulmonary parenchyma. As noted above, biopsy of peripheral nodules originating in the bronchial wall does not represent BLB. Nevertheless, the term BLB is loosely used in clinical practice as well as the literature to describe biopsy of any bronchoscopically invisible lesion. As a result, the interpretation of diagnostic yield from "BLB" of diffuse and localized lesions is difficult. The diagnostic accuracy also depends on the pathologist's understanding of the clinical features. Therefore, clear communication (preferably before BLB is obtained) between the bronchoscopist and the pathologist is important (70). The diagnostic rates of BLB can be considered separately for diffuse and localized lesions.

Diffuse Lesion

Biopsy of uniformly diffuse lung infiltrates are more likely to provide diagnosis than a small (less than 1.0 cm) peripheral nodule. The rate of diagnostic accuracy from BLB depends also on the predetermined criteria for the diagnosis. If nonspecific fibrosis is accepted as a definitive diagnosis in the presence of typical clinical features, then the diagnostic yield can be considered high. A review of several series observed that using such criteria, the overall diagnostic yield from BLB was 72% (71). When more specific diagnostic criteria were applied prospectively to 176 patients with interstitial lung disease, the diagnostic yield was substantially lower (37.7%) (71). In addition, the acceptance of "specific" diagnoses based on nonspecific histologic changes is tenuous and often that diagnosis is not confirmed when patients are further subjected to open lung biopsy (72).

It may be prudent to avoid particular areas when performing BLB. Biopsy of the lingula may be a common site of chronic nonspecific inflammation and might best be avoided when performing BLB in patients with diffuse lung disease (73,74), although this has been challenged by some (75). Areas of greatest involvement have traditionally been preferred sites of BLB, but it may be better to target areas of intermediate involvement because the more severely involved areas may display only end-stage fibrosis, the final common pathway of innumerable diffuse lung diseases.

In patients who are immunocompromised and develop diffuse pulmonary infiltrates, BLB is reported to provide a diagnostic rate of 28% to 68% (15,76). In renal transplant patients who develop lung infiltrates, BLB has been shown to provide a diagnostic rate of 54% (77). In patients with AIDS, BLB has been shown to provide a diagnostic yield of 88% to 97% in *P. carinii* pneumonia (16, 69,78). The diagnostic accuracy of BLB has been much lower in those with cytomega-lovirus pneumonia (22%), *Mycobacterium avium intracellulare* infection (0 of 11 patients), and pulmonary Kaposi's sarcoma (0 of 11 patients) (78). Others have reported a diagnostic yield of 67% in patients with AIDS and opportunistic infections caused by organisms other than *P. carinii* (79). The same study observed an overall diagnostic accuracy of 73% in patients with AIDS.

Localized Lesion

Because many bronchoscopists do not differentiate between the biopsy of a peripheral (bronchoscopically invisible) endobronchial lesion and a true BLB, we assess this issue here. Bronchoscopic biopsy of very localized lesions should be performed under fluoroscopic guidance. The biopsy is reported to yield approximately a 60% diagnostic rate in primary lung cancer and a 50% diagnostic yield in metastatic cancer, when these tumors present as peripheral lung nodules (80). Cytologic brushing increases the diagnostic yield in both conditions. An important determinant of diagnostic yield is the size of the nodule. Biopsy of lesions larger than 2.0 cm provides a greater than 60% diagnostic yield, whereas lesions less than 2.0 cm in diameter yield a diagnosis in less than 25% of cases (80). The diagnostic rates are likely to be lower if nodular or localized lesions are caused by nonmalignant processes. Bronchial washings, brushings, and curettage add to the diagnostic yield in both malignant and nonmalignant processes.

Mechanical Ventilation

Mechanical ventilation is not an absolute contraindication to BLB although the incidence of pneumothorax is reported to be increased (43,81). A study of BLB in 15 patients with diffuse lung disease on mechanical ventilation reported a 7% incidence of post-BLB tension pneumothorax (43). The same study observed a diagnostic yield of 47% and significant alterations in management in 53%; there was a 20% occurrence of self-limiting hemorrhage (43). The institution of positive end-expiratory pressure (PEEP) may increase the risk of pneumothorax.

During BLB, it is advisable to remove the PEEP and support ventilation with a hand-held Ambu-bag and continue ventilatory support without PEEP for 30 to 45 minutes so that PEEP-induced barotrauma can be avoided during and soon after BLB. If BLB is planned in a mechanically ventilated patient, facilities should be immediately available to control the pleural space with thoracostomy tube if necessary (82). Because most of these patients are in critical care units, it may not be possible to easily move them to the bronchoscopy suite for BLB. If the procedure is to be performed in the critical care unit, every effort should be made to obtain a mobile fluoroscopy unit to facilitate optimal BLB.

Lung Transplant

Lung transplant recipients undergo BLB more frequently than any other group of patients. Multiple biopsies are often necessary. Because the patient with a transplanted lung loses the ability to perceive pain when the biopsy forceps touches the visceral pleura of the transplanted lung, the patient may not be able to indicate if the biopsy forceps is close to the visceral pleura or pierces it. This may increase the risk of pneumothorax if fluoroscopy is not used. The perception of pain by the patient may indeed indicate that the biopsy forceps has come in contact with the parietal pleura and that a pneumothorax has occurred. The loss of ability of the transplanted lung to react to stimulation of stretch receptors or tracheobronchial mucosa is an advantage in that the patients do not cough as much. Because bronchial arterial blood supply is absent in the transplanted lung, brisk hemorrhage following BLB is uncommon.

The diagnostic yield from BLB in this group of patients is high if the procedure is performed to diagnose acute rejection or infection. However, the diagnostic rate is low (15%) in the diagnosis of bronchiolitis obliterans (83). In a study of 55 lung transplant recipients who underwent 203 BLBs (clinical indications in 88, routine surveillance in 90, and follow-up of previous biopsy in 25), a specific histologic diagnosis was detected in 57% of surveillance procedures and 64% of the follow-up procedures (84). The overall complication rate was 9%.

Pediatric Patients

Pediatric patients have undergone BLB (85,86) although the procedure is not used as often as in adults. The main impediment to obtaining BLB in children is the inability to insert a biopsy forceps through the narrow channel of pediatric flexible bronchoscope. This can be overcome by using rigid bronchoscope through which a regular flexible biopsy forceps can be inserted to obtain BLB. Another method is to use the pediatric (or ultrathin) flexible bronchoscope through an endotracheal tube and pass the flexible biopsy forceps along the external aspect of the bronchoscope. The tip of the bronchoscope can be used to guide the biopsy forceps into the segmental bronchus leading to the roentgenographic abnormality. Fluoroscopic guidance should be used. Extra sedation or general anesthesia is usually necessary because of the inability of the child to totally cooperate during the procedure.

A study of 12 pediatric patients (median age of 14.5 years) with diffuse pulmonary processes who underwent BLB reported a diagnostic yield of 50% (85). BLB has also been used in children who have undergone lung transplantation (87). Adequate lung tissue has been obtained in more than 84% of the procedures (88,89). A study of 19 children who underwent 25 BLBs (19 procedures using rigid bronchoscope) reported a 12.5% incidence of pneumothorax (88).

Other Issues

Many bronchoscopists recommend the use of an endotracheal tube to obtain BLB (27,31). This enables the bronchoscopist to effectively control post-BLB hemorrhage. Others have reported that BLB can be safely performed using a transnasal approach without an endotracheal tube (90,91). Because of the extremely low incidence of bacteremia associated with bronchoscopic procedures (39,92–95), many publications have advised against endocarditis prophylaxis for BLB (96). Nevertheless, we use endocarditis prophylaxis in patients susceptible to this complication (97,98).

Inability to obtain optimal lung specimens is a common problem even when fluoroscopic guidance is used. Proper functioning of biopsy forceps and good technique will enhance the chance of collecting good biopsy specimens. Opening the biopsy forceps closer to the area of parenchymal abnormality will prevent biopsy of the bronchial wall (52). If biopsy forceps fail to obtain adequate samples, a new or different forceps should be used or a new anatomic area should be selected for biopsy.

It is unclear whether the biopsy forceps pierces the bronchial wall to enter the lung parenchyma to obtain the biopsy or the cups of the biopsy forceps pinch the lung tissue located between the two walls of the bronchioles as shown in Figure 9.2. The presence of bronchial tissue in a significant number of BLB specimens suggests that the latter mechanism may prevail in most attempts to obtain BLB.

The role of BLB in the diagnosis of respiratory vasculitis is unclear. An important part of BLB is to prevent post-BLB hemorrhage by avoiding biopsy of the vascular structures (99). Yet, it is essential to obtain vascular tissue to document the presence of vascular inflammation. It is unclear if biopsy of vessels affected by a vasculitic process increases the risk of BLB-induced bleeding. In our opinion, suspected respiratory vasculitis is not a good indication for BLB.

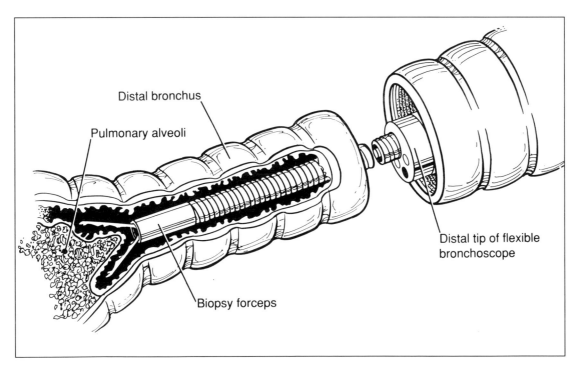

Figure 9.2. Diagrammatic representation of the technique of BLB. The biopsy forceps obtains lung tissue located between the two walls of branching terminal bronchioles. It is unclear if the biopsy forceps actually pierces the wall of the bronchioles to obtain lung specimen.

Reproduced by permission from McDougall JC, Cortese DA. Bronchoscopic lung biopsy. In: Prakash UBS, ed. Bronchoscopy. New York: Raven Press, 1994:141–146.

Complications

Minor complications are the same as those associated with any bronchoscopic procedure. A report based on postal survey of 231 British bronchoscopists noted that the overall complication rate from bronchoscopy increased from 0.12% to 2.7% and the mortality rate went from 0.04% to 0.12% if BLB was included in the procedure (53). Among 540 patients reported in one study, the rate of complication in those who did not undergo BLB was 0.18% and was 2.0% in those who underwent BLB (39).

The two major complications of BLB are hemorrhage and pneumothorax. An earlier study, based on a questionnaire survey of 5450 cases of BLB, reported a 1.2% incidence of post-BLB hemorrhage (greater than 50 mL) and 13 (0.24%) deaths (100). Another study of 438 patients who underwent BLB observed mild to severe hemorrhage in 9% of patients, but the incidence of post-BLB hemorrhage was 29% in immunocompromised patients and 45% in uremic patients; there was one death (31). Andersen and colleagues reported a series of 939 patients who underwent BLB and less than 1% (6 patients) had greater than 50 mL of BLB-associated bleeding (11). Gaensler reviewed a series of studies comprising 1289 cases of BLB and only 3 (0.2%) deaths were recorded (73). Prevention and treatment of BLB-induced hemorrhage is discussed above (see Technique).

The incidence of post-BLB pneumothorax is between 1% and 4% (14,40,49,51,55, 101–103). The risk of pneumothorax can be decreased, as discussed above, by the use of fluoroscopic guidance (53), cough suppression, and proper biopsy techniques.

Current Status of Bronchoscopic Lung Biopsy

In a survey of 1800 North American bronchoscopists, nearly 70% reported that they performed BLB routinely in diffuse lung disease in nonimmunocompromised patients (42). It is our impression from our review of the literature and our experience at the Mayo Clinic that the number of BLB procedures performed in clinical practice has decreased as a result of increasing application of BAL, HRCT of the thorax, and availability of video-assisted thoracoscopic lung biopsy in the diagnosis of diffuse lung disease. The decline in the need for BLB is likely to continue with the introduction of newer sophisticated imaging procedures and further accumulation of knowledge derived from BAL (sometimes described as "liquid lung biopsy") studies in the evaluation of diffuse lung diseases. Presently, the role of BAL in the diagnosis of noninfectious and nonmalignant diffuse lung processes is limited to research protocols. For now, BLB will remain an important diagnostic tool for the evaluation of a myriad of diffuse lung diseases.

REFERENCES

1. Andersen HA, Miller WE, Bernatz PE. Lung biopsy: transbronchoscopic, percutaneous, and open. Surg Clin North Am 1973;53: 785–793.
2. Forrest JV, Sagel SS. Cutting needle biopsies. Chest 1976;69:244–245.
3. Norenberg R, Claxton CP Jr, Takaro T. Percutaneous needle biopsy of the lung: report of two fatal complications. Chest 1974;66:216–218.
4. Zavala DC, Bedell GN. Percutaneous lung biopsy with a cutting needle: an analysis of 40 cases and comparison with other biopsy techniques. Am Rev Respir Dis 1972;106:186–193.
5. Vitums VC. Percutaneous needle biopsy of the lung with a new disposable needle. Chest 1972;62:717–719.
6. Mehnert JH, Brown MJ. Percutaneous needle core biopsy of peripheral pulmonary masses. Am J Surg 1978;136:151–156.
7. Andersen HA, Fontana RS, Harrison EG Jr. Transbronchoscopic lung biopsy in diffuse lung disease. Dis Chest 1965;48:187–192.

8. Andersen HA, Fontana RS. Transbroncho-scopic lung biopsy for diffuse lung diseases: technique and results in 450 cases. Chest 1972;62:125–128.

9. Palojoki A, Sutinen S. Transbronchoscopic lung biopsy as aid in pulmonary diagnostics. Scand J Respir Dis 1972;53:120–124.

10. Andersen HA. Transbronchoscopic lung biopsy in diffuse pulmonary disease. Ann Thorac Surg 1977;24:1.

11. Andersen HA. Transbronchoscopic lung biopsy for diffuse pulmonary disease: Results in 939 patients. Chest 1978;73 (suppl):734–736.

12. Levin DC, Wicks AB, Ellis JH. Trans-bronchial lung biopsy via fiberoptic bron-choscope. Am Rev Respir Dis 1974; 110:4–12.

13. Scheinhorn DJ, Joyner LR, Whitcomb ME. Transbronchial forceps lung biopsy through the fiberoptic bronchoscope in *Pneumocystis carinii* pneumonia. Chest 1974;66:294–295.

14. Hanson RR, Zavala DC, Rhodes ML, et al. Transbronchial biopsy via flexible fiberoptic bronchoscope: results in 164 cases. Am Rev Respir Dis 1976;114:67–72.

15. Haponik EF, Summer WQR, Terry PB, et al. Clinical decision making with transbronchial lung biopsies. The value of non-specific his-tologic examination. Am Rev Respir Dis 1982;125:524–529.

16. Broaddus C, Dake MD, Stulbarg MS, et al. Bronchoalveolar lavage and transbronchial biopsy for the diagnosis of pulmonary infec-tion in the acquired immunodeficiency syn-drome. Ann Intern Med 1985;102:747–752.

17. McCabe RE, Brooks RG, Mark JBD, et al. Open lung biopsy in patients with acute leukemia. Am J Med 1985;78:609–616.

18. Rennard SI. Bronchoalveolar lavage in the diagnosis of lung cancer. Lung 1990;168 (suppl):1035.

19. Rennard SI. Bronchoalveolar lavage in the diagnosis of lung cancer. Chest 1992;102: 331–332.

20. Gracia JD, Bravo C, Miravittles M, et al. Diagnostic value of bronchoalveolar lavage in peripheral lung cancer. Am Rev Respir Dis 1993;147:649–652.

21. Prakash UBS. Pulmonary eosinophilic granu-loma. In: Lynch JP III, DeRemee RA, eds. Immunologically mediated pulmonary dis-eases. Philadelphia: JB Lippincott, 1991: 432–448.

22. Prakash UBS, Barham SS, Carpenter HA, et al. Pulmonary alveolar phospholipopro-teinosis. Experience with 34 cases and a review. Mayo Clin Proc 1987;62:499–518.

23. Linder J, Radio SJ, Robbins RA, et al. Bronchoalveolar lavage in the cytologic diag-nosis of carcinoma of the lung. Acta Cytol 1987;31:796–797.

24. Bellmont J, DeGracia J, Morales S, Orriols R, Tallado S. Cytologic diagnosis in bron-choalveolar lavage specimens. Chest 1990; 98:513–514.

25. McDougall JC, Cortese DA. Bronchoscopic lung biopsy. In: Prakash UBS, ed. Bronchoscopy. New York: Raven Press, 1994:141–146.

26. Prakash UBS, Stubbs SE. The bronchoscopy survey: some reflections. Chest 1991;100: 1660–1667.

27. Prakash UBS, Stubbs SE. Optimal bron-choscopy. In: Prakash UBS, ed. Bronchos-copy. New York: Raven Press, 1994: 415–431.

28. Rodgers RPC, Levin J. A critical appraisal of the bleeding time. Semin Thromb Hemost 1990;16:1–20.

29. Lind SE. The bleeding time does not predict surgical bleeding. Blood 1991;77:2547–2552.

30. George JN, Shattil SJ. The clinical importance of acquired abnormalities of platelet function. N Engl J Med 1991;324:27–39.

31. Zavala DC. Pulmonary hemorrhage in fiberoptic transbronchial bronchoscopy. Chest 1976;70:584–588.

32. Zavala DC. Transbronchial biopsy in diffuse lung disease. Chest 1978;73:727–733.

33. Matsushima Y, Jones RL, King EG, et al. Alterations in pulmonary mechanics and gas exchange during routine fiberoptic bron-choscopy. Chest 1984;86:184–188.

34. Belen J, Neuhaus A, Markowitz D, Rotman HH. Modification of the effect of fiberoptic bronchoscopy on pulmonary mechanics. Chest 1981;79:516–519.

35. Peacock AJ, Benson-Mitchell R, Godfrey R. Effect of fibreoptic bronchoscopy on pul-monary function. Thorax 1990;45:38–41.

36. Oho K, Amemiya R. Open tube broncho-scope or flexible bronchoscope? In: Oho K, Amemiya K, eds. Practical fiberoptic bron-choscopy. Igaku-Shoin; 1984:1.

37. Bernatt TE. Lung biopsy: transthoracic, percutaneous, open. Surg Clin North Am 1973; 53:785–793.

38. Prakash UBS, Freitag L. Hemoptysis and bronchoscopy-induced hemorrhage. In: Prakash UBS, ed. Bronchoscopy. New York: Raven Press, 1994:227–251.

39. Ahmad M, Livingston DR, Golish JA, et al. The safety of outpatient transbronchial biopsy. Chest 1986;90:403–405.

40. Frazier WD, Pope TL Jr, Findley LJ. Pneumothorax following transbronchial lung biopsy. Low diagnostic yield with routine chest roentgenograms. Chest 1990; 97:539–540.

41. Milam MG, Evins AE, Sahn SA. Immediate chest roentgenography following fiberoptic bronchoscopy. Chest 1989;96:477.

42. Prakash UBS, Offord KP, Stubbs SE. Bronchoscopy in North America: The ACCP survey. Chest 1991;100:1668–1675.

43. Papin TA, Grum CM, Weg JG. Transbronchial biopsy during mechanical ventilation. Chest 1986;89:168–170.

44. Cordasco EM Jr, Mehta AC, Ahmad M. Bronchoscopically-induced bleeding. A summary of nine years' Cleveland Clinic experience and review of the literature. Chest 1991;100:1141–1147.

45. Cunningham JH, Zavala DC, Corry RJ, et al. Trephine air drill, bronchial brush, and fiberoptic transbronchial lung biopsies in immunosupressed patients. Am Rev Respir Dis 1977;115:213–220.

46. Mannucci PM, Remozzi MD, Pusineri F, et al. Deamino 8D arginine vasopressin shortens the bleeding time in uremia. N Engl J Med 1983;308:8–11.

47. Mannucci PM, Vicente V, Vianello L, et al. Controlled trial of desmopresin in liver cirrhosis and other conditions associated with a prolonged bleeding time. Blood 1986; 67:1148–1153.

48. Gerristen SW, Akkerman JW, Sixma JJ. Correction of the bleeding time in patients with storage pool deficiency by infusion of cryoprecipitate. Br J Haematol 1978;40:153–160.

49. de Fenoyl O, Capron F, Lebeau B, et al. Transbronchial lung biopsy: a five year experience in outpatients. Thorax 1989; 44:956–959.

50. Puar HS, Young RC, Armstrong RC. Bronchial and transbronchial lung biopsy without fluoroscopy in sarcoidosis. Chest 1985;87:303–306.

51. Anders GT, Johnson JE, Bush BA, et al. Transbronchial lung biopsy without fluoroscopy. A seven year perspective. Chest 1988;94:557–560.

52. Prakash UBS, Cortese DA, Stubbs SE. Technical solutions to common problems in bronchoscopy. In: Prakash UBS, ed. Bronchoscopy. New York: Raven Press, 1994:111–133.

53. Simpson FG, Arnold AG, Purvis A, et al. Postal survey of bronchoscopic practice by physicians in the United Kingdom. Thorax 1986;41:311–317.

54. Fraire AE, Cooper SP, Greenberg SD, et al. Morphometric/histopathologic assessment of transbronchial lung biopsies: diagnostic utility. Chest 1990;98(suppl):727–733.

55. Shure D. Transbronchial biopsy and needle aspiration. Chest 1989;95:1130–1138.

56. Smith LS, Seaquist M, Schillaci RF. Comparison of forceps used for transbronchial lung biopsy: bigger may not be better. Chest 1985;87:574–576.

57. Loube DI, Johnson JE, Wiener D, et al. The effect of forceps size on the adequacy of specimens obtained by transbronchial biopsy. Am Rev Respir Dis 1993;148:1411–1413.

58. Fraire AE, Cooper SP, Greenberg SD, et al. Transbronchial lung biopsy. Histopathologic and morphometric assessment of diagnostic utility. Chest 1992;102:748–752.

59. Anders GT, Linville KC, Johnson JE, Blanton HM. Evaluation of the float sign for determining adequacy of specimens obtained with transbronchial biopsy. Am Rev Respir Dis 1991;144:1406–1407.

60. Kvale PA. Flexible bronchoscopy with brush and forceps biopsy. In: Wang KP, ed. Biopsy techniques in pulmonary disorders. New York: Raven Press, 1989:45–62.

61. Whitcomb ME, Hawley PC, Kataria YP, et al. The role of the fiberoptic bronchoscope in the diagnosis of sarcoidosis. Chest 1978; 74:205–208.

62. Gilman MJ, Wang KP. Transbronchial lung biopsy in sarcoidosis. An approach to determine the optimal number of biopsies. Am Rev Respir Dis 1980;122:721–724.

63. Kvale PA, Popovich J Jr, Radke JR, et al. (unpublished data quoted in reference no. 35).

64. Koontz CH, Joyner LR, Nelson RA. Transbronchial lung biopsy via the fiberoptic bronchoscope in sarcoidosis. Ann Intern Med 1976;85:64–66.

65. Koerner SK, Sakowitz AJ, Appelman RI, et al. Transbronchial lung biopsy of the diagnosis of sarcoidosis. N Engl J Med 1975; 293:268–270.

66. Poe RH, Israel RH, Utell MJ, Hall WJ. Probability of a positive transbronchial lung biopsy results in sarcoidosis. Arch Intern Med 1979;139:761–763.

67. Roethe RA, Fuller PB, Byrd RB, et al. Transbronchoscopic lung biopsy in sarcoidosis. Optimal number and sites for diagnosis. Chest 1980;77:400–402.

68. Armstrong JR, Radke JR, Kvale PA, et al. Endoscopic findings in sarcoidosis. Characteristics and correlations with radiographic staging and bronchial mucosal biopsy. Ann Otol 1981;90:339–343.

69. Mones JM, Salvana MJ, Oldham SA. Diagnosis of *Pneumocystis carinii* pneumonia. Roentgenographic-pathologic correlates based on fiberoptic bronchoscopy specimens from patients with the acquired immunodefiency syndrome. Chest 1986;89:522–526.

70. Fechner RE, Greenberg FZ, Wilson RA, et al. Evaluation of transbronchial biopsy of the lung. Am J Clin Pathol 1977;68:17–20.

71. Wall CP, Gaensler EA, Carrington CB, et al. Comparison of transbronchial and open biopsies in chronic infiltrative lung diseases. Am Rev Respir Dis 1981;123:280–285.

72. Nishio JN, Lynch JP III. Fiberoptic bronchoscopy in the immunocompromised host: the significance of a "nonspecific" transbronchial biopsy. Am Rev Respir Dis 1980; 121:307–312.

73. Gaensler EA. Open and closed lung biopsy. In: Sackner MA, ed. Diagnostic techniques in pulmonary disease, part II. New York: Marcel Dekker, 1980:579–622.

74. Wilson RK, Fechner RE, Greenberg SD, et al. Clinical implications of a "nonspecific" transbronchial biopsy. Am J Med 1978; 65:252–256.

75. Newman SL, Michel RP, Wang N-S. Lingular lung biopsy: is it representative? Am Rev Respir Dis 1985;132:1084–1086.

76. Matthay RA, Farmer WC, Odero D. Diagnostic fiberoptic bronchoscopy in the immunocompromised host with pulmonary infiltrates. Thorax 1977;32:539–545.

77. Hedemark LL, Kronenberg RS, Rasp FL, et al. The value of bronchoscopy in establishing the etiology of pneumonia in renal transplant recipients. Am Rev Respir Dis 1982;126: 981–985.

78. Stover DE, White DA, Romano PA, et al. Diagnosis of pulmonary disease in acquired immune deficiency syndrome (AIDS). Role of bronchoscopy and bronchoalveolar lavage. Am Rev Respir Dis 1984;130: 659–662.

79. Chopra SK, Mohsenifar Z. Fiberoptic bronchoscopy in diagnosis of opportunistic lung infection. Assessment of sputa, washings, brushings, and biopsy specimens. West J Med 1979;141:4–7.

80. Cortese DA, McDougall JC. Bronchoscopy in peripheral and central lung lesions. In: Prakash UBS, ed. Bronchoscopy. New York: Raven Press, 1994:135–140.

81. Pincus PS, Kallenbach JM, Hurwitz MD, et al. Transbronchial biopsy during mechanical ventilation. Crit Care Med 1987;15: 1136–1139.

82. Stubbs SE, Brutinel WM. Complications of bronchoscopy. In: Prakash UBS, ed. Bronchoscopy. New York: Raven Press, 1994: 357–366.

83. Kramer MR, Stoehr C, Whang JL, et al. The diagnosis of obliterative bronchiolitis after heart-lung transplantation. J Heart Lung Transplant 1993;12:675–681.

84. Trulock EP, Ettinger NA, Brunt EM, et al. The role of transbronchial lung biopsy in the treatment of lung transplant recipients. An analysis of 200 consecutive procedures. Chest 1992;102:1049–1054.

85. Fitzpatrick SB, Stokes DC, Marsh B, et al. Transbronchial lung biopsy in pediatric and adolescent patient. Am J Dis Child 1985;139:46–49.

86. Levy M, Glick B, Springer C, et al. Bronchoscopy and bronchography in children. Experience with 110 investigations. Am J Dis Child 1983;137:14–16.

87. Whitehead B, Scott JP, Helms P, et al. Technique and use of transbronchial biopsy in children and adolescents. Pediatr Pulmonol 1992;12:240–246.

88. Muntz HR, Wallace M, Lusk RP. Pediatric transbronchial lung biopsy. Ann Otol Rhinol Laryngol 1992;101:135–137.

89. Scott JP, Higenbottom TW, Smyth RL, et al. Transbronchial biopsies in children after

heart-lung transplantation. Pediatrics 1990; 86:698–702.

90. Kvale PA, Bode FR, Kini S. Diagnostic accuracy in lung cancer. Comparison of techniques used in association with flexible fiberoptic bronchoscopy. Chest 1976;69:752–757.

91. Feldman NT, Pennington JE, Ehrie MG. Transbronchial lung biopsy in the compromised host. JAMA 1977;238:1377–1379.

92. Watts JW, Green RA. Bacteremia following transbronchial needle aspiration. Chest 1984;85:295.

93. Conte JE Jr. Prophylaxis of endocarditis during surgical and dental procedures. West J Med 1980;133:141–147.

94. Kane RC, Cohen MH, Fossieck BE Jr, et al. Absent bacteremia after bronchoscopy. Am Rev Respir Dis 1975;111:102–104.

95. Pereira W, Kovnat DM, Kahn MA, et al. Fever and pneumonia after flexible fiberoptic bronchoscopy. Am Rev Respir Dis 1975; 112:59–64.

96. Witte MC, Opal SM, Gilbert JG, et al. Incidence of bacteremia following transbronchial needle aspiration. Chest 1986; 89:85–87.

97. Dajani AS, Bisno AL, Chung KJ, et al.

Prevention of bacterial endocarditis. Recommendations by the American Heart Association. JAMA 1990;264:2919–2924.

98. Working Party of the British Society for Antimicrobial Chemotherapy. Lancet 1983; 2:1323.

99. Flick MR, Wasson K, Dunn LJ, et al. Fatal pulmonary hemorrhage after transbronchial lung biopsy through the fiberoptic bronchoscope. Am Rev Respir Dis 1975;111: 853–856.

100. Herf SM, Suratt PM, Arora NS. Deaths and complications associated with transbronchial lung biopsy. Am Rev Respir Dis 1977; 115:708–711.

101. Joyner LR, Scheinhorn DJ. Transbronchial forceps through the fiberoptic bronchoscope. Diagnosis of diffuse pulmonary disease. Chest 1975;67:532–535.

102. Hernandez-Blasco L, Sanchez-Hernandez IM, Villena-Garrido V, et al. Safety of the transbronchial biopsy in outpatients. Chest 1991; 99:562–565.

103. Zavala DC. Diagnostic fiberoptic bronchoscopy: techniques and results of biopsy in 600 patients. Chest 1975;68:12–19.

Bronchoscopy for Airway Lesions | 10

Heinrich D. Becker

"Although hardly any scientific progress may be expected resulting from Killian's work, it appears to me of such outstanding practical importance that I am considering it to be worthy of the Nobel prize." (1)
     — G. Holmgren, 1920
"Everything we see hides another thing, we always want to see what is hidden by what we see. There is an interest in that which is hidden and which the visible doesn't show us." (2)
     — Rene Magritte, Painter (1898–1967)

In 1898 Gustav Killian of Freiburg University stated in his first report on direct bronchoscopy, which he gave on May 29th of that year at the fifth annual meeting of the South German Laryngological Society at Heidelberg, "The practical relevance of bronchoscopy cannot be assessed accurately at the moment. I hope that, apart from foreign bodies and bronchial diseases, it may also be applied to diagnosis and therapy of affections of the lung." (3) Today, almost 100 years after Killian's invention of direct bronchoscopy in 1897, it has become one of the most important diagnostic and therapeutic tools in pulmonary medicine.

The possibility of direct visualization of the central airways through the rigid bronchoscope was further improved by the development of lens optics (Hopkins and Lumina optic), providing a much better field of view and visualization of details. The introduction of the fully flexible bronchofiberscope by Ikeda in 1967 has made the peripheral bronchial system and even every part of the lung parenchyma easily accessible for the endoscopist. By its comparatively easy handling and comfortable application for the patient it has provided a strong impetus for the spreading of bronchoscopic technique to many institutions. Furthermore, because of improvements in technique and pharmacology of general and local anesthesia, risks of complications have become so few (4) that bronchoscopy, despite its invasive nature, belongs to the basic procedures in pulmonary medicine of today and is applied early in the diagnostic process.

This is all the more important for lesions of the central airways because these are located deeply inside the thoracic cavity and are surrounded by a complexity of mediastinal organs and are poorly visualized by radiologic examination despite profound technical revolutions such as the computed tomography (CT) scan and magnetic resonance imaging (MRI). Early consideration of endoscopy of the airways is further enhanced by the fact that most diseases involving the central airways are producing uncharacteristic clinical symptoms that are often not pathognomonic for the underlying process.

In this short overview on bronchoscopy for airway lesions we shall point out a few aspects of the technical approach and systematization of endoscopic findings in the airways that, in our experience, seem to be important.

Technical Considerations

The general technical considerations concerning instrumental equipment, operational approach, and anesthesiologic management are dealt with elsewhere in this book. Here we offer special considerations on the approach in airway diseases.

Systematic Inspection

The first consideration is the systematization of bronchoscopic examination. Because many diseases of the airways are not strictly localized to only one site but rather frequently tend to be part of a more systemic spread, one should always strictly adhere to a scheme of systematic inspection of the whole airway tract during the procedure. This will frequently include the upper airways above the larynx as well (Plate 8).

The attention of the examiner is easily drawn toward obvious pathologies of the airways, so we examine first those areas of the airways that do not seem to be involved by the pathologic process radiologically or endoscopically. Additional alterations that stayed occult may be discovered early during the diagnostic procedure and are not missed after attention has been distracted by the exploration of the obviously pathologic process. This may happen easily if difficulties arise due to obscured vision caused by mucus, purulent secretions, and bleeding or by technical problems in providing specimens for laboratory examinations (5).

Documentation

All endoscopic findings must be meticulously documented by verbal and graphic description together with the resultant diagnostic and therapeutic conclusions. Additional diagnostic, documentary, and therapeutic measures must be noted. Video documentation may be useful in longitudinal follow-up of diseases and information of colleagues. But one should always keep in mind that on the video we just see sequences that have been documented and important additional information may be missed or lost. Direct communication among the physicians involved is still indispensable.

Instrumentation

The second consideration involves the instrument and approach chosen by the examiner. The examination by flexible fiberscope under local anesthesia obviously needs much less staff and instrumental equipment and seems to be comfortable for the patient. Furthermore, a detailed functional analysis of the pharyngeal space, the vocal cords, and the stability of the tracheobronchial system under almost physiologic conditions is only possible under local anesthesia.

Visualization of details and management under conditions of poor compliance and obstruction of view by excessive secretions or bleeding are not so easily managed under local anesthesia. Sometimes even under local anesthesia after inspection of the larynx and the upper trachea, it seems advisable to insert a tracheal tube if the instrument has to be withdrawn frequently for cleansing. This prevents excessive coughing due to repeated passage of the larynx.

Under these conditions, we still regard the rigid bronchoscope as an ideal instrument because it provides an optimal overview and a much safer airway for ventilation in all circumstances. For gaining large and reliable biopsy specimens, for most therapeutic procedures such as removal of large foreign bodies, especially in children, for laser treatment, dilatation of stenoses and stenting, and for optimal photographic and video documentation, we still use the rigid bronchoscope.

The rates of complications of flexible bronchoscopy under local anesthesia as compared to rigid bronchoscopy under general anesthesia and high-frequency jet ventilation, according to major comparative studies and in our personal experience, seem to be almost equal. Whereas in rigid bronchoscopy traumatic lesions due to instrumentation and larger biopsies are more frequent, in flexible bronchoscopy side effects of local anesthetics and problems in ventilation are more common (6).

Because the general risk of bronchoscopy is higher as compared to gastroenterologic endoscopy and the time for examination is limited due to the vanishing effect of anesthesia, meticulous planning and preparation for the procedure are necessary.

Prerequisites

History and Physical Examination

Because the amount of information from endoscopic examination is limited and frequently may also be ambiguous, some information before starting the procedure is essential. History of symptoms and physical examination of the patient must be established. Frequently signs of central airway disease are subtle but pathognomonic, and diagnosis may be suspected by careful examination. Anamnesis of smoking for decades, progressive dyspnea and coughing, hemoptysis or purulent secretions, acute persistent hoarseness, or a history of traumatic lesions of the airways such as prolonged intubation or tracheotomy may give the first hint of airways involvement.

On clinical examination, asymmetrical excursions of the thorax and one-sided "asthmatic" wheezing or reduction of breathing sounds are typical for obstruction of a main stem bronchus, especially if the onset of symptoms occurs in adults without a prior history of asthma. Signs of overinflation or of impaired ventilation of parts of the lungs can be pathognomonic for localized airway obstruction, rales, and signs of pleurisy for postobstructive infiltration.

Laboratory Tests and Radiologic Examination

These findings may be further quantified by lung function tests, giving an idea of the stability of the airways and especially of organic obstruction. A preoperative analysis of the blood gases will help in taking special precautions for safe ventilation during the procedure.

Laboratory blood tests usually do not give much information about airway pathology. However, they are needed for assessment of risks prior to bronchoscopy.

Because during bronchoscopy frequently only indirect signs of central airway problems may be visualized, it is essential to establish an orienting survey on the thoracic organs to establish a diagnosis. Therefore, radiologic exploration before bronchoscopy is essential. Plain frontal and lateral x-rays are indispensable prerequisites. On these areas of impaired ventilation, malformations of respiratory organs and tumorous lesions of the lung, the bronchi, or neighboring organs may be suspected, if not already diagnosed.

Depending on these findings and according to the urgency of endoscopic examination, further investigations may be necessary for exact localization of a pathologic process. Fluoroscopy with examination of the esophagus is helpful in assessing dynamic alterations of the great vessels, heart and lungs, and of the esophageal passage.

Because even by CT scan and MRI, visualization of the central airways and the hilar region still is unsatisfactory for details, we frequently perform hilar tomography with filters whenever a lesion of these structures is suspected.

Safety Measures

For early recognition and prevention of complications, safety precautions have to be taken—a safe intravenous access, oxygen insufflation, electrocardiographic and blood pressure monitoring, and percutaneous pulse oximetry. All instruments for intervention in the case of complications must be readily available and must be regularly tested for function.

Anatomic Considerations

Every textbook of pulmonary medicine and every atlas of bronchoscopy contains ample information on the endoscopic appearance of the normal bronchial tree and nomenclature of its ramifications. Looking at the complexity of the bronchopulmonary system one will always marvel at the constancy of the basic anatomic structure that is found in most patients.

For example, there is a constant number of 22 tracheal cartilage rings and the well-known asymmetry of lobes on both sides with 19 segmental bronchi. The pulmonary vessels cross at definite regions so that inadvertent puncture during transbronchial needle biopsy of the regional lymph nodes and tumor masses can be avoided. The regional lymph nodes have been numbered according to their regular distribution along the bronchial tree, which is essential for the staging of involvement in bronchial carcinoma. The pulmonary fissures are a fairly safe guideline to assess the segmental localization of intrapulmonary lesions.

By these examples, without having mentioned the close anatomic relation of the tracheobronchial tree to neighboring organs of the mediastinum, we demonstrate the importance of a thorough knowledge of the anatomy. Table 10.1 lists five aspects that deserve further discussion (7).

Anatomic Orientation

To the beginner the number and nomenclature of the bronchi will appear to be confusing. But once used to it, orientation will be comparatively easy because the tracheobronchial system is not as easily deformed and has no motility in itself as compared to the gastrointestinal tract.

An obstacle to orientation is its confinement, especially if vision is further impaired by mucus, blood, or tumor infiltration. This will be experienced more frequently in flexible bronchoscopy under local anesthesia than during rigid bronchoscopy under general anesthesia because the mucosa may be damaged easily due to forced maneuvers and coughing. Repeated withdrawal for cleansing of the lens of the fiberscope and reintroduction of the instrument will not be too readily tolerated by the patient.

Once one has lost the anatomic orientation during the procedure one should withdraw the instrument to a distinct landmark such as the main bifurcation of the trachea or into the trachea itself and start the examination from there again. Many of the suspected "anatomic variations" will become clear as misinterpretation of the actual region that is inspected.

Normal Anatomy

During development of the embryonal lung, the tracheobronchial system has adopted its definite structure by the sixteenth gestational week. In the newborn and child up to the age of about 4 to 6 years, the trachea has an almost round shape and the dorsal ends of the cartilages may almost meet, especially during forced breathing and coughing, which must not be mistaken for complete cartilage rings. It

Table 10.1. Anatomic Aspects in Bronchoscopy

1. Anatomic orientation
2. Normal anatomy
3. Variations without clinical relevance
4. Pathologic malformations
5. Considerations regarding resectability

is only at the age of about 8 to 10 years that the typical horseshoe shape is completed. In children also the bifurcation of the trachea appears blunt and the angle wider than in the adult (8), in whom this would be a sign of displacement by extraluminal infracarinal masses (Plate 9).

Because the cartilages still are very soft at that age, total tracheal and bronchial collapse during coughing and forced breathing maneuvers in smaller children is physiologic as long as the airways remain open in the resting or inspirating position. The diameter of the trachea varies according to size and physical condition of the child. Instead of using tables as a guideline to choose the appropriate diameter of the bronchoscope, we prefer to use the little finger of the individual child, the caliber of which usually closely resembles that of the trachea ("rule of the little finger") (Figure 10.1).

In the young adult the trachea has grown in length and diameter and has adopted the typical horseshoe form. Only during coughing does the paries membranaceus bulge toward the anterior wall; otherwise the trachea is stable under physiologic conditions. The main carina usually is sharp and the angulation of the main bronchi narrow.

Although the branching of the lobar and segmental bronchi is astonishingly consistent, some variations are so frequent that they may be considered as harmless variations. However, because severe pathologic malformations may be similar, some experience is required for their discrimination.

Anatomic Variations without Clinical Relevance

Many variations are seen in the branching of the segmental bronchi. Early branching of the subsegments may mimic additional segmentation. On the other hand, segmental bronchi that normally are separated may arise from a common stem. This should not be confused with agenesis of segments. These variations can cause difficulties in localization and access to peripheral lesions by transbronchial biopsy. Sometimes segmental or even lobar bronchi may be found as an "anlage" only, that is, bronchial buds, forming diverticulous excavations of the bronchial system (Plate 10). This will be most frequently found with the paracardial segment in the lower lobe of the right side.

The most frequent surplus variation is an additional bronchus of the apical segments of both lower lobes, the so-called subapical segments. An additional, completely developed lobus cardiacus on the left side is comparatively rare. On the right side the apicodorsal segments of the upper lobe may branch separately from the main bronchus, thus producing a double upper lobe carina. These segments or even the whole upper lobe bronchus may separate from the distal trachea as a so-called tra-

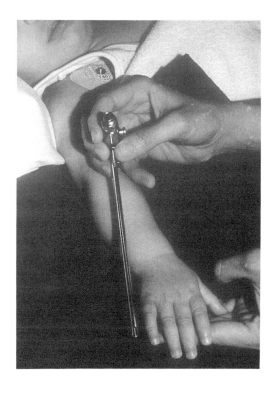

Figure 10.1. Choosing a bronchoscope somewhat smaller than the little finger will always provide the right size for the individual child.

cheal bronchus. We have found this far more frequently on the right side than on the left (Plate 11). On the left side sometimes there is no common upper lobe bronchus if the lingula arises directly from the main bronchus. A trifurcation may be formed or even a short intermediate bronchus if the branching occurs at the level of the apical segment of the lower lobe.

These branching varieties cause clinical symptoms only if the bronchus is hypoplastic or shows some kinking due to its abnormal course, leading to impairment of ventilation or clearing of secretions of the corresponding part of the lungs.

In cartilage development, fusions of branchings or whole rings may be found as variations. A common variation is the finding of ecchondromas, harmless protrusions of normal cartilaginous tissue, resembling compression by expansive extraluminal tumor growth. They may easily be distinguished due to their garland-like appearance being restricted to the cartilages only and leaving the intercartilaginous spaces unharmed (Plate 12). At biopsy the tissue will be very hard and after removal of the mucosa white cartilage will lay bare.

This is not to be confused with the so-called tracheobronchopathia chondro sive osteoplastica, a condition of excessive exophytic tumor-like growth of cartilaginous and mostly ossified tissue in the mucosa and submucosa without anatomic restriction to the cartilages. The inflammatory etiology of this disease is still debated; rarely is mechanical or laser removal used if it is obstructing the large airways.

Pathologic Malformations of the Bronchial System

Many of the pathologic malformations can be explained as developmental disorders at different stages of fetal organ formation. They may be solitary lesions restricted to the bronchial tree only or they may be part of complex disorders of the bronchopulmonary system, which in themselves again may be part of a multiple organ malformation syndrome.

Because the complex history of embryologic organ formation still is not completely understood, the classification of developmental malformations is arbitrary to some extent. Nevertheless a systematic overview will help the understanding (9), and because it will enhance orientation, we shall discuss the most important malformations as they are encountered passing the tracheobronchial tree.

Larynx

By far the most frequent anomaly and cause of stridor in the newborn is laryngomalacia due to immature soft cartilages (85%), causing a "flabby larynx" with excess folding of the epiglottis and shortness with inward bending of the aryepiglottic folds. The larynx most frequently will stabilize spontaneously after some time of stabilization by a tracheal tube. The diameter of the tube should be rather small to not cause further damage to the mucosal lining and to the cartilages by exertion of pressure.

Laryngeal stenoses due to supraglottic, glottic, or subglottic webs much more frequently are the sequelae to intubation trauma during neonatal intensive care than a congenital anomaly. They can be treated by endoscopic mechanical removal or laser resection.

Laryngotracheal clefts and fistulas are rare events caused by a defect in development of the tracheoesophageal septum (Plate 13). They require surgery because they cause symptoms of repeated aspiration. Endoscopic closure by fibrin application will rarely be successful and may only be considered in very small hair fistulas.

The involvement in hemangiomas or hamartomas, such as in familial neurofibromatosis, causes symptoms of upper airway obstruction due to submucosal tumors protruding into the lumen of the larynx and the upper trachea. Hemangiomas may frequently be coagulated by neodymium:yttrium-aluminum-garnet (Nd:YAG) laser if they do not resolve spontaneously (Plates 14 and 15).

Trachea

Mechanical instability of the trachea is so common in early childhood that it can be regarded as an almost normal finding as long as the airways are regaining their normal diameter during the resting position. It takes several years for the cartilages to gain their definite stability. Complete rings and complete agenesis of the cartilages are rare malformations causing life-threatening symptoms due to chronic obstruction and inflammation. Surgical management using grafts of cartilages or pericardium still is restricted and not always successful.

It is especially in combination with other developmental disorders of the vascular system, aberrant bronchi, or malformations of the esophagus that tracheal stenosis due to chondromalacia may become pathologic. In these instances, the cartilages can be softened due to chronic pressure or partially absent as fistulas, or aberrant bronchi may cause defects in the structures of the tracheal wall (Figure 10.2,A,B).

Congenital tracheobronchomegaly (Mounier-Kuhn) usually becomes symptomatic in adulthood only because the sequelae of chronic inflammation develop gradually over the years.

Tracheal diverticula will be either formed by rudimentary accessory bronchi or rudimentary tracheoesophageal fistulas. Sometimes they are found as the result of traction by scars from healed lymph nodes after specific inflammation or after perforation.

Esophagotracheal fistulas cause symptoms of aspiration in early infancy and most frequently are associated with esophageal atresia. Closure by endoscopic means, such as laser obliteration or application of fibrin glue, are frequently unsuccessful and surgical repair must be performed (Plate 16) (10).

Bronchi

Branching abnormalities of the bronchi cause symptoms only if they are associated with problems of ventilation or drainage of secretions from the parts of the lung parenchyma to which they lead. Accessory bronchi frequently have narrow ostia due to malformations of the corresponding cartilages causing retention of secretions due to their instability. Abnormal cartilage spurs or complete rings at the branching levels lead to major stenoses of the large airways, which is especially common in aberrant tracheal bronchi (Figure 10.3).

Aberrant branching is most common in the right upper lobe, either arising from the main

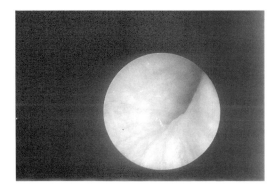
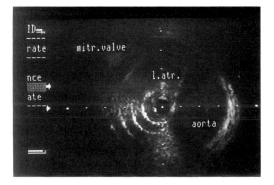

Figure 10.2. *A,* Bronchial compression. Elastic compression stenosis of the left main bronchus was found in a 7-year-old child suffering from severe kyphoscoliosis. *B,* Ultrasonography demonstrates compression of the bronchus by the left atrium (ventrally) and the descending aorta (dorsally).

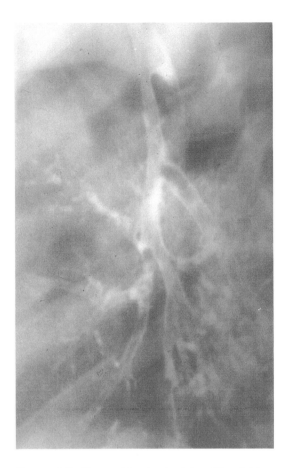

Figure 10.3. Aberrant tracheal origin of the right upper lobe bronchus. Note the significant narrowing of the lower third of the trachea close to the bifurcation. Because of recurrent pneumonic infiltrations and recurrent bouts of dyspnea, resection of the stenotic tracheal segment with end-to-end anastomosis and resection of the infiltrated upper lobe was performed, resulting in persistent relief of symptoms.

bronchus or from the trachea. Repeated inflammatory infiltration in the dependent lung tissue due to retention of secretions is not uncommon.

On the medial wall of the intermediate bronchus one occasionally sees a fistulous opening, which is the ostium of an accessory lobus cardiacus. This is also the most common location for bronchogenic cysts if the accessory lobe has not fully developed into a pulmonary segment.

Stenoses of the bronchi by webs usually are secondary due to inflammation during early childhood. They probably are the most common cause of isolated bronchiectasis. Bronchiectasis due to agenesis of cartilages in the segmental bronchi resulting in localized bronchial stenosis or due to complete malformation of the "anlage" is far less frequent.

Membranes or complete atresia of bronchi are rare events. We have found these in two cases of lobar sequestration. The hyperlucent lung tissue on the x-ray in these cases obviously was inflated via Kohn's pores from adjacent areas.

The syndromes associated with immotile cilia, specifically, Kartagener's disease or Young syndrome, are always associated with diseases of the bronchi, mostly chronic inflammation or bronchiectasis.

Whether the syndrome of unilateral hyperlucency (Swyer-James or Macleod syndrome) is caused by primary hypoplasia of the pulmonary artery or is due to peripheral obliterative bronchiolitis of viral origin is still debated. Any malformations of the lung parenchyma, especially those associated with regional hypo- or hyperinflation, may lead to displacement or obstruction of the central bronchial system.

Pulmonary vascular disorders are only visible to the bronchoscopist if the bronchial circulatory system is involved or if they are part of systemic malformation syndromes. The latter are rarely found in arteriovenous fistulas (as, for example, in Osler's disease), the former in cardiac vitia that are causing redistribution of the intrathoracic blood flow to the bronchial vessels (Plate 17) (11). In these instances we have found bronchial varicosis that resolved after surgical repair of the cardiac vitium.

Anatomic Considerations Regarding Resectability

This is one of the most important anatomic aspects for the bronchoscopist in daily routine work. In the presurgical staging procedures to assess the resectability of lesions of the central airways, accurate assessment to the millimeter of the structures involved is essential. The distances of lesions to structures marking crucial limitations for standard surgical procedures have to be watched closely because involvement of central parts of the tracheobronchial system proximal to the pulmonary lesion will usually only be manageable by extensive surgical procedures. In these situations bronchoplastic operations must be considered in favor of the conservation of healthy functioning lung tissue (12).

This is most important at the level of the right and left main bronchus for so-called sleeve lobectomy and at the level of the main carina and bifurcation for sleeve pneumonectomy, when resection of the bifurcation and reimplantation of the remaining main bronchus has to be planned. In a large prospective study for the evaluation of staging and therapeutic procedures in bronchogenic carcinoma, we could show, however, that routine biopsy of macroscopically normal carinas proximal to the lesion hardly ever produced positive results.

Because the resectability of tracheal lesions is limited, it is essential that the bronchoscopist exactly measures not only the dimensions of the lesion itself but also its distances to crucial landmarks, especially the carina, the cricoid cartilage, and the vocal cords. Counting the number of cartilage rings involved may be helpful.

The involvement of mediastinal structures surrounding the central airways, that is, the mediastinal lymph nodes, the esophagus, or the major blood vessels, may be suspected due to displacement or direct involvement of the central airways at the corresponding level. In these cases the bronchoscopist can induce further investigational studies such as esophagoscopy, exploration by ultrasound and radiology, or even mediastinoscopy for the staging procedure.

Semiotics

To establish a diagnosis by endoscopy of the airways we have to consider the structures that can be seen and the changes due to pathologic processes as compared to the normal situation.

As in every kind of morphologic diagnosis in medicine, interpretation of bronchoscopic findings and establishment of a diagnosis is based on a synopsis of changes of the morphologic structures, which is finally integrated into the clinical context. This procedure, the art of interpretation of appearances of diseases, is called semiotics (from the Greek word: "to semeion," the sign) (13).

In contrast to the complex information through all our senses that we obtain at the bedside, in endoscopy we have to rely mainly on visual information, rarely on additional indirect palpation. A diagnosis by bronchoscopic examination is achieved by interpreting the alterations of the visible structures of the tracheobronchial structures. Table 10.2 lists the structures that should be recognized in relation to their anatomy.

We shall discuss each of these items in some detail and try to show how they may be set into a clinical context in establishing a diagnosis. Although the discussion covers the different aspects separately in some arbitrary arrangement, it must be stressed that in most instances various combinations of several

Table 10.2. Structures as Diagnostic Guidelines in Bronchoscopy

1. Contents of bronchi
2. Coloration and surface of mucosa
3. Blood vessels
4. Lymph vessels
5. Integrity of the mucosa
6. Integrity of the bronchial wall
7. Involvement by surrounding structures
8. Clinical context

components will be found and only the complete mosaic will make the diagnosis. Obviously some structures will be discussed under more than one category.

Contents of the Bronchi

Physiologically, in the normal subject the bronchi are filled mainly by air. The mucosal lining is covered by a thin layer of translucent fluid that is transported orally in a well-coordinated, mostly clockwise, spiral movement by the mucosal cilia (Plate 18). Because of pathologic changes in the bronchial mucous glands or of the alveolar fluid formation, the composition of secretions may be altered in quantity and quality, consistency, and color.

Abundant clear liquid, sometimes foamy fluid secretions are pathognomonic for bronchioalveolar carcinoma. The abundant secretions in alveolar proteinosis and the not always copious secretions in *Pneumocystis carinii* pneumonia usually are more opaque due to the high protein content. In pulmonary edema the foamy secretions frequently are stained by traces of blood.

The sticky clear secretions in the asthmatic patient are well known and may even be so viscous that they form casts of the smaller bronchi, known as Curshmann's spirals. Larger agglomerations may form mucoid impactions, causing the obstruction of segmental or even larger bronchi. The resulting shadows on the plain x-ray will mimic obstructive pneumonia due to bronchial carcinoma.

The grayish brown sticky secretions, which are full of macrophages loaded with condensed remnants of tobacco smoke at cytologic examination, are pathognomonic for the smoking patient suffering from chronic bronchitis. During episodes of bacterial infection they may turn more yellowish.

Severely purulent secretions will be found in bacterial pneumonia, especially in its obstructive form and in patients with abscess formation. The abundant purulent secretions with "mouthful expectorations" are patho-

gnomonic for bronchiectasis, which is found in its most extensive form in mucoviscidosis due to chronic infection by pseudomonas. The secretions will settle in three layers of foam on top, cloudy fluid in the middle, and sediments of leukocytes at the bottom of a vessel when recovered for bacteriologic examination (Figure 10.4). The purulent secretions may also form thick plugs, causing bronchial obstruction by mucoid impactions and thereby further aggravating the distention of the peripheral bronchi. Tomography frequently shows "sausage formed" shadows that are suggestive of the diagnosis.

Superinfection of those plugs by *Aspergillus fumigatus* makes the secretions even more sticky, almost rubber-like, causing the clinical picture of allergic bronchopulmonary

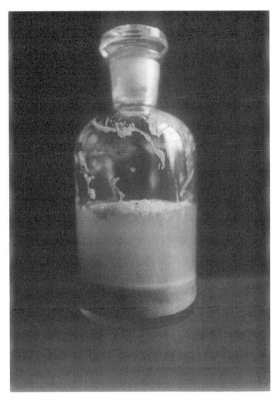

Figure 10.4. Secretions from bronchiectasis. Typical three-layered purulent sputum of a patient suffering from mucoviscidosis: foamy secretions on top, opaque infected material in the middle, and a thick layer of leukeocytic sediments at the bottom of the vessel.

aspergillosis, a hypersensitivity reaction to the pathologic agent (14).

In all these diseases, cytologic and microbiologic examination of the bronchoscopically gained secretions will yield further information on the nature of the underlying pathogenic cause. The samples may be obtained by special sheathed catheters or microbiology brushes. In our experience, asservation by simple suction through the biopsy channel of the fiberscope will yield reliable results for most routine clinical purposes (15). Bronchoalveolar lavage (BAL) is the method of choice in the diagnosis of infections of the alveolar space, which have become the most important pneumologic problem in the im-munocompromised patient, especially in the acquired immunodeficiency syndrome (16).

Frequently under various conditions, blood staining of different degrees will be mixed with the secretions. If these stains accompany clinical symptoms of chronic bronchitis with the endoscopic findings of distended mucosal blood vessels, they are readily interpreted as benign.

Unfortunately the same patients, that is, the chronic smokers, also run a high risk of bronchial carcinoma. Therefore, one should always insist on visualizing the actual site of bleeding because this may be the early sign of an otherwise occult bronchial carcinoma.

In our opinion, every patient with hemoptysis, apart from the obvious clinical picture of pulmonary embolism, should undergo bronchoscopic examination immediately during the episode of bleeding. Thus, at least the site of bleeding may be assessed and further investigations (bronchography, angiography, etc.) can be focused on the potential source of bleeding. Sometimes acribic sequential lavage of each lobar bronchus may be necessary for localization. In some cases of episodic hemoptysis the procedure has to be repeated. Every patient with an unexplained source of hemop-

tysis must be regarded as carrying an occult bronchogenic carcinoma and must be kept under close observation.

Malignant diseases make up 25% of the sources of bleeding in our patients. In 50%, chronic inflammatory processes are the source of bleeding of which chronic bronchitis (15%), bronchiectasis (8%), and tuberculous caverns (8%) are the most frequent underlying causes. In about 70% of our cases the source of bleeding could be established by bronchoscopy. Adding positive results of conventional radiology, bronchography, and angiography, in only 10% were we not able to establish a definite diagnosis of the bleeding source. This has been especially true for catamenial hemoptysis, if the ectopic uterine mucosa is not to be found endobronchially nor showing on the plain x-ray film in the lung parenchyma (17).

Coloration and Surface of the Mucosa

The normal bronchial mucosa is a pink colored glistening layer smoothly covering all the structures of the bronchial wall. Only the cartilages are yellow whitish in color. The nourishing capillary vessels are clearly seen as a delicate network. In the normal bronchial mucosa the lymph vessels are not seen nor are the openings of the mucous glands visible. The submucosal longitudinal bundles of connective tissue may be somewhat prominent, giving a washboard-like appearance to the paries membranaceus, especially during forced breathing or coughing, but they cannot be seen themselves through healthy mucosa.

Many of the factors causing changes in the secretions also influence the bronchial mucosa, thereby changing its color and the structures described above.

Acute inflammatory reactions due to infectious or toxic agents frequently cause diffuse bright or dark reddening of the mucosa, according to the extent of vascular congestion. In this situation, the capillary network no longer can be discriminated. By a concomitant edematous swelling, the mucosa may be thickened, leveling the contours of the bronchial wall.

Especially in the asthmatic patient edematous swelling is the main feature of mucosal alteration, whereas the vascular injection may be much less prominent. In these patients the mucosa appears pale and has a cushion-like swelling, which may cause mechanical bronchial obstruction on top of the functional bronchospasm.

In the most common form of chronic bronchitis, the mucosa appears thinned and rather pale. The underlying structures of the bronchial wall are prominent. This is conspicuous in the elastic layers of connective tissue on the dorsal parts of the larger airways. Longitudinal strands of white color, sometimes branching, can be seen lying directly beneath the thinned mucosa (Plate 19).

The mucosa and submucosal tissue may sag between the fiber bundles because the chronic inflammatory process and the continuous mechanical stress of coughing cause the elastica to be distended as in the cutaneous striae due to pregnancy. Typical changes in the mucous glands are found; because of the formation of viscous bronchial secretions, the ducts become distended by mucous retention and their normally invisible openings appear as small holes in the mucosa. All of these features make up the picture of chronic deforming bronchitis.

During episodes of acute inflammation due to viral or bacterial superinfection there may be some reddening but the blood vessels will be still visible and even more prominent due to the congestion.

In the rarer form of chronic hypertrophic bronchitis there is marked swelling of the pale mucosa by an excessive lymphocytic infiltration of the submucosal layers, which produces thickened folds that can even mimic amyloidosis of the bronchial wall or submucosal tumor infiltration. This also may cause mechanical obliteration of the bronchial lumina.

The transparent nodular lesions in sarcoidosis are easily recognized. Frequently in these lesions, as in discontinuous lymphangic tumor spreading on close view, small capillary vessels may be seen extending into the nodular lesions (Plate 20). Sometimes patchy mucous collections may appear in a similar pattern but in contrast they can be removed easily by gentle suctioning.

Blood Vessels

The normal bronchial mucosa is nourished by a delicate network of arterial blood vessels that can be seen clearly. In the trachea these vessels are entering the mucosa in a segmental array between the cartilages, spreading like small trees upward and downward to the adjacent segment where they form anastomoses (Plate 21). It is in the dorsal membranaceous wall only that they take a longitudinal course covering several segments. In the larger bronchi the vascularization is arranged longitudinally, covering larger areas. Here anastomoses are scarce, so they have to be regarded as end arteries. The postcapillary venous blood is collected in an intra- and submucosal plexus from where it is carried directly to the pulmonary venous system (18). In contrast to the blood vessels, the lymphatics are not seen in the normal bronchial mucosa.

In acute bacterial and especially in viral infections of the lower respiratory tract, the mucosa frequently is dark red so that the capillary network is completely blurred. Although in these cases the discoloration is spread evenly over the whole mucosa, in localized types of inflammatory reactions like sarcoidosis the reddening may be patchy, sometimes arranged around granulomas, leaving spaces of completely normal vascular structure in between.

It is especially in sarcoidosis that we see the phenomenon of vascular engorgement due to enhanced blood flow in the inflammatory process and impairment of venous drainage due to compression of the vessels by enlargement of the hilar lymph nodes adjacent to the bronchial wall.

Most frequently, vascular engorgement is due to swelling of the lymph nodes by malignant infiltration. Especially if a lymph node is penetrating the bronchial wall or if lymphangic tumor is spreading submucosally, the blood vessels have an irregular corkscrew-like appearance and the mucosal tumor nodules also show an irregular structure with a tendency to confluence.

In chronic bronchitis the mucosal blood vessels become more prominent as the inflammatory reddening of the mucosa is much less conspicuous than in acute bronchitis and the mucosa due to chronic edema and scar formation becomes pale. In chronic bronchitis with a rise of pressure in the pulmonary circulation, marked distention of the bronchial blood vessels may develop because there are many anastomoses between the bronchial and pulmonary circulation. This is also true for chronic congestive cardiovascular disease, where in severe cases we even have seen bleeding bronchial mucosal varices that were treated by laser coagulation.

Acute bacterial infection in chronic bronchitis may cause further distention of blood vessels by an enhancement of blood flow, and additional inflammatory damage to the mucosal lining can lead to hemoptysis. This is a most common complication of bronchiectatic lung disease and may even be life threatening because in bronchiectasis the source of bleeding usually is the bronchial artery with high systemic pressure that may be distended to the caliber of a knitting needle due to the chronic inflammatory process.

The vascular pattern in chronic inflammation may also become fairly irregular, even forming small angiomatous structures. Rarely we have seen true spider nevi of the bronchial mucosa in liver cirrhosis. Hemangiomas in Osler's disease in contrast are smaller, more

evenly distributed, and regular (Plate 22). True submucosal hemangiomas of the bronchial wall mostly show a cushion-like appearance and especially in children one will often find further lesions on the body surface.

Lymphatic Vessels

In contrast to the blood vessels the lymphatics are not seen in the normal bronchial mucosa. Only if there is marked obstruction of the lymphatic drainage due to malignant invasion of lymph nodes, scar formation, or postoperative lymphedema after surgical interruption of lymph drainage are the mucosal lymphatic vessels prominent and visible. Due to the congestion by lymphatic edema, the mucosa may then be markedly swollen and show a cobblestone pattern on its surface. The distended lymph vessels then are seen as a fine whitish network between the polypoid formations (Plate 23). If enlarged lymph nodes adjacent to the bronchi are obstructing the lymphatic drainage, the distended larger mucosal lymph vessels may become visible as milky streaks, resembling "glass noodles," running parallel to the blood vessels.

Lymphatic cysts of the mucosa, as we have seen due to malignant occlusion of the lymph ducts in the mediastinum, never occur in benign inflammatory disease.

Foreign material, such as anthracotic pigment that is inhaled into the alveolar space, may be carried by the intra- and interlobular lymphatics toward the hilar lymph nodes and to the bronchial mucosa where it then is deposited and may become visible as black streaks, especially if the lymph vessels are further distended by lymphangic tumor invasion.

Integrity of the Mucosa

Ordinary acute viral and bacterial infections leave the macroscopic structure of the mucosa intact, showing only the secondary reactions described above. The inflammatory process is seen on the microscopic level only.

However, in some instances of nonspecific

viral and nonviral infections (*Mycoplasma pneumoniae* and some strains of streptococci among others), a granulomatous reaction can develop and may lead to polypoid and ulcerative formations (Plate 24). If this reaction is progressive and inflammatory destruction of the bronchial wall becomes invasive, severe scar formation may set in afterward during the process of healing with consecutive obliteration of the lumina, which may be one of the causes of bronchocentric granulomatosis. This kind of etiology, besides scar formation due to perforation of specific lymph nodes, is believed to be the most common cause of secondary isolated bronchiectasis in single lobes.

Rapid and extensive granuloma formation occurs after impaction of foreign bodies. If foreign bodies are not removed soon after accidental aspiration, inflammatory pseudotumors may develop with consecutive complete bronchial obstruction, resulting in chronic atelectasis or poststenotic bronchiectasis. The same can be true for penetrating lymph nodes in tuberculosis or anthracosilicosis.

Granulomatous inflammatory reaction is the typical form of bronchial involvement in sarcoidosis and tuberculosis. Whereas granulomata in sarcoidosis usually are clearly separated pinhead-sized glassy nodules, in mycobacterial disease there is a tendency to confluence of the lesions and superficial necrosis of the mucosa, showing the picture of specific bronchitis. This is either due to bronchogenic propagation from the lung or specific lymph node invasion.

Besides tuberculous inflammation, ulcerative bronchitis may also be found in bronchial involvement of Wegener's granulomatosis and other forms of vasculitis. The same will happen if pulmonary granulomata invade the adjacent bronchial wall. Biopsy will show granulomatous destruction of the blood vessels by histologic examination. Chronic relapsing polychondritis may have the appearance of ulcerative bronchitis, most frequently involving proximal parts of the airways as

well, especially the region of the cricoid cartilage, the arytenoids, and the cartilages of the nose (Plate 25) (19).

The most common cause of ulcerative bronchitis is malignant infiltration of the bronchial wall, which must always be excluded by sufficient biopsies.

The inflammatory process of common chronic bronchitis gradually affects the mucosa itself and the underlying structures of the bronchial wall. The recurrent infiltration by polymorphonuclear leukocytes with the liberation of destructive substances like elastase causes atrophy of the mucosa and distention of the underlying layers of elastic connective tissue leading to the morphologic changes described above. Due to the altered viscosity of the secretions, mucus is retained in the glands, which gradually leads to distention of orifices of the ducts that are seen as small holes in the mucosa, forming one of the distinctive features of chronic deforming bronchitis. Over years of duration the chronic inflammatory process also involves the deeper structures, thereby affecting the bronchial wall as a whole.

Integrity of the Bronchial Wall

In chronic nonspecific bronchitis the destruction of the elastic connective tissue of the bronchial wall gradually is followed by a loss of stability, leaving the larger airways even more susceptible to the damaging effects of excessive chronic recurring changes in pressure from attacks of coughing. The result of these ongoing combined destructive processes is a relaxation and prolapse of the paries membranaceus and chondromalacia of the larger airways. These cause further mechanical obstruction, thereby closing the vicious circle.

The most extensive kind of destruction in nonspecific chronic inflammation is found in bronchiectasis. Here the destruction of the bronchial wall leads to saccular excavations between the cartilages and membranaceous scars in between (Plate 26). The accumulation of the sticky secretions causes further distention. The most severe form of this disease can be seen in patients suffering from mucoviscidosis.

The deep-reaching destructive processes of chronic relapsing polychondritis have been mentioned above. Healing after immunosuppressive therapy may leave extensive scar formation and malacic stenosis after destruction of the supporting cartilages. Even more extensive scar formation is seen after inhalation injury due to toxic agents.

Similar reactions may also be seen in the long term after high-dose radiotherapy, especially after endobronchial brachytherapy. After this treatment chondromalacia and chondroradionecrosis may develop with sequestration of the necrotic cartilages. After 6 months or longer, extensive scar formation may result in strictures that are difficult to treat.

The same may also be true for the destruction of the bronchial wall by invasion of inflammatory lymph nodes. Tumor invasion will be the most common reason for the destruction of the bronchial wall. One of the specific features in contrast, however, is the rare involvement of the cartilages. Even in extensive and deep malignant necrosis the cartilaginous structures may frequently be seen fairly intact. To our knowledge there is no satisfactory explanation for this.

Because of the tremendous progress in intensive care procedures, many iatrogenic traumas are seen involving the tracheobronchial wall. Tracheomalacia and granulomatous inflammatory destruction at the site of mechanical alteration are the most serious sequelae of this kind of damage.

Involvement by Diseases of the Surrounding Structures

The central airways are surrounded by the complex anatomy of the organs in the mediastinum. A vast variety of pathologic processes of these organs may go along with involvement of the trachea and bronchi. In the newborn and young child, congenital malformations of the foregut and larger vessels are the most common causes of compression of the central airways. During later life, enlargement of the thymus, then the thyroid gland and the mediastinal lymph nodes due to their proximity to the central airways, is frequently followed by breathing impairment.

Lymph node invasion is never seen in ordinary sarcoidosis nor in anthracosis. Only if there is additional involvement in silicosis or tuberculosis will penetration or even perforation occur. If the lymph node is still covered by intact mucosa, the typical bronchial pseudotumor is formed that macroscopically cannot be differentiated from malignant disease. Calcified specific lymph nodes that are not evacuated after perforation will remain inside the bronchial lumen as broncholiths and cause postobstructive bronchiectasis (Figure 10.5) (20).

The most frequent penetration of lymph nodes is caused by malignant infiltration. Endoscopically it can be difficult to assess the depth of penetration from the outer layers of the bronchial wall. We currently are investigating whether endobronchial sonography in this situation is helpful in guiding the needle for transbronchial needle biopsy (Figure 10.6), so that in the future it may become a routine procedure in staging of bronchial carcinoma.

Deviation of the spinal column in severe kyphoscoliosis or Bechterew's disease as well as pectus excavatum can involve the trachea by compression or distortion. Differentiation from impression by aortic aneurysms is easy as in the latter pulsation of the mass is obvious. Only in small children are the airways still so soft that it may be difficult to discriminate intrinsic instability from extrinsic compression. Also in this situation, according to our preliminary experience, endobronchial ultrasonography may be helpful.

All pathologic processes causing deviation or enlargement of the mediastinal organs, such

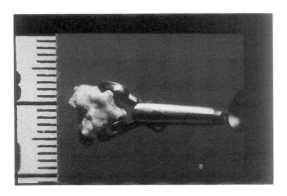

Figure 10.5. Broncholith. This calcified formerly lymphatic tissue was removed from the intermediate bronchus of an elderly lady who suffered from repeat postobstructive pneumonia of the lower lobe, which had been caused by mechanical obstruction. On the chest x-ray an old primary complex was noted.

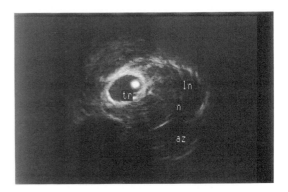

Figure 10.6. Sonography of paratracheal mass. The ultrasonic probe of 12 MHz is placed to the right wall of the trachea (tr). Adjacent is a large para tracheal, not very echodense mass, caused by enlarged lymph nodes (ln). The mass has been punctured by a Wang needle for asservation of cytology and the exact position is documented by the ultrasonic probe (bright streak pointing toward n).

as lymphomas, thymomas, cardial distention or pericardial effusions, esophageal diverticula and tumors, mesothelioma, or pleural effusions, may cause extrinsic compression of the central airways.

Clinical Context

Because the repertoire of reactions to different noxes is limited, the diagnosis is not always clear from the endoscopic aspect by itself. Before any final conclusions can be drawn, all the clinical and technical information achieved by anamnesis, physical examination, and technical investigations before and after the endoscopic examination must be considered. In the whole context of this information the diagnosis is finally established.

Findings in Airway Lesions

Upper Airways

Although the upper airways, nose and nasopharynx, are not exactly the domain of bronchoscopy, one always should keep in mind

that they are an integral part of the airway system. Because diseases of the airways frequently are systemic, involvement of the upper airways should always be considered. This especially applies to systemic diseases such as Wegener's granulomatosis, chronic relapsing polychondritis, and bronchiectasis in Kartagener's syndrome. Not uncommonly malignant tumors of the upper and the lower airways are associated because the impact of noxes, especially cigarette smoke, is affecting both. Organic obstruction of the upper airways due to conchal hyperplasia or deformation and functional obstruction like airway collapse in sleep apnea may cause secondary afflictions of the bronchial system such as chronic inflammation or aspiration pneumonia. A source of hemoptysis should always be excluded in the upper airways if it cannot be found in the tracheobronchial system or in the lung itself.

Larynx

The larynx is the most complicated and sensitive structure of the tracheobronchial system and thorough knowledge of its anatomic and functional properties is essential for diagnosis (21).

The most frequent functional disorder to be diagnosed is paralysis of a vocal cord, which is mainly caused by compression or destruction of the recurrent laryngeal nerve due to malignancies either of the thyroid gland or more frequently by bronchial carcinomas as a sign of tumor spreading to the aortopulmonary window beneath the aortic arch. Secondary paralysis after resection of goiter or bronchial carcinoma with extensive lymph node resection is not uncommon. For accurate assessment of laryngeal function visualization under local anesthesia is required. In small children this can easily be performed under sedation, for example, by propofol, and additional local anesthesia while breathing spontaneously.

In early infancy, developmental malformations or delay of maturation are frequent causes of breathing problems. Whereas instability of the cartilaginous support of the epiglottis and the cricoid are frequent especially in the premature infant, laryngeal clefts or fistulas between the pharynx and esophagus are comparatively rare. Hemangiomatous obstructing lesions in the larynx may be found in children with cutaneous hemangiomas. Spontaneous resolution is seen frequently, but in severe cases laser destruction may give immediate relief.

In later childhood and in the adult, traumatic and inflammatory lesions are the most frequent besides neoplasias. Since diphtheria has become a rare disease, it is unspecific bacterial or viral infection, causing even necrotic inflammation of the larynx, that may result in membranes and synechiae after resolution. Specific tuberculous inflammation of the vocal cords with its typical nodular aspect has become extremely rare in our patients. Chronic inflammatory processes like relapsing polychondritis or Wegener's granulomatosis involve the mucosa as well as the cartilages and result in severe stenotic scars if not treated aggressively from the beginning (Plate 27). Ankylosis of the arytenoid cartilages due to inflammatory processes at the joints may be diagnosed by gently moving the cartilages with a forceps (Plate 28).

In the larynx the most frequent benign neoplasias are cysts of the epiglottis and the vocal cords. In the latter, differentiation from chronic Reinke's edema may be difficult and is only possibly by biopsy. Polyps due to strain or postintubational trauma have a smooth and shiny surface as compared to the more villous aspect of papillomas (Plate 29).

Primary malignant neoplasias of the larynx frequently arise from the vocal cords. If the lumen is compromised by extensive tumor growth, passage with the endoscope may result in severe swelling with imminent suffocation. Thus, preparations for an emergency intubation should always be made. Because treatment will usually be performed by the laryngologist, exact estimation of the extent of these tumors will not be necessary for the bronchoscopist. Synchronous tumors of the lower airways are not uncommon, so thorough examination of these should be performed.

Secondary malignancies mostly arise from direct invasion of hypopharyngeal carcinomas, of neoplasias of the thyroid gland, or of metastatic lymph node involvement.

The larynx is sensitive to trauma. Today iatrogenic trauma during resuscitation and intensive care is much more frequent than lesions by accidents. Due to improved materials for intubation and improved methods of intensive care therapy, lesions are no longer induced as easily as formerly. But trauma due to intubation in an emergency situation still is common. Damage will mostly hurt the subglottic area at the level of the cricoid cartilage because it is the narrowest part for intubation. Lesions or damage due to prolonged intubation are hard to treat because they are combined lesions of endoluminal granulomata and invasive inflammatory reactions with chondromalacia.

Trachea

Although the trachea and its bifurcation are part of the central airways, it assumes a special role in airway pathology. Owing to its position and structure, it is subject to major functional and organic changes under physiologic and pathologic conditions. Because it is a single organ, vital to survival, severe impairment of air passage at this level will always be life threatening. The position of the trachea makes it especially prone to involvement in diseases of adjacent organs such as the esophagus, the great vessels, the heart, thymus, lymph nodes, and spinal column. Owing to its both intrathoracic and extrathoracic position, it is subject to considerable changes in pressure, up to 300 mm Hg, causing major changes in diameter. During forced respiratory maneuvers it also may undergo a change of several centimeters in length. These high functional demands are met by its intricate structure, combining rigid and flexible structures in the most delicate arrangement.

Functional impairment of the trachea is mostly due to loss of its stability. As the mechanical stability gradually develops during maturation in early infancy, comparative instability with nearly total collapse during coughing is almost physiologic in this age. Only if the collapse persists during normal ventilation, does prolonged intubation using atraumatic material become necessary. In the adult instability most frequently is caused by chronic inflammatory damage. Destruction of the collagen fibers by elastase of polymorphonuclear leukocytes and weakening of the cartilages by chronic coughing finally results in total collapse of the stabilizing tracheal structures (Plate 30).

Congenital malformations will usually become symptomatic during childhood. The most frequent is esophagotracheal fistula causing chronic aspiration. In our experience, tracheal stenosis due to complete rings of the tracheal cartilages is a rare event. Because in early childhood the cartilages are almost completely round in shape and the dorsal ends almost meet dorsally in the midline, especially during forced respiratory maneuvers and coughing, it may be easily misdiagnosed. Surgical repair by splinting and insertion of cartilaginous or pericardial flaps is a risky procedure; therefore, the diagnosis should be established by further radiologic studies before taking any such measures. Aberrant tracheal bronchi usually cause problems only if they are combined with malformations of the cartilages and additional tracheal stenosis or if narrowing of their ostia interferes with ventilation or drainage of the secretions.

Viral and bacterial inflammation is the most common disease of the airways and usually will not be an indication for bronchoscopy. Sometimes, however, staphylococci or other bacterial infections result in ulcerative lesions and if unrecognized may cause severe scar formation and tracheal stenosis. Chronic inflammatory processes, caused by immunologic disorders such as Wegener's granulomatosis, chronic relapsing polychondritis, and rheumatoid arthritis involve the deeper structures, especially the cartilages, eventually resulting in strictures and instability. Diagnosis frequently can only be established by the clinical synopsis and not only by histologic examination of biopsy specimens. Inflammatory granulomatous reactions or invasion by specific lymph nodes may appear as pseudotumors and can only be proven as of benign origin by biopsy.

True benign neoplasias of the trachea are not frequent. Whether tracheopathia chondrosive osteoplastica is regarded as true neoplasia or an inflammatory reaction is still debated. By its typical macroscopic appearance and hard consistency, it may be diagnosed easily. As in the larynx, polypoid lesions such as fibrolipomas may be distinguished from papillomas due to viral infection by their smooth shiny surface.

The most common primary malignant neoplasias of the trachea are squamous cell carcinomas and adenoid cystic carcinomas. The latter are remarkable because they commonly grow slowly and metastasize at late stages only. There are two types of this tumor, the one localized in a polypoid fashion (Plate 31), the other expanding submucosally over a large portion of the central airways so that its boundaries are not clear by macroscopic appearance.

Much more frequent is secondary neoplastic involvement of the trachea. Because the trachea is adjacent to many structures in the mediastinum, it may easily become involved in malignancies of the neighboring organs such as neoplasias of the thyroid gland, the esophagus, the thymus, or the mediastinal lymph nodes. Direct infiltration by bronchial carcinomas or invasion of lymph node metastases as well as continuous lymphangic tumor spreading will usually represent a barrier to radical surgical therapy that can only rarely be overcome. Endotracheal metastasis in the mucosa from distal endobronchial carcinomas is an extremely rare event, which in our opinion is an argument against the induction of metastatic tumor implantation by bronchoscopic biopsy, the theoretical risk of which is surely overcome by the advantage of establishing a definitive diagnosis for further treatment.

Frequently patients with obstructing tracheal tumors present as emergency cases. Even high-grade stenosis of the trachea may remain unrecognized for a long time, or misinterpreted as "asthma," because the radiographic density of the surrounding structures of the mediastinum does not provide a good contrast of the trachea on the routine chest radiograph, and tomography of the trachea may be obscured by sectional artefacts. Stenosis may be compensated down to a minimal lumen of 3 to 5 mm until acute obstruction is caused by retention of sticky secretions. For this reason bronchoscopy is the principal diagnostic tool in this area of the airways and should always

be considered in otherwise unexplained symptoms as stated above (22).

Because the trachea is surrounded by many organs in its extrathoracic and intrathoracic course, not being covered by protecting tissues, it is easily afflicted by pathologic processes of these surrounding structures. Processes causing an increase in volume or deviation will involve the trachea frequently because due to the narrow space it may not easily give way. In its cervical portion one of the most frequent causes is enlargement of the thyroid gland, which if not treated effectively may eventually lead to almost total compression and asphyxia. And in long-standing compression simple surgical removal is no longer sufficient because tracheomalacia requires segmental tracheal resection as well. The compression by goiters may reach deep into the mediastinum, almost down to the carinal region.

In the upper and middle mediastinum the trachea may even more easily be compressed; its confinement between the spinal column and the sternum means giving way is more difficult. In contrast to displacement by deviations of the spinal column and pectus excavatum, which rarely cause problems of the central airways, abnormal vessels or enlargement of the heart are common causes of displacement and even obstruction. But the most frequent causes are tumors of the esophagus, the thymus gland, or the mediastinal lymph nodes. The most devastating affliction is esophagotracheal fistula due to necrotic invading tumors, the treatment of which is difficult.

Trauma is inflicted to the trachea as easily as to the larynx. The cartilages are extremely sensitive to mechanical (intubation trauma), thermal (laser treatment), or radiation trauma. Even if primarily only the mucosa is damaged, secondary inflammatory reactions frequently involve the deeper submucosal layers and the cartilages as well. This will lead to chronification of the process, which eventually will result in a combined stenosis due to malacia and strictures. The true extent of these lesions will always be larger than it appears by endoscopy.

For assessment of operability, exact measurement of the extent of a tumor or traumatic lesion is essential. Distances to the main carina, to the cricoid cartilage, and the vocal cords as well as total extent of the lesion must be measured exactly to calculate the possibility of segmental resection. The rigid or flexible endoscope is passed down to the carina and during successive withdrawal the respective distances may easily be measured by marking the level of the teeth (fiberscope) or the proximal end of the bronchoscope (on the rigid optic). Diameters of the airways may be calculated by the diameter of the bronchoscope that can be introduced through a stenosis or by placing an opened forceps close to the lesion and measuring the distance of the cups. For the exact intraoperative assessment of the tracheal segment to be resected we found marking of the proximal and distal end by needles under bronchoscopic control useful (Plate 32).

Bronchi

Localized functional disorders of the bronchi obviously will cause less severe symptoms than is the case in the larynx or trachea. Bronchial collapse will cause segmental or lobar symptoms of disturbances in ventilation such as atelectasis or overinflation.

Acute nonspecific inflammation due to viral and bacterial agents is the most common affliction of the airways but will rarely be an indication for bronchoscopy. The mucosa is diffusely reddened, sometimes even hemorrhagic, and heavy more or less purulent secretions are seen. The most frequent community-acquired bacterial agents found in our probes are nonhemolytic streptococci, *Diplococcus pneumoniae, Hemophilus influenzae,* and in some populations also *Legionella* species, whereas in nosocomial infections staphylococci, *Pseudomonas* species,

Klebsiella, and enterococci are the most frequent pathogens.

Several sampling devices have been proposed that are supposed to avoid contamination. Results of accuracy are inconclusive so far. In a comparative study in 60 patients we were not able to demonstrate a significant difference in the results of bacteriologic sampling, whether we used different devices of protected microbiology brushes or simple suction through the biopsy channel of the fiberscope. The negative influence of some local anesthetics on bacterial growth, though, must be considered. In special cases, as in the immunocompromised host, the additional cost of these devices may be worthwhile to establish a definite diagnosis. The value of special laboratory tests such as the polymerase chain reaction for the detection of *Mycobacteria tuberculosis* or cytomegalovirus has yet to be established.

Much more frequently we will be confronted with diagnosis of persistent or recurrent purulent infections due to resistant bacteria or to abnormalities such as localized bronchiectases or abscesses. In these cases besides establishing a diagnosis of the pathologic agent, exact description of the anatomic cause and extent of the lesion is necessary. This is one of the comparatively rare cases besides stenoses, cysts, or fistulas where bronchography is still needed in addition to conventional radiologic analysis and CT scanning. In localized bronchiectasis or cavitational lesions the colonization by fungi, mostly *Aspergillus fumigatus,* has always to be considered, which may cause asthmatic symptoms such as allergic bronchopulmonary aspergillosis.

The most common inflammatory finding is chronic bronchitis mostly caused by chronic cigarette smoke inhalation. The macroscopic aspect and sequelae of this disease have been described in some detail above.

The most common specific form of inflammation of the bronchi today is sarcoidosis. Diagnosis is easy if the typical granulomas are seen (Plate 33), especially if further symptoms such as enlargement of the parabronchial lymph nodes are present and if the radiologic picture is consistent with the diagnosis. But positive endobronchial histology will also be achieved in up to 20% to 30% of the cases even if no granulomas are visible at bronchoscopy. The most reliable histologic confirmation, however, will be found by transbronchial biopsy, the diagnostic yield of which in our experience is over 95% even if granulomatous intrapulmonary lesions are not seen radiologically.

Regarding technique of transbronchial biopsy in disseminated interstitial lung diseases, we could find a significant improvement in diagnostic results if we performed more than 8 biopsies (usually 10 to 15) from different parts of one lung and if we avoided damage to the biopsy specimens by not pulling the biopsy forceps through the biopsy channel of the fiberscope. Instead we remove the fiberscope completely, leaving the tip of the forceps outside in front of the tip of the endoscope for recovery of the biopsy specimen. Irritation by frequent passage of the airways under local anesthesia can be avoided if a tube is inserted over the bronchoscope. Complications in our series are comparatively rare (2.5% of pneumothoraces, no severe bleeding) although in disseminated interstitial lung disease we normally do not apply fluoroscopy and we routinely use large forceps to obtain large biopsy specimens.

Primary specific tuberculous bronchitis due to bronchogenic spreading has become comparatively rare. Specific ulcerating tuberculous bronchitis is mostly caused by penetration of lymph nodes. All stages from invasion of the outer layers of the bronchial wall with still intact mucosal covering to intramural penetration and finally ulceration and resulting scar formation may be seen if the disease is taking its spontaneous course.

If calcified specific lymph nodes are penetrating into the bronchi and if the masses are not evacuated due to bronchial stenosis, broncholiths will be seen, which frequently cause postobstructive atelectasis or bronchiectasis. Occlusion by specific lymph nodes has been the most frequent reason for the so-called middle lobe syndrome before the epidemic progress of bronchogenic carcinoma.

Immunologic inflammatory processes such as vasculitis in Wegener's granulomatosis or in chronic relapsing polychondritis are comparatively rare and may only be discerned by histology. Whether tumor-like bronchial amyloidosis is due to chronic inflammatory processes or whether it is caused by the production and deposition of pathologic immunoglobulins in the bronchial mucosa is still debated (Plate 34).

True benign neoplasias of the bronchi are rare as compared to primary bronchial carcinoma. Metaplastic polyps and chondrofibrolipomas are the most frequent, whereas true benign adenomas are rare. Papillomas of the tracheobronchial tree may be due to chronic infection by papilloma viruses type 11 and 16 and there are descriptions of malignant transformation as we have also seen ourselves. The so-called micropapillomatosis may be regarded as a precancerous lesion.

Against frequent common opinion, carcinoid tumors have to be regarded and treated as true malignancies because they show all signs of malignant growth such as infiltration, recurrence after local treatment, and metastasis. We have seen metastatic lymph node skipping in very young adults as well as late distant mucosal metastases and local recurrences after insufficient local treatment of these tumors (Plate 35).

The most common bronchial neoplasia is primary bronchial carcinoma. The prognosis of bronchial carcinomas is influenced by its histologic differentiation and by its extent, which are the main influences on therapeutic procedures. By bronchoscopy we are able to give the decisive answers to these questions in over 80% of all cases. In endobronchially visible tumors the accuracy of endoscopic staging is about 95%, which makes bronchoscopy the most important diagnostic procedure. For the bronchoscopist there exist clear definitions of the TNM classification (Tables 10.3 and 10.4) regarding extension of the primary tumor, lymph node involvement, and metastases (17).

Endoscopists must be completely familiar with the TNM staging criteria and all macroscopic aspects of lung tumors and with all conventional and surgical therapeutic options. They should be acquainted with the surgical resection procedures to ascertain bioptically that prospective lines of resection are free of

Table 10.3. TNM Classification of the Primary Tumor in Non–Small-Cell Carcinoma Using Bronchoscopy

T1: The tumor is not visible endoscopically or has not yet extended proximally beyond the respective lobar bronchus.

T2: The main bronchus is involved but the lesion is still at least 2 cm distal to the main carina.

T3: The tumor is within 2 cm distance to but it has not yet involved the main carina; or there is atelectasis or obstructive inflammation of one entire lung.

T4: The main carina is involved or the tumor is even infiltrating the trachea.

Table 10.4. TNM Classification of Lymph Node Involvement and Metastasis of Non–Small-Cell Carcinoma Using Bronchoscopy

N1: Involvement of the ipsilateral peribronchial and hilar lymph nodes

N2: Involvement of the ipsilateral mediastinal and/or subcarinal lymph nodes

N3: Extension of tumor to the contralateral hilar or mediastinal lymph nodes

M1: Intrabronchial or intrapulmonary metastases or lymphangiosis carcinomatosa of the lung

tumor growth before operation. Routine biopsy from macroscopically unsuspect regions in a study at our institution did not yield enough positive results to advise it as a standard procedure.

Bronchoscopists must be familiar with the appearance of bronchial carcinoma from its earliest manifestations to its latest stages and be aware of all the complications that may be caused by the primary tumor and its metastases. They must be familiar with indirect signs of spreading of the neoplasia and with routes of hematogenous and lymphogenous metastatic dissemination. They must know about typical surgical procedures and their endoscopic appearance to assess the postoperative result and to recognize and prevent imminent complications. Results and complications of conservative therapy have to be distinguished from tumor relapse. Lastly, a large number of patients suffering from severe complications of advanced tumor growth may benefit from palliative therapeutic bronchoscopic procedures.

Secondary neoplasias involving the lung and bronchi have become a field of special interest in pulmonary medicine because the therapeutic approach has changed tremendously during the last 10 years. It has been shown that surgical resection of isolated pulmonary metastases of tumors from other organs showed an even better prognosis than many cases of primary lung carcinoma. This has been proved especially when they could be successfully treated in a multidisciplinary concept of preoperative chemotherapy, operation, and, if necessary, postoperative chemotherapeutic consolidation. In some tumors, such as metastasizing testicular tumors or osteosarcoma, 5-year survival rates of more than 50% could be achieved. Because involvement of the central bronchial system in these cases means a much more extensive resection of lung parenchyma, preoperative bronchoscopy is indispensable (Plate 36).

In metastases of a primary tumor of unknown localization and unknown histology, bronchoscopic biopsy may give the decisive histologic information for the original tumor. Involvement of the central airways or the lung itself in systemic malignancies as lymphomas will have an enormous influence on staging and therapy. Every patient with suspicion of involvement of the airways or lung should undergo bronchoscopy in these cases.

Because the sensitivity of clinical assessment of hilar or mediastinal lymph node involvement in malignancies by conventional radiology, CT scan, or MRI still is not better than 60%, we are currently investigating the potentials of external mediastinal and endobronchial ultrasonography. Despite encouraging preliminary results, it is still too early to draw final conclusions on the additional benefit of these procedures (see Figure 10.6).

Because the bronchi are deep inside the thorax, they are protected much better against traumatic lesions from internal iatrogenic or accidental external impact than are the larynx and trachea. Unrecognized damage to the central airways such as bronchial rupture can cause devastating secondary complications; therefore, early meticulous bronchoscopic examination should exclude such damage in every patient with severe thoracic trauma. This may be difficult because signs of bronchial rupture or perforation may be discreet, especially if the rupture has occurred submucosally and severe mucosal swelling with obliteration of vision has set in.

Aspiration of foreign bodies is still frequently unrecognized and extraction delayed for weeks and months when endoscopic removal is much more complicated than early after the accident. This is especially the case in small children who cannot tell their history. Early sequelae are marked mucosal swelling and reddening with retention and bacterial infection of secretions. Later granuloma formation and in severe scar formation with post-obstructive atelectasis, bronchiectasis, or abscess formation will result.

Summary

This concise overview on the aspects of bronchoscopy in airway lesions should demonstrate the ever-growing potential and central diagnostic position of bronchoscopy in pulmonary medicine. Far from being at its limits, by continuous introduction of new methods and tools for application, bronchoscopy seems just at the verge of a renaissance in its utility. This is clearly shown by the number of procedures being done throughout the world and also at our institution. We perform almost 5000 procedures annually and the numbers are increasing. This is especially due to the progress in diagnostic and therapeutic procedures introduced during the last 5 years. The growing interest shown by specialists of other disciplines, such as internists, anesthesiologists, surgeons, and pediatricians, expressed in the growing number of participants in training courses and the growing demand for textbooks, is encouraging enough to look for further applications of this already 100-year-old but still young procedure.

REFERENCES

1. Holmgren G. In: Killian H. Gustav Killian. Sein Leben—Sein Werk. Remscheid-Lennep: Dustri-Verlag, 1958:250–254.
2. Sylvester D. Magritte. The silence of the world. New York: The Menil Foundation. Harry N. Abrams, Inc., 1992:24.
3. Killian G. Über directe Bronchoskopie. MMW 1898;27:844–847.
4. Becker HD, Kayser K, Schulz V, Tuengerthal S, Vollhaber H-H. Atlas of bronchoscopy. Philadelphia, Hamilton: BC Decker, 1991.
5. Prakash UBS, Cortese DA, Stubbs SE. Technical solutions to common problems in bronchoscopy. In: Prakash UBS, ed. Bron-

choscopy. New York: Raven Press, 1994: 111–133.

6. Lukomsky GI, Ovchinnikov AA, Bilal A. Complications of bronchoscopy. Comparison of rigid bronchoscopy under general anesthesia and flexible fiberoptic bronchoscopy under topical anesthesia. Chest 1981;79: 316–321.

7. Becker HD, di Rienzo G. Anatomical considerations in bronchoscopy. Atti I. Corso internationale di bronchoscopia. Editrice Roma, 1990:13–18.

8. Thal W. Kinderbronchologie. Leipzig: JA Barth, 1972:93–105.

9. Clements BS, Warner JO. Pulmonary sequestration and related congenital bronchopulmonary-vascular malformations: nomenclature and classification based on anatomical and embryonical considerations. Thorax 1987;42:401–408.

10. Holder TM, Ashcraft KW, Sharp RJ, Armoury RA. Care of infants with esophageal atresia, tracheoesophageal fistula and associated anomalies. J Thorac Cardio-vasc Surg 1987;94:828–835.

11. Schäfers HJ, Luhmer I, Oehlert H. Pulmonary venous obstruction following repair of total anomalous pulmonary venous drainage. Ann Thorac Surg 1987;43: 432–434.

12. Bülzebruck H, Bopp R, Drings P, et al. New aspects in the staging of lung cancer. Cancer 1992;70:1102–1110.

13. Becker HD, di Rienzo G. On semiotics in bronchology. The interpretation of bronchoscopic findings by the example of inflamma-

tory diseases. Atti I. Corso internationale di bronchoscopia. Editrice Roma, 1990:58–64.

14. Katzenstein AA, Liebow A, Freidmann P. Bronchocentric granulomatosis, mucoid impaction and hypersensitivity reactions to fungi. Am Rev Respir Dis 1975;11:497–537.

15. Torres A. Accuracy of diagnostic tools for the management of nosocomial respiratory infections in mechanically ventilated patients. Eur Respir J 1991;4:1010–1019.

16. Klech H, Hutter C, Costabel U, eds. Clinical guidelines and indications for bronchoalveolar lavage (BAL). Eur Respir Rev 1992;2:8.

17. Cahill BC, Ingbar DH. Massive hemoptysis. Assessment and management. Clin Chest Med 1994;15:147–168.

18. Murata K, Ito H, Todo G, Kanaoka M, Furita M, Torizuka K. Bronchial venous plexus and its communication with pulmonary circulation. Invest Radiol 1986;21:24–30.

19. Dolan D, Lemmon GB Jr, Teitelbaum SL. Relapsing polychondritis. Analytical literature review and studies of pathogenesis. Am J Med 1966;41:285–298.

20. Igoe D, Lynch V, McNicholas WT. Broncholithiasis: bronchoscopic vs. surgical management. Respir Med 1990;84:163–165.

21. Hanafee WH, Ward PH. The larynx. Radiology, surgery, pathology. New York: Thieme Medical Publishers, 1990.

22. Becker HD, Blersch E, Vogt-Moykopf I. Urgent treatment of tracheal obstruction. In: Grillo H, Eschapasse H, eds. Major challenges. International trends in general thoracic surgery, vol. 2. Philadelphia, London, Toronto: WB Saunders, 1987.

Bronchoalveolar Lavage | 11

Richard A. Helmers and Gary W. Hunninghake

Although the technique of washing the lung with physiologic saline to remove accumulated material and cells from the air space has been used therapeutically for many years, it was with the advent of widespread use of flexible fiberoptic bronchoscopy (FOB) in the 1970s that instillation of smaller quantities of saline directly into the distal airways and recovering the aspirate for analysis—bronchoalveolar lavage (BAL)—became an important clinical and investigational tool (1,2). BAL allows the recovery of both cellular and noncellular components from the epithelial surface of the lower respiratory tract and differs significantly from bronchial washings, which refer to aspiration of either secretions or small amounts of instilled saline from the large airways (3). The conceptual basis of BAL is that cells and noncellular components present on the epithelial surface of the alveoli are representative of the inflammatory and immune system of the entire lower respiratory tract. In addition, BAL allows sampling of various components of the inflammatory and immune system at their site of action (1,4). BAL has become a widely used technique applied to virtually every area of pulmonary medicine.

Techniques and Processing

The techniques for performing BAL and processing the fluid are not standardized from one institution to another, which may account, in part, for the variability in reported results. The techniques we describe are identical to our routine bronchoscopies, with the exception that the lavage procedure is also performed. BAL is performed after routine inspection/ examination of the tracheobronchial tree and before biopsy or brushings to avoid contamination of the recovered fluid with excess blood, which would alter the concentrations of cellular and noncellular components. The suction channel of the bronchoscope is thoroughly rinsed with saline, the suction trap is changed, and the tip of the bronchoscope is advanced distally until it is wedged into a subsegmental bronchus, usually at the level of the fourth to fifth branching. Care should be taken to avoid trauma and coughing because these may lead to excessive contamination of the recovered fluid with mucus and blood (5). Passing the bronchoscope through a previously inserted endotracheal tube has been shown to reduce oropharyngeal contamination when BAL specimens are cultured (6). There are no absolute contraindications to BAL, but one should be aware of high-risk situations and *relative* contraindications. These include an uncooperative patient, a forced expiratory volume in one second (FEV_1) less than 800 to 1000 cc, moderate to severe asthma, hypercapnia, hypoxemia uncorrected to an oxygen saturation of 90% with supplemental oxygen, serious cardiac dysrhythmia, myocardial infarction within 6 weeks, uncorrected bleeding diathesis, and hemodynamic instability (3).

In most cases, both segments of the lingula

A modified version of this chapter originally appeare in Bronchoscopy, edited by U.B.S. Prakash. Raven Pres 1994. Reprinted by permis sion of The Mayo Foundati and the right middle lobe are routinely lavaged and analyzed separately. Other lobes may be lavaged (especially if radiographically abnormal); however, because of the upper lobe bronchial anatomy, returns from lavage of the upper lobe are significantly less than that from the middle or lower lobes (1,2,7).

In normal patients, the cell counts, cell differentials, and lavage proteins are similar between the right middle lobe, lingula, and lower lobes (7). However, when localized disease is apparent radiographically, lavage should be carried out in multiple sites, including the area with focal radiographic abnormalities, because the BAL results may be most abnormal from these areas (4,8,9). There is not uniform agreement regarding interlobar variation in BAL results when the chest radiograph shows diffuse changes and, consequently, we routinely lavage both the right middle lobe and lingula. Garcia and colleagues (10) found significant interlobar variation in BAL cell differentials between the right middle lobe and lingula obtained from patients with idiopathic pulmonary fibrosis (IPF), pulmonary fibrosis associated with collagen vascular disease (PF-CVD), and in a small group of mixed interstitial lung disorders; patients with sarcoidosis, however, had excellent bilobar agreement. In this study, the chest x-ray was markedly insensitive to lavage interlobar variation (10). In contrast, a study in our laboratory (11) found no significant differences in BAL cell concentration or differential from side to side (right middle lobe versus lingula) in patients with sarcoidosis, IPF, or PF-CVD with nonfocal disease on chest radiograph.

In an average-sized person at total lung capacity (TLC), the typical lavaged zone represents about 165 mL and the residual volume of this zone is approximately 45 mL (12). It might be argued that pockets of residual gas may prevent BAL fluid from reaching some alveolar spaces and that BAL, in these sites, might be more bronchiolar than alveolar; however, animal studies have shown that, although lavage of an air-free lobe recovers a larger number of cells than an air-filled lobe, the cell differentials remain the same (13).

After the bronchoscope is wedged, 20 mL of 0.9% sterile saline, preferably at 37°C, is infused with a syringe with or without a three-way stopcock into the suction port of the bronchoscope. The fluid is then removed from the lung by the use of 50 to 80 mm Hg of negative pressure from a usual suction apparatus and collected into 50- to 100-mL specimen traps. Prewarming the lavage fluid to 37°C may help prevent coughing and bronchospasm, especially in patients with hyperresponsive airways, and may increase fluid recovery and cellular yield in comparison to instillations of fluid at room temperature (3,5,9). The traps should be made of material to which the cells are poorly adherent, such as polyethylene or polycarbonate; unsiliconized glass materials should not be used (5,9). The lavage procedure is repeated a total of five times in each site for a total of 100 mL per site. One should instruct the patient to inhale and exhale deeply during fluid aspiration and maintain the suction channel of the bronchoscope in the center of the airway lumen. If an adequate "wedge" is maintained throughout the lavage, the patient should not experience cough because the lavage fluid should not "leak" proximal to the tip of the bronchoscope (4). Levels of applied suction greater than 50 to 80 mm Hg may cause distal airway collapse and lead to inadequate returns. Both during and for 2 hours following the BAL, all patients are routinely administered 2 L nasal oxygen (12).

The lavage of a normal adult with 100 mL saline yields 40 to 60 mL fluid containing 5 to 10 x 10^6 cells and 1 to 10 mg protein (1). It has been estimated that a 100-mL lavage of a bronchial subsegment represents the sampling of about 10^6 alveoli (2,12). Lavage results are, in general, not considered valid if: 1) the patient has purulent secretions in the airways, 2) the bronchoscope is not maintained in the "wedge" position during the lavage procedure, and 3) the volume of fluid recovery is less than 40% of the volume infused (4). In general, 40% to 60% of the infused volume is recovered and cell viability is generally greater than 80% (1,7,14). In patients with loss of elastic recoil, the recovery of fluid is usually less since the bronchial walls collapse when suction is applied (1,2,5). In general, the volume of fluid recovered decreases also with advancing age and with cigarette smoking; at least in normals, the percent of fluid recovery is greatest in young never-smokers (15). It has also been noted that the percentage of fluid recovered and total cell counts are significantly lower if the procedure is performed using general anesthesia versus local/topical anesthesia; the cell concentrations, proportions of various cells, and cell viability are not affected (16). Excessive lidocaine should be avoided primarily because of the theoretical argument that it may impair the in vitro function of the inflammatory and immune effector cells recovered; it is thought, however, that this effect is reversible by cell washing (17–19). BAL specimens have also been shown to *not* contain lidocaine concentrations high enough to inhibit the culture and growth of pathogens that may be inhibited by lidocaine (20).

The volume of fluid infused is an important variable between institutions. Often larger amounts of lavage fluid (up to 240 to 300 mL) have been used, particularly if a larger number of inflammatory cells is required; but it is generally agreed increased patient morbidity may result, particularly local atelectasis and transient fevers (1,4,5). Smaller amounts of BAL fluid, in contrast, may sample only small bronchi or relatively few alveoli. Kelly and colleagues (21), by a digital subtraction imaging technique in normal volunteers, demonstrated that lavage volumes of 60 mL sampled only proximal airways, but that a volume of 120 mL instilled into a single segment appeared to perfuse the entire segment (including distal airways and alveoli) and aspiration of this volume produced fluid movement from within the

whole of the segment. Similar preliminary observations by magnetic resonance imaging (MRI) in patients with interstitial lung disease (after lavage with 100 mL saline instilled into either the right middle lobe or lingula) support the concept that volumes of 100 to 120 mL adequately sample the alveolar surface (22). We examined 55 patients with nonfocal interstitial lung disease (ILD) and performed both a 100-mL (20 cc × 5) and a 250-mL (50 cc × 5) BAL in the same lobe of the lung along with a 100 mL BAL on the contralateral side (11). Although the percent fluid return was slightly higher with the large-volume BAL, there were no significant differences in cell differentials or cell concentrations between 100-mL and 250-mL BAL. For clinical purposes, then, a small-volume BAL of 100 to 150 mL is preferable because large-volume lavage may be associated with increased morbidity (see below).

Several investigators have evaluated cell differentials on sequential aliquots of recovered lavage fluid and have concluded that the initial aliquot (if the volume of infused fluid is small, i.e., 20 mL) is different from subsequent aliquots in that the initial aliquot is likely to recover cells and proteins from distal bronchi and not alveoli (5,23–26). For this reason, some suggest the return from the initial aliquot should be discarded. Merrill and associates (27) evaluated protein recovery in successive aliquots of BAL fluid in normals and noted a decrease in the absolute concentration of all proteins in serial aliquots; however, the ratio of various proteins to an albumin standard did not change. They concluded that lung proteins are efficiently and homogeneously sampled with 100 mL of lavage instillate. Rennard and colleagues (26) processed the first 20-mL aliquot ("bronchial") separately from the return of the subsequent four 20-mL aliquots ("alveolar") in 109 patients and 18 normals. They found that pooling the "bronchial" and "alveolar" material resulted in a sample that was mostly "alveolar" and concluded it is unlikely that including the first aliquot, which represents 10% or less of the total recovered cells, will affect the cellular analysis in the absence of significant inflammation. But if a patient has obvious airway inflammation, the analysis may be heavily influenced by bronchial airway secretions.

The problem of data standardization is also apparent with the quantification in lavage fluid of soluble, noncellular constituents of the lower respiratory tract such as proteins, lipids, and carbohydrates. The concentration of a soluble substance recovered with BAL depends on the lavage volume. However, as the lavage volume increased, the concentration of soluble factors decreases in a way that is not predicted by simple dilution (12). Quantitative expression of the noncellular constituents of BAL fluid is complex and controversial because of the variability of BAL return and the unavailability of satisfactory reference standards to control for the dilution of soluble components by the lavage fluid (3). Comparison to a standard substance may be necessary, however, if: 1) a substance is present in the serum and also derived from local lung production and 2) the percentage of recovery is markedly reduced by the underlying disease (9). Many investigators at present use albumin as the standard to normalize the concentration of soluble factors in BAL fluid. This relies on the assumption that the amounts of albumin on the alveolar surface are not altered by various disease processes; this is clearly not the case in various interstitial lung diseases or in acute respiratory distress syndrome (ARDS) (14,28,29). If albumin is used as a standard in certain disease states, the concentration of certain components of lavage fluid may be underestimated (14). The use of urea or methylene blue as markers remains controversial (3,9,30). There is general agreement that no ideal denominator or method of calculation exists to quantitate the dilution factor; currently soluble components of the lower respiratory tract are expressed either as units per milliliter albumin or as units per milliliter of lavage fluid (3,9).

Kelly and colleagues (31), using tritiated water, technetium colloid, and methylene blue, performed a quantitative analysis of the complex fluid dynamics of a standardized BAL. They demonstrated a bidirectional flux of water occurred across the alveolar membrane. With the 5×20-mL technique, the net dilution of the aspirate was 20%; a 3×60-mL BAL produced a net dilution of 25%. But the final dilution was the net effect of fluid loss and gain and the total water gained contributed 45% of the total aspirated volume. Thus, for example, for every 180 mL of fluid introduced into a middle lobe segment, about 60 mL effluxed into the circulation, countered by an influx of about 105 mL from the circulation, giving a net dilutional volume of 225 mL (31).

The concentration of glucose in BAL fluid is approximately 40 μg/mL and of protein is about 0.06 mg/μL, of which 30% is albumin (32). Rankin and associates (33) found that the viability of cells obtained by BAL was maintained when the lavage fluid was maintained at 25°C for up to 4 hours and that it is not necessary to add either culture medium or antibiotics to lavage specimens for transport to a centralized laboratory.

Sample Processing

Lavage samples (4) are processed as follows. Immediately following lavage, the fluid is strained through two layers of surgical 4×4 gauze into 50-mL conical tubes. The volume is measured and the tube is centrifuged for 5 minutes at 200g. The supernatant fluid is then frozen at -80°C for later use. The residual pellet of cells is resuspended and washed twice in Hanks' balanced salt solution (without calcium or magnesium). After a second wash, a small aliquot of the sample is taken for cell count using a hemocytometer or a Coulter Counter (Model FN, Coulter Electronics, Hialeah, FL). The cells are then washed once more and resuspended in RPMI-1640 medium so that the final concentration gives a cell count of 1×10^7 cells/mL. The cells that are present in 10 μL of the cell suspension are placed in a cytocentrifuge (Cytospin-2, Shanden Southern Instruments, Sewickey, PA). The cytospin is set for 5 minutes of centrifugation at 120 rpm, after which time the slide is removed and dried for one or 2 minutes. Staining is carried out using either Wright-Giemsa or an analogous stain such as DiffQuick Stain Set (Harleco, Gibbstown, NJ). After the slide is dried, one drop of optically clear immersion oil is placed over the cells and a coverslip is placed on top. The characteristics of a satisfactory cytocentrifuge preparation include negligible staining artifacts, uniform dispersal of the cells without clumping, essentially no disruption of cells, and less than 3% airway epithelial cells. The cells are not counted unless a cytocentrifuge preparation meets these criteria. In our laboratory, using these criteria, there is less than 3% intraobserver and interobserver variability in reading a cytocentrifuge preparation for each type of cell that is present.

Some important differences exist between various methods of processing lavage samples. For example, routinely filtering the sample through fine gauze to remove mucus may, in some situations, lead to a loss of potentially useful information, that is, ferruginous bodies in patients with asbestos exposure, and, possibly, cells with increased adherence such as activated neutrophils (5). Studies by Saltini and colleagues (34) suggested that the cytocentrifuge preparations, in general, underestimate the actual numbers of lymphocytes recovered by lavage and the "washing" procedure itself may lead to significant loss of all types of cells. To avoid this problem, they developed a method using Millipore filters. This finding has not been duplicated, however, by all investigators. Cytocentrifuge preparations also provide a clearer evaluation of the cytologic features of cells. The filter technique takes longer to perform and is more expensive than the cytocentrifuge technique. In addition, filter preparations are not suitable for further analysis of cells such as determination of lymphocyte subpopulations (35). The filter preparation also underestimates neutrophil counts, most likely due to neutrophil loss during membrane filtration (35,36). Some suggest lavage fluid should be processed by both centrifugation and membrane filtration (33). Recently, Laviollette and colleagues (32) described a glass cover technique that avoids several of these problems and does not diminish lymphocyte counts.

When the results of a lavage cell analysis are reported, BAL fluid cells should be expressed both as number/mL and as a percentage of the total cell population (plus an estimate of total cell numbers should be given). These numbers provide complementary information (1,15). A normal cell differential does not always indicate that the lung is free of inflammation; that is, a markedly increased number of cells with a normal differential may be associated with an inflammatory process in the lung (14).

Safety and Complications

Lavage is a relatively safe procedure that adds about 15 minutes to a routine flexible fiberoptic bronchoscopic examination. Strumpf and associates (37) reviewed 281 BAL procedures performed on 141 individuals. In more than 95% of the procedures, no complications or adverse reactions occurred. In the remaining procedures, only minor complications developed, none of which significantly compromised patient care. There were no episodes of pneumothorax, significant dysrhythmia, respiratory arrest, or mortality. The most frequently seen complication was post-BAL fever, which occurred in 7 (2.5%) patients and resolved with no therapy. Other studies have demonstrated that a delayed febrile response may occur in up to 10% to 50% of patients who undergo BAL; usually this does not represent pulmonary infection but a transient pyrogen effect that can be treated with antipyretics (32). Cole and colleagues (38) noted fever in approximately 20% of patients who underwent large-volume (300 to 500 mL) BAL and Pingleton and coworkers (7) noted fevers, chills, and myalgias in nearly 50% of normal volunteers who underwent extensive lavage of four lobes. The incidence of post-BAL fever thus seems to be related to both the number of lobes lavaged and the total volume of fluid instilled into each lavage site. Post-BAL fever may be related to elevated serum levels of tumor necrosis factor (39). Bronchoscopy with BAL has also recently been shown to induce both alveolar and peripheral blood neutrophilia in normals which resolves over 72 hours (40).

Tilles and colleagues (41) examined changes in pulmonary function 30 minutes after small-volume (175 mL) and large-volume (500 mL) BAL in normals and after small-volume lavage in patients with sarcoidosis. In normals, small-volume lavage produced no change in pulmonary function except for a small fall in peak expiratory flow; large-volume lavage resulted in a significant fall in FEV_1, forced vital capacity (FVC), and peak expiratory flow rate (PEFR). In patients with sarcoidosis, FEV_1, FVC, and PEFR declined by 20% ± 4.8%, 26.7% ± 7.3%, and 15.2% ± 4.1%, respectively. Although these changes are greater than those found in our experience, they indicate that it is necessary to be cautious in performing BAL on patients with interstitial lung disease when this degree of reduction in pulmonary functions would be poorly tolerated (41). Ettensohn and coworkers (42) recently reported that pulmonary function in normals remains unchanged after multiple small-volume (120 mL) BAL procedures and concluded it was safe to perform repeated BAL in normal volunteers.

Lavage may also result in a decrease in PaO_2. Cole and colleagues (38) noted an average fall in PaO_2 of 22.7 mm Hg, which persisted for at least 2 hours. Pirozynski and associates (43) noted that the degree of desaturation associated with BAL was related to the volume of fluid instilled. Lin and coworkers (44) performed 200-mL BAL in 27 young healthy individuals and found one to 2 hours following BAL that the PaO_2 fell 28.42 ± 6.2 mm Hg and a significant fall in forced expiratory flow, mid-expiratory phase (FEF_{25-75}) when room temperature saline was instilled, but a fall in PaO_2 of 14.91 ± 5.04 mm Hg (and no change in FEF_{25-75}) if the saline instilled was 37°C.

Stover and colleagues (45) reviewed their results in 97 immunocompromised patients who underwent BAL in the evaluation of diffuse infiltrates. Eighteen patients were on assisted ventilation and 35 had severe thrombocytopenia at the time of BAL. There were no major complications; two thrombocytopenic patients had an increased amount of blood in their BAL fluid, but there was no persistent hemorrhage. Fifty percent of their patients had an increase in temperature post-BAL as well as a slight worsening of infiltrate in the area of lavage, but blood cultures were consistently negative and there were no adverse sequelae.

Multiple studies have looked at the safety of diagnostic BAL in patients with acquired immunodeficiency syndrome (AIDS). In general, most AIDS patients experience a transient increase in oxygen requirements, a transient increase in pulmonary infiltrates, and transient elevation in temperature post-BAL (46–48). In AIDS patients who were thrombocytopenic or who required mechanical ventilation, there was no significant morbidity or mortality with BAL and no episodes of serious hemorrhage. Similarly, in bone marrow transplant patients (even if thrombocytopenic or requiring mechanical ventilation) BAL has been judged to be safe (49). In studies of the adult respiratory distress syndrome, BAL has also been well tolerated. In summary, multiple studies at different institutions have examined immunosuppressed and thrombocytopenic patients, in some cases requiring mechanical ventilation, and have concluded that BAL has an acceptable morbidity as a diagnostic tool.

Gurney and coworkers (50) prospectively evaluated the radiographic manifestations of lavage. In their study, 30 minutes after lavage, 90% (47 of 52) of lobes lavaged revealed homogenous areas of new or increased consolidation, most often in the peripheral portion of the lobe. Usually, the margins were indistinct, and prominent air bronchograms were not present. Resolution of these opacities was gradual, with opacities remaining in 91% (of the 47) at 90 minutes, 73% at 240 minutes, and all had cleared by 24 hours. The presence of these opacities correlated with the amount of retained saline solution, was limited to the area lavaged, and was not associated with clinical complications. The authors concluded that, following BAL, these benign fleeting opacities related to BAL should be considered in the differential diagnosis of new findings on chest x-ray (50).

Normal Values

Bronchoalveolar lavage fluid in a normal adult will be comprised of approximately 92% ± 5% macrophages, 7% ± 1% lymphocytes, and less than 1% neutrophils, eosinophils, basophils, or mast cells (1,14). The high normal percentage of lymphocytes in lavage fluid is considered to be in the 10% to 15% range, with most normal individuals falling under 10%. However, Laviollette (51) reported 5 of 42 normal healthy nonsmoking volunteers who had a lymphocyte count greater than 20%, which then normalized to below 14% on follow-up BAL in 4 of the 5. Ettensohn and coworkers (42) reported similar findings. These observations suggest normal subjects may have a transient increase in BAL lymphocytes with no clinically apparent reason.

Recently a multicenter cooperative study (15) was conducted to evaluate the range of cellular and protein constituents of BAL fluid in healthy individuals. The findings were as follows:

1. Age, gender, and race had no significant effect on BAL fluid cell quantity or cell differential.
2. There were no significant differences in total cells in BAL fluid between ex-smokers and never-smokers (whether the results were expressed as total cells recovered or as cells/mL BAL fluid). The total number of cells obtained, however, were three times as high in current smokers.
3. The number of macrophages from current smokers was four times that of never-smokers and the increase in macrophages exceeded the increase in total cells so that the percentage of macrophages (92.5%) in smokers was significantly greater than that of never-smokers (85.2%). There were no differences between ex-smokers and never-smokers.
4. The number of neutrophils/mL in current smokers was approximately six times that in never-smokers, and in ex-smokers neutrophils were also significantly increased (twice that of never-smokers). But, when expressed as a percentage of total cells recovered, only the ex-smokers differed significantly from never-smokers. Also, the neutrophils remained significantly elevated in ex-smokers who had stopped smoking for more than 10 years, suggesting the impact of smoking on the cell populations in the lung may not be entirely reversible. Smoking must be considered when comparing groups of subjects or patients with various diseases and ex-smokers should be differentiated from never-smokers.

In normals, the subtypes of lymphocytes found within the alveolar structures are similar to those of blood. Using surface marker criteria, approximately 73% of alveolar lymphocytes are T cells, 7% are B cells, and the remaining 19% do not react with conventional agents and are thus classified as "null cells"

(1,14). T-helper cells are reported to represent 39% to 48% of lymphocytes and T-suppressor cells between 23% and 28%, so that the normal ratio of T-helper cells to T-suppressor cells (H/S) is 1.6:1.8 (15,52). The National Institutes of Health (NIH) cooperative study findings included:

1. The percentage of T-helper cells in individuals greater than 50 years old was, on the average, more than 10% higher than that in individuals under 37 years old.
2. Total T cells, T-suppressor cells, and B cell percentages were significantly higher in men than in women and the H/S ratio was significantly lower in men.
3. T-helper cells were significantly lower (32.2%) in current smokers than in ex-smokers (46%) and in never-smokers (44.4%), and T-suppressor cells were higher in current smokers (29.2%) than in ex-smokers (20.7%) and never-smokers (20.7%). Thus, the H/S ratio was significantly lower in current smokers than in either ex-smokers or never-smokers.

Ciliated or squamous epithelial cells from the bronchi may also be present but usually do not exceed 3% of the total number of cells; higher counts may indicate bronchial inflammation (5). Again, polymorphonuclear (PMN) leukocytes are rare in the alveoli of normal individuals and represent less than 1% of the total. When PMN cells (particularly neutrophils) are in higher numbers in BAL fluid, one of the following is suggested:

1. There is blood contamination secondary to bronchoscopic trauma.
2. The patient is a smoker.
3. The patient has a chronic lung disease characterized by increased neutrophils in the alveolar structures (see below).
4. Inflammatory airway disease is present and the source of neutrophils is the bronchi and not the alveoli (1,4).

Clinical Utility of Bronchoalveolar Lavage

In most situations, BAL, by itself, does not provide information to make specific diagnoses with absolute certainty. However, the BAL cell profile has important diagnostic value when considered in conjunction with other information. If patients cannot safely undergo open lung biopsy, BAL can provide supportive evidence for a diagnosis, and if a patient has respiratory symptoms but near normal pulmonary functions and a normal chest x-ray, an abnormal BAL result facilitates the decision to proceed with open lung biopsy (53).

Interstitial Lung Diseases

The interstitial lung diseases (ILDs) are a group of greater than 100 different disorders that are often disabling, sometimes fatal, and characterized morphologically by an increase in the number of inflammatory and immune effector cells within the lung parenchyma, that is, a chronic alveolitis. It is believed that the alveolitis may precede and modulate the derangement of alveolar structures, including thickening and fibrosis of the adjacent interstitium, which may eventually lead to sufficient damage to the alveolar capillary membrane to interfere with proper gas exchange (1,54). If this observation is valid, knowledge of the presence and the intensity of the alveolitis is important in understanding these illnesses and may be of benefit in planning and evaluating therapeutic strategies, and the data that currently exist to address these questions in specific diseases are discussed below. Conventional studies, including chest x-ray and pulmonary functions, do not specifically assess the alveolitis. The classical approach to evaluate the alveolitis of ILD has been to biopsy the lung parenchyma and describe qualitatively the inflammatory and immune effector cells within the alveoli and the amount of fibrosis (55). However, this does not give information regarding type and function of the cells comprising the alveolitis and practically cannot be performed serially during a patient's clinical course.

Bronchoalveolar lavage is ideally suited to evaluate the alveolitis of ILDs. Patients with ILD usually have little associated inflammatory airway disease and the cells obtained by BAL are reflective of alveolar rather than airway processes. In addition, BAL permits functional evaluation of the inflammatory and immune effector cells involved in chronic lung diseases and is easily repeated. Thus, it can be used to follow the status of the alveolitis and its response to therapy (55).

It is essential that the inflammatory and immune effector cells collected by lavage accurately represent the effector cell within the alveolar structures; multiple studies illustrate this point. Haslam and colleagues (53) compared yields of cells obtained from BAL fluid with those observed using quantitative counts of cells extracted from open lung biopsy specimens in patients with idiopathic pulmonary fibrosis (IPF) and found that there was a correlation between the proportion of neutrophils obtained from lung lavage and tissue extraction ($P < 0.02$), but this correlation did not exist for eosinophils ($P < 0.07$) or lymphocytes ($P < 0.08$). They concluded that their data suggested that lung lavage reflects the cellularity of the peripheral parts of the lung in IPF patients without overt bronchial disease (53). Similarly, Hunninghake and coworkers (55) found that the proportions of BAL macrophages, neutrophils, eosinophils, baso-phils, and T and B lymphocytes were similar to those extracted from lung tissue in normal subjects and patients with either sarcoidosis or IPF. Similarly, Semenzato and coworkers (56) used monoclonal antibodies to compare cells in tissue sections to cells recovered by BAL in patients with sarcoidosis and hypersensitivity pneumonitis. A significant correlation between percentages

of lymphocytes and macrophages in BAL and lung biopsies was found, supporting the concept that BAL correctly samples the alveolitis of these disorders (56).

Implications for Diagnosis and Management: Specific Interstitial Lung Diseases

Sarcoidosis

Although BAL cannot be used to make a definitive diagnosis of sarcoidosis, analysis of helper (CD4) and suppressor (CD8) T lymphocytes may be of benefit in distinguishing sarcoidosis from other granulomatous diseases such as hypersensitivity pneumonitis. In sarcoidosis, the H/S T cell ratio may be as high as 10 to 20:1; in hypersensitivity pneumonitis, the H/S ratio is decreased (14,57,58). An elevated neutrophil count (with or without an increased lymphocyte count) may also be present in the BAL fluid of patients with advanced sarcoidosis, but usually only in those whose disease has progressed to an extensively fibrotic or bullous radiographic pattern (59).

Although the clinical course of most sarcoid patients is relatively benign, 20% to 25% may suffer permanent loss of lung function, and in 5% to 10% of patients the disease may eventually be fatal (50,58). The ability to predict by BAL which patients will have an unstable course would be clinically useful in decisions regarding therapy.

Keogh and colleagues (60) evaluated 19 untreated sarcoid patients without extrapulmonary manifestations and found subjects with a "high-intensity" alveolitis (defined as lavage T lymphocytes greater than 28% and a positive gallium scan) had a greater (87% deteriorated) propensity to suffer significant deterioration in lung function over a 6-month period than did subjects with a "low-intensity" alveolitis (8% deteriorated). Similar results would have been obtained if lavage itself had been used as the only criterion for active disease. However, the results of this study should be interpreted with caution since: 1) "deteriorated" was defined as a 10% fall in only one pulmonary function parameter (TLC, FVC, FEV_1, or single-breath diffusing capacity [Dsb]); 2) there was a significant difference in both the age and the duration of symptoms between the "high-" and "low-intensity" alveolitis patients—the "high-intensity" groups were younger and had disease of shorter duration, both important factors in the prognosis of sarcoidosis; 3) 75% of the episodes of "high-intensity" alveolitis spontaneously reverted to "low-intensity," whereas 12% of all episodes of "low-intensity" alveolitis spontaneously reverted to "high-intensity"; and 4) the study was short term.

In contrast, Israel-Biet and coworkers (61) performed BAL on 94 untreated sarcoidosis patients with "recent onset of the disease." All patients underwent repeat BAL at one year and 18 patients at 2 years. These investigators concluded that initial lymphocyte counts were "devoid of any predictive value" in predicting spontaneous "cure." However, to be considered "cured" in this study, all pulmonary functions as well as chest radiographs had to be considered totally normal on follow-up.

Foley and associates (62) evaluated 67 patients with sarcoidosis with a mean duration of disease of 60 months, none of whom had received corticosteroids for at least 6 months. Twenty-four subsequently required treatment with corticosteroids. The mean follow-up period was 25 (range 13 to 37) months. Repeat BAL at a mean of 8.4 months (range 4 to 20 months) was performed in 34 patients. On the basis of the initial lavage fluid, 42 patients had a total lymphocyte count of 28% or more of total cells, 25 patients had less than 28% total lymphocytes. There was no significant relation between initial lavage lymphocyte count and final outcome, whether judged by FVC_1, diffusing capacity of the lung for carbon monoxide (D_LCO), or radiologic score. Most patients with chronic sarcoidosis

who had pulmonary functional or radiographic deterioration belonged to the "low-intensity" alveolitis group at the initial assessment, so that the absence of lymphocytes *did not* indicate "burned out" disease (62). Repeat BAL found a significant correlation between the fall in BAL fluid lymphocyte percentage and improvement in FVC (the more the lymphocytes fell, the greater improvement in FVC), but appeared "to have little to add" to standard pulmonary function tests and chest radiograph in patient management.

Costabel and colleagues (63) examined 31 untreated sarcoid patients with disease of varying duration (range 0 to 108 months) and defined deterioration as the occurrence of any *one* of the following conditions: 1) new symptoms developed or old symptoms progressed; 2) values for *one* pulmonary function (vital capacity [VC], TLC, Dsb, or PaO_2 with exercise) fell 10%; or 3) successive radiographs indicated the disease was progressive. With these criteria, lavage lymphocytes did not predict subsequent deterioration, but the T lymphocyte H/S cell ratio did. A normal H/S cell ratio was highly predictive of a stable clinical course, whereas an elevated ratio was associated with deterioration during a one-year follow-up period. In contrast Cueppens and colleagues (64) found in 9 untreated patients followed up from 2 to 16 months that the initial H/S T cell ratio had no predictive value regarding spontaneous improvement of the disease. The same group more recently (28) examined 28 untreated patients with sarcoidosis after 22 to 36 months of follow-up. They found a significantly lower lymphocyte count in patients with stage III rather than stage I or II disease. The T4/T8 (H/S) ratio was highest in stage I disease and correlated negatively with the radiologic stage. No correlation was found between the total cell count or the percentage of lymphocytes in the baseline BAL fluid and the evolution of any of the lung volumes or the D_LCO. But, the evolution of the D_LCO correlated positively with the proportion of BAL T4 cells (as a percentage of lymphocytes) and with the BAL T4/T8 ratio and negatively with the proportion of BAL T8 cells (as a percentage of lymphocytes) in the BAL sample obtained at the start of follow-up. The authors concluded that the total cell count and lymphocyte cell count in BAL fluid of untreated patients with sarcoidosis are not predictive of the evolution of the disease and that a high T4/T8 ratio is not an indicator of poor prognosis and may even be associated with a better prognosis (28).

Although there is not uniform agreement, BAL findings in sarcoidosis do not seem to correlate with disease duration. However, Ward and colleagues (29) found that two groups of patients with sarcoidosis presenting with acute inflammatory events (erythema nodosum or uveitis) had higher lavage T-lymphocyte percentages, T-helper cell percentages and H/S ratios than patients with other presentations of sarcoidosis. They also found a progressive diminution over time in lavage T-lymphocyte percentage and H/S ratio for erythema nodosum patients not seen with patients with uveitis or respiratory symptoms, which is interesting because erythema nodosum is generally associated with a good prognosis. The authors concluded that the category of disease presentation may be crucial in the interpretation of individual lavage results and may explain the diversity of results in the literature. Widely varying results may be due to differences in the study population: if a particular study population has a large number of patients studied soon after an acute onset with erythema nodosum or uveitis, results may tend to show high lymphocyte counts and H/S ratios plus find them associated with a good prognosis.

In addition to the potential role of lavage lymphocyte counts in the management of patients with sarcoidosis, Bjermer and colleagues (65,66) have examined lavage fluid mast cells. A significant increase in mast cells is 0.5% or more of the total cells recovered. In 69 untreated sarcoid patients, they found: 1) a significant relationship between mast cell counts and both absolute and relative lymphocyte counts, 2) mast cells in lavage fluid were inversely related to lung function, and 3) mast cell counts tended to increase with radiographic stages. Hyaluronate (a potential marker for activated pulmonary fibroblasts) concentrations were also found to be strongly correlated with mast cell counts. In 45 newly diagnosed patients with sarcoidosis followed over a 2-year period, they found both the lymphocyte counts and the neutrophil count had limited prognostic value. In contrast, lavage mastocytosis was associated in general with lung disease deterioration, and lymphocytosis or neutrophilia plus mastocytosis had the highest specificity for prediction of deterioration. Increased mast cell counts were seen in 15 of 16 patients with more active and progressive disease, but in only 8 of 23 patients with inactive disease ($P < 0.02$). How exactly the recruitment of mast cells would be linked to the established cellular immune events in the lung is not clear.

Bronchoalveolar lavage has also been postulated to be of benefit to predict steroid responsiveness in sarcoidosis. Lawrence and associates (67) treated 12 patients with "clinically active disease" independent of the results of BAL and found no relationship between subsequent improvements and initial BAL lymphocyte counts. Hollinger and coworkers (68) followed up 21 treated patients for a mean of 22 weeks. They defined improvement as an increase in FVC. All patients with a pretreatment lavage lymphocyte count of 35% or greater were stable or improved, whereas one half of patients with a pretreatment lavage lymphocyte count less than 35% worsened. In contrast, Baughman and colleagues (69) found no relationship in 16 patients treated for pulmonary symptoms between the percentage of lymphocytes obtained in initial lavage and the change in VC after 2 months of therapy. There was a positive correlation, however, between the change in VC and both the H/S T cell ratio and the absolute numbers of helper cells in the BAL fluid. However, this group did not find the H/S ratio useful in predicting long-term (2-year) prognosis (70). Similarly, Turner-Warwick and coworkers (71) found that initial lavage lymphocyte counts were not predictive of radiographic improvement in 32 sarcoid patients. Thus, currently, no conclusive data demonstrate that lavage can accurately predict steroid responsiveness in sarcoidosis. There are also no published studies to our knowledge to determine whether lavage cellular analysis can predict when therapy may be safely tapered or discontinued in sarcoidosis patients.

Others have recently evaluated the potential utility of noncellular substances in BAL fluid of patients with sarcoidosis. Ward and colleagues (72,73) measured initial BAL collagenase and subsequent disease course in 84 untreated sarcoidosis patients. Those with significant collagenase activity in their BAL fluid had more severe physiologic and radiographic impairments, were less likely to improve spontaneously, had a more prolonged disease duration, and had a greater need for steroid intervention than in the collagenase negative group. The same group (74) also examined type 3 procollagen peptide concentrations in BAL fluid of 84 nontreated sarcoidosis patients. Procollagen type 3 is synthesized by fibroblasts as a precursor of collagen type 3 and thus type 3 procollagen peptides are potential markers of collagen secretion (75). Type 3 procollagen peptide levels were significantly elevated in this group compared to normals and usually correlated with increased T lymphocytes, but had no correlation with pulmonary function, mode of presentation, length of disease, or subsequent functional deterioration. Blaschke and colleagues (76) reported similar findings. Type 3 procollagen peptide levels thus do not appear to be of prognostic significance in sarcoidosis. Lavage lymphocyte activation markers also have not shown any correlation with disease duration or results of pulmonary function tests (77).

In summary, at the current time no BAL cellular or noncellular parameter has been shown to definitely be predictive in determining prognosis or making therapeutic decisions for individual patients with sarcoidosis.

Idiopathic Pulmonary Fibrosis/Cryptogenic Fibrosing Alveolitis

In many patients, IPF is usually fatal an average of 3 to 6 years after the onset of symptoms (52). IPF is a difficult disorder to manage because of its variable prognosis plus in some patients corticosteroids or cytotoxic agents can induce substantial subjective and objective improvement, whereas others show no improvement or deteriorate despite therapy (78,79). Due to potentially serious side effects of these medications, the ability to predict which patients would respond to therapy would be very beneficial. In contrast to sarcoidosis, there are no prospective studies of lavage in untreated IPF patients. Several studies suggest that BAL can predict response to therapy and prognosis in this disorder. Rudd and associates (79) studied 120 patients with IPF/cryptogenic fibrosing alveolitis (CFA), 74 with histologic confirmation, and 26 with an associated systemic disorder. All living patients were followed up for at least 12 months and for a mean of 38 months; 79 patients were treated with corticosteroids and 12 were treated with various cytotoxic drugs; response was defined as a 10% increase in FVC. Increased proportions of lymphocytes were associated with responsiveness to corticosteroids, whereas increased eosinophils or increased neutrophils without increased lymphocytes were associated with failure to respond. Increased eosinophils were also associated with a greater likelihood of progressive deterioration. Turner-Warwick and Haslam (80) showed, by repeated lavage analysis in 32 patients with CFA (6 with associated systemic disorders), that falls in neutrophils were significant in patients responding to prednisone, whereas falls in eosinophils were significant in those responding to cyclophosphamide. In patients who failed to improve, neutrophil and eosinophil counts tended to remain elevated. Interestingly, 6 patients with asymptomatic stable disease were not treated; 4 had raised neutrophil counts. Two of these remained completely stable although their neutrophil counts remained substantially elevated.

In contrast, O'Donnell and coworkers (81) found that cyclophosphamide was much more effective than corticosteroids in suppressing the neutrophil component of the alveolitis (as assessed by BAL) despite the fact that the functional response to each drug was similar. Those patients treated with corticosteroids alone showed no suppression in the neutrophil components of the alveolitis after 3 to 6 months of therapy, whereas the cyclophosphamide group showed a marked reduction in the neutrophilic alveolitis at 3 months.

Recently, Watters and associates (82) reported that in 26 patients with IPF/CFA pretreatment lavage neutrophils or eosinophils were *not* related to the clinical response of patients after one year of corticosteroid therapy and would be an unreliable marker on which to base therapeutic decisions. There was an association, though, between the presence of BAL lymphocytosis prior to therapy and clinical improvement after 6 months of corticosteroid therapy. BAL lymphocytosis was also positively associated with biopsy findings of moderate-to-severe alveolar septal inflammation and negatively correlated with honeycombing and smooth muscle hypertrophy (advanced fibrosis). BAL neutrophil and eosinophil content did not correlate significantly with any of the histopathologic architectural abnormalities. The absence of BAL lymphocytosis did not entirely preclude improvement with therapy because 2 patients without this finding also improved. Lavage eosinophilia is frequently associated with more advanced IPF/CFA clinically, but does not always predict a lack of responsiveness to therapy, especially if BAL lymphocytosis is also present. Interestingly, this

group also followed 3 patients with neutrophil counts ranging from 1% to 25% and eosinophil counts ranging from 0% to 8% who remained stable 6 and 12 months after open lung biopsy without therapy.

Other more recent investigations have focused on noncellular components in the BAL fluid of patients with IPF/CFA and their potential usefulness, for example, phospholipids. Pulmonary surfactant, which mainly consists of phospholipids such as dipalmitoyl phosphatidylcholine (DPPC) and phosphatidylglycerol (PG), is synthesized in alveolar type II cells and secreted into alveolar spaces where it stabilizes the pulmonary alveoli against collapse (83). Thus, phospholipid analysis of BAL fluid may be important in evaluating alveolar type II cells and metabolic changes in pulmonary surfactant (83). Phosphatidylinositol (PI) is formed from the same precursor as PG, CDP-diacylglycerol (DG) (83). The phospholipid profiles of BAL fluid are significantly altered in IPF (83–85). The prominent changes are: 1) an overall decrease in the total phospholipid content and concentration; 2) a significant decrease in the PG/PI ratio; and 3) a relative decrease in DPPC, a main phospholipid component of pulmonary surfactant synthesized in alveolar type II cells (83,84). Robinson and colleagues (84) found no significant correlation between BAL fluid cellular constituents or pulmonary function tests and BAL phospholipid content or composition. They did find that IPF patients with relatively prominent alveolar septal inflammation tended to have a higher (more nearly normal) amount of phospholipid in BAL fluid plus the PG/PI ratio correlated better with histologic alterations than total phospholipid amounts: PG/PI correlated negatively (was lower and more abnormal) with alveolar septal fibrosis and honeycombing and was higher (closer to normal) in patients with more cellularity and less fibrosis and honeycombing (84). There was a significant increase in BAL total phospholipid content after 3 months of high-dose corticosteroids, which fell again as the steroids were tapered. This increase in phospholipid content was not necessarily associated with clinical improvement. But, the higher the *pretherapy* BAL phospholipid content, the greater the improvement in exercise gas exchange induced by 6 months of corticosteroid therapy, and a low pretherapy BAL phospholipid content was associated with a poor clinical outcome. The PG/PI ratio, on the other hand, did not predict clinical response nor did this ratio change with corticosteroid therapy in a statistically significant manner (84). In contrast, Hughes and coworkers (85) reported that although PG proportions were frequently reduced in the lavage of untreated IPF/CFA patients, an early and sustained increase in this component was associated with clinical improvement after corticosteroid therapy was instituted, whereas it did not increase in those who failed to improve. Thus, near normal phospholipid levels and ratios in IPF/CFA may be representative of lung parenchyma not yet irreversibly damaged and thus more responsive to corticosteroid therapy (84,85).

As mentioned earlier, hyaluronate and type 3 procollagen peptide concentrations may be potential markers of activated fibroblasts or an expanded fibroblast mass associated with interstitial fibrosis (75). Bjermer and associates (75) found higher concentrations of hyaluronate and type III procollagen peptide in patients with IPF/CFA than in normal controls. Neutrophil and lymphocyte counts correlated with hyaluronate but not type 3 procollagen peptide levels. Diffusing capacity was inversely correlated with hyaluronate concentration. Patients who had deterioration in lung function and radiographic progression over 6 months had higher lavage fluid concentrations of hyaluronate and type 3 procollagen peptide levels than patients whose disease was stable. Increased levels of these substance may be linked to severity and activity of the lung disease.

All of these above studies clearly demonstrate that additional studies of both the cellular and noncellular components of BAL fluid are necessary to define the appropriate clinical use of BAL in patients with IPF/CFA.

Pulmonary Fibrosis Associated with Collagen Vascular Disease

The inflammatory process that develops in the lung in many of the collagen vascular diseases usually results in a diffuse interstitial disease similar to IPF/CFA (54). The findings in BAL fluid in patients with interstitial lung disease associated with collagen vascular disease (PF-CVD) are also similar to those of patients with IPF/CFA (4). In general, in PF-CVD, when there are increased numbers of lymphocytes present in BAL fluid, the lung disease is associated with a relatively good prognosis and response to therapy, whereas the presence of a predominantly neutrophilic or eosinophilic alveolitis is associated with a higher risk of functional and radiographic deterioration and a poor response to therapy (54,79,86–88).

Casale and colleagues (89), in patients with rheumatoid arthritis and PF-CVD, found a good association between BAL histamine levels, BAL neutrophil and eosinophil numbers, pulmonary function tests, and chest radiographic findings. Similar to findings in IPF discussed above, Gilligan and associates (90) found increased neutrophils, collagenase levels, and increased concentrations of type 3 procollagen peptide in the BAL fluid of patients with rheumatoid arthritis and advanced PF-CVD.

Silver and coworkers (91) examined 43 patients with systemic sclerosis. Nearly 50% had an alveolitis, usually characterized by increased numbers of macrophages and granulocytes (neutrophils and eosinophils), but without a lymphocytosis. The alveolitis persisted on serial studies. Those with an abnormal BAL had more dyspnea and greater abnormalities in pulmonary function and chest radiographs and a faster rate of deterioration in pulmonary function than those with a normal BAL.

Several investigators have also evaluated "subclinical" pulmonary involvement in the collagen vascular diseases. Wallaert (92,93) performed BAL on 61 patients with various CVDs free of pulmonary symptoms with normal chest radiographs. Eight of 61 had abnormal pulmonary functions on entry into the study; 29 of 61 patients were found to have an abnormal BAL. A lymphocytic alveolitis was found in 11 of 25 patients with primary Sjögren's syndrome and 4 of 8 patients with Sjögren's associated with another CVD. A neutrophilic alveolitis with or without increased lymphocytes was found in patients with scleroderma (6 of 10), rheumatoid arthritis (1 of 4), dermatomyositis (2 of 3), and mixed connective tissue disease (3 of 8). Abnormalities in BAL were more common in patients with active and severe extrapulmonary disease. On 12 month follow-up, patients with either a normal BAL or a lymphocytic alveolitis had no functional deterioration, whereas 6 of 7 patients with an untreated neutrophilic alveolitis had deterioration in pulmonary function tests. Four steroid-treated patients with a neutrophilic alveolitis did not deteriorate. The authors concluded that BAL allows early detection of a subclinical inflammatory alveolitis in CVD and that a neutrophilic alveolitis is associated with a higher risk of functional deterioration (92). Garcia and associates (94) in a similar manner examined BAL in patients with rheumatoid arthritis and found three distinct groups: 1) patients with definite interstitial involvement clinically; 2) patients with a normal chest x-ray and pulmonary function tests but an abnormal BAL; and 3) patients with a normal chest x-ray, pulmonary function tests, and BAL. Group 1 patients, in general, had increased BAL neutrophils, and group 2 patients had elevated lymphocytes. The above observations suggest BAL may be useful in managing patients with PF-CVD, but the exact manner in which it should be used is still not well defined (4).

Hypersensitivity Pneumonitis/Extrinsic Allergic Alveolitis

Hypersensitivity pneumonitis/extrinsic allergic alveolitis (HSP/EAA) is an inflammatory granulomatous response of the lungs to antigens in a wide range of inhaled organic dusts (95). The characteristic feature of BAL in HSP/EAA is increased numbers of lymphocytes, particularly suppressor T lymphocytes (in contrast to sarcoidosis). The percentage of lymphocytes may be strikingly increased (often above 60%) compared to normal controls (96). Some of the lymphocytes have an atypical appearance suggestive of blast cells having markedly indented multiclefted nuclei and increased cytoplasmic area (95). By the time of clinical presentation, patients with HSP/EAA invariably show increased BAL lymphocytes. Macrophages account for a lower percentage of the total cells obtained by BAL in HSP/EAA (often less than 40%), but the actual numbers are comparable to controls (96). Neutrophils and eosinophils may also be present in the BAL in HSP/EAA, especially if there has been a recent exposure to antigen. Fournier and colleagues (97) found a marked increase in neutrophils in BAL of patients with HSP/EAA who underwent antigen inhalation in an experimental setting. Twenty-four hours after exposure, 41.2% of the BAL cells were neutrophils compared to 8.3% prior to antigen challenge. The increased numbers of neutrophils returned to baseline 5 to 8 days later. In this study, the presence of neutrophils in BAL was associated with clinical symptoms. BAL samples from exposed patients with HSP/EAA also contain mast cells in increased numbers (as much as 10-fold higher) in addition to lymphocytes (95,98). In most patients, the increased mast cells occur when individuals are currently or have been recently exposed and fall soon after removal from exposure, but the lymphocyte increase may (including the atypical forms) persist, often for years (95). Mast cells and neutrophils may remain elevated with continued exposure and symptoms (95). In this manner, serial studies of BAL mast cells and neutrophils may be useful in monitoring removal from exposure (95). During an acute episode of farmer's lung disease, markedly elevated concentrations of hyaluronate and type 3 procollagen peptide are recovered in BAL fluid and are closely related to mast cell levels.

The lymphocyte counts are high in patients with episodic and chronic symptoms; even those who recover and become asymptomatic after removal of the antigen retain persistently increased counts of total BAL lymphocytes (96). It remains unclear what the role of lung lymphocytes is in such asymptomatic patients with previous HSP/EAA; but an elevated percentage of BAL lymphocytes is a persistent finding for at least 2 years in patients with a history of previous farmer's lung disease who stay in contact with the farm environment (99). BAL lymphocytes are not a sign of active disease and do not predict outcome or prognosis in patients with an established diagnosis of HSP/EAA (99). In this regard, increased levels of BAL lymphocytes and mast cells are also found in asymptomatic dairy farmers with positive serum precipitins who subsequently have not developed HSP/EAA over 6 to 7 years of follow-up: increased lymphocytes and mast cells are thus not a sign of lung disease nor a predictor of eventual development of HSP/EAA (100).

Pneumoconioses

Asbestos-related Interstitial Lung Disease

The assessment of asbestos exposure is often difficult because of the numerous jobs and hobbies in which asbestos is used and because the patient is usually unaware of its risk (101). The assessment of prior occupational exposure to asbestos can usually be accomplished through the clinical history; however, considering the large numbers of occupations in which asbestos is used and the long latency period between exposure and the development of disease, some patients may not be aware of or may fail to recall such exposure (102).

Asbestos body (AB) formation is an intracellular process that occurs as one or more alveolar macrophages engulfs an asbestos fiber. The fiber then becomes incorporated into an intracytoplasmic vacuole and is coated with an acid mucopolysaccharide (103). Iron accumulates in the coating initially as hemosiderin. Only a small portion of asbestos fibers in the lung become coated as ferruginous bodies (103,104). Ferroprotein rarely develops on chrysotile and other short fibers; therefore, ABs are formed primarily on long fibers (e.g., amphibole) and represent only a fraction of the total asbestos burden in the lung and thus in BAL (103,105). The presence of ABs thus reflects primarily the burden of long amphibole fibers, which are considered to be most frequently associated with asbestosis and mesothelioma (101,105). In the population without occupational asbestos exposure, but exposed to urban pollution, chrysotile constitutes the bulk of the asbestos fibers (106,107). These small fibers do not form ABs, which explains why finding ABs in BAL usually correlates well with occupational exposure, implying inhalation of long industrial fibers (106).

Measurement of ABs in lung parenchyma obtained at autopsy or surgery is a useful way of assessing exposure to asbestos, and a parenchymal concentration of greater than 1000 AB/g dried lung tissue is generally associated with past specific exposure to asbestos (106,107). Data from both Sebastien and coworkers (108) and DeVuyst and colleagues (105) demonstrate that measuring the concentrations of ABs in BAL fluid constitutes a useful test for predicting parenchymal concentrations: a measured BAL concentration of one AB/mL would predict a parenchymal concentration ranging between 1050 and 3010 AB/g (107). Thus, all measured BAL concentrations one AB/mL or greater would correspond to lung concentrations in excess of 1000 AB/g and thus indicate nontrivial and significant asbestos exposure (107).

DeVuyst and associates (105,106) recently published their experience in 563 subjects who underwent analysis of BAL for ABs. Of 215 patients, 84.3% with a definite exposure to asbestos had more than one AB/mL; 53.5% of 116 patients with probable or suspected asbestos exposure had more than one AB/mL; and 17.8% of 117 blue-collar workers with no known asbestos exposure and 6.9% of 115 white-collar workers with no known asbestos exposure had more than one AB/mL. All patients who had more than 1000 AB/mL of BAL fluid and 36 of 37 with more than 100 AB/mL were in the definite exposure group. Their study also indicated that there is a definite relationship between asbestos exposure and BAL fluid AB counts: the greater or more definite the exposure, in general, the higher the number of ABs per mL of lavage fluid (101,106). Repeated lavages in 10 patients showed that the ABs remain at roughly the same concentration from one BAL to another. When ABs were compared to the categories of asbestos-related disease, in patients with radiographic findings consistent with asbestosis, 93.3% had more than one AB/mL; 70.4% of patients with asbestos-related pleural disease had more than one AB/mL; 62.5% of patients with malignant mesothelioma had more than one AB/mL; 78.3% of patients with lung cancer and occupational asbestos exposure had more than one AB/mL; and 63.5% of patients with occupational asbestos and no evidence of lung cancer or asbestos-related disease had more than one AB/mL. The mean AB/mL recovery was significantly higher in the subjects with asbestosis (mean 120.5 AB/mL) than in subjects with benign pleural disease (mean 4.77 AB/mL, $P < 0.001$) or in workers with negative chest x-rays (mean 3.57 AB/mL, $P < 0.001$). The presence or absence of ABs in BAL is most likely not a reliable indication of sub-

pleurally deposited fibers involved in the development of asbestos-related pleural disease (effusion, fibrosis, malignancy). Of patients with an ill-defined occupational exposure and radiographic lesions consistent with an asbestos etiology, 83% (65 of 78) had a positive BAL for AB. There were also significant correlations between AB counts and duration of exposure (positive) and AB counts and time since the end of the last exposure (negative).

Recently, Schwartz and colleagues (109) have suggested that the relationship between AB counts and indices of exposure to asbestos may not be this strong in the United States because of the lower exposure to amphibole instead of chrysotile in workers in this country. However, in another study of 93 asbestos-exposed patients, Garcia and coworkers (110) noted that ABs in BAL were significantly and inversely correlated with the diffusing capacity and directly correlated with profusion score abnormalities and BAL eosinophil levels.

The following can be concluded regarding ABs in BAL:

1. AB analysis of BAL fluid is probably of most value in patients with radiographic changes suggestive of an asbestos-related disease with an ill-defined exposure history (106).
2. Finding ABs in BAL fluid correlates with the occupational risk and can disclose unknown or forgotten exposure better than a questionnaire (101,104). AB in BAL is an excellent objective measure of asbestos exposure but, in itself, is not a good marker or proof of disease (101, 104,106).
3. The absence of ABs in a correctly performed BAL does not exclude asbestos-related pleural disease but is significant evidence against the diagnosis of asbestosis (106).
4. In the presence of ILD, the finding in BAL of numerous ABs tilts the balance of probabilities toward a diagnosis of

asbestosis because ABs are not usually found in patients with other ILDs and, when they are found in patients who do not have asbestosis, they do so in smaller numbers than are seen in asbestosis (102,111).

5. The concentration of ABs in BAL may positively correlate with length and intensity of exposure and may negatively correlate with time since last exposure.

6. AB concentration in BAL correlates well with the lung tissue burden.

Lavage fluid cellular analysis in patients with asbestosis is similar to that of patients with IPF/CFA. Geller and colleagues (111) evaluated 32 patients with documented previous occupational asbestos exposure and clinical and radiographic features of asbestosis. Forty-six percent (13 of 31) of the patients showed an increase in the percentage of neutrophils with or without an increase in the percentage of eosinophils; 29% (8 of 31) showed an increased proportion of lymphocytes. Multiple subsequent studies demonstrate that the H/S ratio of the T lymphocytes in the BAL fluid of patients with asbestosis probably is elevated (111). The numbers of neutrophils correlated positively with the length of history of the disease and higher percentages were associated with more severe impairment of lung function. Smokers more frequently had increased numbers of neutrophils than did non-smokers. In non-smokers, a negative correlation was found between the diffusing capacity and the percentages of PMN cells, and a positive correlation between the diffusing capacity and the proportion of lymphocytes.

In a review of 27 patients with asbestosis, Robinson and coworkers (112) found that 70% had increased numbers of neutrophils in lavage fluid and 52% had increased numbers of eosinophils. They also found that there was no difference in the severity of the alveolitis in patients with radiographic and physiologic evidence of asbestosis compared to those with asbestos exposure and crackles but no radiologic or physiologic evidence of asbestosis, suggesting that radiologic or functional parameters do not reflect the severity of the alveolitis (112). Xaubet and coworkers (113), in contrast, found that the proportion of neutrophils in BAL correlated with the PaO_2 and PAO_2–PaO_2.

Several studies have also suggested that a "subclinical" pulmonary involvement occurs in some asbestos-exposed workers. Begin and colleagues (114) found a significant increase in numbers of total cells, neutrophils, and lymphocytes in BAL of 17 of 42 exposed workers without the criteria for asbestosis; several of them developed full criteria for asbestosis within 3 to 5 years. The authors concluded that evidence of alveolitis on BAL should strongly argue against any further exposure to asbestos dust at any levels in such patients (114). Gellert and associates (111,115,116) have also reported the presence of increased numbers of lymphocytes in BAL fluid in asbestos workers without clinical and radiographic evidence of asbestosis. Garcia and coworkers (110) also found that non-smoking asbestos-exposed subjects without asbestosis had higher numbers of neutrophils in BAL than did non-exposed workers. Further follow-up, both functionally and by BAL, in this group with "subclinical" involvement will determine if these abnormalities do indeed represent the early stages in the development of asbestosis.

Silicosis

Begin and colleagues (117) evaluated with BAL 22 silica-exposed (average of 31 years of exposure) workers: 7 had no evidence of silicosis (group 1), 9 (group 2) had simple silicosis (no coalescence or large opacities), and 6 had silicosis with coalescence or large opacities. In all three groups there were twice as many total cells as controls with a prominent increase in macrophages and some increases in lymphocytes and neutrophils. The BAL cellularity did not differentiate the three groups of silica-exposed workers with different severity of disease. These data are not in agreement with those of Schuyler and associates (118) who noted *only* an increase in type II pneumocytes in the BAL of 6 silicotics compared to normal controls.

Christman and coworkers (119) evaluated 9 healthy Vermont granite workers with normal spirometry and chest radiographs with BAL. Five of the 9 workers had increased lymphocytes in BAL, significantly greater than controls, which was thought to represent a subclinical chronic inflammatory process (119). Polarizing particles were present in 5.8% of the alveolar macrophages in the controls compared with 75.7% of the workers' cells. There was also an increase in the percentage of alveolar macrophages that contained particulates with increasing duration of granite dust exposure, and the percentage of lymphocytes in BAL also increased with longer duration of granite dust exposure. When clinical and radiographic data are consistent with silicosis, BAL is a noninvasive means to document silica exposure because birefringent particles are easily detected by polarized microscopy (109).

Bronchiolitis

Kindt and coworkers (120) performed BAL on 16 adult patients with bronchiolitis both before and after 3 months of corticosteroid therapy. These patients had: 1) severe obstruction on pulmonary function testing, 2) hyperinflation on chest radiograph with no interstitial lung disease, 3) minimal smoking history, and 4) biopsy evidence of prominent bronchiolar inflammation. Neutrophils initially comprised 54% ± 10% of the cells re-covered by BAL from the patients with bronchiolitis compared with 3.9% ± 1% in smokers with chronic bronchitis ($n = 8$) and 0.8% ± 0.5% in normal non-smoking volunteers ($n = 6$) ($P < 0.01$, both comparisons). BAL

performed after 3 months of cortico-steroids in 8 of 16 patients with bronchiolitis demonstrated a significant decrease in the percentage of BAL neutrophils (before: 57% ± 11% versus post: 26% ± 13%, $P < 0.05$). Of this group, the responder subset ($n = 5$) had a marked reduction in BAL neutrophil percentage after corticosteroids (46% ± 15% to 6% ± 3%, $P < 0.05$), whereas the nonresponder subset ($n = 3$) did not (76% ± 11% to 59% ± 26%, $P = 0.391$). This study suggests that BAL is useful for evaluating the inflammatory response at the level of the bronchioles in these patients. In addition, in patients for whom a high clinical suspicion of bronchiolitis exists, the finding of an elevated (greater than 25%) percentage of neutrophils by BAL may be sufficient for a presumptive diagnosis of bronchiolitis (120).

In the separate clinical entity of bronchiolitis obliterans organizing pneumonia/cryptogenic organizing pneumonia, the data on lavage findings reveal that either lymphocytes or neutrophils may be elevated (121,122). In diffuse panbronchiolitis, another clinical entity described in Japan (123), neutrophils have been shown to comprise 55.3% ± 24.4% of recovered cells by BAL (124).

Wegener's Granulomatosis

The NIH recently reviewed their experience with BAL in Wegener's granulomatosis (125). In active, untreated disease there was a marked increase in neutrophils and eosinophils, which usually fell when the patients went into remission. The antineutrophil cytoplasmic antibody (ANCA) was present in lavage fluid in patients with active disease and serum ANCA reactivity and the titers of ANCA in BAL fluid correlated with the presence or absence of active Wegener's granulomatosis.

Drug-Induced Lung Disease

Pulmonary drug toxicity can be suspected from the finding of bronchial and alveolar cell atypia (cytotoxic changes) in BAL fluid; however, these changes need to be interpreted with caution because they can appear similar to changes seen in some cases of malignancy (37,126). Consequently, the diagnosis of drug toxicity cannot be definitively made by BAL alone.

However, BAL has potential as an important adjunctive test in the evaluation of suspected amiodarone lung toxicity (127). Phospholipid accumulation in alveolar macrophages results in lamellar body formation, which gives the macrophages a "foamy" appearance because of these characteristic cytoplasmic inclusions (127). This is relatively characteristic for drug effect secondary to amiodarone. Lavage provides excellent cellular material for assessment of the "foamy" inclusions in alveolar macrophages. However, since its presence can be detected in up to 50% of patients receiving amiodarone, it is not diagnostic of toxicity—but its absence makes the diagnosis of amiodarone pulmonary toxicity unlikely (127).

In a review of 14 subjects with amiodarone pulmonary toxicity from the Mayo Clinic, the cell differential counts from BAL grouped into three categories: 1) normal cell differential, 2) lymphocyte predominant, and 3) PMN leukocyte predominant (127). The lymphocyte typing in the lymphocyte-predominant pattern showed a marked increase in CD8-positive lymphocytes (CD4/CD8 ratio of 0.4:1). Similar findings were noted by Israel-Biet and colleagues (128). When present, the finding of increased numbers of T-suppressor lymphocytes with or without PMN leukocytes strongly supports the diagnosis of amiodarone pulmonary toxicity; a normal cell differential neither supports nor excludes the diagnosis (127).

Implications for Diagnosis and Management—Rarer Lung Disorders

Berylliosis

Beryllium has found widespread application in modern industry because of its physical properties, and it is used in the manufacture of products such as thermal coating nuclear reactors, rocket heat shields, and brakes (129). Inhaled beryllium metal dusts, beryllium oxide, or beryllium salts can cause either acute or chronic lung disease. The acute form appears to be a toxic dose-related effect on the lungs and has largely been eliminated by controls on environmental exposure. The chronic form develops over one to 20 years in 1% to 3% of exposed persons and is a granulomatous interstitial disease remarkably similar, histopathologically and clinically, to sarcoidosis (14,129). The diagnosis of chronic berylliosis is usually based on a history of beryllium exposure, typical clinical and histologic abnormalities, and elevated lung beryllium levels (14,129).

Bronchoalveolar lavage may be extremely valuable in the evaluation of a patient with suspected berylliosis. BAL cells from patients with berylliosis are remarkably similar to those with sarcoidosis: the total numbers of macrophages and T cells are increased. The percentage of lymphocytes is increased, and most of these cells are helper T cells (14,129). BAL in berylliosis has its greatest use in showing a local immunologic response to beryllium. Lymphocytes from the BAL of berylliosis patients proliferate when stimulated in vitro with soluble beryllium salts, with a sensitivity and specificity approaching 100% (14,129, 130). This has become a valuable diagnostic tool in berylliosis and may replace open lung biopsy as a way to make a definitive diagnosis of chronic berylliosis (14,129,130).

Histiocytosis X (Eosinophilic Granuloma)

Histiocytosis X (HX) is a chronic granulomatous disorder that involves the mononuclear phagocytes of the reticuloendothelial system. With pulmonary involvement, reticulonodular infiltrates progress to cystic changes and honeycombing, primarily in the upper lobes. Pathologically, there is an interstitial accumulation of atypical histiocytes similar to

Langerhans' cells (14). Electron microscopic examination of these tissue histiocytes reveals an indented nucleus and small (40 to 45 nm diameter) elongated bodies scattered throughout the cytoplasm termed "X bodies" (1,14,131). Identification of HX cells by transmission electron microscopy is often time consuming and expensive (4).

Lavage may be useful in the diagnosis of HX. In these patients, there is usually an increased total number of cells, the percentage of lymphocytes may be normal or elevated, and there may be a small increase in neutrophils and eosinophils (4). Chollet and colleagues (132) evaluated the use of immunofluorescence of Langerhans' cells using monoclonal antibodies to these cells (OKT6 monoclonal antibody) in BAL specimens. BAL from 131 patients with a variety of pulmonary diseases including HX (18 patients) were examined; fluorescent (OKT6-positive) cells were found in all patients with biopsy-confirmed HX (range 1.8% to 25% of all BAL cells). In the other 113 patients, the fluorescent cells constituted only 0.2% of the total number of cells, significantly fewer than in the HX patients.

Casolero and associates (133) evaluated BAL fluid from 5 normal non-smokers and 10 normal smokers for the presence of Langerhans' cells as identified by the OKT6 monoclonal antibody and by transmission electron microscopy. The OKT6 antibody identified 0.1% ± 0.1% of the cells from non-smokers but labeled 1.1% ± 0.3% of the cells recovered from smokers ($P < 0.01$). By electron microscopy, no Langerhans' cells were demonstrated in non-smokers while 0.4% ± 0.1% of the cells recovered from smokers contained the characteristic intracytoplasmic inclusions of Langerhans' cells. Xaubet and coworkers (134) evaluated BAL fluid for OKT6-positive cells in 70 subjects: 18 normal smokers, 14 normal non-smokers, 15 patients with sarcoidosis, 12 patients with IPF, 3 patients with HX, and 8 patients with lung neoplasms. OKT6-positive cells were observed in 41 of 77

lavages (53.2%), accounting for 0.25% to 7% of alveolar macrophages. OKT6 positive cells were present in BAL from 12 of 18 control smokers, 7 of 14 control non-smokers, 5 of 15 patients with sarcoidosis, 8 of 12 patients with IPF, and 3 of 8 patients with lung neoplasm. The percentage of positive cells was significantly higher in smokers than non-smokers. In all of these groups, though, the OKT6-positive cells comprised less than 1% of alveolar macrophages, except in one case of IPF with 2% OKT6-positive cells. In contrast, OKT6-positive cells accounted for 3% to 7% of the alveolar macrophages in six BALs performed in the 3 patients with HX. These authors concluded that normal smokers and non-smokers as well as patients with various lung disorders rarely have more than 1% of positive cells in BAL fluid and that a percentage of OKT6-positive cells equal to or greater than 3% suggests the diagnosis of histiocytosis X (134). Whereas these are probably appropriate general guidelines, further studies with quantitative evaluation of Langerhans' cells in BAL fluid are needed before there can be *clearly defined* criteria for the diagnosis of HX by BAL fluid analysis (3).

Pulmonary Alveolar Proteinosis

Pulmonary alveolar proteinosis (PAP) involves widespread filling of alveoli with a lipoprotein material that stains with a periodic acid-Schiff (PAS) reagent. Electron microscopic examination of the lipid material shows characteristic whorled lamellar bodies (14). In addition, the lipoprotein material has been demonstrated to stain with specific antibodies to surfactant apoprotein (14,135). Analysis of BAL may obviate the need for a diagnostic open lung biopsy in patients with PAP (3,136). The findings by BAL which have been reported in BAL in PAP include: 1) the gross appearance is opaque or milky; 2) few alveolar macrophages and a normal cell differential; 3) alveolar macrophages occasionally contain eosinophilic granules identical to that seen in lung biopsies in PAP; 4) large acellular eosinophilic bodies against a background of small eosinophilic granules and amorphous debris; and 5) predominant PAS staining of the proteinaceous material with a lack of significant alcian blue staining (5,137). It is important that all of these conditions be satisfied before a diagnosis of PAP is considered because milky appearance and lipoprotein aggregates may only occasionally occur in lavage fluid from patients with a variety of other interstitial lung disease; however, they are ultrastructurally and biochemically different than those from PAP (3,138). BAL may provide important diagnostic information in PAP, but an open lung biopsy may still be necessary, in some instances, for a definitive diagnosis.

Chronic Eosinophilic Pneumonia

Bronchoalveolar lavage of patients with chronic eosinophilic pneumonia usually shows a marked increase in eosinophils (14,139,140). Dejaegher and Demendts (141) found that patients treated with steroids normalized their BAL along with improvements in clinical and radiologic features of the disease.

Alveolar Hemorrhage

Bronchoalveolar lavage may also be clinically useful in the diagnosis of occult pulmonary hemorrhage, which may cause radiographic abnormalities simulating other interstitial or infectious disorders. This is a particularly difficult problem in immunocompromised patients, and hemoptysis is often absent. A grossly bloody appearance to BAL is not always diagnostic because it may be secondary to bronchoscopy-induced trauma, especially in the anticoagulated patient (4). Gold and colleagues (142), Finley and coworkers (143), and Drew and associates (144) reported that alveolar hemorrhage could be diagnosed safely in both immunocompromised, thrombocytopenic, and anticoagulated patients by staining alveolar macrophages obtained by BAL for the presence of hemosiderin. The

episode of acute pulmonary hemorrhage probably has to occur at least 48 hours before BAL for the alveolar macrophages to demonstrate increased amounts of hemosiderin (42,145). Although the utility of BAL in the diagnosis of occult pulmonary hemorrhage has been recognized for some time, two important points must be remembered: 1) the cause of pulmonary hemorrhage is not diagnosed by BAL; that is, other important pulmonary processes may be associated with occult pulmonary hemorrhage such as infection, particularly in immunocompromised patients, and 2) hemosiderin-laden macrophages have been found in a variety of other lung diseases including IPF, cardiac disease, sarcoidosis, carcinoma, vasculitis, PAP, and HX (4,14,143). Hemorrhage should be assumed to be the sole cause for pulmonary infiltrates if hemosiderin-laden macrophages predominate in lavage, pulmonary edema has been excluded, therapy is not altered, and the alveolar disease clears within one to 3 days (147).

Fat Embolism

The identification of neutral fat droplets by staining with oil red O within cells recovered by BAL in patients with recent trauma may be a rapid and specific method for establishing the diagnosis of the fat embolism syndrome (146). Lipid staining of BAL specimens may also be useful in the diagnosis of lipoid pneumonia (149,150).

Use of Bronchoalveolar Lavage in the Diagnosis of Malignancy

Bronchoalveolar lavage may also be a useful adjunct along with other diagnostic techniques in the diagnosis of malignancy involving the lung. BAL usefulness in primary lung cancer is primarily limited to peripheral lesions not endoscopically visible. The diagnostic yield of BAL varies from series to series and may be as high as 69% (151) when all lesions are included; however, BAL cytology is positive in approximately 25% of patients with peripheral lesions eventually proved to have malignancy (140, 152). Lavage is probably particularly useful in diffuse lesions, such as those found with bronchoalveolar cell carcinoma; the diagnostic yield of BAL is probably higher for bronchoalveolar cell carcinoma than for other cell types of primary pulmonary malignancy with a positive cytology frequency approaching 90% (153,154). However, the cytologic diagnosis of malignancy does not always correspond to the histologic pattern; in the series of Linder and colleagues cytology agreed with biopsy in only 80% of cases (151,153). In addition, severe dysplastic changes that may develop in airway epithelial cells in clinical circumstances such as pneumonia, viral infections, and following chemotherapy can be difficult to distinguish from malignant changes (153). Diagnostic yield may also be diminished if the lavage fluid is filtered through gauze to remove mucus prior to cytologic examination: malignant cells are often removed by such filtration procedures. A number of tumor markers and other BAL measurements such as immunoglobulins or prostaglandins have been studied in BAL (153,155–157), but none have proved to be diagnostic and reliable enough to justify routine clinical use. At present, use of these markers must be considered investigational. Overall, in cases of suspected bronchogenic carcinoma, especially with peripheral distal lesions, performing BAL in the involved segment adds little time or risk to the bronchoscopic procedure, but may give valuable diagnostic information.

Metastatic disease may also be occasionally detected by BAL cytology, particularly in metastatic breast cancer and in patients with lymphangitic carcinoma (158,159).

Numerous case reports confirm the ability of BAL to diagnose leukemia and lymphomatous pulmonary involvement as well as plasma cell dyscrasias (160–165). BAL lymphocyte percentages greater than 20% were seen in all

reports of pulmonary lymphoma diagnosed by BAL; Hodgkin's disease can be diagnosed by the identification of Reed-Sternberg cells in BAL cytology specimens (161).

Bronchoalveolar Lavage in the Diagnosis of Infectious Diseases

Bacterial/Nosocomial Pneumonia

The primary difficulty in obtaining samples of lower respiratory tract secretions by FOB with BAL is contamination of the bronchoscope as it passes through the naso-oropharynx. Administration of lidocaine by inhalation rather than bolus injection and performance of BAL through a previously inserted endotracheal tube have been shown to reduce the incidence of contamination (6). In eight normal volunteers, Kirkpatrick and Bass (166) found BAL to yield sterile growth in only one specimen; however, quantitative cultures revealed less than 10^4 cfu/mL (colony forming units) in all specimens. Henceforth, quantitative cultures of BAL fluid have been used in multiple studies, with conflicting results. This may, in large part, be due to the difficulty in defining bacterial/nosocomial pneumonia. Fever, pulmonary infiltrates, and purulent tracheal secretions, for example, can be associated with a variety of other pathologic processes (167).

Thorpe and colleagues (168) performed semiquantitative cultures of BAL fluid in 77 patients with a variety of pulmonary disorders (e.g., carcinoma, tuberculosis, sarcoidosis, bronchitis, and histoplasmosis) and 15 patients believed to have bacterial pneumonia (active or progressive infiltrate with fever and leukocytosis). Bronchoscopy was performed either transnasally or through an endotracheal tube. In 13 of 15 pneumonia patients, various bacteria grew at densities of 10^5 cfu/mL or greater. Four patients with cultures 10^5 cfu/mL or greater also had positive blood cultures for the same organism as that recovered from the BAL fluid. Gram stains of cytocentrifuged

BAL specimens also showed a high degree of correlation with the BAL culture results and were good predictors of the organism subsequently cultured. None of the 77 patients without acute pneumonia had BAL cultures that showed 10^5 cfu/mL or more and only 4 of 77 had BAL cultures that showed 10^4 cfu/mL or greater.

Kahn and Jones (169) in a similar fashion examined 57 patients with fever and a new pulmonary infiltrate. Most patients, however, were immunocompromised. They observed that quantitative BAL cultures (with a transnasal approach) was 100% sensitive (13 of 13) in diagnosing bacterial pneumonia when BAL bacteria counts exceeded 10^5 cfu/mL *with* less than 1% squamous epithelial cells on differential count of the lavage pellet. Eight with bacterial infection had received antibiotics for one to 7 days prior to bronchoscopy and still had 10^5 cfu/mL or more of bacteria.

Johansen and coworkers (170), using an intubated baboon model, which also allowed the investigators to culture lung homogenates and review lung histology, concluded that in nosocomial pneumonia occurring in the setting of mechanical ventilation, BAL provides the best reflection of the lung's bacterial burden. Using a "bacterial index" (BI) (converting the bacterial concentration of the separate bacterial species to log 10), all animals with moderate to severe pneumonia had at least one BAL BI value of greater than 6.0 /mL. BAL recovered 74% of all bacterial species found in lung tissue compared with 41% by protected specimen brush (PSB) and 56% for direct lung needle aspirates. The BI values of BAL were linearly related to tissue values, whether the BAL was performed in the same lobe or a different lobe.

Torres and associates (171) compared the diagnostic yield of BAL and PSB in 34 mechanically ventilated subjects suspected of having bacterial pneumonia and found the culture results of each technique agreed 89% of the time. Guerra and Baughman (172) performed BAL on 54 patients on mechanical ventilators who underwent bronchoscopy for clinical pneumonia (30 patients) or a noninfection process (14 patients). Eighteen patients were felt to have bacterial pneumonia. A large number of cfu/mL were seen in 16 of 18 patients with pneumonia and none of those without pneumonia had greater than 10^4 cfu/mL. Seventy percent of the patients with bacterial pneumonia were receiving antibiotics and none of the significant organisms was sensitive to an antibiotic the patient was already receiving.

Chastre and coworkers (167) examined 21 patients who had received mechanical ventilation for more than 3 days, had not been treated with antibiotics for 10 days, and clinically were suspected to have nosocomial bacterial pneumonia. Lung tissue specimens were available at autopsy in 6 of these patients. Five patients were thought to definitely have pneumonia and in 13 patients it was thought to be definitely excluded by clinical course. The authors found quantification of intracellular organisms in cells recovered from BAL (greater than 25% of cells with intracellular organisms in pneumonia patients versus less than 15% of cells with intracellular organisms in patients without pneumonia) useful in distinguishing pneumonia patients. They did not find quantitative culture of BAL fluid helpful because they could find no clear threshold that clearly separated patients with pneumonia from those without, although the number of organisms recovered per mL of BAL fluid from patients with pneumonia was higher than that recovered from patients without pneumonia ($P < 0.05$). However, one year later, they no longer considered 15% to 25% as a suitable cutoff (for quantification of intracellular organisms in cells recovered from BAL) for distinguishing pneumonia patients, and dropped the cutoff to 7% of cells containing intracellular bacteria to identify patients with pneumonia (173).

Meduri and colleagues (174,175) most recently described a technique of protected bronchoalveolar lavage (pBAL), performed through a protected transbronchoscopic balloon-tipped catheter, designed to minimize oropharyngeal and tracheobronchial contamination. In 46 patients with lung disease, pBAL had fewer than 1% squamous epithelial cells in 91% of specimens and no growth in 59% of specimens from patients without pneumonia. With a diagnostic threshold of 10^4 cfu/mL, 1 of 33 patients without pneumonia had a false positive result, and 1 of 13 patients with pneumonia had a false negative finding. The presence of intracellular organisms in 2% or greater of the recovered BAL cells was seen in all but 2 patients with pneumonia and in none of the patients without pneumonia. Gram stains of the pBAL specimens were positive in all but one patient with pneumonia and negative in all but one patient without infection. The time off antibiotic therapy before bronchoscopy did not affect the result of pBAL cultures (175).

Thus, in summary, in bacterial/nosocomial pneumonia quantitative cultures of BAL fluid may be clinically helpful, even if the patient is already taking antibiotics. The presence of intracellular organisms in recovered cells may be helpful as well. However, there is no clear consensus currently on the use of BAL in this group of patients.

Bronchoalveolar Lavage in the Immunocompromised Host

Numerous reviews confirm the diagnostic utility and safety of BAL in the immunocompromised host (176–180). The utility of BAL in several specific categories of immunocompromised patients is discussed below.

Human Immunodeficiency Virus and AIDS

The largest study examining the utility of BAL in AIDS involved 276 bronchoscopies in 171 patients with AIDS and respiratory symptoms or an abnormal chest x-ray, gallium scan, or diffusing capacity (47). BAL and transbronchial biopsy had sensitivities of 86% and

87%, respectively. When both techniques were used, the yield for all pathogens was 98% and the sensitivity for *Pneumocystis carinii* infections was 100% with a negative predictive value of 92% to 100%. Weldon-Linne and colleagues (181) more recently found in 183 patients that BAL was more sensitive for *P. carinii* than transbronchial biopsy. These two studies showed quite similar results: *P. carinii* was present in 50% to 57% of specimens, cytomegalovirus in 43% to 50%, and *Mycobacterium avium-intracellulare* in 10%, with all other pathogens seen in frequencies less than 5%. Weldon-Linne and coworkers concluded that in the work-up of nonneoplastic pulmonary disease in AIDS patients, transbronchial biopsy is not necessary as a routine procedure when both BAL cytology and culture are performed at bronchoscopy (181).

Johnson and associates (182) evaluated 39 HIV-positive patients without AIDS, some with blood CD4 counts less than $400/mm^3$. There was no difference in macrophage or lymphocyte percentages compared to controls. There was no difference in BAL CD4 numbers or the CD4/CD8 ratio in patients with blood CD4 counts above or below 400 mm^3. Opportunistic organisms such as *P. carinii* were not found in any of the 35 BAL fluids sent for cultures and special stains. The authors concluded that opportunistic pulmonary infection is unlikely in HIV-seropositive patients with normal chest x-rays despite symptoms of dyspnea on exertion.

In patients with AIDS, BAL fluid tends to have more lymphocytes and neutrophils, a lower T4/T8 ratio due to an increase in total T8 cells, and normal T4 cell counts, despite a significant decrease in numbers of T4 cells in peripheral blood (183).

Leukemia

Tenholder and Hooper (184) reported that the etiology of pulmonary infiltrates in leukemic patients depends on the radiographic pattern and the timing of the infiltrate appearance.

Infiltrates before or within 72 hours of the initiation of treatment are usually not caused by opportunistic infections. Focal infiltrates appearing later tend to be caused by bacterial infection. Diffuse lung infiltrates appearing later are likely to be of noninfectious etiology, but when caused by infection (35% of cases) opportunistic infections were the cause in 93%. BAL is helpful in the diagnosis of such infections.

Bone Marrow Transplant

As many as one half of bone marrow transplant (BMT) patients suffer from a major pulmonary problem in the 6 months immediately after transplantation (186). The organisms most commonly identified by BAL in BMT patients are cytomegalovirus, bacteria, and aspergillus (187). A syndrome of diffuse alveolar hemorrhage unique to BMT patients developing about 2 weeks after transplant has been described (188). This is associated with fever, renal failure, central nervous system dysfunction, thrombocytopenia, and diffuse infiltrates. The BAL findings include little or no blood on bronchial wash but each successive aliquot of fluid lavaged at a single wedged site yields returns that are progressively bloodier. BAL is a safe and well-tolerated procedure in BMT patients and often will be the only bronchoscopic procedure which can be safely performed; the diagnostic yield overall was 52% in one study and 80% in another (186,187).

Summary

In conclusion, the appropriate clinical role of BAL in the various aspects of pulmonary medicine is continually evolving. In ILDs such as sarcoidosis, IPF, and PF-CVD, the precise role of BAL in determining therapeutic decisions or predicting response to therapy is currently unclear. In occupational lung diseases, particularly asbestos-related lung disease and berylliosis, BAL may give important information in assessing exposure. In malignancy, performing

a BAL adds little risk or time to the bronchoscopic procedure and may give valuable diagnostic information that may not be provided by forceps biopsy or brushings (8). More studies are clearly needed to develop a clear consensus on the use of BAL in the diagnosis of nosocomial/bacterial pneumonia, but it is a valuable technique in immunocompromised patients, particularly AIDS.

In the future, hopefully, the role of BAL, especially in ILD and bacterial/nosocomial pneumonia, will be more clearly elucidated. BAL will also in the future allow experimental manipulations of the lower respiratory tract and may even be used therapeutically: cells obtained by BAL could be subjected to "repair" mechanisms and reinfused into the lungs (189). For example, some methods to alter cellular functions in cells obtained from the lung include selection, activation, or expansion of specific subpopulations of lung cells (189). Immune and inflammatory effector cells could be activated and reinfused in diseases such as malignancy, or specific suppressor cells could be activated and reintroduced in diseases like asthma characterized by inappropriate activation of inflammatory effector cells (189). BAL is one procedure where its potential will be most fully realized with continued cooperation between cellular and molecular biologists and clinicians.

ACKNOWLEDGMENT: The authors would like to thank Karen Schuldies for her expert secretarial assistance in the preparation of this manuscript.

REFERENCES

1. Hunninghake GW, Gadek JE, Kawanami O, Ferrans VJ, Crystal RG. Inflammatory and immune processes in the human in health and disease: evaluation by bronchoalveolar lavage. Am J Pathol 1979;97:149–198.
2. Reynolds HY, Newball HH. Analysis of proteins and respiratory cells from human lungs by bronchial lavage. J Lab Clin Med 1974;84:559–573.

3. American Thoracic Society. Clinical role of bronchoalveolar lavage in adults with pulmonary disease. Am Rev Respir Dis 1990;142:481–486.

4. Helmers RA, Hunninghake GW. Bronchoalveolar lavage. In: Wang KP, ed. Biopsy techniques in pulmonary disorders. New York: Raven Press, 1989:15–28.

5. Haslam, PL. Bronchoalveolar lavage. Sem Respir Med 1984;6:55–70.

6. Pang JA, Cheng AFB, Chan HS, French GL. Special precautions reduce oropharyngeal contamination in bronchoalveolar lavage for bacteriologic studies. Lung 1989;167: 261–267.

7. Pingleton SK, Harrison GF, Stechschulte DJ, Wesselius LJ, Kerby GR, Ruth WE. Effect of location, pH, and temperature of instillate in bronchoalveolar lavage in normal volunteer. Am Rev Respir Dis 1983;128:1035–1037.

8. Helmers RA, Hunninghake GW. Bronchoscopy: bronchoalveolar lavage in the nonimmunocompromised patient. Chest 1989; 96:1184–1190.

9. European Society of Pneumology Task Group on BAL. Technical recommendations and guidelines for bronchoalveolar lavage (BAL). Eur Respir J 1989;2:561–585.

10. Garcia JGN, Wolven RG, Garcia PL, Keogh BA. Assessment of interlobar variation of bronchoalveolar lavage cellular differentials in interstitial lung diseases. Am Rev Respir Dis 1986;133:444–449.

11. Helmers RA, Dayton CS, Floerchunger C, Hunninghake GW. Bronchoalveolar lavage in interstitial lung disease: effect of volume of fluid infused. J Appl Physiol 1989;67:1443–1446.

12. Davis GS, Giancola MS, Constanza MC, Low RB. Analyses of sequential bronchoalveolar lavage samples from healthy human volunteers. Am Rev Respir Dis 1982;126:611–616.

13. Carre PH, Laviolette M, Belanger J, Cormier Y. Technical variations in bronchoalveolar lavage (BAL): influence of atelectasis and the lung region lavaged. Lung 1985; 163:117–125.

14. Daniele RP, Elias JA, Epstein PE, Rossman MD. Bronchoalveolar lavage: role in the pathogenesis, diagnosis, and management of interstitial lung disease. Ann Intern Med 1985;102:93–108.

15. The BAL Cooperative Group Steering Committee. Bronchoalveolar lavage constituents in healthy individuals, idiopathic pulmonary fibrosis, and selected comparison groups. Ann Rev Respir Dis 1990;141: S169–S202.

16. Kuylenstiern R, Hernbrand R, Eklund A. Comparison of bronchoalveolar lavage fluid recovered during bronchoscopy with local or general anesthesia. Arch Otolaryngol 1988; 144:443–445.

17. Hoidal JR, White JG, Repine JE. Impairment of human alveolar macrophage oxygen consumption, and superoxide anion production by local anesthetics used in bronchoscopy. Chest 1979;755(suppl):2435–2465.

18. Rabinovitch M, DeStefano MJ. Cell shape changes induced by cationic anesthetics. J Exp Med 1976;143:290–304.

19. Hold PG. Alveolar macrophages. I. Simple technique for the preparation of high numbers of viable alveolar macrophages from small laboratory animals. J Immunol Methods 1979;27:189–198.

20. Strange C, Barbarash RA, Heffner JE. Lidocaine concentrations in bronchoscopic specimens. Chest 1988;93:547–549.

21. Kelly CA, Kotre CJ, Ward C, Hendrick DJ, Walters EH. Anatomical distribution of bronchoalveolar lavage fluid as assessed by digitalsubtraction radiography. Thorax 1987;42: 624–628.

22. Helmers RA, Galvin J, Dayton CS, Yuh W, Stanford W, Hunninghake GW. Small volume bronchoalveolar lavage (BAL) uniformly perfuses the lung segment in interstitial lung disease as assessed by magnetic resonance imaging (MRI). Am Rev Respir Dis 1989; 139:A472.

23. Crystal RG, Reynolds HY, Kalica AR. Bronchoalveolar lavage. The report of an international conference. Chest 1986; 90:122–131.

24. Dohn MN, Baughman RP. Effect of changing instilled volume for bronchoalveolar lavage in patients with interstitial lung disease. Am Rev Respir Dis 1985;132:390–392.

25. Lam S, Leriche JC, Kijek K, Phillips D. Effect of bronchial lavage volume on cellular and protein recovery. Chest 1985;88:856–859.

26. Rennard SI, Ghafouri M, Thompson AB, et al. Fractional processing of sequential

bronchial and alveolar samples. Am Rev Respir Dis 1990;141:208–217.

27. Merrill W, O'Hearn E, Rankin J, Naegel G, Matthay RA, Reynolds HY. Kinetic analysis of respiratory tract proteins recovered during a sequential lavage protocol. Ann Rev Respir Dis 1982;126:617–620.

28. Reynolds HY. Bronchoalveolar lavage. Am Rev Respir Dis 1987;135:250–263.

29. Rankin JA, Naegel GP, Reynolds HY. Use of a central laboratory for analysis of bronchoalveolar lavage fluid. Am Rev Respir Dis 1986;133:186–190.

30. Kelly CA, Fenwick JD, Corris PA, Fleetwood A, Hendrick DJ, Walters EH. Fluid dynamics during bronchoalveolar lavage. Am Rev Respir Dis 1988;138:81–84.

31. Saltini C, Hance AJ, Ferrans VJ, Bassett F, Bitterman PB, Crystal RG. Accurate quantification of cells recovered by bronchoalveolar lavage. Am Rev Respir Dis 1984; 130:650–658.

32. Laviolette M, Carreau M, Coulombe R. Bronchoalveolar lavage cell differential on microscope glass cover: a simple and accurate technique. Am Rev Respir Dis 1988; 138:451–457.

33. Thompson AB, Robbins RA, Ghasfouri MA, et al. Bronchoalveolar lavage fluid processing: effect of membrane filtration preparation on neutrophil recovery. Acta Cytol 1989; 33:544–549.

34. Strumpf IJ, Feld MK, Cornelius MJ, Keogh BA, Crystal RG. Safety of fiberoptic bronchoalveolar lavage in evaluation of interstitial lung disease. Chest 1981;80:268–271.

35. Cole P, Twiton C, Lanyon H, Collins J. Bronchoalveolar lavage for the preparation of free lung cells: techniques and complications. Br J Chest 1980;74:273–278.

36. Standiford TJ, Kunkel SL, Strieter RM. Elevated serum levels of tumor necrosis factor-α after bronchoscopy and bronchoalveolar lavage. Chest 1991;99:1529–1530.

37. Vonessen SG, Robbins RA, Spurzem JR, et al. Bronchoscopy with bronchoalveolar lavage causes neutrophil recruitment to the lower respiratory tract. Am Rev Respir Dis 1991;144:848–854.

38. Tilles DS, Goldheim PD, Ginns LC, Hales CA. Pulmonary function in normal subjects and patients with sarcoidosis after bronchoalveolar lavage. Chest 1986;89:244–248.

39. Ettensohn DB, Jankowski MJ, Redondo AA, Duncan PG. Bronchoalveolar lavage in the normal volunteer subject. 2. Safety and results of repeated BAL, and use in the assessment of intrasubject variability. Chest 1988;94:281–285.

40. Pirozynski M, Sliwinski P, Zielinski J. Effect of different volumes of BAL fluid on arterial oxygen saturation. Eur Respir J 1988;1:943–947.

41. Lin C, Jen-Liang W, Huang W. Pulmonary function in normal subjects after bronchoalveolar lavage. Chest 1988;93:1049–1053.

42. Stover DE, Zaman MB, Hajdu SI, Lange M, Gold J, Armstrong D. Bronchoalveolar lavage in the diagnosis of diffuse pulmonary infiltrates in the immunocompromised host. Ann Intern Med 1984;101:1–7.

43. Ognibene FP, Shelhamer J, Giu V, et al. The diagnosis of *Pneumocystis carinii* pneumonia in patients with the acquired immunodeficiency syndrome using subsegmental bronchoalveolar lavage. Am Rev Respir Dis 1984;129:929–932.

44. Broaddus C, Dake MD, Stulbarg MS, et al. Bronchoalveolar lavage and transbronchial biopsy for the diagnosis of pulmonary infection in the acquired immunodeficiency syndrome. Ann Intern Med 1985;102:747–752.

45. Stover DE, White DA, Romano PA, Gelleue RA. Diagnosis of pulmonary disease in the acquired immune deficiency syndrome (AIDS): role of bronchoscopy and bronchoalveolar lavage. Am Rev Respir Dis 1984;130:659–662.

46. Cordonnier C, Bomaddin JF, Fleury J, et al. Diagnostic yield of bronchoalveolar lavage in pneumonitis occurring after allogeneic bone marrow transplantation. Am Rev Respir Dis 1985;132:1118–1123.

47. Gurney JW, Harrison WC, Sears K, Robbins RA, Dobry CA, Rennard SI. Bronchoalveolar lavage: radiographic manifestation. Radiology 1987;163:71–74.

48. Marcy TW, Merrill WW, Rankin JA, Reynolds HY. Limitations of using urea to quantify epithelial lining fluid recovered by bronchoalveolar lavage. Am Rev Respir Dis 1987;135:1276–1280.

49. Laviolette M. Lymphocyte fluctuation in bronchoalveolar lavage fluid in normal volunteers. Thorax 1985;40:651–656.

50. Crystal RG, Bitterman PB, Rennard SI, Hance AJ, Keogh BA. Interstitial lung disease of unknown cause—disorders characterized by chronic inflammation of the lower respiratory tract. N Engl J Med 1984;310: 154–166, 235–244.

51. Haslam PL, Turton GWG, Heard B, et al. Bronchoalveolar lavage in pulmonary fibrosis: comparison of cells obtained with lung biopsy and clinical features. Thorax 1980;35:9–18.

52. Hunninghake GW, Gadek JE. Immunological aspects of chronic noninfectious pulmonary diseases of the lower respiratory tract in man. Clin Immunol Rev 1981–1982;1:337–374.

53. Hunninghake GW, Kawanai O, Ferrans VJ, Young RC, Robert WC, Crystal RG. Characterization of the inflammatory and immune effect on cells in the lung parenchyma of patients with interstitial lung disease. Am Rev Respir Dis 1981;123:401–412.

54. Semenzato G, Chilosi M, Ossi E, et al. Bronchoalveolar lavage and lung histology—comparative analysis of inflammatory and immunocompetent cells in patients with sarcoidosis and hypersensitivity pneumonitis. Am Rev Respir Dis 1985;132:400–404.

55. Hunninghake GW, Crystal RG. Pulmonary sarcoidosis—a disorder mediated by excess helper T-lymphocyte activity at sites of disease activity. N Eng J Med 1981;305: 429–434.

56. Leathermann JW, Michael AF, Schwartz BA, Hoidal JR. Lung T-cells in hypersensitivity pneumonitis. Ann Intern Med 1984;100:390–392.

57. Lin YN, Haslam PL, Turner-Warwick M. Chronic pulmonary sarcoidosis: relationship between lung lavage cell counts, chest radiograph, and results of standard lung function test. Thorax 1985;40:501–507.

58. Keogh BA, Hunninghake GW, Line BR, Crystal RG. The alveolitis of pulmonary sarcoidosis—evaluation of natural history and alveolitis-dependent changes in lung function. Am Rev Respir Dis 1983;128:256–265.

59. Israel-Biet D, Venet A, Chretien J. Persistent high alveolar lymphocytosis as a predictive criterion of chronic pulmonary sarcoidosis. Ann N Y Acad Sci 1986;465:395–406.

60. Foley NM, Coral AP, Tung K, Hudspith BN, James DG, Johnson NM. Bronchoalveolar lavage cell counts as a predictor of short-term outcome in pulmonary sarcoidosis. Thorax 1989;44:732–738.

61. Costabel U, Bross KJ, Guzman J, Nilles A, Ruhle KH, Matthys H. Predictive value of bronchoalveolar T-cell subsets for the course of pulmonary sarcoidosis. Ann N Y Acad Sci 1986;465:418–426.

62. Cueppens JL, Lacquet LM, Marien G, Demedts M, van den Eeckhout A, Stevens E. Alveolar T-cell subsets in pulmonary sarcoidosis—correlation with disease activity and effect of steroid treatments. Am Rev Respir Dis 1984;129:563–568.

63. Verstraeten A, Demedts M, Verwilghen J, et al. Predictive value of bronchoalveolar lavage in pulmonary sarcoidosis. Chest 1990;98: 560–567.

64. Ward K, O'Connor C, Odlum C, Fitzgerald M. Prognostic value of bronchoalveolar lavage in sarcoidosis: the critical influence of disease presentation. Thorax 1989;44:6–12.

65. Bjermer L, Engstrom-Laurent A, Thune UM, Hallgren R. Hyaluronic acid in bronchoalveolar lavage fluid in patients with sarcoidosis: relationship to lavage mast cells. Thorax 1987;42:933–938.

66. Bjermer L, Rosenhall L, Angstrom T, Hallgren R. Predictive value of bronchoalveolar lavage cell analysis in sarcoidosis. Thorax 1988;43:284–288.

67. Lawrence ED, Teague RB, Gottlieb MS, Jhingran SG, Liebermann J. Serial changes in markers of disease activity with corticosteroid treatment in sarcoidosis. Am J Med 1983; 74:747–756.

68. Hollinger WM, Staton GW, Fajman WA, Gilman MJ, Pine JR, Check IJ. Prediction of therapeutic response in steroid-treated pulmonary sarcoidosis—evaluation of clinical parameters, bronchoalveolar lavage, gallium-67 lung scanning, and serum angiotensin-converting enzyme levels. Am Rev Respir Dis 1985;132:65–69.

69. Baughman RP, Fernandez M, Bosken CH, Mantil J, Hurtubise P. Comparison of gallium-67 scanning, bronchoalveolar lavage, and serum angiotensin-converting enzyme levels in pulmonary sarcoidosis. Am Rev Respir Dis 1984;129:676–681.

70. Baughman RP, Shipley R, Eisentrout CE.

Predictive value of gallium scan, angiotensin-converting enzyme level, and bronchoalveolar lavage in two-year follow-up of pulmonary sarcoidosis. Lung 1987;165:371–377.

71. Turner-Warwick M, McAllister W, Lawrence R, Britten A, Haslam PL. Corticosteroid treatment in pulmonary sarcoidosis: do serial lavage lymphocyte counts, serum angiotensin-converting enzyme measurements, and gallium-67 scans help management? Thorax 1986;41:903–913.

72. O'Connor C, Odlum C, Van Breda A, Power C, Fitzgerald MX. Collagenase and fibronectin in bronchoalveolar lavage fluid in patients with sarcoidosis. Thorax 1988; 43:393–400.

73. Ward K, O'Connor CM, Odlum C, Power C, Fitzgerald MX. Pulmonary disease progress in sarcoid patients with and without bronchoalveolar lavage collagenase. Am Rev Respir Dis 1990;142:636–641.

74. O'Connor C, Ward K, Van Breda A, McIlgorn A, Fitzgerald MX. Type 3 procollagen peptide in bronchoalveolar lavage fluid: poor indicator of course and prognosis in sarcoidosis. Chest 1989;96:339–344.

75. Bjermer L, Lundgren R, Hallgren R. Hyaluron and type III procollagen peptide concentrations in bronchoalveolar lavage fluid in idiopathic pulmonary fibrosis. Thorax 1989;44:126–131.

76. Blaschke E, Eklund A, Hembrand R. Extracellular matrix components in bronchoalveolar lavage fluid in sarcoidosis and their relationship to signs of alveolitis. Am Rev Respir Dis 1990;141:1020–1025.

77. Ainslie GM, Poulter LW, duBois RM. Relation between immunocytological features of bronchoalveolar lavage fluid and clinical indices of sarcoidosis. Thorax 1989;44:501–509.

78. Haslam PL, Turton CWG, Lukoszek A, et al. Bronchoalveolar lavage fluid cell count in cryptogenic fibrosing alveolitis and their relation to therapy. Thorax 1980;35:328–339.

79. Rudd RM, Haslam PL, Turner-Warwick M. Cryptogenic fibrosing alveolitis relationships of pulmonary physiology and bronchoalveolar lavage to response to treatment and prognosis. Am Rev Respir Dis 1981; 124:1–8.

80. Turner-Warwick M, Haslam PL. The value of serial bronchoalveolar lavages in assessing the clinical progress of patients with cryptogenic fibrosing alveolitis. Am Rev Respir Dis 1987;135:26–34.

81. O'Donnell K, Keogh B, Cantin A, Crystal RG. Pharmacologic suppression of the neutrophil component of the alveolitis in idiopathic pulmonary fibrosis. Am Rev Respir Dis 1987;136:288–292.

82. Watters LC, Schwarz MI, Cherniack RM, et al. Idiopathic pulmonary fibrosis: pretreatment bronchoalveolar lavage cellular constituents and their relationships with lungs to pathology and clinical response to therapy. Am Rev Respir Dis 1987;135:696–704.

83. Honda Y, Tsunematsu K, Suzuki A, Akino T. Changes in phospholipids in bronchoalveolar lavage fluid of patients with interstitial lung diseases. Lung 1988;166:293–301.

84. Robinson PC, Walters LC, King TE, Maron RJ. Idiopathic pulmonary fibrosis: abnormalities in bronchoalveolar lavage fluid phospholipids. Am Rev Respir Dis 1988; 137:585–591.

85. Hughes DA, Haslam PL. Changes in phosphatidylglycerol in bronchoalveolar lavage fluids from patients with cryptogenic fibrosing alveolitis. Chest 1989;95:82–89.

86. Silver RM, Metcalf JF, Stanley JH, LeRoy EC. Interstitial lung disease in scleroderma—analysis by bronchoalveolar lavage. Arthritis Rheum 1984;27:1254–1262.

87. Kallenberg CGM, Jansen HM, Elema JD, The TH. Steroid-responsive interstitial pulmonary disease in systemic sclerosis—monitoring by bronchoalveolar lavage. Chest 1984;86: 489–491.

88. Greene NB, Solinger AM, Baughman RP. Patients with collagen vascular disease and dyspnea: the value of gallium scanning and bronchoalveolar lavage in predicting response to steroid therapy and clinical outcome. Chest 1987;91:698–703.

89. Casale TB, Little MM, Furst D, Wood D, Hunninghake GW. Elevated BAL fluid histamine levels and parenchymal pulmonary disease in rheumatoid arthritis. Chest 1989; 96:1016–1021.

90. Gilligan DM, O'Connor CM, Ward K, Moloney D, Bresnihan B, Fitzgerald MX. Bronchoalveolar lavage in patients with mild and severe rheumatoid lung disease. Thorax 1990;45:591–596.

91. Silver RM, Miller KS, Kinsella MB, Smith

EA, Schabel SI. Evaluation and management of scleroderma lung disease using bronchoalveolar lavage. Am J Med 1990;88: 470–476.

92. Wallaert B, Hatron P, Grosbois J, Tonnel A, Devulder B, Voisin C. Subclinical pulmonary involvements in collagen vascular diseases assessed by bronchoalveolar lavage—relationship between alveolitis and subsequent changes in lung function. Am Rev Respir Dis 1986;133:574–580.

93. Wallaert B, Prin L, Hatron P, Ramon P, Tommel A, Voisin C. Lymphocyte subpopulations in bronchoalveolar lavage in Sjögren's syndrome: evidence for an expansion of cytotoxic/suppressor subset in patients with alveolar neutrophilia. Chest 1987; 92:1025–1031.

94. Garcia JGN, Parhami N, Killam D, Garcia PL, Keogh BA. Bronchoalveolar lavage fluid evaluation in rheumatoid arthritis. Am Rev Respir Dis 1986;133:450–454.

95. Haslam PL, Dewar A, Butcher P, Primett ZS, Newman-Taylor A, Turner-Warwick M. Mast cells, atypical lymphocytes and neutrophils in bronchoalveolar lavage in extrinsic allergic alveolitis. Am Rev Respir Dis 1987;135:35–47.

96. Haslam PL. Bronchoalveolar lavage in extrinsic allergic alveolitis. Eur J Respir Dis 1987;154(suppl):120–135.

97. Fournier E, Tonnel AB, Gossett P, Wallaert B, Ameisen JL, Voisin C. Early neutrophil alveolitis after antigen inhalation in hypersensitivity pneumonitis. Chest 1985;88:563–566.

98. Bjermer L, Engstrom-Laurent A, Hallgren R, Rosenhall L. Bronchoalveolar lavage in persons acutely exposed to dust in the farm environment. Am J Ind Med 1990;17:106.

99. Cormier Y, Belandger J, Laviollette M. Prognostic significance of bronchoalveolar lymphocytosis in farmer's lung. Am Rev Respir Dis 1987;135:692–695.

100. Gariepy L, Cormier Y, Laviollette M, Tardif A. Predictive value of bronchoalveolar lavage cells and serum perceptive in asymptomatic dairy farms. Am Rev Respir Dis 1989;140:1386–1389.

101. DeVuyst P, Jedaub J, Dumortier P, Vandermoten G, Vande Meyer R, Yernault JC. Asbestos bodies in bronchoalveolar lavage. Am Rev Respir Dis 1982;126: 972–976.

102. Roggli VL, Piantadosi CA, Bell DY.

Asbestos bodies in bronchoalveolar lavage fluid: a study of 20 asbestos-exposed individuals and comparison to patients with other chronic interstitial lung diseases. Acta Cytol 1986;30:470–476.

103. Rebuck AS, Brande AC. Bronchoalveolar lavage in asbestosis. Arch Intern Med 1983;143:950–952.

104. DuMortier P, DeVuyst P, Yernault JC. Mineralogical analysis of bronchoalveolar lavage fluids. Z Erkrank Atmorg 1988; 171:50–58.

105. DeVuyst P, DuMortier P, Moulin E. Yourassowski N, Roomans P, Yernault JC. Asbestos bodies in bronchoalveolar lavage reflect lung asbestos body concentration. Eur Respir J 1988;1:362–367.

106. DeVuyst P, DuMortier P, Moulin E, Yourassowski N, Yernault R. Diagnostic value of asbestos bodies in bronchoalveolar lavage fluid. Am Rev Respir Dis 1987; 136:1219–1224.

107. Churg A. Fiber counting and analysis in the diagnosis of asbestos-related disease. Hum Pathol 1982;13:381–392.

108. Sebastien P, Armstrong B, Monchaux G, Bignon J. Asbestos bodies in bronchoalveolar lavage fluid and in lung parenchyma. Am Rev Respir Dis 1988;137:75–78.

109. Schwartz DA, Galvin JR, Burmeister LF, et al. The clinical utility and reliability of asbestos bodies in bronchoalveolar fluid. Am Rev Respir Dis 1991;144:684–688.

110. Garcia JGN, Griffith DE, Cohen AB, Callahan KS. Alveolar macrophages from patients with asbestos exposure release increased levels of leukotriene By. Am Rev Respir Dis 1989;139:1494–1501.

111. Gellert AR, Langford JA, Winter RJD, Uthayakumar S, Sinha G, Rudd RM. Asbestosis: assessment by bronchoalveolar lavage and measurement of pulmonary epithelial permeability. Thorax 1985;40:508–514.

112. Robinson BWS, Rose AH, James A, Whitaker D, Musk AW. Alveolitis of pulmonary asbestosis-bronchoalveolar lavage studies in crocidolite- and chrysotile-exposed individuals. Chest 1986;90:396–402.

113. Xaubet A, Rodriquez-Roisin R, Bombi JA, Marin A, Roca J, Agusti-Vidal A. Correlation of bronchoalveolar lavage and clinical and functional findings in asbestosis. Am Rev Respir Dis 1986;133:848–854.

114. Begin R, Bisson G, Boileau R, Masse S. Assessment of disease activity by gallium-67 scan and lung lavage in the pneumoconioses. Semin Respir Med 1986;7:271–280.

115. Gellert AR, Langford JA, Uthayakumar S, Rudd RM. Bronchoalveolar lavage and clearance of 99mTc-labelled DTPA in asbestos workers without evidence of asbestosis. Thorax 1985;40:221.

116. Gellert AR, Macey MG, Uthayakumar S, Newland AC, Rudd RM. Lymphocyte subpopulations in bronchoalveolar lavage fluid in asbestos workers. Am Rev Respir Dis 1985;132:824–828.

117. Begin RO, Cantin AM, Boileau RD, Bisson GY. Spectrum of alveolitis in quartz-exposed human subjects. Chest 1987;92:1061–1067.

118. Schuyler MR, Gaumer HR, Stankus RP, Kaimal J, Hoffman E, Salvaggio JE. Bronchoalveolar lavage in silicosis—evidence of type II hyperplasia. Lung 1980;157:95–102.

119. Christman JW, Emerson RJ, Graham WGB, Davis GS. Mineral dust and cell recovery from the bronchoalveolar lavage of healthy Vermont granite workers. Am Rev Respir Dis 1985;132:393–399.

120. Kindt GC, Weiland JE, Davis WB, Gadek JE, Dorinsky PM. Bronchiolitis in adults: a reversible cause of airway obstruction associated with airway neutrophils. Am Rev Respir Dis 1989;140:483–492.

121. Davison AG, Heard BE, McAllister WA, Turner-Warwick MEH. Cryptogenic organizing pneumonitis. Q J Med 1983;52:382–394.

122. Cordier J, Loire R, Brune J. Idiopathic bronchiolitis obliterans organizing pneumonia: definition of characteristic clinical profiles in a series of 16 patients. Chest 1989; 96:999–1004.

123. Homma H, Yamanaka A, Tanimoto S, et al. Diffuse panbronchiolitis: a disease of the transitional zone of the lung. Chest 1983; 83:63–69.

124. Ichikawa Y, Koga H, Tanaka M, et al. Neutrophilia in bronchoalveolar lavage fluid of diffuse panbronchiolitis. Chest 1990; 98:917–923.

125. Hoffman GS, Sechler JMG, Gallin JI, et al. Bronchoalveolar lavage analysis in Wegener's granulomatosis: a method to study disease pathogenesis. Am Rev Respir Dis 1991; 143:401–407.

126. Huang M, Colby TV, Goellner JR, Martin WJ II. Utility of bronchoalveolar lavage in the diagnosis of drug-induced pulmonary toxicity. Acta Cytol 1989;33:533–538.

127. Martin WJ II, Rosenow EC III. Amiodarone pulmonary toxicity; recognition and pathogenesis. Chest 1988;93:1067–1075, 1242–1248.

128. Israel-Biet D, Venet A, Caubarrere I, et al. Bronchoalveolar lavage in amiodarone pneumonitis: cellular abnormalities and their relevance to pathogenesis. Chest 1987;91:214–221.

129. Epstein PE, Dauber JH, Rossman MD, Daniele RP. Bronchoalveolar lavage in a patient with chronic berylliosis: evidence for hypersensitivity pneumonitis. Ann Intern Med 1982;97:213–216.

130. Rossman MD, Kern JA, Elias JA, et al. Proliferative response of bronchoalveolar lymphocytes to beryllium: a test for chronic beryllium disease. Ann Intern Med 1988;108:687–693.

131. Basset F, Soler P, Jaurand MC, Bignon J. Ultra-structural examination of bronchoalveolar lavage for the diagnosis of pulmonary histiocytosis X: preliminary report on 4 cases. Thorax 1977;32:303–306.

132. Chollet S, Soler P, Dournoro P, Richard MS, Ferraus VJ, Basset F. Diagnosis of pulmonary histiocytosis X by immunodetection of Langerhans' cells in bronchoalveolar lavage fluid. Am J Pathol 1984;115:225–232.

133. Casolaro MA, Bernaudin J, Saltini C, Ferraus VJ, Crystal RG. Accumulation of Langerhans cells on the epithelial surface of the lower respiratory tract in normal subjects in association with cigarette smoking. Am Rev Respir Dis 1988;137:406–411.

134. Xaubet A, Agusti C, Picado C, et al. Bronchoalveolar lavage analysis with anti-T6 monoclonal antibody in the evaluation of diffuse lung diseases. Respiration 1989; 56:161–166.

135. Singh G, Katyal SL, Bedrossian CWM, Rogers RM. Pulmonary alveolar proteinosis: staining for surfactant apoprotein in alveolar proteinosis and in conditions simulating it. Chest 1983;83:82–86.

136. Prakash UBS, Barham SS, Carpenter HA, Dines DE, Marsh HM. Pulmonary alveolar phospholipoproteinosis: experience with 34 cases and a review. Mayo Clinic Proc 1987;62:499–518.

137. Martin RJ, Coalson JJ, Rogers RM, Horton FO, Manous IE. Pulmonary alveolar proteinosis: the diagnosis by segmented lavage. Am Rev Respir Dis 1980;121:819–825.

138. Haslam PL, Hughes DA, Dewar A, Pantin CFA. Lipoprotein macroaggregates in bronchoalveolar lavage fluid from patients with diffuse interstitial lung disease: comparison with idiopathic alveolar lipoproteinosis. Thorax 1988;43:140–146.

139. Lieske TR, Sunderrajan EV, Passamonte PM. Bronchoalveolar lavage and technetium-99m glucoheptonate imaging in chronic eosinophilic pneumonia. Chest 1984;85:282–284.

140. Dejaegher P, Demendts M. Bronchoalveolar lavage in eosinophilic pneumonia before and during corticosteroid therapy. Am Rev Respir Dis 1984;129:631–632.

141. Golde DW, Drew WL, Klein HZ, Finley TN, Cline MJ. Occult pulmonary hemorrhage in leukemia. Br Med J 1975;2:166–168.

142. Finley TN, Aronow A, Cosentino AM, Golde DW. Occult pulmonary hemorrhage in anticoagulated patients. Am Rev Respir Dis 1977;166:215–221.

143. Drew WL, Finley TN, Golde DW. Diagnostic lavage and occult pulmonary hemorrhage in thrombocytopenic immunocompromised patients. Am Rev Respir Dis 1977;166:215–221.

144. Sherman JM, Winnie G, Thomasseu MJ, Abdul-Karin FW, Boat TF. Time course of hemosiderin production and clearance by human pulmonary macrophages. Chest 1984;86:409–411.

145. Springmeyer SC, Hoges J, Hammar SP. Significance of hemosiderin-laden macrophages in bronchoalveolar lavage fluid. Am Rev Respir Dis 1984;131:A76.

146. Tenholder MF. Pulmonary infections in the immunocrompromised host: perspective on procedure. Chest 1988;94:676–678.

147. Chastre J, Fagon J, Soler P, et al. Bronchoalveolar lavage for rapid diagnosis of the fat embolism syndrome in trauma patients. Ann Intern Med 1990;113:583–588.

148. Silverman JF, Turner RC, West RL, Dillard TA. Bronchoalveolar lavage in the diagnosis of lipoid pneumonia. Diagn Cytopathol 1989;5:3–8.

149. Spatafora M, Bellia V, Ferrara G, Genova G. Diagnosis of a case of lipoid pneumonia by bronchoalveolar lavage. Respiration 1987;52:154–156.

150. Linder J, Radio SJ, Robbins RA, Ghafouri M, Rennard SI. Bronchoalveolar lavage in the cytologic diagnosis of carcinoma of the lung. Acta Cytol 1987;31:796–797.

151. Bellmunt J, DeGracia J, Morales S, Orriols R, Tallada S. Cytologic diagnosis in bronchoalveolar lavage specimens. Chest 1990;98:513–514.

152. Shiner RJ, Rosenman J, Katz I, Reichart N, Hershko E, Yellin A. Bronchoscopic evaluation of peripheral lung tumors. Thorax 1988;43:887–889.

153. Rennard SI. Bronchoalveolar lavage in the diagnosis of cancer. Lung 1990;168(suppl):1035–1040.

154. Springmeyer SC, Hackman R, Carlson JJ, McClellan E. Bronchoalveolar cell carcinoma diagnosed by bronchoalveolar lavage. Chest 1983;83:278–279.

155. LeFever A, Funahashi A. Elevated prostaglandin E$_2$ levels in bronchoalveolar lavage fluid of patients with bronchogenic carcinoma. Chest 1990;98:1397–1402.

156. deDiego A, Compte L, Sanchis J, et al. Diagnostic value of carcinoembryonic antigen in bronchoalveolar lavage fluid of peripheral lung cancer. Chest 1990;97:767–768.

157. Pisani RJ, Cortese DA, Homburger HA, Grambsch PM. A prospective pilot study evaluating the effectiveness of secretory IgA measurements in bronchoalveolar lavage to detect non-small cell lung cancer. Chest 1990;97:586–589.

158. Radio SJ, Rennard SI, Kessinger A, Vaughan WP, Linder J. Breast carcinoma in bronchoalveolar lavage. Arch Pathol Lab Med 1989;113:333–334.

159. Levy H, Horak DA, Lewis MI. The value of bronchial washings and bronchoalveolar lavage in the diagnosis of lymphangitic carcinomatosis. Chest 1988;94:1028–1030.

160. Pisani RJ, Witzig TE, Li CY, Morris MA, Thibodeau SN. Confirmation of lymphomatous pulmonary involvement by immunophenotypic and gene rearrangement analysis of bronchoalveolar lavage fluid. Mayo Clin Proc 1990;65:651–656.

161. Wisecarver J, Ness MJ, Rennard SI, Thompson AB, Armitage JO, Linder J. Bronchoalveolar lavage in the assessment of

pulmonary Hodgkin's disease. Acta Cytol 1989;33:528–529.

162. Morales FM, Matthews JI. Diagnosis of parenchymal Hodgkin's disease using bronchoalveolar lavage. Chest 1987;91:785–787.

163. Davis WB, Gadek JR. Detection of pulmonary lymphoma by bronchoalveolar lavage. Chest 1987;91:787–791.

164. Menashe P, Stenson W, Reynoso G, et al. Bronchoalveolar lavage plasmacytosis in a patient with a plasma cell dyscrasia. Chest 1989;95:226–231.

165. Rossi GA, Balbi B, Risso M, Repetto M, Ravazzoni C. Acute myelomonocytic leukemia. Demonstration of pulmonary involvement by bronchoalveolar lavage. Chest 1985;87:259.

166. Kirkpatrick MB, Bass JB Jr. Quantitative bacterial cultures of bronchoalveolar lavage fluids and protected brush catheter specimens from normal subjects. Am Rev Respir Dis 1989;139:546–548.

167. Chastre J, Fagon JY, Soler P, et al. Diagnosis of nosocomial bacterial pneumonia in intubated patients undergoing ventilation: comparison of the usefulness of bronchoalveolar lavage and the protected specimen brush. Am J Med 1988;85:499.

168. Thorpe JE, Baughman RP, Frame BT, Wessler TA, Staneck JL. Bronchoalveolar lavage for diagnosing acute bacterial pneumonia. J Infect Dis 1987;155:855–861.

169. Kahn FW, Jones JM. Diagnosing bacterial respiratory infection by bronchoalveolar lavage. J Infect Dis 1987;155:862.

170. Johanson WG, Seidenfeld JJ, Gomez P, et al. Bacteriologic diagnosis of nosocomial pneumonia following prolonged mechanical ventilation. Am Rev Respir Dis 1988; 137:259–264.

171. Torres A, De La Bellacasa JP, Xaubet A, et al. Diagnostic value of quantitative cultures of bronchoalveolar lavage and telescoping plugged catheters in mechanically ventilated patients with bacterial pneumonia. Am Rev Respir Dis 1989;140:306–310.

172. Guerra LF, Baughman RP. Use of bronchoalveolar lavage to diagnose bacterial pneumonia in mechanically ventilated patients. Crit Care Med 1990;18:169–173.

173. Chastre J, Fagon JY, Soler P, et al. Quantification of BAL cells containing intracellular bacteria rapidly identifies ventilated

patients with nosocomial pneumonia. Chest 1989;95(suppl):190S.

174. Meduri GU, Baselski V. The role of bronchoalveolar lavage in diagnosing nonopportunistic bacterial pneumonia. Chest 1991; 100:179–190.

175. Meduri GU, Beals DH, Maijub AG, Baselski V. Protected bronchoalveolar lavage: a new bronchoscopic technique to retrieve uncontaminated distal airway secretions. Am Rev Respir Dis 1991;143:855–864.

176. Martin WJ II, Smith TF, Brutinel WM, Cockerill FR III, Douglas WW. Role of bronchoalveolar lavage in the assessment of opportunistic pulmonary infections: utility and complications. Mayo Clin Proc 1987; 62:549–557.

177. Kahn FW, Jones JM. Analysis of bronchoalveolar lavage specimens from immunocompromised patients with a protocol applicable in the microbiology laboratory. J Clin Microb 1988;26:1150–1155.

178. Xaubet A, Torres A, Marco F, Puig-de la Bellacasa J, Faus R, Agusti-Vidal A. Pulmonary infiltrates in immunocrompromised patients. Diagnostic value of telescoping plugged catheter and bronchoalveolar lavage. Chest 1989;95:130–135.

179. Pisani R, Dupras DM. Clinical utility of BAL in non-AIDS immunocompromised host. Chest 1990;98:1015.

180. Johnson PC, Hogg KM, Sarosi GA. The rapid diagnosis of pulmonary infections in solid organ transplant recipients. Sem Respir Infect 1990;5:2–9.

181. Weldon-Linne CM, Rhone DP, Bourassa R. Bronchoscopy specimens in adults with AIDS. Comparative yields of cytology, histology and culture for diagnosis of infectious agents. Chest 1990;98:24–28.

182. Johnson JE, Anders GT, Hawkes CF, LaHatte LJ, Blanton HM. Bronchoalveolar lavage findings in patients seropositive for the human immunodeficiency virus HIV. Chest 1990;97:1066–1071.

183. Young KR, Rankin JA, Naegel GP, et al. Bronchoalveolar lavage cells and proteins in patients with the acquired immunodeficiency syndrome: an immunologic analysis. Ann Intern Med 1985;103:522–533.

184. Tenholder MF, Hooper RG. Pulmonary infiltrates in leukemia. Chest 1980;78:468–469.

185. Saito H, Anaissie EJ, Morice RC, Dekmezian

R, Bodey GP. Bronchoalveolar lavage in the diagnosis of pulmonary infiltrates in patients with acute leukemia. Chest 1988:94:745–749.

186. Milburn HJ, Prentice HG, DuBois RM. Role of bronchoalveolar lavage in the evaluation of interstitial pneumonitis in recipients of bone marrow transplants. Thorax 1987;42: 766–772.

187. Cordonnier C, Bernaudin J-F, Bierling P, Huet Y, Vernant J-P. Pulmonary complications occurring after allogeneic bone marrow transplantation. Cancer 1986;58:1047–1054.

188. Rennard SI. Role of bronchoalveolar lavage in the assessment of pulmonary complications following bone marrow and organ transplantation. Eur Respir J 1990;3:373–375.

189. Rennard SI. Future directions for bronchoalveolar lavage. Lung 1990;168(suppl): 1050–1056.

12 | Transbronchial Needle Aspiration for Cytology Specimens

Ko-Pen Wang

Transbronchial needle aspiration (TBNA) for diagnosing and staging of bronchogenic carcinoma was developed in the late 1970s in the United States (1). Initial reports advised that the aspirated specimen be flushed into a container by normal saline or Hank's solution (2–5). This specimen in the fluid form is processed by Millipore and other techniques in the cytology laboratory. A highly sophisticated cytology laboratory is the key to the success of this procedure. We evaluated the efficacy of a newly designed spring transbronchial needle and assessed a direct smear technique. The data in this chapter have been previously presented (6) and also printed in our hospital journal, *Harbor Medical Review* (7). This discussion emphasizes the instrument selection and technique of specimen preparation to help readers avoid some of the problems that occur in selection and usage of transbronchial needles.

Materials and Methods

During a 3-month period, 40 consecutive TBNA procedures were performed on 34 patients referred to the Chest Diagnostic Center. Seventy-two paired direct smear and fluid specimens were collected for cytologic examination. Biopsy sites included mediastinum (37), hilar (14), and lung nodules or masses (21). For mediastinum and hilar lesions, a central transbronchial needle was used (MW-122 or SW-121). For a lung nodule

or mass, a peripheral transbronchial needle was used, which is more flexible than a central needle (MW-522 or SW-521). At each biopsy site at least two punctures were made; one each by smear needle (SW-121 or SW-521) and regular transbronchial needle (MW-122 or MW-522). The difference between the smear needle and a regular needle is the smear needle's central core. It blocks the flow so that the specimen obtained stays in the distal lumen of the needle, which allows the specimen to be easily expelled onto a slide.

The TBNA techniques used were as previously reported, except that in the smear technique, the negative pressure in the syringe is released by momentarily detaching the syringe from the proximal side lure of the transbronchial needle before the needle is pulled out of the biopsy site. The needle is pulled out of the biopsy site without suction and withdrawn from the scope. The tip of the needle is held close and vertical to a glass slide. The specimen collected and stored at the lumen of the needle is rapidly blown onto the slide by air in the syringe. Another glass slide is used to press and smear the specimen, which is then immediately fixed in the 95% alcohol jar. Paired specimens, one in the slide and the other in fluid form, were sent to the cytology laboratory. Smears were stained without further preparation. Fluid specimens were processed by Millipore filtration technique and other techniques, such as centrifuge smear, cytospin, and cell block, then stained by the Papanicolaou method.

Results

Twenty-six patients had a final diagnosis of malignancy, 4 had benign diseases, and 4 were without a final diagnosis at the time this chapter was prepared. Analyses of the 72 paired specimens were both negative in 50 pairs, both positive in 15 pairs, and discrepant in 7 pairs. In 6 pairs the only positive report was from the smear specimen. In only one paired specimen was the Millipore technique the sole diagnostic specimen.

Discussion

The use of TBNA for staging of bronchogenic carcinoma through flexible bronchoscopy was first reported by Wang and colleagues in 1982 (3). Follow-up reports by Schenk and coworkers (4) and Shure and Fedullo (5) provided information about the insignificant possibility of false positive results and the potential financial saving on the care of lung cancer patients. A report by Harrow and associates (8) first described the application and success of using this procedure in private practice. Each group used the technique to collect specimens into a fluid, which was then processed by a cytology laboratory, usually by Millipore filtration technique and other techniques. A report by Rosenthal and Wallace (9) first used the smear technique only for TBNA specimens.

In our study a comparison between these two techniques indicates that the smear technique is better than the Millipore and other techniques. The lumen of the smear transbronchial needle we used is partially blocked at its proximal end by a guidewire. In addition, releasing the suction before the needle is pulled out of the biopsy site prevents the specimen from being moved into the plastic catheter, which makes expelling the specimen harder and the smear technique difficult. Using this instrument and technique, the specimen collected will be stored inside the distal lumen

of the needle. It can easily be blown onto a glass slide, smeared, and immediately dropped into a jar of 95% alcohol. This fixes the cells so that they can be stained shortly after or much later without risk of cellular deterioration. The quantity of a positive smear specimen usually having abundant tumor cells makes preliminary screening almost unnecessary. The quality of a positive smear specimen, usually containing cancer cells with lymphocytes or clusters of cancer cells and microfragments of tumor tissue, resembles a histology specimen. Often, tissue fragments or the arrangement of cells provide the diagnosis when each individual cell does not look too malignant. In a negative specimen, the presence of lymphoid tissue confirms accurate placement of the needle, indicating true negative reactive lymphadenopathy.

Dividing the transbronchial needle to the central and peripheral needle is simpler to use and less confusing than the original (MW-222) versatile needle (10) (Table 12.1). The disadvantage of the MW-222 needle is that it is more complex than the central or peripheral needle (Figure 12.1) because the proximal end has three parts rather than just two parts. If the operator tried to adjust the flexibility of the needle in vivo, retracting the guidewire when the distal end of the catheter is bent, then the inner catheter might follow. As a result, the tip of the needle is withdrawn proximal to the metal hub. If this occurs, advancing and locking of the needle will cause

Table 12.1. Wang Transbronchial Needles

	Cytology Specimen		
	C	C+P	P
22 gauge	MW–122	MW–222	MW–522
21 gauge	SW–121	SW–221	SW–521

W, Wang; MW, modified Wang or Mill-Rose Wang; SW, spring Wang; 1;C, central: mediastinal and hilar lymph node; 2;C+P, combined central and peripheral; 5;P, peripheral: lung nodules or mass

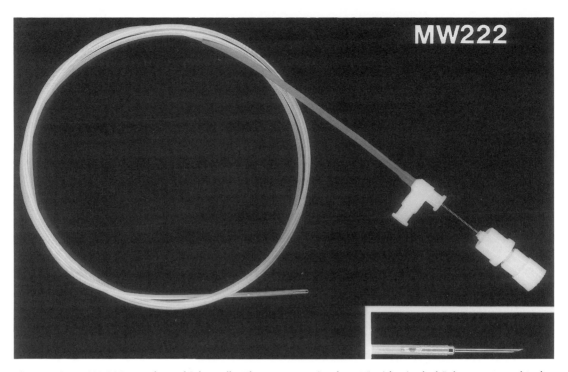

Figure 12.1. MW-222 transbronchial needle. The most proximal part "guidewire hub" does not need to be retracted for suction. However, it can be retracted partially to increase flexibility for peripheral lesions. This should be done before the instrument is introduced through the scope. In this instance, it is not necessary to readvance the guidewire cap for suction.

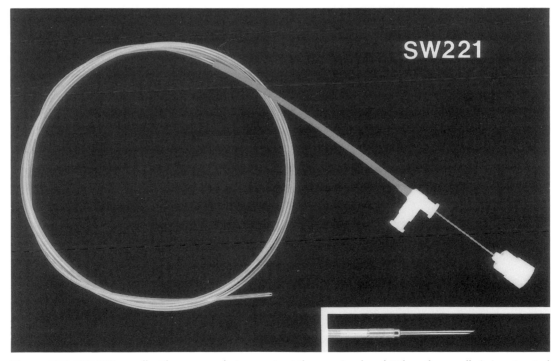

Figure 12.2. SW-221 needle. There are only two parts at the proximal end. When the needle is in retracted position, the distal end is flexible. When the needle is advanced and locked for puncture, the distal end is stiffer. All the rest of the cytology needles, central (MW-122 and SW-121) or peripheral (MW-522 and SW-521) are similar in appearance to this needle. In all spring needles, if the tip of the needle is still exposed when in retracted position, simply push it back against a hard sterile surface before use.

puncturing of the outer catheter or failure of the needle to advance. In fact, this is the most frequent complaint. This was the only reason we designed a peripheral needle. A combined needle (MW-222) should be used when the patient has both central and peripheral lesions to be sampled; otherwise either a central or peripheral needle can be used. The new combined spring needle (SW-221) is automatically versatile (Figure 12.2). In this needle, there are only two parts at the proximal end. When in retracted position, the distal end of the catheter is flexible so it can easily be directed toward and reach the lesion to be punctured. When the needle is advanced for puncture, the spring is compressed, the guidewire enters into the proximal lumen of the needle, and stiffens the catheter. This has become our most preferred needle. In using spring needles, sometimes it is necessary to push the needle tip against a sterile hard surface to retract the needle into the metal hub.

Transbronchial needle aspiration has become a useful procedure for the diagnosis and staging of bronchogenic carcinoma. Continuous effort to improve the instrument and methodology will increase the sensitivity and specificity of this relatively new procedure.

For TBNA specimens, making a direct smear at the bedside is better than putting the specimen in a fluid, then processing it by the Millipore filtration and other techniques. The simplicity and effectiveness of using the smear needles will be readily appreciated and accepted by bronchoscopists.

REFERENCES

1. Wang KP, Terry PB, Marsh B. Bronchoscopic needle aspiration biopsy of paratracheal tumors. Am Rev Respir Dis 1978;118:17–21.
2. Wang KP, Terry PB. Transbronchial needle aspiration for staging of bronchogenic carcinoma. Am Rev Respir Dis 1983;127:344–347.
3. Wang KP, Brower R, Haponik EF, Siegelman SS. Flexible transbronchial needle aspiration for staging of bronchogenic carcinoma. Chest 1983;84:571–576.
4. Schenk DA, Bower JH, Bryan CL, et al. Transbronchial needle aspiration staging of bronchogenic carcinoma. Am Rev Respir Dis 1986;134:146–148.
5. Shure D, Fedullo PF. The role of transcarinal needle aspiration in the staging of bronchogenic carcinoma. Chest 1984;86:693–696.
6. Ndukwu I, Wang KP, Davis D, Welk P, Sutula M. Direct smear for cytological examination of transbronchial needle aspiration specimens. Chest 1991;100:888. Abstract.
7. Wang KP, Ndukwu I, Davis D, Welk P, Sutula M. Direct smear by cytological examination of transbronchial needle aspiration specimens. Harbor Medical Review 1991;2:10–11.
8. Harrow EM, Oldenburg FA, Smith AM. Transbronchial needle aspiration in clinical practice. Thorax 1985;40:756–759.
9. Rosenthal DL, Wallace JM. Fine needle aspiration of pulmonary lesions via fiber-optic bronchoscope. Acta Cytol 1984;28(3):203–210.
10. Gittlen SD, Erozan Y, Wang KP. A new versatile transbronchial cytology needle for the staging and diagnosis of bronchogenic carcinoma. Chest 1988;94:561–564.

13 | Transbronchial Needle Aspiration for Histology Specimens

Atul C. Mehta and David P. Meeker

The role of fine-gauge (21-gauge, 22-gauge) flexible transbronchial needle aspiration (TBNA) in obtaining specimens through the flexible fiberoptic bronchoscope for cytologic examination is well established. Indications extend from the staging of bronchogenic carcinoma to the diagnosis of a bronchogenic cyst (1–12). However, the procedure has certain limitations (13–17) (Table 13.1). Cytologic interpretation requires optimally prepared specimens and experienced personnel. Fine-gauge TBNA is further complicated by the problem of false positive results and overinterpretation that may occur when the mediastinal aspirate is contaminated by tumor cells from respiratory secretions, or a malignant but noninvasive lesion close to the mediastinum is aspirated and thereby falsely interpreted as N_2

disease (13,14). A micrometastasis from an ipsilateral paratracheal area can be interpreted as unresectable disease in a patient with squamous cell carcinoma, where surgery could still be beneficial (3). On occasion the differential diagnosis of small cell carcinoma, carcinoid tumor, and lymphoma is difficult even for an experienced cytopathologist. Furthermore the diagnosis of benign conditions is seldom made by fine-gauge TBNA examination (18).

Diagnostic accuracy is improved with histologic examination of tissue obtained from the mediastinum or hilar areas. Tissue was previously available only by mediastinoscopy or thoracotomy, both invasive procedures requiring general anesthesia and hospitalization. In 1985, Wang and colleagues (19) demonstrated that a core of extrabronchial tissue can be safely obtained for histologic examination from either the mediastinum or hilar areas using a modified Turner's needle through a rigid scope. Accurate diagnosis of malignant and benign conditions was established in 70% of cases by histologic examination. An earlier study from France, using a similar needle through the rigid scope, reported a 53% yield in diagnosing various stages of sarcoidosis (20). However, rigid bronchoscopy has limited applicability because it most often requires general anesthesia and the majority of pulmonologists are not trained in its use.

Recently Wang introduced flexible versions of this needle for use with the flexible bronchoscope. In his preliminary study, he

---

Table 13.1. Drawbacks of Cytologic Studies of TBNA Specimens

Procedural

Requires laboratory sophistication
Damage to fiberoptic bronchoscope (16,17)
Hemomediastinum (15)

Interpretation

Requires qualified personnel
False positive results (staging) (13,14)
Overinterpretation (staging) (3)
Misinterpretation
Limited to malignant conditions

successfully obtained specimens for histologic examination from mediastinal and hilar areas in a majority of patients without complications (21). This chapter describes this device and updates the Cleveland Clinic experience with TBNA (22,23).

Needle Assembly

The flexible needle (MW319-1 Mill-Rose Lab, Inc., Mentor, OH) can be divided into three sections: 1) distal metal needle, 2) middle flexible catheter, and 3) proximal suction port.

The distal end of this instrument is comprised of a 15-mm long, 19-gauge retractable metal needle that is connected to a 110-cm long thin hollow spring, which controls the movement of the 19-gauge needle (Figure 13.1). A 21-gauge, 5-mm long, beveled, retractable needle attached to a guidewire is housed within the 19-gauge needle. The guidewire lies inside the lumen of the hollow spring and controls the movement of the 21-gauge needle. Both needles along with the metal spring and guidewire are arranged inside a 120-cm long, 2-mm diameter flexible catheter. The proximal end of the hollow spring is attached to a thin, metal tubing to facilitate movement of the 19-gauge needle. Communication between the lumen of the 19-gauge needle and the catheter is maintained through a small opening located on the proximal portion of the body of the 19-gauge needle. The proximal suction port of the device consists of a connector that opens laterally to accommodate the syringe used to apply suction and an exit port for the metal tubing attached to the inner hollow spring. This thin metal tubing in turn provides an exit for the guidewire connected to the 21-gauge needle. Separate mechanisms lock the 19-gauge and 21-gauge needles into place once they are in an extended position.

The design of the original 18-gauge flexible needle used by Wang to obtain histology specimens was described in our initial report (23). The modified version of this device, which is described above, is now available. A 19-gauge retractable needle has replaced the fixed 18-gauge needle, although the inner diameter of both needles remains the same. This modification is an effort to reduce trauma to the inner channel of the flexible bronchoscope without compromising the size of the specimen (17). The beveled tip of the 19-gauge needle instead of the flat tip facilitates insertion through the tracheobronchial wall (22,23).

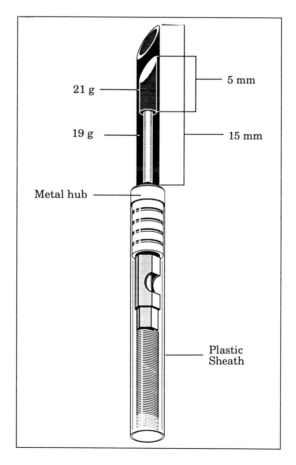

Figure 13.1. Schematic diagram of distal end of transbronchial aspiration needle for histology specimen.

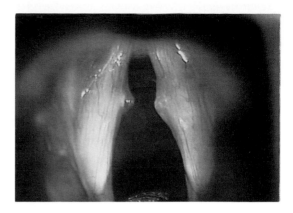

Plate 1. Amyloidosis involving the larynx.

Photo courtesy of Atul Mehta, MB.

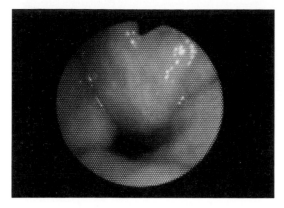

Plate 2. Reinke's edema.

Photo courtesy of Eiji Yanagisawa, MD.

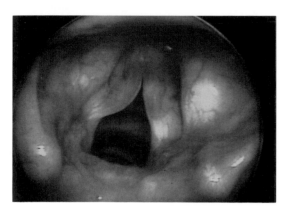

Plate 3. Right vocal cord polyp.

Photo courtesy of Eiji Yanagisawa, MD.

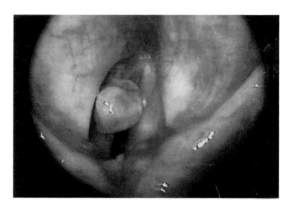

Plate 4. Vocal cord nodules.

Photo courtesy of Eiji Yanagisawa, MD.

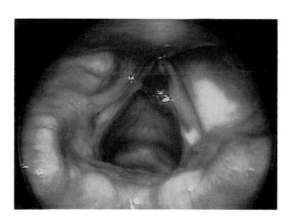

Plate 5. Left vocal cord granuloma.

Photo courtesy of Eiji Yanagisawa, MD.

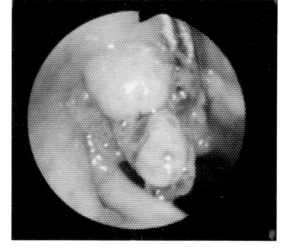

Plate 6. Laryngeal papilloma.

Photo courtesy of Atul Mehta, MB.

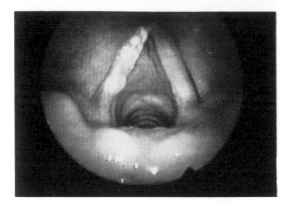

Plate 7. Squamous cell carcinoma of the left vocal cord.

Photo courtesy of Eiji Yanagisawa, MD.

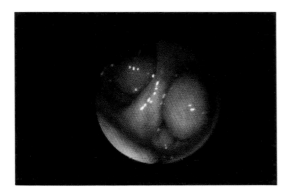

Plate 8. Choanal Polyps. Retrograde view to the choanae of a 4-year-old child. Hyperplastic polypoid conchae occlude the airways imitating symptoms of central airway stenosis.

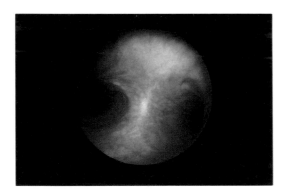

Plate 9. Normal bifurcation of a 6-year-old boy. Note the apparently blunt carina that in an adult would be suspicious for subcarinal lymph node enlargement.

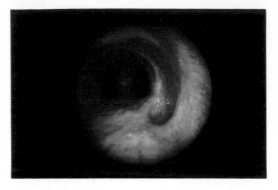

Plate 10. Tracheal diverticulum. A rudimentary bronchial bud is found at the lower third of the dorsal trachea. There was no additional lung tissue.

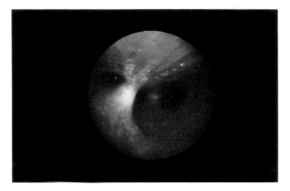

Plate 11. Tracheal bronchus. An accessory tracheal bronchus leads to a displaced apical segment of the right upper lobe. Narrowing and kinking of the bronchus caused repeated postobstructive pneumonia.

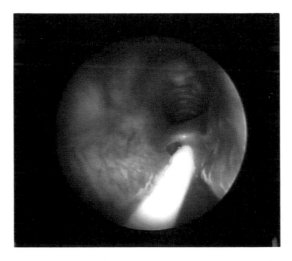

Plate 12. Ecchondromas. View to the right intermediate bronchus. Garland-like protrusions strictly related to the cartilages are typical for multiple ecchondromas.

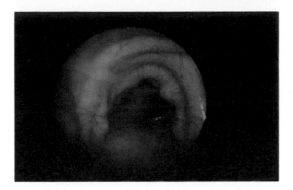

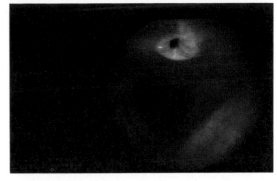

Plate 13. Laryngeal cleft. The view into the larynx shows a large gap on the posterior wall extending down to the level of the cricoid cartilage. The entrance to the esophagus is marked by the nutritional tube. After surgery for esophagotracheal fistula this four-month-old girl still showed symptoms of severe aspiration pneumonia, which was due to the laryngeal cleft that had been unnoticed despite previous bronchoscopy.

Plate 16. Congenital esophagotracheal fistula in the upper trachea. Note the bright color of the esophageal mucosa prolapsing through the gap in the posterior tracheal wall.

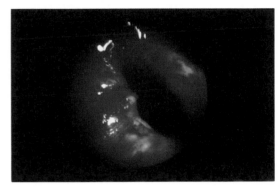

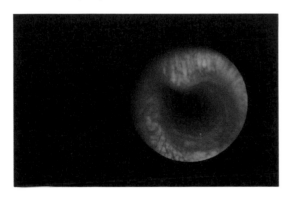

Plate 17. Bronchial varicosis. Polypoid spontaneously bleeding protuberances of the bronchial wall at the entrance of the left upper lobe caused by bronchial varicosis due to congestion by a complex cardiac vitium. The varices were coagulated by Nd:YAG laser. Four years later bronchoscopy for pneumonic infiltrate in the 18-year-old man showed stable scar formation without any residual varices at the site of laser treatment.

Plate 14. Tracheal hemangioma. The picture shows a hypervascularized protrusion of the dorsal wall of the subglottic trachea in a one-year-old child.

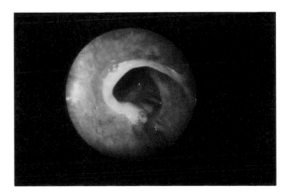

Plate 18. Transport of secretions. Note the spiral transport of purulent secretions in postobstructive pneumonia.

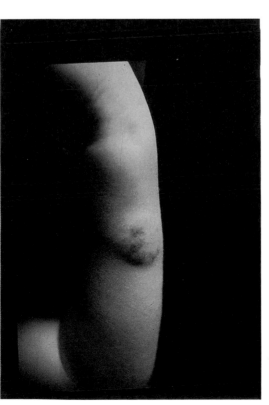

◀ **Plate 15.** Hemangioma on forearm. The simultaneous hemangioma on the forearm of the child arouses suspicion of a hemangiomatous lesion.

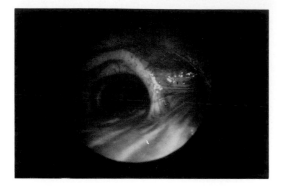

Plate 19. Chronic deforming bronchitis. The mucosa shows enlarged orifices of the mucous gland ducts at the entrance of the right upper lobe bronchus and distended washboard-like strands of elastic tissue on the dorsal wall of the bronchi.

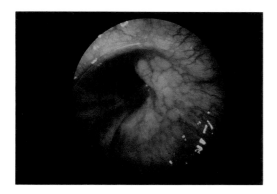

Plate 20. Granulomata in sarcoidosis. Note the vascularization of the nodular lesions at the right wall of the intermediate bronchus.

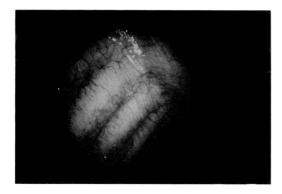

Plate 21. Normal vascularization of the trachea. Between the cartilages the vessels enter the mucosa and spread upward and downward, whereas in the dorsal parts of the tracheal wall there is a continuous network of capillary vessels.

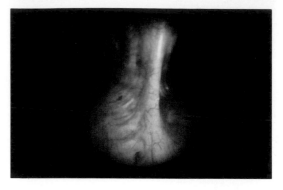

Plate 22. Hemangiomas in Osler's disease. On the left side of the main carina are three capillary convolutes of blood vessels. The patient was referred to our clinic for a coin lesion that by angiography proved to be an arteriovenous fistula. More hemangiomas were seen on the skin, the oral mucosa, and the larynx.

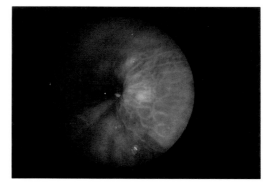

Plate 23. Lymphedema due to lymph node metastasis. The view of the right main bronchus shows an impression of the lateral wall by extrinsic tumor. The mucosa shows a cobblestone feature and a delicate network of whitish streaks, which represents the enlarged lymphatic vessels.

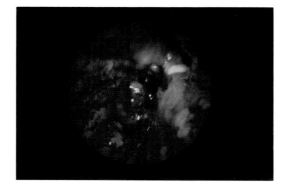

Plate 24. Bronchocentric granulomatous inflammation. In a little girl suffering from infection by *eibenella corrodens*, ulcerative and polypoid lesions are seen in the intermediate bronchus, causing obstruction of the middle lobe and especially the lower lobe ostia. The lesion resolved completely after treatment with antibiotics.

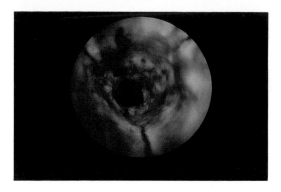

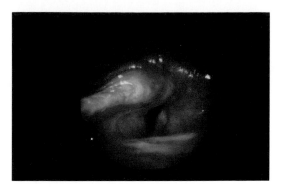

Plate 25. Laryngitis in chronic relapsing polychondritis. Below the vocal cords at the level of the cricoid cartilage there is marked swelling of the mucosa, superficial exulcerations, and fissures extending upward to the glottis. Immunosuppressive treatment and even local injection of corticosteroids could not prevent severe progressive stenosis. The patient had to have a Montgomery-T prosthesis.

Plate 28. Luxation of the arytenoid cartilage. The right arytenoid cartilage together with the aryepiglottic fold bulges forward into the rima glottidis, causing severe obstruction as by forced respiratory maneuvers it is drawn further inside the larynx. Lateral fixation was accomplished by surgery.

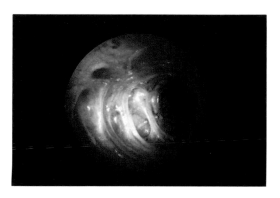

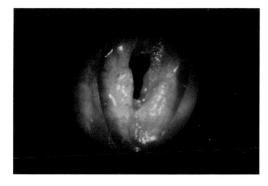

Plate 29. Papillomas of the vocal cords. The normally shiny and very smooth surface has a rough nodular appearance and the reflection of the flashlight is fragmented. Small vessels protrude into the nodular lesions.

Plate 26. Bronchiectasis. The view of the middle lobe bronchus shows an outward bulging mucosa between webs of elastic fiber bundles, producing the radiologic picture of varicose bronchiectasis on bronchography.

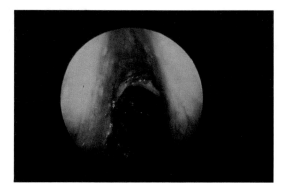

Plate 27. Laryngitis in Wegener's granulomatosis. In a 12-year-old girl presenting with severe dyspnea due to complete atelectasis of the left lung caused by complete cicatric obstruction of the main bronchus surprisingly additional involvement of the larynx was found during bronchoscopy. Below the vocal cords there is an ulcerative laryngitis with extensive fibrin deposition. Renal involvement was proven by biopsy. Due to the laryngeal involvement, it was decided to perform conservative therapy by aggressive immunosuppression. The bronchial stenosis was bronchoscopically dilated and an expandable metallic stent inserted. The lung has been reventilated for almost 3 years and the girl is leading an almost normal life.

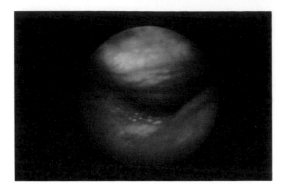

Plate 30. Collapse of the trachea. Due to chronic inflammation and pressure changes during coughing, the cartilages have become weak and lost their horseshoe shape. There is also marked relaxation of the membranaceous wall that is bulging to the anterior wall of the trachea.

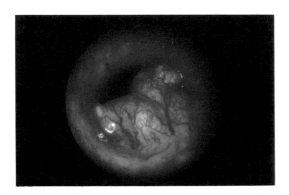

Plate 31. Adenoid cystic carcinoma of the trachea. A typical polypoid tumor extends from the anterior tracheal wall to the lumen, causing an obstruction of nearly 80%.

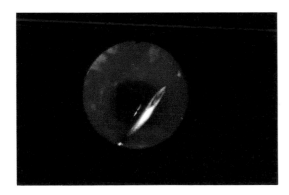

Plate 32. Intraoperative marking of a tracheal stenosis. The upper and lower end of a postintubation stenosis that has been endoscopically dilated for safe ventilation is marked by the surgeon. The endoscopist asserts exact positioning according to the internal aspect.

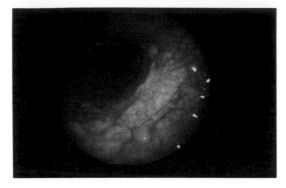

Plate 33. Granulomas in sarcoidosis. At the entrance of the left upper lobe the hyper-vascularized mucosa shows multiple nodular lesions that cause fragmentation of the light reflection.

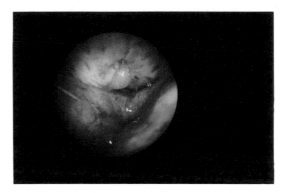

Plate 34. Tumor-like amyloidosis at the branching of the left main bronchus. The entrance to the upper and lower lobe bronchus is almost totally occluded by a tumor-like mucosal swelling. The entrance to the S-6 bronchus appears as a small crater. The amyloid masses were removed by Nd:YAG laser after immunosuppressive therapy failed. Recanalization has been successful for 5 years.

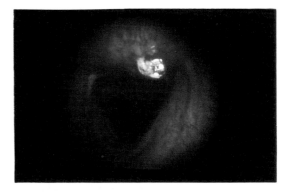

Plate 35. Metastasizing carcinoid. On the dorsal wall of the upper trachea there is a whitish nodular lesion. The primary tumor was localized at the left upper lobe. The traces of blood led to bronchoscopic examination.

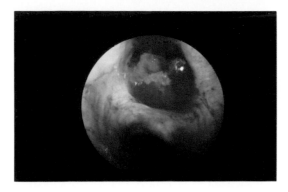

Plate 36. Intrabronchial metastasis. S-6 of the left lower lobe is occluded by a spontaneously bleeding villous tumor. Bronchoscopy was performed for hemoptysis and multiple intrapulmonary nodular lesions. The histologic examination confirmed macroscopic suspicion of a chorion carcinoma. The patient had been hospitalized for abortion previously.

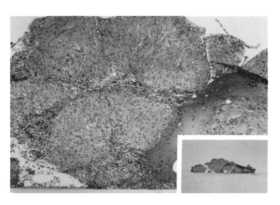

Plate 37. Histology specimen obtained via 19-gauge TBNA demonstrating nonnecrotizing granuloma compatible with the diagnosis of sarcoidosis, ×80. (Inset 10× magnification of the actual specimen.)

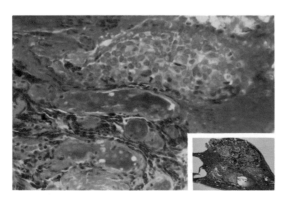

Plate 38. Histology specimen obtained via 19-gauge TBNA demonstrating small cell carcinoma, ×400. (Inset 40× magnification of the actual specimen.)

Reproduced by permission from Mehta AC, Kavuru M, Meeker DP, Gephardt GN, Nunez C. Transbronchial needle aspiration for histology specimens. Chest 1989;96: 1228–1232.

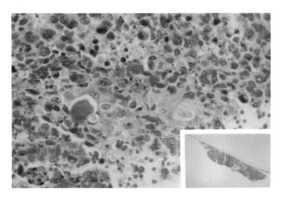

Plate 39. Histology specimen obtained via 19-gauge TBNA diagnostic of squamous cell carcinoma, ×128. (Inset 10× magnification of the actual specimen.)

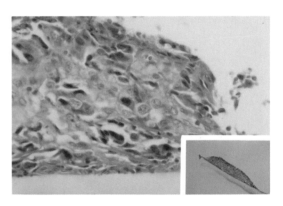

Plate 40. Histology specimen obtained via 19-gauge TBNA diagnostic of adenocarcinoma, ×128. (Inset 25× magnification of the actual specimen.)

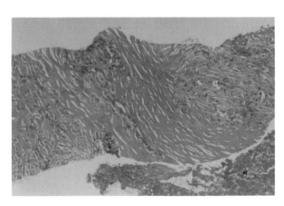

Plate 41. Histology specimen obtained via 19-gauge TBNA demonstrating nondiagnostic lymph node segment, ×32. Note fibrosis as well as necrosis (N) involving the lymph node.

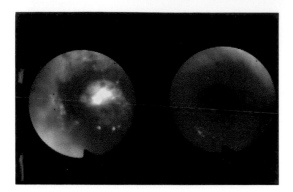

Plate 42. "Ideal" endobronchial lesion for Nd:YAG laser photoresection (see text), before *(A)* and after *(B)* resection.

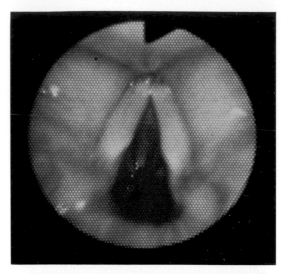

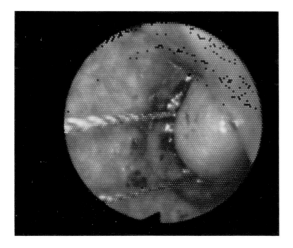

Plate 43. Hemorrhagic lesion. Hemostasis is achieved by firing the Nd:YAG beam in a rosette pattern around an arteriovenous malformation on the nasal septum of a patient with hereditary hemorrhagic telangiectasia.

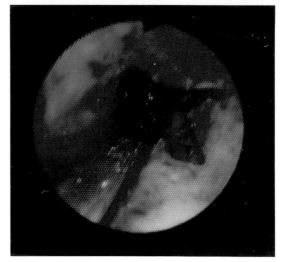

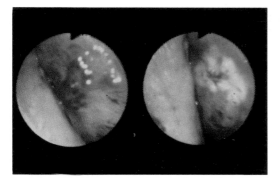

Plate 44. Polypoid lesion. Shown with a polypectomy snare encircling the base.

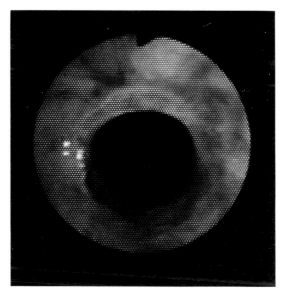

Plates 45, 46, 47. Tracheal stenosis before *(top)*, during *(middle)*, and after *(bottom)* Nd:YAG LPR.

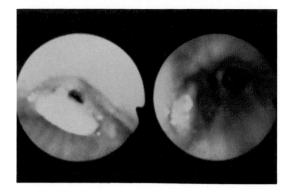

Plate 48. Pill lodged in main stem bronchus (left) and after its removal with alligator forceps.

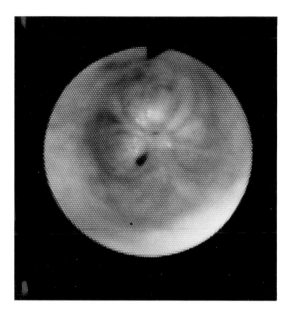

Plate 49. Endoscopic visualization of severe airway stenosis.

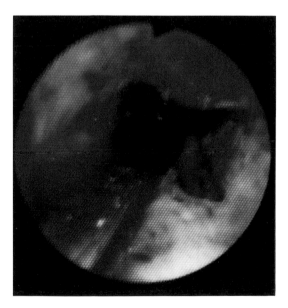

Plate 50. Laser radial incision technique allowing for rapid reepithelialization.

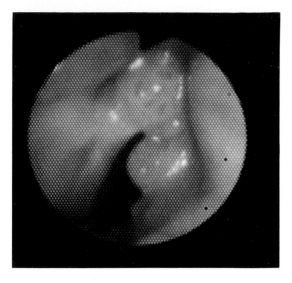

Plate 51. Benign laryngotracheobronchial papillo-matosis supraglottic lesions.

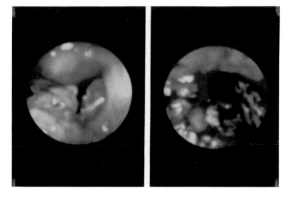

Plate 52. Endobronchial lesions before and during laser therapy.

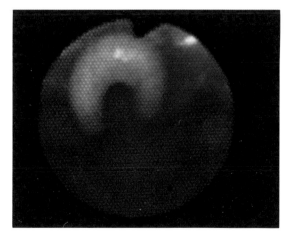

Plate 53. Normal-appearing omega-shaped epiglottis of a 3-month-old child.

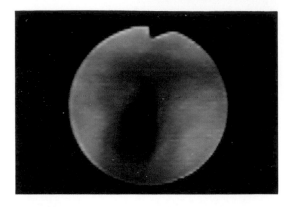
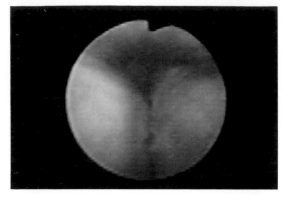

Plate 54. Laryngomalacia in an 8-month-old child. *Left,* Normal-appearing larynx during exhalation. *Right,* Involution of laryngeal structures during inspiration.

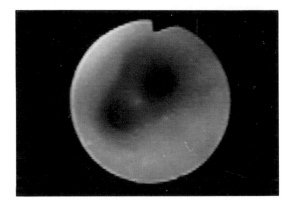
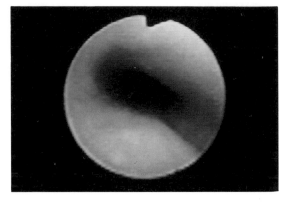

Plate 55. Tracheomalacia in an 8-month-old child (same child with laryngomalacia). *Left,* Normal-appearing trachea during exhalation. *Right,* Moderate, subtotal collapse of tracheal walls during inspiration.

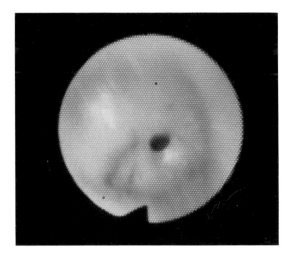
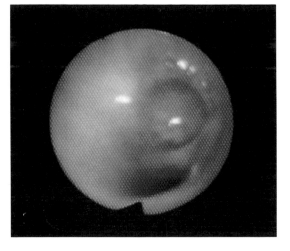

Plate 56. Subglottic stenosis caused by neonatal intubation in a 15-month-old child.

Plate 57. Foreign body (a toy peg covered with mucus) in the right main stem bronchus of a 2-year-old child who presented with recurrent pneumonia. The peg was successfully removed by rigid bronchoscopy.

Specimen Retrieval

Before the insertion of the assembly through the working channel of the scope, the 21-gauge needle is retracted inside the 19-gauge needle and the 19-gauge needle inside the plastic catheter, protecting the distal end of the needle inside the metal hub (Figure 13.2, Step 1). During the insertion of the device the distal end of the bronchoscope is kept in a neutral forward viewing position maintaining the entire body of the scope as straight as possible. These measures are mandatory to prevent damage to the inner channel of the instrument (17). At the target site, the distal end of the needle assembly is positioned beyond that of the scope. The 19-gauge needle, followed by a 21-gauge needle, is pushed out of the catheter and locked in place (Figure 13.2, Step 2). The 21-gauge needle is then inserted through the tracheobronchial wall and suction is applied at the proximal end using a 60-mL syringe containing 3 mL of normal saline solution (Figure 13.2, Step 3). This is to ascertain that the needle is not entering a major intrathoracic vessel. Once this is confirmed, the suction is released and the 19-gauge needle is advanced by a few millimeters through the tracheobronchial wall and the 21-gauge needle is withdrawn. The 21-gauge needle thereby prevents plugging of the 19-gauge needle by a piece of tissue from the tracheobronchial wall. The 19-gauge needle is then thrust out to its fullest length (15 mm) (Figure 13.2, Step 4).

Although the 19-gauge needle has been modified to facilitate insertion, problems may still be encountered with this part of the procedure. A few simple maneuvers may prove useful. The plastic catheter can be stabilized at the proximal end of the bronchoscope channel by using one finger, and then the entire scope is advanced, thereby advancing the needle. The proximal end of the metal needle can also be kept within the distal end of the channel, using

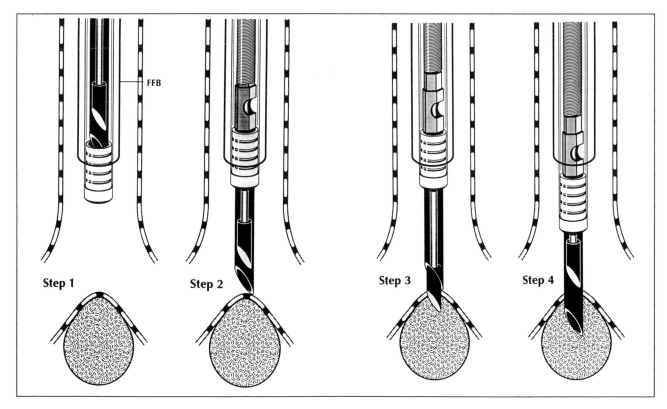

Figure 13.2. Schematic representation of histology specimen retrieval by 19–gauge TBNA.

the working channel of the scope to splint the needle–catheter junction. If fine-gauge needle aspiration is performed prior to the procedure, then the same track can be used to obtain the histology specimen. One can also ask the patient to cough while the needle is held firmly at the target site to achieve spontaneous penetration of tracheobronchial wall by the 19-gauge needle (24). Once the needle is inserted, suction is reapplied and tissue for histology is obtained by moving the 19-gauge needle in and out (partially) through the tracheobronchial wall. Once the assembly is removed from the scope, the specimen is collected by flushing the needle assembly with normal saline solution from the syringe. On occasion the 21-gauge needle is used to push the core tissue out of the 19-gauge needle for histologic examination. Two passes are made at each site using a single disposable needle. Either histologic or cytologic examination is performed depending on the size of the specimen.

Using a similar technique, Wang (21) successfully obtained tissue for histologic examination in 21 of 25 patients, establishing a diagnosis in 18. Overall the diagnostic yield was 72%. In patients in whom tissue was obtained the yield was 85%. Specimens were obtained from the carinal, paratracheal, and hilar areas. Diagnoses of malignant as well as benign conditions, including lymphoma and sarcoidosis, were successfully made. There were no complications and the study proved the safety and efficacy of the 19-gauge TBNA.

Cleveland Clinic Experience

Our initial experience with TBNA has been published (22,23). Flexible fiberoptic bronchoscopy (FOB) was performed in patients with radiographic evidence of hilar, subcarinal, or paratracheal abnormalities. In these patients, 18-gauge or 19-gauge TBNA was performed if there was no obvious exophytic or submucosal abnormality and evidence of extrinsic compression was present. The pri-

mary purpose of TBNA was diagnostic. Where applicable this information was used for staging; however, the procedure was not performed or repeated solely for the purpose of staging either suspected or documented bronchogenic carcinoma. Computed tomography (CT) scan of the chest was not a prerequisite; however, if available, this information was used to select the insertion site. In addition to 18-gauge or 19-gauge TBNA, samples were obtained by 22-gauge TBNA, bronchial washings, brush biopsy, or transbronchial biopsy where applicable. Percutaneous needle aspiration, mediastinoscopy, or thoracotomy was performed if the bronchoscopy was nondiagnostic. In the absence of a tissue diagnosis, the benignity of certain conditions was established by review of old chest radiographs or by close follow-up of the old radiographic abnormality until its resolution or proven stability over time.

Fifty patients were studied with either the original 18-gauge fixed needle or the modified 19-gauge retractable beveled needle. Samples were obtained from hilar, subcarinal, or paratracheal areas depending on the radiographic abnormality. Adequate specimens for histologic examination were obtained in 25 patients. In 17 patients, the specimen either was too small or fragmented immediately after retrieval, and therefore only cytologic examination could be performed. Material was insufficient for either histologic or cytologic examination in 3 patients. In 5 patients insertion of the 18-gauge TBNA needle through the tracheobronchial wall was unsuccessful (22,23).

Of 25 patients in whom adequate histology specimens were obtained, the procedure was diagnostic in 16 and nondiagnostic in 9 (Table 13.2). Eleven malignant and five benign conditions were diagnosed in this fashion. In one patient with adenocarcinoma, TBNA established the diagnosis and staged the cancer as unresectable. The histologic examination was exclusively diagnostic in 2 patients with sar-

Table 13.2. TBNA for Histology Specimens

Conditions	Diagnostic	Nondiagnostic
Adenocarcinoma	3	2
Squamous cell carcinoma	3	0
Small cell carcinoma	5	1
Large cell carcinoma	0	2
Sarcoidosis	4	1
Granulomatous inflammation (Histoplasmosis)*	1	0
Mesothelioma	0	1+
Silicosis	0	1+
Empyema	0	1+
TOTAL	16	9

Patients studied, 50; specimens obtained, 25
*Confirmed by mediastinoscopy
+True negatives

coidosis. In 3 of the 9 nondiagnostic cases, the test was a true negative in 3, whereas in the remaining 6 it was falsely negative. Nondiagnostic histology specimens usually demonstrated a normal lymph node with some histiocytes with anthracosis or necrosis (23) (Plate 41).

Material for cytologic examination only was obtained in 17 patients and proved diagnostic in 5. In 2 of these patients, the test was exclusively diagnostic. No benign conditions were diagnosed in this fashion.

Thus the overall diagnostic yield of 18-gauge and 19-gauge TBNA in our hands was 44%, 32% by histologic and 12% by cytologic examination. If we exclude the cases with an unsuccessful insertion or insufficient material obtained, the diagnostic yield increases to 52%. In four patients TBNA was exclusively diagnostic (histology two, cytology two) increasing the overall diagnostic yield from 56% to 64% in patients with no exophytic or submucosal process. Although the test was exclusively diagnostic in two others, further confirmation by mediastinoscopy was required, in one to rule

out lymphoma and in the other to confirm the type of lymphoma (23). There were no false positives. The specificity and positive predictive value of the test was 100%. The sensitivity and the negative predictive value of the test were 61% and 30%, respectively.

Several difficulties were encountered (Table 13.3). All patients felt some discomfort during the insertion of the histology needle, complaining of pressure in the chest, discomfort in the nose, or coughing. The discomfort appeared less severe when the beveled 19-gauge retractable needle was used. Insertion of the 18-gauge needle was unsuccessful in five patients because of kinking of the catheter by the force used for insertion, either inside the endobronchial tree or proximally outside the scope. This reflected our lack of experience and a design flaw in the original 18-gauge nonbeveled needle in that the needle was too blunt to readily penetrate the tracheobronchial wall (22,23). Indeed, insertion was much easier with the 19-gauge beveled needle as compared to the 18-gauge needle. In our hands insertion of the 19-gauge beveled needle through the tracheobronchial wall was uniformly successful. Three patients experienced bleeding of less than 50 mL, including aspiration of frank blood in the syringe or endobronchial bleeding from the insertion site. No instances of hemomedia-stinum were encountered (15).

Fine-needle aspiration did not add to the diagnostic yield of FOB provided that two successful passes were made with the 18-gauge or 19-gauge needle through the tracheobronchial wall. If the fine-needle aspiration specimen was

Table 13.3. Drawbacks of TBNA for Histology Specimens

Patient discomfort	–all
Unsuccessful insertion	–5
Bleeding < 50 mL	–3
Damage to bronchoscope	–1
Hemomediastinum	–0

positive, the 18-gauge or 19-gauge TBNA specimen was also positive. Conversely, cytologic specimens obtained through 18-gauge or 19-gauge TBNA provided a higher diagnostic yield than those obtained by 22-gauge TBNA. Of five patients in whom insertion of the 18-gauge needle was unsuccessful, 22-gauge TBNA was exclusively diagnostic in two. No benign conditions were diagnosed in this fashion. In one patient in whom only a single pass of the 18-gauge needle was successful, histologic as well as cytologic examination were both negative, whereas the 22-gauge TBNA was positive for adenocarcinoma.

Seven patients did not have CT scans performed prior to bronchoscopy. In 3 patients, the needle aspiration was unsuccessful. A diagnosis of sarcoidosis in 2 patients and small cell carcinoma in one was made successfully from the histology specimens. The remaining patient had no pulmonary pathology. Of the 27 patients in whom CT scans were available, insertion was unsuccessful in 2, while TBNA was nondiagnostic or failed to provide sufficient material in 14 patients.

Summary

The 18-gauge and 19-gauge TBNA proved effective in obtaining specimens for histologic examination from the mediastinal and hilar areas in at least 50% of attempts and provided material for cytologic examination in the majority of remaining cases. Malignant and benign conditions were diagnosed successfully by TBNA. In selected cases, 18-gauge and 19-gauge TBNA increased the diagnostic yield of FOB; moreover, the problem of false positivity and overinterpretation associated with use of the fine-gauge needle was eliminated. Prior CT scanning of the chest is desirable, but not mandatory. At our institution CT scanning of the chest is generally not performed for staging prior to FOB in patients with suspected bronchogenic carcinoma. However, it is likely that we would have performed TBNA more frequently if all patients undergoing FOB had had prior CT scans of the chest because CT may identify subtle mediastinal masses not seen on the chest radiograph. The 22-gauge TBNA adds to the diagnostic yield of FOB only if two passes with 18-gauge or 19-gauge TBNA remain unsuccessful.

Prior experience with fine-gauge TBNA is helpful in learning to use the 18-gauge or 19-gauge needle. As with any procedure, there is a learning curve. A pulmonologist needs to perform the procedure about 10 times before feeling comfortable with it. Paratracheal insertion is somewhat more difficult than subcarinal or hilar insertion. The 19-gauge beveled needle provides maximum ease of insertion when compared to the 18-gauge flat-tipped needle. Of note, the new Olympus BFIT20-OES fiberoptic bronchoscope does not admit the 18-gauge needle (25).

Even though our experience with 18-gauge and 19-gauge TBNA for histology is limited, we believe that it has great potential for acceptance as a routine staging procedure for bronchogenic carcinoma. It may become the procedure of choice for conditions such as type I and II sarcoidosis, lymphoma, and other conditions presenting with a mediastinal mass, thereby limiting the need for mediastinoscopy. It is also likely to limit the use of the fine-gauge needle to conditions such as peripheral nodules. The success achieved by Pauli and colleagues (20) in making the diagnosis of sarcoidosis by TBNA using rigid needles will surely be reproduced using flexible histology needles as further experience is acquired with this technique. The number of mediastinoscopies at Wang's hospital has decreased since he started using fine-gauge TBNA (26). Even further reductions in the number of mediastinoscopies can be expected at institutions adopting the 18-gauge or 19-gauge TBNA technique for obtaining histology specimens.

REFERENCES

1. Shure D, Fedullo PF. The role of transcarinal needle aspiration in the staging of bronchogenic carcinoma. Chest 1984;86:693–696.

2. Schenk DA, Bower JH, Bryan CL, et al. Transbronchial needle aspiration staging of bronchogenic carcinoma. Am Rev Resp Dis 1986;134:146–148.

3. Wang KP, Brower R, Haponik EF, Siegelman S. Flexible transbronchial needle aspiration for staging of bronchogenic carcinoma. Chest 1983;84:571–576.

4. Shure D, Fedullo PF. Transbronchial needle aspiration in the diagnosis of submucosal and peribronchial bronchogenic carcinoma. Chest 1985;88:49–51.

5. Mehta AC, Ahmad M, Nunez C. Golish JA. Newer procedures using the fiberoptic bronchoscope in the diagnosing of lung cancer. Cleve Clin J Med 1987;54:195–1203.

6. Shure D, Fedullo PF. Transbronchial needle aspiration of peripheral masses. Am Rev Resp Dis 1982;128:1090–1092.

7. Wang KP, Haponik EF, Britt EF, Khouri N, Erozan Y. Transbronchial needle aspiration of peripheral pulmonary nodules. Chest 1984; 86:819–823.

8. Wang KP, Terry PB. Transbronchial needle aspiration in the diagnosis and staging of bronchogenic carcinoma. Am Rev Resp Dis 1983; 127:344–347.

9. Givens CD Jr, Marini JJ. Transbronchial needle aspiration of a bronchial carcinoid tumor. Chest 1985;88:152–153.

10. Ketai L, Chauncey J, Duque R. Combination of flow cytometry and transbronchial needle aspiration in the diagnosis of mediastinal lymphoma. Chest 1985;88:936. Letter.

11. Barzo P. Transbronchial mediastinal cystography. Chest 1988;93:431–432.

12. Schwartz AR, Fishman EK, Wang KP. Diagnosing and treatment of bronchogenic cyst using transbronchial needle aspiration. Thorax 1986;41:326–327.

13. Schenk DA, Chasen MH, McCarthy MJ, Duncan CA, Christian CA. Potential false positive mediastinal transbronchial needle aspiration in bronchogenic carcinoma. Chest 1984; 86:649–650.

14. Cropp AJ, Dimarco AF, Laukerani M. False positive transbronchial needle aspiration in bronchogenic carcinoma. Chest 1985; 5:696–697.

15. Kucera RF, Wolfe GK, Perry ME. Hemomediastinum after transbronchial needle aspiration. Chest 1986;90:466. Letter.

16. Kelly SJ, Wang KP. Transbronchial needle aspiration. J Thorac Imaging 1987;2:33–40.

17. Mehta AC, Curtis PS, Scalzitti ML, Meeker DP. The high price of bronchoscopy: maintenance and repair of the flexible fiberoptic bronchoscope. Chest 1990;98:448–454.

18. Anzaki Y, Asahi Y, Kiyatake K, et al. A case of small pulmonary hamartoma diagnosed by transbronchial needle aspiration cytology. Jpn J Thorac Dis 1986;24:692–697.

19. Wang KP, Britt EJ, Haponik EF, Fishman EK, Siegelman SS, Erozan YS. Rigid transbronchial needle aspiration biopsy for histological specimens. Ann Otol Rhinol Laryngol 1985; 94:382–385.

20. Pauli G, Pelletier A, Bohner C, Roeslin N, Warter A, Roegel E. Transbronchial needle aspiration in the diagnosis of sarcoidosis. Chest 1984;85:482–484.

21. Wang KP. Flexible transbronchial needle aspiration biopsy for histology specimens. Chest 1985;88:860–863.

22. Mehta AC, Nunez C. Stoller JK, Ahmad M. Diagnostic usefulness of transbronchial aspiration with an 18 gauge needle. Chest 1987; 92:148(S).

23. Mehta AC, Kavuru M, Meeker DP, Gephardt GN, Nunez C. Transbronchial needle aspiration for histology specimens. Chest 1989; 96:1228–1232.

24. Olsen JD, Thomas DA, Young MB, Perry ME. Cough and transbronchial needle aspiration. Chest 1986;89:315. Letter.

25. Curtis P, Mehta AC, Kavuru MS. Inability of the Olympus BF-IT20 fiberopticbronchoscope to incorporate the flexible 18 gauge transbronchial needle for histology specimen. Chest 1989;95(5):1172.

26. Wang KP, Haponik EF, Gupta PK, Erozan YS. Flexible transbronchial needle aspiration: technical considerations. Ann Otol Rhinol Laryngol 1984;93:233–236.

Staging of Bronchogenic Carcinoma by Bronchoscopy | 14

Ko-Pen Wang

Since the development of computed tomography (CT) scanning and the transbronchial needle aspiration (TBNA) technique, staging of bronchogenic carcinoma has been changed. Previous staging mainly by plain chest x-ray and surgery had been developed and used since the early 1970s by the American Joint Committee on Cancer (AJCC) (1,2). Current modifications of the AJCC system to reflect modern treatment philosophies and to resolve differences between the AJCC system, the Union International Contre Cancer (UICC) (widely used in Europe), and the Japan Joint Committee of lung cancer have provided an opportunity for an international unified system (3–7). It is the intent of this chapter to stimulate the development of an international bronchoscopy staging system and to incorporate it into the new AJCC system.

In the past, bronchoscopy played a limited role in staging of bronchogenic carcinoma; its major use was to assess the T (tumor) status. Lesions beyond the lobar bronchus were considered as T1. Tumors involving the main bronchus, however, 2 cm or more distal to the carina were considered as T2. Tumors in the main bronchus within the 2 cm distance from the carina but without involvement of the carina were considered T3. Finally, tumors invading the carina were considered as T4.

Development of the CT scan has expanded the role of radiology for the staging of bronchogenic carcinoma compared with the limited use and value of routine plain chest x-ray and tomography. Numerous reports on staging of lung cancer, in particular about its value in evaluating the nodal status, have been published (8–10). In general, it is concluded that CT scanning to evaluate the mediastinum is sensitive but not too specific. Since the development of the flexible bronchoscopic TBNA technique, its value in staging bronchogenic carcinoma has also been reported. In general, it is sensitive and specific for the diagnosis of lymph node involvement (10–12). Combined use of these two relatively new techniques, CT scan and TBNA, provided us with an opportunity for noninvasive staging of bronchogenic carcinoma. Bronchoscopy without TBNA has only limited value in evaluating the intrabronchial extent of tumor and has no role for evaluating lymph node status. This limited the use of bronchoscopy mainly for diagnostic purposes, by evaluating the airway.

Development of TBNA has markedly expanded the role of bronchoscopy from diagnosis to staging. Its ability to sample mediastinum and hilar lymph nodes potentially can replace mediastinoscopy for right paratrachea lesions, mediastinotomy for left paratrachea or aortic pulmonary window lesions, and open thoracotomy for posterior, subcarina, and hilar lesions. The noninvasive nature of this technique is most promising for staging of bronchogenic carcinoma. Its combined use with CT scanning can have a major impact on the management of patients with lung cancer. However, one major problem of TBNA is that it has not been used as widely as it should mainly because it is relatively new with unpredictable results. TBNA sensitivity could be improved with proper knowledge of anatomy and technique. This chapter describes the relevant anatomy and technique in using TBNA to assess the mediastinum and hilar lymph nodes to evaluate the "N" status in bronchogenic carcinoma. CT scanning and bronchoscopy are used together to retain the sensitivity of CT scanning in discovering abnormal lymph nodes and the specificity of TBNA to diagnose the cell type of metastatic lesions in the lymph nodes.

Definitions and nomenclature of the lymph nodes and their relationship to the AJCC and American Thoracic Society (ATS) systems have been described (13,14). The intent here is not to create a new system, but rather to use CT and TBNA to describe the mediastinum and hilar lymph node anatomy in a simple, practical manner. The value and definitions of the AJCC and ATS lymph node mapping systems are accepted and recognized; this numbering system is changed to accommodate the TBNA technique. Only the most commonly involved lymph nodes and those nodes on airway branching that can be used as landmarks to be accurately sampled by the TBNA technique are described. Following these landmarks, it is possible to sample even normal-sized lymph node tissue from mediastinum and hilar areas.

Four bronchoscopy views or sections for CT scans are used as key reference points.

I. At the lower trachea near the carina
II. At the right main bronchus near the right upper lobe orifice
III. Bronchus intermedius near the middle lobe orifice
IV. Left main bronchus, near the lower or upper lobe spur

Eleven nodal stations were named (Figure 14.1). The locations of the lymph node by CT image and TBNA puncture site are described in detail (Figures 14.2 and 14.3) (Tables 14.1 and 14.2).

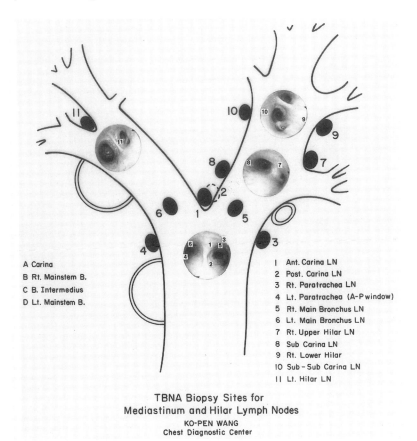

Figure 14.1. Nomenclature of mediastinum and hilar lymph nodes for TBNA.

A Carina
B Rt. Mainstem B.
C B. Intermedius
D Lt. Mainstem B.

1 Ant. Carina LN
2 Post. Carina LN
3 Rt. Paratrachea LN
4 Lt. Paratrachea (A-P window)
5 Rt. Main Bronchus LN
6 Lt. Main Bronchus LN
7 Rt. Upper Hilar LN
8 Sub Carina LN
9 Rt. Lower Hilar
10 Sub – Sub Carina LN
11 Lt. Hilar LN

TBNA Biopsy Sites for
Mediastinum and Hilar Lymph Nodes
KO-PEN WANG
Chest Diagnostic Center

Nodal Stations One through Six

At the first level, from the lower end of the trachea viewing the carina and both main bronchi, six nodal stations can be identified: 1) anterior carina, 2) posterior carina, 3) right paratrachea, 4) left paratrachea, 5) right main bronchus, and 6) left main bronchus lymph node (Figure 14.4A through c).

Carina lymph nodes are divided into anterior and posterior. At this level, the anterior carina is defined as the lymph node in front and between the proximal end of the right and left main bronchus. The posterior carina node is defined as behind and in between the proximal portion of the right and left main bronchus or often directly behind the right main bronchus (Figure 14.4b). For selection of a TBNA puncture site, the length of the needle and angle of entrance should be considered because, despite the attempt to puncture the airway as perpendicular as possible, a

certain degree of angulation will result. The needle should be long enough (1.3 to 1.5 cm) to compensate for the loss from angulation and the tip of the needle should reach the node to be sampled. For anterior carina nodule station 1, the first intercartilage space at about 12 to 1 o'clock is punctured (Figure 14.2, 1). For the posterior carina node, puncture directly opposite to the anterior carina puncture site is recommended, which will be about 5 to 6 o'clock in the posterior trachea wall (Figure 14.2, 2). Although puncturing the anterior carina lymph node occasionally results in bloody aspiration, there are no other complications. Biopsy of the posterior carina lymph node should only be performed when CT scan demonstrates an enlarged lymph node at that area to avoid puncturing the azygoesophageal recess and the potential possibility of pneumothorax.

The right paratrachea lymph node is much more commonly involved compared to the

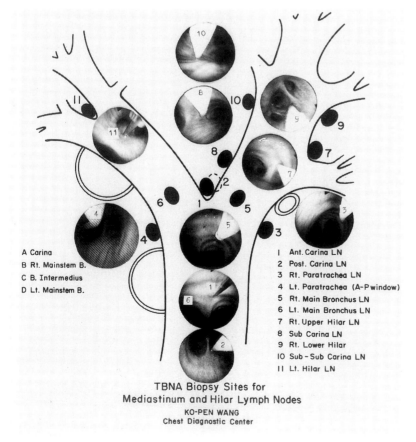

Figure 14.2. TBNA site for mediastinum and hilar lymph nodes (defined by bronchoscopy).

A Carina
B Rt. Mainstem B.
C B. Intermedius
D Lt. Mainstem B.

1 Ant. Carina LN
2 Post. Carina LN
3 Rt. Paratrachea LN
4 Lt. Paratrachea (A-P window)
5 Rt. Main Bronchus LN
6 Lt. Main Bronchus LN
7 Rt. Upper Hilar LN
8 Sub Carina LN
9 Rt. Lower Hilar
10 Sub-Sub Carina LN
11 Lt. Hilar LN

TBNA Biopsy Sites for
Mediastinum and Hilar Lymph Nodes
KO-PEN WANG
Chest Diagnostic Center

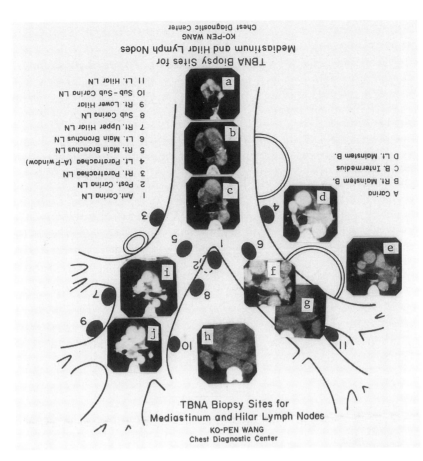

TBNA Biopsy Sites for
Mediastinum and Hilar Lymph Nodes
KO-PEN WANG
Chest Diagnostic Center

1 Ant. Carina LN
2 Post. Carina LN
3 Rt. Paratrachea LN
4 Lt. Paratrachea (A-P window)
5 Rt. Main Bronchus LN
6 Lt. Main Bronchus LN
7 Rt. Upper Hilar LN
8 Sub Carina LN
9 Rt. Lower Hilar
10 Sub-Sub Carina LN
11 Lt. Hilar LN

A Carina
B Rt. Mainstem B.
C B. Intermedius
D Lt. Mainstem B.

TBNA Biopsy Sites for
Mediastinum and Hilar Lymph Nodes
KO-PEN WANG
Chest Diagnostic Center

Figure 14.3. CT scan of the chest. Traditionally, CT scan is viewed from the abdomen toward the head in supine position. When performing TBNA in front of the patient, the bronchoscopist must invert the image (make it upside down) in his or her mind. When performing TBNA behind the patient, the right and left should be inverted.

more proximal lymph nodes such as higher paratrachea lymph node (group 2 in the AJCC system), pre- and retrotracheal lymph node (group 3 in the AJCC system), and highest mediastinum lymph node (group 1 in the AJCC system). In those 1, 2, 3, 4, AJCC system lymph node groups, only group 4, lower right paratrachea, was selected in this system as number 3 for the right paratrachea lymph node. It is most frequently involved and its location can be accurately identified and sampled by using the carina or intercartilage space of the trachea and tracheobronchial angulation as a landmark for TBNA. It is located under or above the level of the azygous arch and anterior lateral aspect of the lower trachea or behind the superior vena cava (ATS) (Figure 14.3b; Figure 14.4a). It should be sampled by puncturing at the 1 to 2 o'clock position of the second to fourth intercartilage space of the lower trachea by counting the lower most intercartilage space from the carina as

the first, then coming up proximally to the larynx (Figure 14.2, 3). This node is most commonly involved in malignant processes and even sarcoidosis. The more proximal node, adjacent to the trachea, groups 1, 2, and 3 (AJCC), is less involved in general. Even if it is involved, it is difficult to identify its exact level of location through bronchoscopy unless there is external compression. In the presence of extrinsic compression, the needle is placed from the upper border of extrinsic compression. In the absence of extrinsic compression, when only higher trachea lymph nodes are involved without lower right paratrachea involvement, fluoroscopic guidance is used to ensure the exact level of needle placement.

The left paratrachea lymph node was defined as nodal 4, which includes left lower paratrachea nodes and some of the aortic pulmonary window lymph nodes (which includes subaortic or suprapulmonic lymph nodes). Both groups can be sampled by TBNA; those nodes usually are around the lateral aspect of lower trachea near the tracheobronchial angulation and below the aortic arch, above the pulmonary artery (Figure 14.3d and e; Figure 14.4b). The puncture site is identified as 9 o'clock around the left lower trachea at the same level of the tip of carina or it can be performed one intercartilage space above or below the tracheobronchial angulation (Figure 14.2, 4). Puncture of this group of lymph nodes is technically more difficult and more fearsome because of proximity to major vessels, the aorta, and the pulmonary artery. In fact, it does not carry any higher risk for TBNA. Other lymph nodes on the left side such as para-aortic (around the side of aorta) or parapulmonary artery (around the side of pulmonary artery) (Figure 14.3d and f) or anterior mediastinum, either in front of the take off of the major vessels from the aorta or

nodes in front of the ligamentum arteriosum, are ignored in this system because they are beyond the reach of TBNA. Lymph node involvement in those areas is often associated with involvement of the subaortic or lower left paratrachea lymph node in which TBNA is applicable (Figure 14.3d and e). Very seldom are only paravascular or anterior vascular lymph nodes involved, which are beyond the reach of TBNA. Then a percutaneous needle aspiration (PCNA), either under fluoroscopy or CT guidance, is an alternative procedure to mediastinotomy. It is relatively easy to perform because the lesion is nonmobile with respiration and if the needle is placed below the aortic arch above the pulmonary artery and lateral to the ascending aorta and depth is controlled to not reach the descending aorta, then the procedure should be safe. The pulsation of the needle due to the transmission from the aorta

Figure 14.4. Location of mediastinum and hilar lymph nodes for TBNA (defined by CT scan).

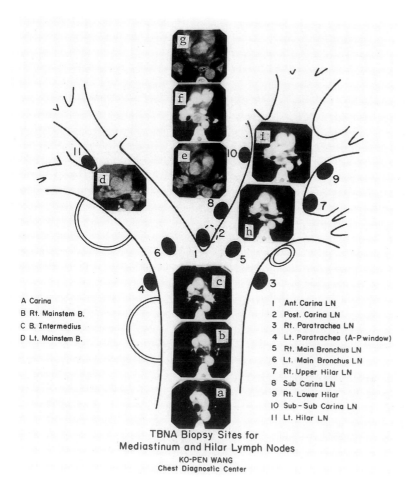

A Carina
B Rt. Mainstem B.
C B. Intermedius
D Lt. Mainstem B.

1   Ant. Carina LN
2   Post. Carina LN
3   Rt. Paratrachea LN
4   Lt. Paratrachea (A-P window)
5   Rt. Main Bronchus LN
6   Lt. Main Bronchus LN
7   Rt. Upper Hilar LN
8   Sub Carina LN
9   Rt. Lower Hilar
10 Sub-Sub Carina LN
11 Lt. Hilar LN

TBNA Biopsy Sites for
Mediastinum and Hilar Lymph Nodes
KO-PEN WANG
Chest Diagnostic Center

is impressive and fearsome, but imposes no real serious risk for the PCNA.

Nodes in front of the right and left main bronchus are defined as stations 5 and 6 (Figure 14.3*f*; Figure 14.4*c*), and the puncture site is at the first or second intercartilage space from 12 o'clock at each main bronchus. The counting of intercartilage space for the main bronchus is from the carina counting distally (Figure 14.2, *5* and *6*).

Nodal Stations Seven through Eleven

In previous reports for TBNA staging, only the right and left paratrachea and carina were emphasized. There is less mention of the main bronchus and different levels of subcarinal or hilar sampling. As experience grows with CT scanning in visualizing mediastinal and hilar lymph nodes, it becomes apparent that lymph nodes in front of the right upper lobe spur and subcarina lymph node are commonly involved. So, a slice near the right upper lobe bronchus is chosen to identify right upper hilar and subcarina nodes as stations 7 and 8 (Figure 14.3*i*). The right upper hilar node is located in front of and in between the right upper lobe bronchus and the bronchus intermedius. It can be sampled by puncturing the anterior aspect of the right upper lobe spur (Figure 14.2, 7). The subcarina lymph node is in between the right

Table 14.1. Location of Mediastinum and Hilar Lymph Nodes for TBNA (Defined by CT Scan)

1. Anterior carina lymph node:	In front and between the proximal portion of the right and left main bronchus
2. Posterior carina lymph node:	Behind and between the proximal portion of the right and left main bronchus, or directly behind the right main bronchus
3. Right paratrachea lymph node:	Behind the superior vena cava and in front of the anterolateral aspect of the lower trachea near the azygous arch
4. Left paratrachea lymph node: (Aortopulmonary window)	Lateral to the trachea near the tracheobronchial angulation, below the aortic arch and above the left main pulmonary artery
5. Right main bronchus lymph node:	In front of the right main bronchus
6. Left main bronchus lymph node:	In front of the left main bronchus
7. Right upper hilar lymph node:	In front and between the right upper lobe bronchus and the bronchus intermedius
8. Subcarina lymph node:	Between the right and left main bronchus, at or near the level of the right upper lobe bronchus
9. Right lower hilar lymph node:	Nodes lateral or in front of the bronchus intermedius, at or near the level of the right middle lobe bronchus
10. Sub-subcarina lymph node:	Between the bronchus intermedius and the left main bronchus, at or near the level of the right middle lobe bronchus
11. Left hilar lymph node:	Between the left upper lobe and left lower lobe bronchus

Table 14.2. TBNA Site for Mediastinum and Hilar Lymph Nodes (Defined by Bronchoscopy)

1. Anterior carina lymph node:	First and second intercartilage interspace from the lower trachea at about the 12–1 o'clock position
2. Posterior carina lymph node:	Posterior portion of the carina at about the 5–6 o'clock position
3. Right paratrachea lymph node:	Second to fourth intercartilage interspace of the lower trachea at about the 1–2 o'clock position
4. Left paratrachea lymph node (AP window):	First or second intercartilage interspace from the lower trachea at about the 9 o'clock position
5. Right main bronchus lymph node:	First or second intercartilage interspace from the proximal right main bronchus at about the 12 o'clock position
6. Left main bronchus lymph node:	First or second intercartilage interspace from the proximal left main bronchus at about the 12 o'clock position
7. Right upper hilar lymph node:	Anterior portion of the right upper lobe spur
8. Subcarina lymph node:	Medial wall of the right main bronchus at about the 9 o'clock position, proximal to the level of the right upper lobe orifice
9. Right lower hilar lymph node:	Lateral or anterior wall of the bronchus intermedius at about the 3 o'clock position and the 12 o'clock position near or at the level of the right middle lobe orifice
10. Sub-subcarina lymph node:	Medial wall of the bronchus intermedius at about the 9 o'clock position, proximal to the level of the right middle lobe orifice
11. Left hilar lymph node:	Lateral wall of the left lower lobe bronchus at about 9 o'clock, at the level of the superior segment orifice of the left lower lobe

and left main bronchus and near the level of the right upper lobe bronchus and can be sampled by puncturing the medial wall of the right main bronchus at about the 9 o'clock position near the right upper lobe bronchus level (Figure 14.2, 8).

At the bronchus intermedius near the right middle lobe bronchus, lymph nodes are around the side of the bronchus intermedius. Occasionally, lymph nodes in front of the bronchus intermedius are noticed, which can push the pulmonary artery forward. Those lymph nodes are defined as station 9, lower

right hilar (Figure 14.3*j* and *h*). They can be sampled around the right lateral aspect of the lower bronchus intermedius (Figure 14.2, *9*). Puncture of this site frequently results in a bloody aspiration but has no increased risk of complication. Directly opposite the right lower hilar lymph node at the medial wall of the bronchus intermedius is the sub-subcarina lymph node group. Puncture should be performed at 9 o'clock at the bronchus intermedius (Figure 14.2, *10*). Often this group of lymph nodes can extend below the right middle lobe orifice. Those nodes are posterior to the heart, so despite its apparent proximity to the left atrium, it poses no increased risk in TBNA (Figure 14.3h). The paraesophageal lymph node and pulmonary ligament lymph node are ignored in this system because of the distance from the airway. Very rarely, the paraesophageal lymph node is the only abnormality; then a transesophageal needle aspiration is performed to sample the specimen. The esophageal needle aspiration is guided by external compression; whether sub- or subsubcarina by our definition represents an enlarged paraesophageal or pulmonary ligament lymph node is unclear.

The final cut by CT scan is the level at the left upper lobe and left lower lobe spur, the lymph node in between upper lobe and lower lobe bronchus defined as left hilar number 11 (Figure 14.3G; Figure 14.4d and e). The puncture site is at the mid-lateral wall of the left lower lobe bronchus at the level of the superior segment orifice to avoid the descending left pulmonary artery and ensure a deeper penetration of the needle into this group of lymph nodes (Figure 14.2, 11). Puncture of the left hilar lymph node can result in bloody aspiration if it is too posterior. However, it occurs much less frequently than the right lower hilar needle aspiration.

Summary

The lower right paratrachea and anterior carina and right main bronchus lymph nodes can be hard to distinguish or often they are all involved (Figure 14.3a through c). The aortopulmonary window lymph node and left main bronchus lymph node can be hard to define or cán both be involved (Figure 14.3d through f). It is exactly for this reason it is important to define the nomenclature and location of lymph nodes and to identify the puncture sites for accurate sampling of the specimen. Despite the overlap, general guidelines are: right paratrachea node should be above the tracheobronchial angulation (Figure 14.3a and b), the right main bronchus node is more in front of the right main bronchus, and anterior carina lymph node is more in between the right and left main bronchus (Figure 14.3c). The left paratrachea or aortopulmonary window lymph node is lateral to the lower trachea or proximal left main bronchus (Figure 14.3d and e). The left main bronchus node is more anterior to the left main bronchus (Figure 14.3f).

This classification is not meant to confuse the issue; it is a response to the development of newer techniques of CT scanning and TBNA. Using CT scanning as a guide to select the most involved group of lymph nodes and the airway as a landmark for TBNA, correct sampling of all mediastinum and hilar lymph nodes is possible for cytologic diagnosis of malignancy and for histologic diagnosis of malignancy and benign disorders. By developing a unified nomenclature and practical anatomy and puncture sites and by increasing education, this procedure can be applied to bronchogenic carcinoma staging.

Although the technique is still in the developmental stage, bronchoscopists can use this system to be more actively involved in lung cancer staging with radiologists and surgeons. This precise and accurate information will guide the proper selection of appropriate treatment or clinical investigation to determine the prognosis.

REFERENCES

1. AJCC. Clinical staging system for carcinoma of the lung. American Joint Committee for Cancer Staging and End Results Reporting. Philadelphia: JB Lippincott, 1973.
2. American Joint Committee on Cancer. Manual for staging of cancer, 2nd ed. Philadelphia: JB Lippincott, 1977:99–105.
3. Mountain CF. A new international staging system for lung cancer. Chest 1986;89(suppl): 225S–233S.
4. AJCC. Staging of cancer, 3rd ed. Philadelphia: JB Lippincott, 1988:115–121.
5. Stitik FP, DiSantis DJ. Lung cancer staging. Seminar Roentgenol 1990;25:34–44.

6. Harmer EM. TNM classification of malignant tumors. Geneva, Switzerland: Union Internationale Contre le Cancer, 1978:41–45.

7. Yoshimura K. A clinical statistical study of lung cancer patients in Japan with special reference to the staging system of TNM classification: a report from the Japan Joint Committee of Lung Cancer associated with the TNM system of clinical classification (UICC). Radiat Med 1983;1:186–195.

8. Zerhouni EA, Stitik FP. Controversies in computed tomography of the thorax. The pulmonary nodule—lung cancer staging. Radiol Clin North Am 1985;23:407–426.

9. Templeton PA, Casekey CI, Zerhouni EA. Current uses of CT and MR imaging in the staging of lung cancer. Radiol Clin North Am 1990;28:631–646.

10. Wang KP, Brower R, Haponik EF, Siegelman S. Flexible transbronchial needle aspiration for staging of bronchogenic carcinoma. Chest 1983;84:671–676.

11. Shure D, Fedullo PF. The role of transcarinal needle aspiration in the staging of bronchogenic carcinoma. Chest 1984;86:693–696.

12. Schenk DA, Bower JH, Bryan CL, et al. Transbronchial needle aspiration staging of bronchogenic carcinoma. Am Rev Respir Dis 1986;134:146–148.

13. Tisi GM, Friedman PJ, Peters RM, et al. Clinical staging of primary lung cancer. Am Rev Resp Dis 1983;127:659.

14. Friedman PJ. Lung cancer: update on staging classifications. AJR Am J Roentgenol 1988;150:261–264.

15 | The Role of Transbronchial Needle Aspiration in Staging of Bronchogenic Carcinoma

David A. Schenk

Most patients who present with bronchogenic carcinoma have surgically unresectable disease for a variety of reasons including the presence of distant metastatic disease, unfavorable histology (small cell undifferentiated carcinoma), or mediastinal extension of the tumor. Before attempting surgical extirpation in patients with non–small-cell carcinoma, accurate pathologic staging must be performed to identify the relatively small number of patients who will benefit from surgical intervention. Accurate mediastinal staging is imperative because survival rates are inversely related to the presence of malignant mediastinal adenopathy (1–3). In addition, therapeutic intervention is often directed by the presence or absence of mediastinal malignancy. To date, the standard for mediastinal staging of bronchogenic carcinoma has been surgical mediastinal exploration. Thirty to 40% of patients who undergo surgical mediastinal exploration have mediastinal extension of their tumor (4–8). Although associated with low morbidity, the cost of surgical mediastinal exploration (surgeon/anesthesiologist fees, operating and recovery room charges, and hospitalization) is significant, ranging from $2000 to $2500. Cervical mediastinal exploration (CME) is limited in its ability to adequately evaluate lymph nodes in the posterior subcarinal, anterior mediastinal, and subaortic lymph node chains. Patients with left upper lobe carcinomas are particularly difficult to stage due to the predilection of metastasis to the aortopulmonic window node chain, an area virtually inaccessible via CME. These patients may require anterior mediastinal surgical exploration for pathologic staging.

Historical Perspectives

Transtracheal needle aspiration of mediastinal tissue was first used by Schieppati over four decades ago (9). Using a 50-cm long, one-mm diameter needle inserted through a rigid bronchoscope, he successfully performed transcarinal aspiration for diagnosis in 69 patients with suspected bronchogenic or esophageal carcinoma. In 216 patients a histologic diagnosis of cancer was established by the needle. No complications occurred (10).

Versteegh and Swierenga performed transcarinal needle puncture using a long, thin needle introduced via rigid bronchoscopy more than 250 times without complication. In a series of 150 patients, there were 25 malignant carinal aspirates (16.6%). In the 25 patients with malignant aspirates the carina was abnormally broadened only 11 times. In 14 cases the malignant carinal puncture was the only indication of the presence of lymph node metastases. He noted that "the carinal puncture . . . does not require an extra operation, but may be carried out during diagnostic bronchoscopy. A positive result of the carinal puncture means that curative resection is excluded" (11).

Fox and colleagues used a modified Vim Biegeleisen biopsy needle, an auger-type instrument with an outside cutting sheath, introduced via a rigid bronchoscope through the medial wall of either main bronchus at or just distal to the carinal spur. At puncture the obturator was removed and the auger biopsy unit introduced and screwed into the hilt. The outer cannula was then rotated and advanced over the auger biopsy unit to cut off the core of tissue. In more than 50 patients there were no complications other than a minimal oozing of blood. In all cases good specimens were reportedly obtained. Carcinoma or lymphoma was diagnosed in 40% of all specimens and thoracotomy was avoided. Lymph node tissue was noted in 65% of the specimens (12).

Having had previous experience with transbronchial left atrial punctures in patients with cardiac valvular lesions, Bridgman and coworkers fastened a Vim-Silverman needle of the standard left atrial puncture apparatus and performed subcarinal lymph node biopsy via rigid bronchoscopy in 50 patients. Inadequate material was obtained in 18 (36%), cancer diagnosed in 12 (24%), silicosis and nonspecific granuloma in 2 (4%), and normal lymph node tissue in 12 (24%). In 4 cases the diagnosis of carcinoma was made solely on the subcarinal node biopsy. As in Versteegh's experience, a normal-appearing carina gave no assurance that subcarinal lymph nodes were normal. When compared to mediastinoscopy, transcarinal needle aspiration proved more valuable. "Obtaining adequate subcarinal lymph node material can be of considerable aid in making a diagnosis, in determining the extent of the disease, and helping us avoid an unnecessary thoracotomy, particularly in patients who are poor operative risks." In 56 additional patients, transcarinal needle biopsies identified malignancy in 29% (13).

Due to the technical skills required to perform transtracheal needle aspiration through a rigid bronchoscope and the emergence of CME, transtracheal needle aspiration failed to gain wide acceptance. Interest in transbronchial needle aspiration (TBNA) was rekindled,

however, in 1978 when Wang and associates demonstrated that paratracheal lymph nodes could be sampled via rigid endoscopy using esophageal varices needles. They obtained diagnostic tissue in three of five patients with paratracheal masses. No complications developed (14).

Initially, TBNA was considered predominantly a diagnostic procedure. In a 1981 study involving 32 patients, a specific diagnosis of carcinoma in the paratracheal or parabronchial tissues was established in 18 of 20 patients proved to have bronchogenic carcinoma by other means (15). Shure and Fedullo demonstrated that TBNA significantly enhanced the diagnosis in 31 patients who presented with endoscopically abnormal airways suggesting submucosal or peribronchial tumors. Forceps biopsy yield was 55% and that of TBNA 71%. The combination of forceps biopsy and TBNA resulted in an 89% diagnostic rate. When brushings and washings were included, the overall diagnostic yield was 97%. TBNA significantly increased the yield over forceps biopsy alone in the detection of submucosal or peribronchial bronchogenic carcinoma (16). In a retrospective review from 1983–1985 involving 68 patients with cancer, TBNA confirmed malignancy in 25 (37%). In 5 patients with peripheral nodules or masses, TBNA under fluoroscopic guidance confirmed malignancy in 3. Overall there were 8 patients in whom only TBNA demonstrated malignancy. It was again noted that TBNA was especially useful in patients presenting with extrinsic bronchial compression, extrabronchial masses, and submucosal infiltration by tumor. Interestingly, TBNA was beneficial in patients who had extrapulmonary malignancies and pulmonary metastases (17).

Harrow and colleagues noted in a study of 70 patients with thoracic cancer that TBNA was positive in 32 (46%) and solely diagnostic in 12 (17%). In 10% of the patients TBNA precluded the need for further diagnostic surgery. There were no complications (18). In a subsequent 5-year review involving 633 patients, they noted malignant mediastinal aspirates in 127 of 547 patients (23%) who had mediastinal TBNA nodal sampling. In 44 of 176 patients (25%) who had mucosal abnormalities that did not appear to be obviously neoplastic on gross inspection, TBNA demonstrated malignancy. In 31 cases (4% of all TBNA procedures performed), TBNA provided the sole cancer diagnosis (19).

Mehta and associates, using both 22- and 18-gauge needles in 34 patients with mediastinal or hilar adenopathy obtained tissue for histologic examination in 17 (50%), which was diagnostic in 11 patients (32%). Three patients had a benign diagnosis confirmed by the 18-gauge needle. The overall diagnostic yield of the 18-gauge needle was 41%. It increased the diagnostic rate of fiberoptic bronchoscopy (FOB) from 50% to 58%. No significant complications were reported (20).

The diagnostic utility of TBNA in patients with peripheral malignant nodules or masses has been demonstrated in two prospective studies. In 42 patients with bronchogenic carcinoma and negative sputum cytology, the addition of TBNA to traditional FOB diagnostic modalities (transbronchial biopsy, brushings, washings) significantly increased the diagnostic yield from 48% to 69%. In 10 patients in whom the brush or biopsy forceps could pass to the border of the lesion but not into it, the needle confirmed malignancy in 8. Overall, TBNA provided the highest diagnostic yield (21). Wang and coworkers studied 20 patients with malignant peripheral nodules or masses and no endobronchial disease. TBNA identified malignancy in 11 and provided the sole diagnosis in 7 patients. It demonstrated a significantly higher yield than the forceps biopsy or brush. One patient suffered a pneumothorax. The yield of TBNA approached that of percutaneous fine-needle aspiration but at a lower complication rate (22).

In a prospective study of 91 consecutive patients who presented with bronchogenic car-

cinoma, Schenk and colleagues compared the diagnostic yields of cytologic examination of sputum, endobronchial brushings and washings, and endobronchial/transbronchial biopsies to TBNA using the Wang 22-gauge needle. The overall diagnostic yield for the conventional modalities combined was 64%. With the addition of TBNA, the yield increased to 71%. Bronchogenic carcinoma was diagnosed solely by TBNA in 6 patients, all with extrabronchial or extratracheal lesions. TBNA failed to significantly contribute to the diagnosis of cancer in patients with lesions readily accessible by conventional bronchoscopic modalities. It was noted, however, that exceptions may include patients with necrotic endobronchial tumors, submucosal lesions, and peripheral masses or nodules (23).

In 1983, Wang and associates assessed the role of TBNA (22-gauge needle) as a staging tool in 39 patients. One patient underwent bronchoscopy with TBNA on two occasions due to an equivocal initial TBNA specimen. The 22-gauge needle demonstrated malignant cytology in 19 patients (48.7%). In the 21 bronchoscopies with negative needle cytology, 15 had no evidence of mediastinal extension of the tumor at the time of surgical staging. There were 6 patients in whom TBNA was falsely negative. The overall sensitivity of TBNA as a staging tool was 76% (24). Shure and Fedullo, using a 20-gauge, one-cm needle obtained carinal biopsies in 110 consecutive patients with bronchogenic carcinoma. Fifteen percent of the aspirates demonstrated malignant cytology. No false positives were encountered. There appeared to be an association between malignant carinal aspirates and the presence of an endobronchial tumor (24%) or an abnormal-appearing carina at the time of bronchoscopy (38%). The incidence of false negative carinal aspirates was not determined, however (25).

As a staging tool, TBNA was initially met with some resistance among surgical colleagues and pulmonologists for a variety of reasons. First, although TBNA using a cytology needle is relatively simple to perform, results are somewhat limited by technique and bronchoscopy time in experienced hands can be prolonged by several minutes. Secondly, concerns arose pertaining to the possibility of obtaining false positive malignant aspirates in patients without mediastinal extension of disease. A malignant aspirate could be obtained by inadvertently suctioning endotracheal secretions containing neoplastic cells from the more distal airways. Thirdly, the initial staging tools, 20- or 22-gauge needles, obtained specimens for cytologic review, requiring the services and support of a sophisticated cytopathology laboratory and cytopathologist. Further studies were necessary to confirm the utility of TBNA in the assessment of patients with bronchogenic carcinoma.

In 1986, Schenk and colleagues reported the results of a prospective study designed to assess the sensitivity, specificity, and accuracy of TBNA using a 22-gauge Wang needle as a staging tool in bronchogenic carcinoma. A total of 88 consecutive patients were enrolled. Each patient underwent chest computed tomography (CT) before bronchoscopy to better localize paratracheal adenopathy to direct TBNA. Disease in 34 patients was determined to be unresectable due to mediastinal extension of tumor via TBNA or surgery. There were 19 malignant mediastinal needle aspirates. Two were false positive aspirates (i.e., malignant cells from patients ultimately demonstrating no mediastinal malignancy at surgical staging). In one patient an aortopulmonary window aspirate was correctly interpreted by the cytopathologist as contaminated by secretions lining the tracheal mucosa. It contained columnar epithelial cells, a scant number of neoplastic cells and an absence of lymphocytes. Surgical staging confirmed reactive lymphadenopathy.

The other false positive aspirate occurred in a patient with a right upper lobe neoplasm that abutted the mediastinum in the right posterior paratracheal area. The mediastinum is a thin structure only 2 to 3 mm in width at this site. The needle apparently exited the mediastinum and entered the parenchymal mass directly. At surgery the tumor fell away from the mediastinum. Despite the two false positive aspirates encountered in this study, the specificity was very high at 96%. Overall, TBNA confirmed mediastinal malignancy in 50% of patients with mediastinal extension of tumor (26).

This experience confirmed the need to use great care to prevent the inadvertent aspiration of material lining the airway. TBNA should be performed prior to brushings, washings, biopsies, and distal airway inspection to minimize the risk of "contaminating" the proximal airway with distal debris or secretions. Secondly, suction should be discontinued prior to withdrawal of the needle from the tracheal wall. This can be ensured by temporary removal of the syringe from the proximal suction port of the catheter. An acceptable cytology specimen should contain a paucity of columnar epithelial cells, a large number of lymphocytes, and an adequate number of malignant cells to confirm the diagnosis.

Due to the concern surrounding mediastinal staging via cytologic methods and to enhance diagnostic yield, Wang pursued modification of the transbronchial needle for histologic sampling. In 1985, he presented his initial experience using an 18-gauge histology needle designed for mediastinal and hilar node aspiration. In 25 patients studied, 21 had histologic specimens, with 18 specific diagnoses (27). The histology needle, designed to obtain a small core of tissue, was a 1.5-cm, 18-gauge needle at the end of a plastic catheter with an inner wire stylet attached to a 5-mm, 21-gauge needle or trochar that could be extended through or retracted into the 18-gauge shell. The 18-gauge needle was somewhat more difficult to pass through the tracheal wall than the 22-gauge needle. Subsequently, a tapered 19-gauge, retractable histology needle with inner 21-gauge needle/trochar was designed by

Dr. Wang for improved penetration of the tracheobronchial wall.

It was apparent from its inception that appropriate technique must be observed closely when using this instrument. First, the needle must always be passed through the bronchoscope with the needle retracted into the catheter to prevent inadvertent puncture of the suction channel. When the site for aspiration is identified, the needles are advanced and secured. The needle hub should be positioned within the distal suction port of the bronchoscope to prevent bending of the catheter while passing the needle through the trachea. Care must be taken to ensure needle passage between the cartilagenous rings. The needle tip or trochar should first "catch" the tracheal mucosa. The catheter must then be anchored in one hand by the thumb and index finger at the proximal suction port of the bronchoscope. The needle is then pushed through the wall with steady forward pressure of the bronchoscope and catheter as a unit. If unsuccessful, the patient can assist by coughing while forward pressure on the bronchoscope is applied (28). Once penetration of the needle to the hub has occurred, the inner 21-gauge needle is retracted and suction is applied to the catheter using a 30 to 60-mL syringe containing 5 to 10 mL saline or Hank's solution to confirm the absence of blood return. While an assistant provides continuous suction, the needle is carefully withdrawn from the wall 5 to 10 mm and reinserted several times at different angles to "shear-off" small core specimens. Before completely withdrawing the needle from the wall, several small, rapid deflections are made with the needle in place to "pack" the specimen within the tapered needle. Suction is then discontinued, the catheter withdrawn from the bronchoscope, and the needle contents flushed into a specimen cup. The procedure is repeated three or four times in the same general area corresponding with adenopathy localized on the CT scan. All mediastinal specimens are collected together.

The flush solution is subsequently decanted and saved for cytologic evaluation. The remaining core specimens are preserved in formalin for histologic review. Following mediastinal staging, diagnostic procedures (brushings, washings, and biopsies) are performed as indicated.

A prospective study of 29 consecutive patients with bronchogenic carcinoma and mediastinal adenopathy demonstrated on chest CT was conducted by our group using the Wang 18-gauge histology needle. Twenty of the 29 patients had malignant aspirates. Four of the 9 negative aspirates were confirmed to be true negative aspirates by surgical staging. Five patients had false negative aspirates. In 4 patients insufficient tissue was obtained for histologic review. No complications were encountered. The overall sensitivity of the Wang 18-gauge histology needle in the mediastinal staging of patients with bronchogenic carcinoma was 80%. If patients with small cell carcinoma were excluded, sensitivity was 82% (29). These results reflect a significant improvement in sensitivity of the 18-gauge histology needle over the 22-gauge cytology needle.

Recently, 55 patients with bronchogenic carcinoma and mediastinal extension of tumor were prospectively studied to compare the results of TBNA using histology and cytology needles. Twenty-nine of the 55 patients had malignant 22-gauge cytology aspirates, for a sensitivity of 52.7%. In contrast, with the 19-gauge histology needle, 43 patients (78.2%) had malignant core specimens and 35 (63.6%) had malignant cells noted on cytologic examination of the flush solution. The overall sensitivity of the histology needle was 85.5%. No false positive aspirates or complications were encountered. The 19-gauge histology needle is significantly easier to pass through the trachea than the 18-gauge prototype needle. The enhanced yield of this histology needle clearly demonstrates that TBNA can avert the need for a separate surgical staging procedure.

The yield of TBNA now approaches that of CME (30).

Throughout our experience, prebronchoscopic chest CT has been a valuable aid in the staging of lung cancer patients. Although the role of chest CT as a separate staging tool is debated, it has been a valuable guide for TBNA or surgical mediastinal staging through its ability to precisely localize paratracheal adenopathy. Small lymph nodes less than one cm in diameter can harbor micrometastases and enlarged lymph nodes may be free of malignancy. Pathologic confirmation of mediastinal malignancy is therefore imperative. Endobronchial sites for TBNA that correspond with the paratracheal adenopathy can easily be identified during bronchoscopy.

Extensive experience by a multitude of investigators confirms the safety of TBNA. Only a few case reports pertaining to TBNA complications appear in the literature (31–33). Bronchoscope channel damage can be avoided by ensuring that the catheter is never forced through a "flexed" bronchoscope or advanced through the bronchoscope with the needle extended. The incidence of false positive aspirates is likewise rare, especially if the previously noted procedural techniques are followed (34–36).

Transbronchial needle aspiration has been established as an accurate, sensitive tool in the pathologic staging of the mediastinum. The safety of the procedure has been clearly established. The unique value of TBNA lies in the fact that it can be performed at the time of diagnostic bronchoscopy, thereby averting the cost and discomfort of a separate surgical staging procedure in a majority of patients who present with bronchogenic carcinoma. The core specimen provided by the histology needle can obviate the need for evaluation by a cytopathologist, making TBNA more universally practical. As health care expenses continue to soar, more emphasis must be placed on efforts to shorten hospitalization time and to minimize cost of medical care. Outpatient management and alternative procedures for traditional methods of diagnosis, staging, and treatment are demanded. When extrapolated to the general population, the cost savings of TBNA staging could be enormous. If one assumes that the average cost for CME ranges between $2000 and $2500 for surgeon/anesthesiologist fees, operating and recovery room charges, and hospitalization, then it is clear that if TBNA supplants surgical mediastinal exploration, several millions of dollars in health care costs will be saved each year in the United States.

Transbronchial needle aspiration offers an effective, safe, cost-saving alternative to surgical mediastinal exploration. It should be performed as the initial staging procedure in all patients with bronchogenic carcinoma who demonstrate paratracheal/parabronchial adenopathy on chest CT.

REFERENCES

1. Mountain CF. A new international staging system for lung cancer. Chest 1986;89:225S–233S.
2. Mountain CF. Value of the new TNM staging system for lung cancer. Chest 1989;96:47S–49S.
3. Watanabe Y, Hayashi Y, Shimizu J, Oda M, Iwa T. Mediastinal nodal involvement and the prognosis of non-small cell lung cancer. Chest 1991;99:422–428.
4. Ashbaugh DG. Mediastinoscopy. Arch Surg 1970;100:568–573.
5. Carlens E. Mediastinoscopy. Ann Otol 1965;74:1102–1112.
6. Gibbons JRP. The value of mediastinoscopy in assessing operability in carcinoma of the lung. Br J Dis Chest 1972;66:162–166.
7. Inberg MV, Klossner J, Linna MI, et al. The role of mediastinoscopy in the treatment of lung carcinoma. Scand J Thorac Cardiovasc Surg 1972;6:293–296.
8. Coughlin M, Deslaurirs J, Beaulieu M, et al. Role of mediastinoscopy in pretreatment staging of patients with primary lung cancer. Ann Thorac Surg 1985;40:556–560.
9. Schieppati E. La puncion mediastinal traves

del espolon traqueal. Rev AS Med Argent 1949;663:497.

10. Schieppati E. Mediastinal lymph node puncture through the tracheal carina. Surg Gynecol Obstet 1958;107:243–246.

11. Versteegh RM, Swierenga J. Bronchoscopic evaluation of the operability of pulmonary carcinoma. Acta Otolaryngol 1963;56:603–611.

12. Fox RT, Lees WM, Shields TW. Transcarinal bronchoscopic needle biopsy. Ann Thorac Surg 1965;1:92–96.

13. Bridgman AH, Duffield GD, Takaro T. An appraisal of newer diagnostic methods for intrathoracic lesions. Dis Chest 1968; 53:321–327.

14. Wang KP, Terry P, Marsh B. Bronchoscopic needle aspiration biopsy of paratracheal tumors. Am Rev Respir Dis 1978;118:17–21.

15. Wang KP, Marsh BR, Summer WR, Terry PB, Erozan YS, Baker RR. Transbronchial needle aspiration for diagnosis of lung cancer. Chest 1981;80:48–50.

16. Shure D, Fedullo PF. Transbronchial needle aspiration in the diagnosis of submucosal and peribronchial bronchogenic carcinoma. Chest 1985;88:49–51.

17. Gay PC, Brutinel WM. Transbronchial needle aspiration in the practice of bronchoscopy. Mayo Clin Proc 1989;64:158–162.

18. Harrow EM, Oldenburg FA, Smith AM. Transbronchial needle aspiration in clinical practice. Thorax 1985;40:756–759.

19. Harrow EM, Oldenburg FA, Lingenfelter MS, Smith AM. Transbronchial needle aspiration in clinical practice. Chest 1989;96:1268–1272.

20. Mehta AC, Kavuru MS, Meeker DP, Gephardt GN, Nunez C. Transbronchial needle aspiration for histology specimens. Chest 1989; 96:1228–1232.

21. Shure D, Fedullo PF. Transbronchial needle aspiration of peripheral masses. Am Rev Respir Dis 1983;128:1090–1092.

22. Wang KP, Haponik EF, Britt EJ, Khouri N, Erozan Y. Transbronchial needle aspiration of peripheral pulmonary nodules. Chest 1984;86:819–823.

23. Schenk DA, Bryan CL, Bower JH, Myers DL. Transbronchial needle aspiration in the diagnosis of bronchogenic carcinoma. Chest 1987;2:83–85.

24. Wang KP, Brower R, Haponik EF, Siegelman S. Flexible transbronchial needle aspiration for staging of bronchogenic carcinoma. Chest 1983;84:571–576.

25. Shure D, Fedullo PF. The role of transcarinal needle aspiration in the staging of bronchogenic carcinoma. Chest 1984;86:693–696.

26. Schenk DA, Bower JH, Bryan CL, et al. Transbronchial needle aspiration staging of bronchogenic carcinoma. Am Rev Respir Dis 1986;134:146–148.

27. Wang KP. Flexible transbronchial needle aspiration biopsy for histologic specimens. Chest 1985;88:860–863.

28. Olsen JD, Thomas DA, Young MB, Perry ME. Cough and transbronchial needle aspiration. Chest 1986;89:315.

29. Schenk DA, Strollo PJ, Pickard JS, et al. Utility of the Wang 18-gauge transbronchial histology needle in the staging of bronchogenic carcinoma. Chest 1989;96:272–274.

30. Schenk DA, Chambers SL, Derdak S, Komadina KH, et al. Comparison of the Wang 19 gauge and 22 gauge needles for mediastinal staging of lung cancer as a cost effective alternative to surgery. ARRD 1993;147:1251–1258.

31. Witte MC, Opal SM, Gilbert JG, et al. Incidence of fever and bacteremia following transbronchial needle aspiration. Chest 1986; 89:85–87.

32. Kucera RF, Wolfe GK, Perry ME. Hemomediastinum after transbronchial needle aspiration. Chest 1986;90:466.

33. Sherling BE. Complication with a transbronchial histology needle. Chest 1990;98: 783–784.

34. Cropp AJ, DiMarco AF, Lankerani M. False-positive transbronchial needle aspiration in bronchogenic carcinoma. Chest 1984; 85:696–697.

35. Schenk DA, Chasen MH, McCarthy MJ, Duncan CA, Christian CA. Potential false positive mediastinal transbronchial needle aspiration in bronchogenic carcinoma. Chest 1984;86:649–650.

36. Carlin BW, Harrell JH, Fedullo PF. False-positive transcarinal needle aspirate in the evaluation of bronchogenic carcinoma. Am Rev Respir Dis 1989;140:1800–1802.

Transbronchial Needle Aspiration in Clinical Practice | 16

Edward M. Harrow, Frederick A. Oldenburg, Jr., Mark S. Lingenfelter, and A. Marshall Smith, Jr.

Although the preceding chapters of this book have outlined the spectrum of uses of the technique of transbronchial needle aspiration (TBNA), its preeminent role remains its ability to diagnose and stage lung cancer. The epidemic of malignant pulmonary disease that physicians now confront on a daily basis continues to grow. Lung cancer has become the most prevalent and lethal malignancy in our society. The irony remains that it is also the most preventable. Although the surgeon general issued his landmark report regarding the dangers of cigarette smoking in 1964 (1), he had been preceded long before by a number of notable detractors. In 1604, King James I wrote, "Tobacco is a filthy weed, and the custom is loathsome to the eye, hateful to the nose, harmful to the brain, dangerous to the lungs, and in the black, stinking fume thereof nearest resembling the horrible Stygian smoke of the pit that is bottomless" (2). Repeated efforts to encourage people to stop smoking have had only limited success. As a result, physicians continue to expend an enormous effort in trying to cure malignant pulmonary disease, often when it is far too late in the course of the illness for their efforts to be effective.

The era of resectional surgery began in 1932 with the first pneumonectomy performed by Evarts Graham (3) and 60 years later pulmonary resection still remains the best hope for cure. Unfortunately, most patients have inoperable disease at the time of discovery either because of local mediastinal extension or distant metastatic spread. The need to be more discriminating in excluding patients for thoracic surgery who have mediastinal disease resulted in the introduction of mediastinoscopy by Carlens in 1959 (4). The application of this technique clearly represented a major advance in assessing mediastinal lymphatics; however, the time, expense, and potential complications of this surgical procedure are significant. The technique of TBNA, first introduced by Schieppati (5) and more recently adapted by Wang and colleagues (6–8) for use with the fiberoptic bronchoscope, has offered a simpler method by which to determine the extent of midline lymphatic disease. In addition, TBNA is noninvasive and permits the aspiration of a number of lymph node regions not accessible by either mediastinoscopy or mediastinotomy.

The success of any technique, however, must be judged by its general applicability and acceptance by the practicing medical community. Because the majority of patients are cared for by private physicians, the utility of TBNA will ultimately be determined by practitioner acceptance of its ability to stage patients with lung cancer and help select those who will benefit most from surgery. This chapter is intended to convey the experience of a group of privately practicing pulmonologists in its use.

Clinical Experience with TBNA

In 1983, the pulmonologists in Bangor, Maine began using TBNA. Nearly all patients suspected of having malignant disease had TBNA for mediastinal staging performed during their initial bronchoscopic examination. Other areas of the tracheobronchial tree were also sampled as seemed appropriate at the time of the procedure. A summary of the first 5 years of our experience with TBNA is presented in Table 16.1. This represents the collective experience of four pulmonologists and indicates that it was consistently used about 35% to 40% of the time.

Aspiration of mediastinal (N2) nodes was performed in 86% of patients who had TBNA. Subcarinal and paratracheal aspirates were usually pooled and submitted as a single specimen. Other investigators, however, have shown that positive subcarinal nodes and multiple areas of nodal involvement portend a poorer prognosis, suggesting that specimen separation may provide additional prognostic information (14–16). In 29% of cases a sample was taken from a visually abnormal location in the tracheobronchial tree and 14% of patients had aspirates obtained both from mediastinal as well as endobronchial locations during the same procedure. Its use with fluoroscopic guidance to sample a parenchymal lesion was infrequent.

Because the most important application of this technique is to determine N2 disease, these results are reported in Table 16.2. The data show that there were distinct differences among the four physicians using TBNA. Drs. X and Y used the technique more frequently than did either Dr. W or especially Dr. Z. In addition, the degree of positivity was also significant. Dr. Y sampled paratracheal locations less frequently than the other three physicians. The low incidence of use by Dr. Z coupled with the highest rate of positive returns suggests that this individual used it primarily in patients with more obvious mediastinal disease.

Over the course of 5 years, we obtained 173 positive aspirates in 728 TBNA attempts (24%) among all patients, even though approximately one third ultimately proved not to have malignant disease. In N2 locations there were 127 positives in 547 aspirates (24%). A total of 363 patients were actually diagnosed as having lung cancer for the first time and 124 (34%) were shown to have a positive TBNA from a mediastinal lymph node. Three other patients had recurrent disease. The cell types from these mediastinal sites are reported in Table 16.3.

The value of TBNA is particularly evident in those cases in which this technique provides the sole cytopathologic evidence for chest malignancy. In 5 years there were 31 cases,

Table 16.1. Incidence of TBNA Use during Bronchoscopy

Year	Bronchoscopies	TBNA	% TBNA
1983 (6 mo)	155	54	35%
1984	264	124	47%
1985	309	132	43%
1986	332	121	36%
1987	397	146	37%
1988 (6 mo)	173	56	32%
Total	1630	633	39%

Table 16.2. TBNA Use in N2 Disease

	Bronchoscopies	TBNA	% TBNA	Positive	% Positive
Dr. W	363	119	33%	30	25%
Dr. X	575	226	39%	54	24%
Dr. Y	303	122	40%	19	16%
Dr. Z	389	80	21%	24	30%
Total	1630	547	34%	127	23%

4% of all TBNAs performed or 18% of all positive TBNAs, in which this procedure provided the sole means of establishing the diagnosis of cancer. The results are demonstrated in Table 16.4. Two cases of lymphoma were diagnosed with a 21-gauge needle on cytologic grounds alone. Both were patients who had been treated with chemotherapy and were felt to be disease free until the clinical suspicion of recurrence was definitively demonstrated by TBNA. One additional patient with lymphoma is not included in these statistics (Case #2) because his diagnosis was confirmed by thoracotomy at a time when we were first developing familiarity with the technique. One patient had both small and large malignant cells seen on his aspirate (17).

In our total series of 173 positive TBNAs, there were 111 cases in which coexistent biopsy material demonstrated malignant tissue. Thirty-one cases had cytology from another site in the tracheobronchial tree that was confirmatory and in an additional 31, TBNA was the only means of proving the diagnosis. In all but 3 cases the aspirate showed cells that were either identical or compatible with the tissue diagnosis. In 2 of these patients, TBNA showed large cell carcinoma while the biopsy showed small cell in one and mixed large and small cell in the other. In the former, the chemotherapeutic response was good, in the latter poor. In the third case the TBNA showed mixed both small and large cell carcinoma, the biopsy small cell, and the patient responded to chemotherapy. In one other individual the aspirate also showed both small and large malignant cells and was the sole means of making the diagnosis of malignancy. In this patient there was no response to chemotherapy.

Because the treatment of small cell carcinoma is clearly different from that of other types of lung cancer, we were initially reluctant to accept the cytologic results of TBNA in these cases as providing sufficient evidence with which to initiate chemotherapy. Our onco-

Table 16.3. Malignant Transbronchial Aspirates from Mediastinal Nodes

	No.	%
Small cell carcinoma	41	32%
Large cell carcinoma	37	29%
Adenocarcinoma	29	23%
Squamous cell carcinoma	14	11%
Poorly differentiated carcinoma	4	3%
Lymphoma	2	2%
Total	127	100

Table 16.4. TBNA Cytology as Sole Means of Diagnosis

Small cell carcinoma	11
Adenocarcinoma	9
Large cell carcinoma	5
Squamous cell carcinoma	3
Lymphoma	2
Large and small cell carcinoma	1
Total	31

logic colleagues, however, felt that if a patient's response to treatment was not prompt, additional tissue could be obtained. Clinical follow-up of the 11 patients with small cell carcinoma diagnosed by TBNA alone has confirmed that the original cytologic diagnosis was, in fact, correct. On the basis of these findings, we believe that it is reasonable to begin initial chemotherapy for patients with small cell carcinoma diagnosed only by TBNA.

Mindful of the report by Cropp and associates (18) that demonstrated contamination of the mediastinal aspirate by tumor present in the airway, we consider all scanty specimens or suspicious cytologies to be negative and require independent tissue confirmation. Over the course of 5 years, 13 patients had cytologic report interpreted to be suspicious. In each case, additional tissue proved that these individuals did, in fact, have a chest malignancy. Six other patients with TBNA of mediastinal nodes had an aspirate in which there were only a few malignant cells. Two had small cell carcinoma on the bronchial biopsy and did not have further investigation. Two had good clinical evidence for mediastinal disease, one with a paralyzed vocal cord and enlarged lymph nodes on computed tomography (CT) scan while the other also had a paralyzed vocal cord and a nonfunctional ipsilateral diaphragm. Two were felt to be false positives on the basis of negative mediastinal exploration at the time of thoracotomy.

Subsequent to the review of this series, we have changed the way specimens are processed in the bronchoscopy suite and now use the "smear technique" described by Ndukwu and colleagues (19). With this method the cytologic specimen is flushed directly onto a slide rather than diluted in a few milliliters of saline and centrifuged in the laboratory. Our more recent experience indicates enhanced cellularity with fewer equivocal findings.

Survey of TBNA Use

To place our experience in perspective, an informal survey was conducted of 31 pulmonologists who practice in northern New England (Maine, Vermont, and New Hampshire). The great majority of these physicians are in private practice, although a few have positions in teaching hospitals with a pulmonary fellowship program. The survey represented the collective experience of 5800 bronchoscopies and 800 TBNAs over a 3-year period.

Approximately 75% of the physicians queried use TBNA. It was estimated that this technique was used in about 15% to 20% of all bronchoscopies performed. Only one third of the physicians who use TBNA had instruction in its application, either in a formal pulmonary training program or a course they attended to learn the technique. CT scans of the chest were obtained two thirds of the time prior to the bronchoscopic examination and one third of the physicians used fluoroscopy on a routine basis while performing TBNA. The technique was used mainly to sample mediastinal lymph nodes (N2 nodes) or areas of submucosal abnormality. It was occasionally used to sample peripheral lesions under fluoroscopic guidance and only rarely to obtain samples from bronchoscopically visible lesions.

Most of the physicians used the technique during the initial bronchoscopic examination to help determine the operability of patients with pulmonary malignancy. Only 20% of these physicians performed TBNA when there was no evidence on the standard chest x-ray of mediastinal adenopathy. There is, however, convincing justification for this practice, since reports (8,9,20) indicate that TBNA may be positive even if conventional radiographs do not show mediastinal disease. Similarly, TBNAs are often positive even if the tracheobronchial anatomy does not suggest extrinsic compression (8,9,20).

A more formal and comprehensive evaluation of TBNA use was reported by Prakash and coworkers, who submitted questionnaires to 1700 American College of Chest Physicians members and received 871 replies (21). Only 11.8% of respondents used it on a routine basis and of all the individual procedures performed during bronchoscopy, TBNA received the most negative replies. This suggests that a great deal of education and training needs to be accomplished if practitioners are to be convinced of the value of this technique.

Bronchoscopic and Roentgenographic Correlations

We reviewed our experience attempting to correlate the likelihood of a positive mediastinal aspirate with radiographic and bronchoscopic findings (20). In 465 cases, 157 had a positive N2 cytology (34%). A widened carina and visible endobronchial disease, particularly right upper lobe tumors, were associated with a positive TBNA. Mediastinal nodes were positive in 105 of 366 patients (29%) when the carina had a normal appearance and in 52 of 99 patients (53%) when it was abnormal. TBNA of N2 nodes was positive in 43 of 73 right upper lobe tumors (59%), but only in 26 of 82 left upper lobe visible malignant lesions (32%). When endoscopic tumors involved more distal areas of the tracheobronchial tree, mediastinal aspirates were positive 25% to 30% of the time.

In our review of chest roentgenograms and CT scans, progressive degrees of adenopathy were associated with an increasing likelihood of TBNA positivity. If hilar or mediastinal adenopathy was absent on standard chest radiographs, mediastinal TBNA was positive in 16 of 77 cases (21%). The absence of adenopathy on thoracic CT precluded a positive aspirate entirely in our series, a finding also noted by Schenk and coworkers (22); however, a more recent report has indicated that even without lymph node enlargement on CT scan, TBNA was positive in 10% of cases (23). In our cases subcarinal nodes enlarged more than 20 mm were strongly correlated with a positive TBNA (14 of 21); however, the location or size of the parenchymal tumor either on chest roentgenogram or CT scan was not indicative of TBNA results.

Complications

Complications of therapeutic significance were not observed by any of the physicians questioned in our survey. All recalled some minor bleeding; however, no significant dyspnea or ventilatory compromise occurred. In addition, there were no reports of pneumothorax, pneumomediastinum, or bacteremia as had been noted in other studies (8,10,11). One patient who inadvertently had TBNA performed while on Coumadin had some mild swelling of the distal membranous portion of the trachea observed during the course of the bronchoscopy. Postoperative observation, however, failed to reveal any significant bleeding or airway compromise.

The experiences of many other authors have also demonstrated the safety of this technique (7,9,12,13). Particular fears of bleeding when puncture of the great vessels occurs have not materialized. This is not surprising if one recalls that a percutaneous lumbar approach for aortography and needle puncture of the left main stem bronchus to obtain left atrial pressures in patients with mitral stenosis were standard and accepted techniques by physicians of a previous generation. Most notable is that the reassuring findings of our survey occurred among physicians practicing in a variety of different settings and whose technique, training, and familiarity with TBNA are widely disparate. Damage to the bronchoscope has proven to be a vexing problem in some circumstances (24) and false positive aspirates have also been reported (18,22), but careful attention to technique should preclude both of these difficulties.

Cost Effectiveness

Economic considerations are now an integral part of medical practice. As a result, the introduction of any new technique should be judged not only by its benefits and complications, but also by its cost effectiveness. By virtue of its ability to sample mediastinal tissue during the course of the bronchoscopic examination, TBNA appears to satisfy this requirement as well.

Table 16.5 shows the results of the first 110 TBNAs performed in Bangor (9). Of these 110 procedures, 70 patients (64%) were ultimately proven to have chest malignancy and 32 patients (29%) had positive aspirates. Noteworthy are the 12 patients (11% of the group) who had the diagnosis of chest malignancy made solely by this technique. In addition, 14 patients (13%) had an additional procedure precluded because of the positive findings from TBNA. In 11 cases mediastinoscopy became unnecessary. One patient (Case 5) with subcarinal widening on chest x-ray 3 years after lobectomy and postoperative radiotherapy, had another thoracotomy canceled when the subcarinal aspirate returned positive for recurrent tumor. Finally, two individuals with visible tumor had positive needle aspirates of paratracheal nodes while their bronchoscopic biopsies showed only necrotic tissue.

The figures for the cost effectiveness of TBNA in these 110 patients are presented in Table 16.6. These data show that when TBNA was performed as part of the initial diagnostic bronchoscopy in all patients suspected to have malignant disease (positivity rate of 29%), the cost incurred was one fifth of what it would have been if more invasive techniques were used. In a subsequent review, the accuracy of TBNA has fallen from 29% (see Table 16.2) in our initial 110 cases to 24% in our total series of 728 attempts. Nonetheless, even with this reduced accuracy the technique remains highly cost effective. Three of us are routinely using it approximately 35% of the time, which undoubtedly represents an aggressive approach. It is entirely possible, as suggested by the results of Dr. Z that in other hands positivity rates may be higher, particularly if TBNA is reserved for use in patients who have more clinically evident mediastinal disease.

Table 16.5. Results of Initial 110 TBNAs*

	No.	%
TBNA	110	100%
Patients with malignancy	70	64%
TBNA positive	32	29%
TBNA positive as sole means of diagnosis	12	11%
Additional procedures precluded by positive TBNA	14	13%
Mediastinoscopy	11	
Thoracotomy	1	
Repeat bronchoscopy	2	

Adapted from Harrow EM, Oldenburg FA, Smith AM. Transbronchial needle aspiration in clinical practice. Thorax 1985;40:756–759.

Table 16.6. Cost Effectiveness of TBNA

Cost of 110 TBNA	Additional procedures
	Mediastinoscopy 11 x $3100 = $34100
	Thoracotomy 1 x $8000 = $8000
TBNA 110 x $75 = $8250	**Bronchoscopy** 2 x $1100 = $2200
$8250	$44300

Case Reports

Perhaps the best way to demonstrate the clinical applicability of TBNA is to illustrate its usefulness in individual cases.

CASE #1: G. D. was a 60-year-old female smoker who presented with the recent onset of cough. A chest roentgenograph showed a right hilar mass, which was new when compared with previous films. The patient underwent fiberoptic bronchoscopy (FOB) with TBNA and on examination, extrinsic compression of the superior segment of the right lower lobe was apparent. Biopsy and brushings of the area were negative; however, TBNA of both subcarinal and right paratracheal regions was positive for poorly differentiated adenocarcinoma. The patient was then referred for radiotherapy (Figure 16.1).

Comment: On the basis of one outpatient procedure, the diagnosis was established and inoperability determined by virtue of the demonstration of positive aspirates from both subcarinal and paratracheal nodes.

CASE #2: W. S. was a 60-year-old male former smoker who was seen for evaluation of dysphagia. A chest radiograph showed a huge

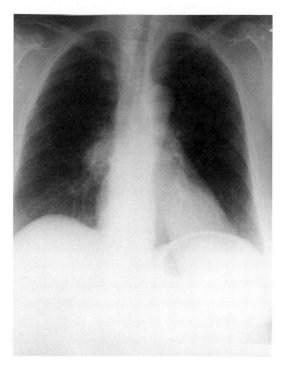

Figure 16.1. Case #1. A 60-year-old with a right hilar mass. Mediastinal TBNA: adenocarcinoma.

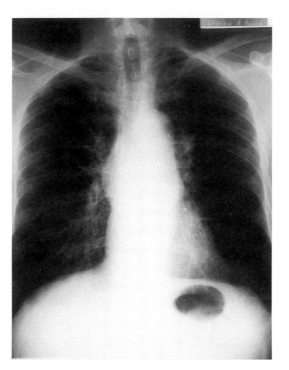

Figure 16.2. Case #2. A 60-year-old with a mediastinal mass. TBNA of mass through the posterior tracheal wall: lymphoma.

middle mediastinal mass. The bronchoscopy showed extrinsic compression of the membranous portion of the trachea. The biopsies were negative; however, needle aspiration into this bulge showed a large number of mononuclear cells consistent with lymphoma. The patient subsequently had an exploratory thoracotomy that confirmed the diagnosis of lymphoma (Figures 16.2 and 16.3).

Comment: This case was evaluated early in our experience with TBNA. As a result, the physicians caring for this patient were not ready to accept a diagnosis of lymphoma on the basis of cytologic material alone. TBNA with a histology needle in this circumstance might have precluded the need for an exploratory thoracotomy.

CASE #3: C. H. was a 77-year-old asymptomatic female smoker who had preoperative screening studies performed prior to a cataract extraction. The chest x-ray showed a normal mediastinum with a right upper lobe coin lesion that was not contiguous with the trachea. A chest radiograph from 3 years previously showed that a small peripheral scar had been present in this location. Because a scar carcinoma was suspected, the patient underwent FOB and transbronchial biopsy of the right upper lobe lesion and TBNA of the ipsilateral paratracheal nodes. The transbronchial biopsy confirmed the presence of adenocarcinoma as did TBNA of the mediastinum on the cytologic aspirate (Figures 16.4 and 16.5).

Comment: In an elderly patient whose chest roentgenograph showed a peripheral lesion and normal mediastinum, one might have considered her to be a candidate for resectional surgery. Because TBNA demonstrated the presence of mediastinal metastases, surgical evaluation was not pursued.

CASE #4: C. B. was a 68-year-old white female who presented with weakness and unsteady begin treatment for carcinoma of the lung in carefully selected patients where chest malignancy is strongly suspected on clinical grounds alone, it is always desirable to obtain a tissue diagnosis. If TBNA had been performed at the time of the initial bronchoscopy, a tissue diagnosis would have been established at the outset and chemotherapeutic treatment for oat cell carcinoma could have been initiated at an earlier date.

CASE #5: T. F. was a 46-year-old white male who had a right upper lobectomy 3 years previously for adenocarcinoma. Because of positive mediastinal nodes, the patient received a postoperative course of radiotherapy. Due to increasing cough, the patient returned and a follow-up chest radiograph showed subcarinal adenopathy. The patient's surgeon scheduled an exploratory right thoracotomy; however, bronchoscopy with TBNA of the

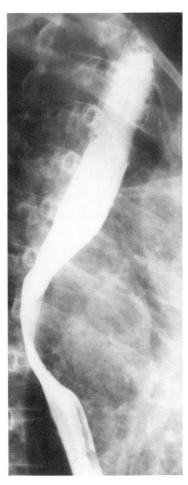

Figure 16.3. Case #2. Barium swallow demonstrating anterior tracheal and posterior esophegeal displacement.

gait. A CT scan of her brain was consistent with multiple cerebral metastases. The chest x-ray demonstrated left paratracheal adenopathy, but the bronchoscopy was negative. The patient was treated with cranial irradiation without a tissue diagnosis. A follow-up chest x-ray several months later showed increasing adenopathy in the area of the aortopulmonary window. This time a repeat bronchoscopy showed a paralyzed left vocal cord and TBNA of the aortopulmonary window demonstrated oat cell carcinoma (Figure 16.6).

Comment: In this individual a tissue diagnosis was not available at the time of initial treatment. Although it is not unreasonable to

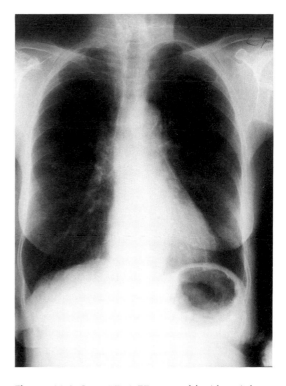

Figure 16.4. Case #3. A 77-year-old with a right upper lobe lesion. Right paratracheal TBNA: adenocarcinoma.

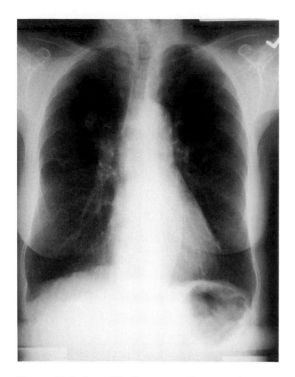

Figure 16.5. Case #3. Chest x-ray 3 years prior to evaluation.

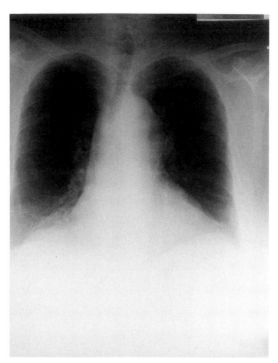

Figure 16.6. Case #4. A 68-year-old with aortopulmonary adenopathy and cerebral metastases. Left paratracheal TBNA: small cell carcinoma.

subcarinal nodes demonstrated the presence of recurrent tumor (Figure 16.7).

Comment: In view of the technical difficulties anticipated by another mediastinoscopy following radiotherapy and the presence of subcarinal adenopathy, a thoracotomy was planned, but precluded by the positive findings on TBNA.

CASE #6: H. O. was a 48-year-old heavy smoker who was seen for malaise and cough. A chest roentgenograph showed a right paratracheal shadow, which was new compared with previous films. FOB and TBNA into the right paratracheal area were negative. A CT scan performed following the bronchoscopic examination showed that the lesion was a vascular shadow (Figure 16.8).

Comment: Although investigation of this right paratracheal shadow proved to be vascular, no complications occurred as a result of the procedure. This experience is consistent

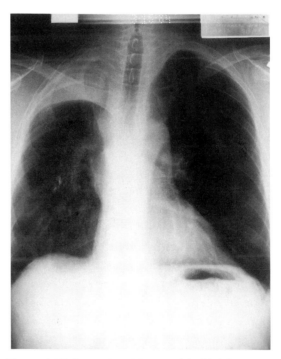

Figure 16.7. Case #5. A 46-year-old with lobectomy 3 years previously for adenocarcinoma. Subcarinal TBNA: recurrent malignancy.

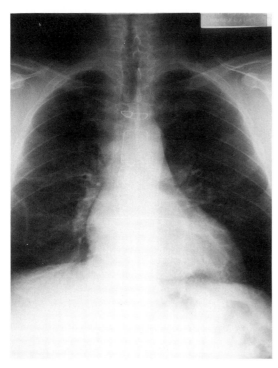

Figure 16.8. Case #6. A 48-year-old with right paratracheal vascular shadow. Right paratracheal TBNA: negative.

with that of many other observers indicating that even when vascular structures are penetrated, there have been no reports of significant bleeding. Superior vena caval obstruction has also proven not to be a contraindication to TBNA.

CASE #7: E. A. was a vigorous 62-year-old woman who presented with a large left upper lobe lesion. CT scan showed a single 15-mm node in the aortopulmonary window. Bronchoscopy with transbronchial biopsy of the parenchymal lesion demonstrated adenocarcinoma and TBNA of the left paratracheal area was also positive. Because of the patient's good physical condition and eagerness to undergo operative treatment, she was further evaluated for surgery. A CT scan of the brain, however, showed two metastatic lesions and the patient was referred for radiotherapy.

Comment: Although the TBNA was positive, the patient was still evaluated for surgery

because of her good physical condition and the presence of only one borderline-sized mediastinal node noted on her chest CT scan. TBNA cannot distinguish between intra- and extracapsular nodal involvement. This case illustrates that TBNA can and should be used only as a guide in the decision-making process regarding surgery, rather than as a definitive determinant of the patient's treatment plan.

Significance of a Positive TBNA

Currently, the diagnostic approach and role of surgery in patients with lung cancer who are suspected of having mediastinal involvement is undergoing reevaluation. The recent modifications of the TNM classification system for lung cancer (25) and the report by the Lung Cancer Study Group (15) are a reflection of this process and emphasize the need for careful mediastinal mapping of all patients. Several observers (26,27) have published data suggesting that CT scans add little to the standard chest radiograph in the staging of lung cancer patients and that individuals with a normal chest x-ray need not have either a thoracic CT scan or mediastinoscopy prior to exploratory thoracotomy. In addition, McLoud and colleagues (28) have suggested that CT scanning may be particularly misleading in underestimating the size of subcarinal nodes. The evaluation of this area is particularly important because these nodes are often unapproachable by mediastinoscopy and if involved with tumor portend a reduced likelihood of patient survival (14). Several authors (16,29,30) feel that patients without conventional radiographic evidence of mediastinal disease, but who are found to have malignant N2 nodes at thoracotomy, may have a better survival than those whose nodes were evident during preoperative evaluation and confirmed positive by mediastinoscopy. They suggest, therefore, that this group need not have a staging procedure prior to thoracotomy. In view of this uncertainty, TBNA, which can be easily performed at the time of initial diagnostic bronchoscopy, has the potential for obtaining important diagnostic and prognostic information.

Although the degree to which mediastinal involvement will predict outcome is not altogether clear, it has been established that a normal chest x-ray or CT scan by no means excludes malignant mediastinal adenopathy (31). In our previous experience, TBNAs were positive 46% of the time when the chest x-ray did not indicate mediastinal disease and 38% of the time when the tracheal anatomy at the time of bronchoscopy was felt to be normal (9). In addition, in 129 patients with a positive TBNA of the mediastinum, small cell carcinoma was present in 41 patients (32%) and was the most common cell type (11 of 31) when TBNA alone established the diagnosis of chest malignancy. In these cases, this information prevented further needless diagnostic evidence. Careful adherence to proper technique in which TBNA of N2 sites precedes the formal bronchoscopic examination is essential to prevent misinterpretation of positive results, particularly if only a few malignant cells are seen. Finally, we are reluctant to preclude surgery on the basis of a positive aspirate alone in patients whose tumors on chest x-ray are adjacent to the trachea because we cannot be sure that the aspirate is truly sampling mediastinal nodes unless lymphocytes are also seen in the aspirate.

What then is the appropriate role for TBNA and what is the significance of a positive aspirate? It is now appreciated that in patients with mediastinal disease four factors indicate a poor prognosis: 1) positive subcarinal nodes, 2) contralateral involvement, 3) multiple levels of nodal involvement, and 4) extracapsular extension of tumor (14–16,32). TBNA provides valuable diagnostic data in three of these four categories and can do so accurately and safely and with minimal additional expense. Whether a positive aspirate in non–small-cell carcinoma in patients without radiographic evidence of N2 involvement is indicative of an improved survival compared with those having obvious roentgenographic mediastinal disease is currently uncertain.

A positive aspirate, therefore, may be interpreted in several ways. In cases of small cell carcinoma, it establishes the diagnosis, precludes surgery and indicates the therapeutic course. Surgery would also appear to be obviated in patients with non–small-cell needle aspirates whose chest x-rays show enlarged mediastinal nodes. In otherwise healthy individuals with a non–small-cell aspirate and roentgenographically normal mediastinum, surgery remains an option. Similarly, in patients with a tumor contiguous with the trachea, mediastinal exploration may still be necessary because one cannot be certain that the mediastinal lymphatics have been sampled. Aspirates, however, that contain lymphocytes and a paucity of epithelial cells along with malignant cytology can reasonably be assumed to be representative of paratracheal nodes. Also, when tumors are located posteriorly even though they may appear adjacent to the trachea on the posteroanterior radiograph, they will not be within reach of the exploring needle and cannot cause a false positive result. In many patients, significant coexistent pulmonary, cardiac, or vascular disease is such that these problems along with the demonstration of frankly malignant cells in the mediastinal lymph nodes are often sufficient to preclude them from further surgery. In all cases, however, we believe that the finding of a positive TBNA should be considered an important contribution to the decision-making process, rather than an absolute arbiter of an individual's fate.

ACKNOWLEDGMENT: The authors wish to acknowledge with thanks Donna Leonard for her assistance in manuscript preparation.

REFERENCES

1. Smoking and Health Report of the Advisory Committee to the Surgeon General. Washington, DC: US Department of Health, Education and Welfare, Publication No. 1103, 1964.
2. Author unknown. "Sold American!"—The first fifty years. Durham: American Tobacco Company, 1954.
3. Graham EA, Singer JJ. Successful removal of an entire lung for carcinoma of the bronchus. JAMA 1933;101:1371.
4. Carlens E. Mediastinoscopy: a method for inspection and tissue biopsy in the superior mediastinum. Dis Chest 1959;36:343.
5. Schieppati E. Mediastinal lymph node puncture through the tracheal carina. Surg Gynecol Obstet 1958;110:243–246.
6. Wang KP, Haponik ER, Gupta PK, Erozan YS. Flexible transbronchial needle aspiration. Ann Otol Rhinol Laryngol 1984;93:233–236.
7. Wang KP, Terry PB. Transbronchial needle aspiration in the diagnosis and staging of bronchogenic carcinoma. Am Rev Respir Dis 1983;127:344–347.
8. Wang KP, Brower R, Haponik EK, Siegelman S. Flexible transbronchial needle aspiration for staging of bronchogenic carcinoma. Chest 1983;84:571–576.
9. Harrow EM, Oldenburg FA, Smith AM. Transbronchial needle aspiration in clinical practice. Thorax 1985;40:756–759.
10. Wang KP, Marsh BR, Summer WR, Terry PB, Erozan YS, Baker RR. Transbronchial needle aspiration for diagnosis of lung cancer. Chest 1981;80:48–50.
11. Watts WJ, Green RA. Bacteremia following transbronchial fine needle aspiration. Chest 1984;85:295.
12. Shure D, Fedullo P. The role of transcarinal needle aspiration in the staging of bronchogenic carcinoma. Chest 1984;86:693–696.
13. Shure D, Fedullo P. Transbronchial needle aspiration in the diagnosis of submucosal and peribronchial bronchogenic carcinoma. Chest 1985;88:49–51.
14. Naruke T, Suemasu K, Ischikawa S. Lymph node mapping and curability at various levels of metastasis in resected lung cancer. J Thorac Cardiovasc Surg 1978;76:832.
15. Lung Cancer Study Group. Should subcarinal lymph nodes be routinely examined in patients with non-small cell lung cancer? Thorac Cardiovasc Surg 1988;95:883–887.
16. Martini N, Flehinger BJ, Zama MB, Beattie EJ. Results of resection in non-oat cell carcinoma of the lung with mediastinal lymph node metastases. Ann Surg 1983;198:386–397.
17. Harrow EM, Oldenburg FA, Smith AM, Lingenfelter MS. Transbronchial needle aspiration in clinical practice—a five year experience. Chest 1989;96:1268–1272.
18. Cropp AJ, DiMarco AF, Lankerani M. False positive transbronchial needle aspiration in bronchogenic carcinoma. Chest 1984;85:696–697.
19. Ndukwu I, Wang KP, David D, Welk P, Sutula M. Direct smear for cytological evaluation of transbronchial needle aspiration specimens. Chest 1991;100(suppl):8859. Abstract.
20. Harrow EM, Oldenburg FA, Lingenfelter MS. Bronchoscopic and roentgenographic correlates of a positive transbronchial needle aspiration in the staging of lung cancer. Chest 1991;100:1592–1596.
21. Prakash UBS, Offord KP, Stubbs SE. Bronchoscopy in North America: the ACCP survey. Chest 1991;100:1668–1675.
22. Schenk DA, Bower JH, Bryan CL, et al. Transbronchial needle aspiration staging of bronchogenic carcinoma. Am Rev Respir Dis 1986;134:146–148.
23. Utz JP, Patel AM, Edell ES. The role of transcarinal needle aspiration in the staging of bronchogenic carcinoma. Chest 1993;104:1012–1016.
24. Mehta AC, Curtis PS, Scolzitti ML, Meeker DP. The high price of bronchoscopy—maintenance and repair of the flexible fiberoptic bronchoscope. Chest 1990;98:448–454.
25. Mountain CF. A new international staging system for lung cancer. Chest 1986;89:225S–233S.
26. McKenna RJ, Libshitz HI, Mountain CE, McMurtrey MJ. Roentgenographic evaluation of mediastinal nodes for preoperative assessment in lung cancer. Chest 1985;88:206–210.
27. Baker CL, Shields TW, Lockhart CG, Vogelzang R, LoCicero J. Selective preoperative evaluation for possible N2 disease in carcinoma of the lung. J Thorac Cardiovasc Surg 1987;93:337–343.

28. McLoud TC, Woldenburg R, Mathiesen DJ, et al. CT in the staging of bronchogenic carcinoma: analysis by correlative lymph node mapping and sampling. Radiology 1987;165:21–22. Abstract.

29. Martini N, Kris MG, Gralla RJ, et al. The effects of preoperative chemotherapy on the resectability of non-small cell lung carcinoma with mediastinal lymph node metastases (N2M0). Ann Thorac Surg 1988; 45:370–379.

30. Pearson FG, Delarue NC, Ilves MD, Todd TRJ, Cooper JD. Significance of positive superior mediastinal nodes identified at mediastinoscopy in patients with resectable cancer of the lung. J Thorac Cardiovasc Surg 1982;83:1–11.

31. Gross BH, Glazer GM, Orringer MB, et al. Bronchogenic carcinoma metastatic to normal-sized lymph nodes: frequency and significance. Radiology 1988;166:71–74.

32. Rotto GB, Mereu C, Motta G. The prognostic significance of preoperative assessment of mediastinal lymph nodes in patients with lung cancer. Chest 1988;93:807–813.

17 | Evaluation of Benign Mediastinal Cysts—Transbronchial and Transesophageal Approach

Akira Kawashima, Janet E. Kuhlman, Elliot K. Fishman, and Ko-Pen Wang

Mediastinal cysts of foregut origin represent a small but important diagnostic group, totaling up to 9% of all primary mediastinal tumors in surgical series (1,2). The challenge for the pulmonary specialist is to diagnose and manage these benign mediastinal lesions without surgical intervention. Mediastinal cysts may present as incidental findings on chest films or routine esophagrams (3). When the patient is symptomatic or the lesion has changed in size, the possibility of mediastinal malignancy requires a more definitive evaluation of the lesion. In the past, this has necessitated either invasive mediastinoscopy or thoracotomy for definitive diagnosis.

A new, less invasive approach to the diagnosis of benign mediastinal lesions is now possible through the combined use of computed tomography (CT) and transtracheal or transesophageal needle aspiration. As a technique, transbronchial needle aspiration in the mediastinum was first used for staging of lung cancer out of a need to reach subcarinal and retrotracheal lymph node groups not accessible by mediastinoscopy (4–6). The technique is now being used successfully to evaluate mediastinal masses such as tumors, abscesses, and benign mediastinal cysts (7,8). Congenital mediastinal cysts are excellent candidates for this type of approach because they are typically found in the paratracheal, subcarinal, and paraesophageal locations, easily accessible by needle aspiration. CT plays an important role in this approach by providing a presumptive diagnosis of benign mediastinal lesion based on CT criteria, by providing a helpful road map for the bronchoscopist, and by providing a means of monitoring the lesion following aspiration.

In this chapter, we discuss the congenital origins and CT characteristics of benign mediastinal cysts. CT scanning techniques and CT criteria for presumptive diagnosis of benign mediastinal cysts are reviewed. A brief description of the transbronchial and transesophageal needle aspiration approach with respect to benign mediastinal cysts is included.

Origins and Types of Benign Mediastinal Cysts

Mediastinal cysts result from embryologic aberrations and anomalous budding of the primitive foregut and early tracheobronchial tree (9). The spectrum of bronchopulmonary malformations includes bronchogenic cysts, esophageal duplications, and neurenteric cysts. Each type of foregut cyst has typical histologic features and characteristic anatomic locations within the chest. Bronchogenic cysts are usually located in the subcarinal or paratracheal area. Esophageal duplication cysts are usually located along the esophagus in the lower posterior mediastinum. Neurenteric cysts are associated with spinal anomalies. Distinction between the various types of congenital cysts is sometimes more difficult, however, when they share overlapping anatomic locations and similar histologic features (10). In addition, when inflammation and hemorrhage occur in the foregut cyst, the type-specific lining may be replaced by nonspecific granulation tissue. Such nonspecific cysts account for 17% to 20% of all foregut cysts (2,11).

Bronchogenic Cysts

Bronchogenic cysts are the most common intrathoracic foregut cysts, accounting for 54% to 63% of cases in surgical series (2,3,11). Early in embryogenesis the lung begins as a ventral diverticulum that arises from the primitive foregut. This diverticulum then undergoes a series of generations of buddings that results in the tracheobronchial tree and alveoli. When the budding process goes awry, aberrant buds give rise to cystic structures that may or may not communicate with the bronchial tree. These cystic structures become bronchogenic cysts, which are typically lined by ciliated columnar epithelium and pseudo-stratified squamous epithelium (3). Histo-logically, bronchogenic cysts may also contain bronchial glands or bronchial cartilage (3,10,11).

Bronchogenic cysts may be either parenchymal or mediastinal in location. Common locations include paratracheal, carinal, hilar, and paraesophageal sites. Bronchogenic cysts occasionally communicate with the bronchial lumen and rarely occur in an endobronchial location (10,11).

Esophageal Duplication Cysts

Esophageal duplication cysts are uncommon and constitute 0.5% to 2.5% of all esophageal masses (12). Esophageal duplication cysts make up 10% to 15% of all alimentary tract duplications, which may occur at any level of the gastrointestinal tract from mouth to anus (12,13). Most esophageal duplication cysts are discovered in children, but up to 25% to 30% are not found until adulthood (12).

The primitive foregut begins to elongate at about the fourth week of embryologic development. At this stage, proliferation of lining cells produces a nearly solid tube. By the sixth week, however, small holes or vacuoles begin to arise in the tube and eventually coalesce to form the lumen of the esophagus. Duplication cysts arise when isolated vacuoles fail to coalesce with the rest of the lumen (1,3,12,13).

Histologically, esophageal duplication cysts contain a double layer of smooth muscle without cartilage (10). They can also contain gastric mucosa that leads to peptic ulceration or hemorrhage (3,10). Technetium 99m sodium pertechnetate scans show uptake of tracer in some duplications, indicating the presence of ectopic gastric mucosa (14). In children, 50% of thoracic duplication cysts are reported to contain ectopic gastric mucosa (12).

Esophageal duplication cysts may be found adjacent to the esophagus throughout its course, with 60% located around the lower third of the esophagus. The remainder are found near the upper or middle thirds of the esophagus in equal numbers (12). Although a paraesophageal location is common for duplication cysts, they may also be intramural in location.

Neurenteric Cysts

Neurenteric cysts are part of the split notochord syndrome (3). At the third week of embryogenesis the notochord appears. If a split in the notochord occurs, a portion of the yolk sac and primitive foregut may herniate through the gap and attach itself to dorsal ectoderm or primitive skin tissue. A number of congenital abnormalities may result: dorsal enterocutaneous fistula, a dorsal sinus, or neurenteric cyst.

Neurenteric cysts have a smooth muscle wall similar to the gastrointestinal tract, but a variable epithelial lining. Associated spinal defects such as hemivertebrae, butterfly vertebrae, and scoliosis are common, usually with the position of the cyst below the vertebral abnormality. This is because the foregut elongates faster than the spinal column during embryogenesis (3,15). A connection may or may not exist between the neurenteric cyst and the thoracic spine meninges, but communication with the actual subarachnoid space is unusual.

Clinical Presentation

Mediastinal cysts can present in a variety of ways. Although they are usually asymptomatic, mediastinal cysts may produce symptoms by compressing adjacent structures, such as the esophagus with resultant dysphagia, or the tracheobronchial tree leading to dyspnea or persistent cough. Bleeding or infection may cause the cyst to enlarge, exacerbating symptoms (12).

Computed Tomography Evaluation of Benign Mediastinal Cysts

Technique

Mediastinal masses are routinely evaluated with CT using 8-mm thick sections taken at one-cm intervals from lung apex to diaphragm. Typical scanning parameters on the Somatom Plus model scanner (Siemens Medical Systems, Iselin, NJ) are 250 mA, 125 kVp, and one-second scan acquisition times; and on the DR3 or DRH model scanners, 230 mA, 125 kVp, and 3-second scans, or 310 mA, 125 kVp, and 4-second scans, respectively. All images are viewed at mediastinal window settings (window width 420; window center 36) and at lung and bone window settings when appropriate. In most cases, intravenously administered contrast is required to confirm the lesions to be nonvascular in nature. Dynamic images may be obtained after a bolus injection of intravenous contrast material. Our current technique is to inject approximately 150 mL of Hypaque-60 (Winthrop Pharmaceuticals, New York, NY) at a rate of

1.0 to 1.5 mL per second with an automated power injector. Use of a barium paste (Esopho-CAT, E-Z-EM, Westbury, NY) is particularly useful in coating the lumen of the esophagus and delineating its position with respect to a mediastinal mass.

Appearances of Benign Mediastinal Cysts

The majority of benign mediastinal cysts have characteristic, identifiable features on CT, which allow their diagnosis with a high degree of certainty. The classic CT appearance of a benign mediastinal cyst is that of a well-defined, cystic mass, with homogenous low CT attenuation in the range of water density (0 to 20 Hounsfield units, HU) (Figures 17.1 through 17.3). The cystic mass shows a thin or imperceptible wall and demonstrates no enhancement with intravenous contrast injection. Common locations of mediastinal cysts identified by CT include the subcarinal, paratracheal, and paraesophageal regions.

A number of other disease processes may produce mediastinal masses with low CT attenuation. They include metastases from testicular tumors, cystic metastases from ovarian or gastric cancer, abscesses, resolving hematomas, treated or untreated lymphoma, hydatid cysts, lymphoceles, seromas, and some neurogenic tumors (16,17). The CT attenuation of these masses is rarely as low as water density, and seldom do these mediastinal masses fulfill the other CT criteria for diagnosing a benign mediastinal cyst (7,8,18).

Although most benign mediastinal cysts demonstrate CT attenuation values in the range of 0 to 20 HU, occasionally a mediastinal cyst will be found with a higher CT density than water. This is most often due to the presence of milk of calcium, proteinaceous fluid, mucus, or blood debris within the cyst (19–21). Thus, high-attenuation cysts may offer a diagnostic dilemma for the radiologist and clinician. One can often suspect the correct diagnosis of benign mediastinal cyst, however, even in these cases because of the characteristic shape and location of the lesion, its homogenous appearance, and the complete absence of contrast enhancement (22).

In symptomatic patients or in problem cases, CT evaluation of benign mediastinal lesions contributes valuable information regarding the cystic nature and size of the lesion and its anatomic location relative to other mediastinal organs. This information is vital for planning more definitive procedures such as fiberoptic bronchoscopy or endoscopy with transbronchial or transesophageal needle aspiration (7,8).

Preliminary reports suggest a promising role for magnetic resonance imaging (MRI) in the evaluation of the mediastinal cysts. MRI

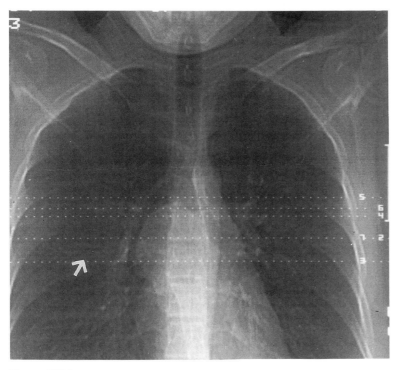

Figure 17.1A

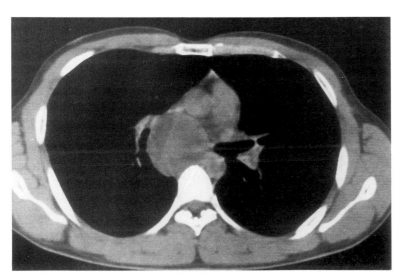

Figure 17.1B

Figure 17.1. Typical CT features of benign mediastinal cyst. A 26-year-old man with subcarinal mass. *A,* Topogram of CT shows a subcarinal mass (*arrow*). *B,* CT examination demonstrates features typical for benign mediastinal cyst. A 6 × 6 cm fluid-filled cyst (*arrow*) with homogenous CT attenuation measuring 10 to 20 HU is identified. CT shows that the mediastinal cyst is large enough that it splays the carina and displaces the bronchus intermedius laterally. *C,* A CT scan obtained after the mediastinal cyst was aspirated by transbronchial needle approach. Clear serous fluid (70 mL) was obtained. CT now shows the cyst to be smaller (*arrow*). *D,* Six months later, reevaluation with CT shows no reaccumulation of cyst fluid. A small soft tissue remnant remains (*arrow*).

Figures 17.1C and D were reproduced by permission from Kuhlman JK, Fishman EK, Wang KP, Zerhouni EA, Siegelman SS. Mediastinal cysts: diagnosis by CT and needle aspiration. AJR Am J Roentgenol 1988;150:75–78.

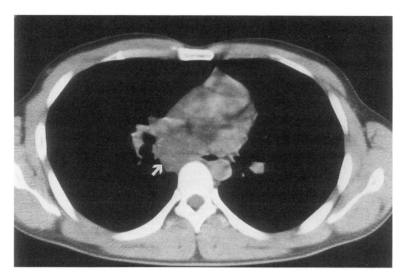

Figure 17.1C

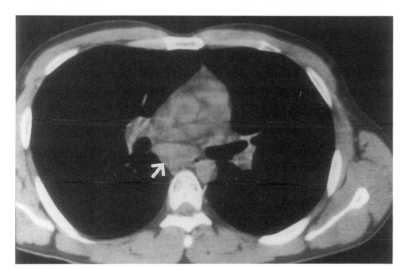

Figure 17.1D

appearances of the mediastinal cysts include the presence of a well-defined, rounded mass in the middle and posterior mediastinum (23,24). Depending on the protein content of the cyst fluid, T1 signal intensity is variable, whereas signal intensity on T2 sequences is quite high, characteristic of fluid. MRI may also demonstrate the presence of hemorrhage in some mediastinal cysts. One advantage of MRI is the ability to outline in multiple imaging planes the anatomic relationships of the mass with its surrounding mediastinal structures.

Transbronchial and Transesophageal Needle Aspiration

On the basis of CT findings, a presumptive diagnosis of a benign mediastinal cyst can often be made. In symptomatic or problem cases, the presumptive CT diagnosis can be confirmed without resorting to thoracotomy or invasive surgery by using the less invasive techniques of transbronchial or transesophageal needle aspiration. The specifics of the technique have been described previously in the literature (4,6–8) and in this textbook.

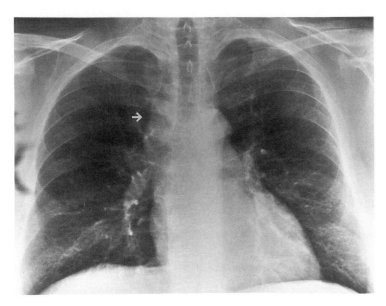

Figure 17.2A

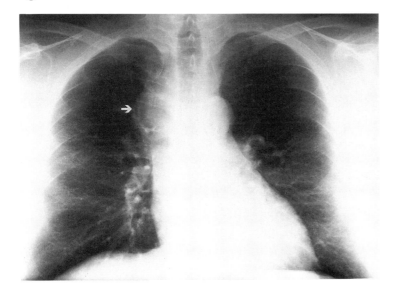

Figure 17.2B

Figure 17.2. An enlarging right paratracheal mass in an otherwise asymptomatic 51-year-old man. Serial chest films in 1982 (*A*) and 1985 (*B*) show increasing size of the lesion (*arrows*). *C*, CT scan demonstrates features suggestive of benign mediastinal cyst. Oval, right paratracheal lesion (*arrow*) with homogenous CT attenuation and a density slightly less than that of soft tissue. *D*, Transtracheal needle aspiration was used to confirm the benign cystic nature of the lesion. Following the procedure an air-fluid appears in the cyst (*arrow*).

Figures 17.2A, B, and D were reproduced by permission from Kuhlman JK, Fishman EK, Wang KP, Zerhouni EA, Siegelman SS. Mediastinal cysts: diagnosis by CT and needle aspiration. AJR Am J Roentgenol 1988;150:75–78.

Only a general outline of the approach will be reviewed here.

Biopsy System

The biopsy system consists of a semitransparent polyethylene sheath 120 cm long with an attached 18-, 21-, or 22-gauge needle, 12 mm in length (Mill-Rose Company, Mentor, OH) (Figure 17.4). The sheath system also includes a retractable inner steel stylet with a blunt tip that provides the necessary rigidity to allow puncture of the bronchial or esophageal wall.

A Luer-lok side port at the proximal end of the sheath allows aspiration of cyst contents without complete removal of the stylet. The sheath system is used in conjunction with a specially designed bronchoscope (Fujinon BRO-Y2S) (6).

Biopsy Procedure

The procedure is performed in the operating room or endoscopy suite without the need for general anesthesia; intramuscular meperidine and atropine premedication, along with sequential topical anesthesia of the nasal cavity, nasopharynx, and oropharynx with 2% Xylocaine are used instead (6).

Based on the CT findings, the flexible bronchoscope or esophageal endoscope is introduced to the appropriate level. The biopsy sheath system is passed through the scope until the needle projects just beyond the end of the scope. The stylet is retracted slightly and the needle aimed at the target site. The stylet is then further retracted and the cyst is aspirated using a 30- or 50-mL syringe containing 3 mL normal saline or Hank's balanced solution attached to the proximal Luer-lok port. Cytopathology and cultures of the aspirated material are obtained (6).

A follow-up CT examination of the mediastinal lesion is used to determine the success of the aspiration procedure and to exclude complications such as bleeding, abscess formation, or pneumomediastinum.

Advantages of the Transtracheal and Transesophageal Approach

Computed tomography followed by transtracheal or transesophageal needle aspiration of benign mediastinal cysts is an alternative to invasive mediastinoscopy or thoracotomy (7,8). It is less expensive, less invasive, and does not require hospitalization or the higher risk of general anesthesia. The transtracheal or transesophageal approach is preferred over a percutaneous thoracic approach because the majority of mediastinal cysts are located intimately close to the tracheobronchial tree or esophagus. The distance that the needle must

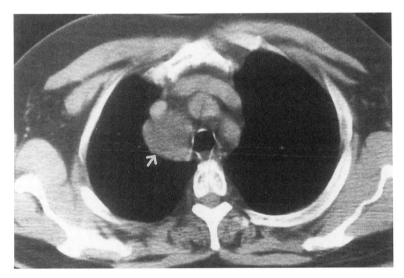

Figure 17.2C

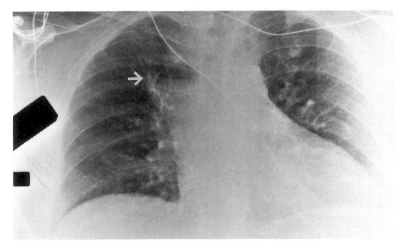

Figure 17.2D

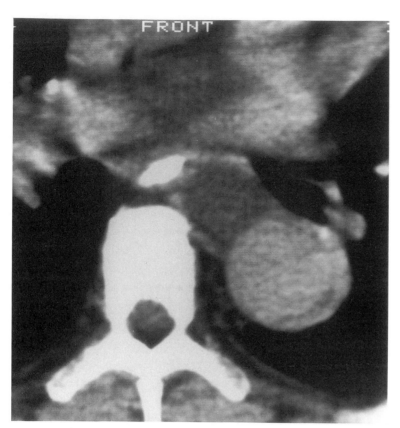

Figure 17.3A

Figure 17.3. A 74-year-old woman with 4-month history of mild dysphagia, anorexia, and chest fullness. *A,* CT identifies a cystic tubular structure with CT attenuation equal to water compatible with an esophageal duplication (a, aorta; e, esophagus). *B,* An off-axis reconstructed CT image delineates the length of the esophageal duplication.

Reproduced by permission from Kuhlman JE, Fishman EK, Wang KP, Siegelman SS. Esophageal duplication cyst: CT and trans-esophageal needle aspiration. AJR Am J Roentgenol 1985;145: 531–532.

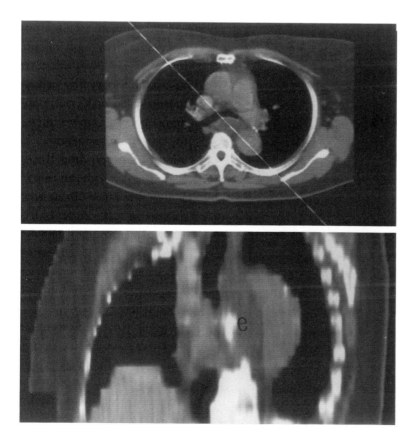

Figure 17.3B

traverse is smaller, the risk of pneumothorax less, and the nearby vascular structures are more easily avoided.

Combined Approach to Mediastinal Cysts

Computed tomography plays a critical role in this nonsurgical approach to mediastinal cysts (7,8). CT confirms the presence of a mediastinal mass and based on CT criteria provides a presumptive diagnosis of benign mediastinal cyst. In the asymptomatic individual or elderly patient, a benign mediastinal cyst can be followed conservatively with serial CT examinations to ensure stability of the size and character of the lesion over time. A more definitive answer is required when the patient is symptomatic, if signs and symptoms suggest possible malignancy, or the lesion changes in size or shape over time. CT findings of a benign mediastinal cyst can still be confirmed without the need for surgery by using transbronchial or transesophageal needle aspiration. The lack of malignant cells or infection in the aspirated fluid substantiates the benign nature of the lesion.

Prior to needle aspiration, CT documents the size of the cyst, its anatomic location, and relationships to other vital mediastinal structures, and confirms the nonvascular nature of the lesion. By identifying these important features, the radiologist assists the endoscopist in planning the approach to the target. Follow-up management of patients with mediastinal cysts is also aided by CT evaluation. CT documents decrease in size of the cyst following needle aspiration, evaluates for complications, and monitors the cyst for reaccumulation of fluid on serial follow-up examinations.

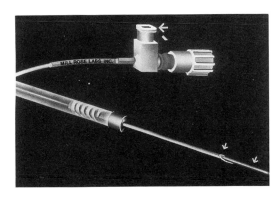

Figure 17.4. The transbronchial or transesophageal needle aspiration system. A beveled needle (*small arrow*) is attached to a semitransparent sheath. An inner steel stylet (*large arrow*) traverses the sheath providing rigidity during aspiration procedure. Proximal side port (*curved arrow*) used for syringe.

Reproduced by permission from Kuhlman JK, Fishman EK, Wang KP, Zerhouni EA, Siegelman SS. Mediastinal cysts: diagnosis by CT and needle aspiration. AJR Am J Roentgenol 1988;150:75–78.

REFERENCES

1. Morrison IM. Tumors and cysts of the mediastinum. Thorax 1958;13:294–307.
2. Wychulis AR, Payne WS, Clagett OT, Woolner LB. Surgical treatment of mediastinal tumors: a 40 year experience. J Thoracic Cardiovasc Surg 1971;62:379–392.
3. Kirwan WO, Walbaum PR, McCormick RJM. Cystic intrathoracic derivatives of the foregut and their complications. Thorax 1973;28:424–428.
4. Wang KP, Terry P, Marsh B. Bronchoscopic needle aspiration biopsy of paratracheal tumors. Am Rev Respir Dis 1978;118:17–21.
5. Lemer J, Malberger E, Konig-Nativ R. Transbronchial fine needle aspiration. Thorax 1982;37:270–274.
6. Scatarige JC, Wang KP, Siegelman SS. Transbronchial needle aspiration biopsy of the mediastinum. In: Siegelman SS, ed. Contemporary issues in computed tomography, vol. 4. Computed tomography of the chest. New York: Churchill Livingstone, 1984:59–79.
7. Kuhlman JE, Fishman EK, Wang KP, Siegelman SS. Esophageal duplication cyst: CT and transesophageal needle aspiration. AJR Am J Roentgenol 1985;145:531–532.
8. Kuhlman JK, Fishman EK, Wang KP, Zerhouni EA, Siegelman SS. Mediastinal cysts: diagnosis by CT and needle aspiration. AJR Am J Roentgenol 1988;150:75–78.
9. Heithoff KB, Sane SM, Williams HJ, et al.

Bronchopulmonary foregut malformations: a unifying etiological concept. AJR Am J Roentgenol 1976;126:46–55.

10. Salyer DC, Salyer WR, Eggleston JC. Benign developmental cysts of the mediastinum. Arch Pathol Lab Med 1977;101:136–139.

11. Sirivella S, Ford WB, Zikria EA, Miller WH, Samadani SR, Sullivan ME. Foregut cysts of the mediastinum: results in 20 consecutive surgically treated cases. J Thorac Cardiovasc Surg 1985;90:776–782.

12. Whitaker JA, Deffenbaugh LD, Cooke AR. Esophageal duplication cyst. Am J Gastroenterol 1980;73:329–332.

13. Hocking M, Young DG. Duplications of the alimentary tract. Br J Surg 1981;68:92–96.

14. Ferguson CC, Young LN, Sutherland JB, Macpherson RI. Intrathoracic gastric cyst: preoperative diagnosis by technetium pertechnetate scan. J Pediatr Surg 1973;8:827–828.

15. Reed JC, Sobonya RE. Morphologic analysis of foregut cysts in the thorax. AJR Am J Roentgenol 1974;120:851–860.

16. Yousem DM, Scatarige JC, Fishman EK, Siegelman SS. Low-attenuation thoracic metastases in testicular malignancy. AJR Am J Roentgenol 1986;146:291–293.

17. Glazer HS, Siegel MJ, Sagel SS. Low-attenuation mediastinal masses on CT. AJR Am J Roentgenol 1989;152:1173–1177.

18. Weiss LM, Fagelman D, Warhit JM. CT demonstration of an esophageal duplication cyst. J Comput Assist Tomogr 1983;7:716–718.

19. Nakata H, Nakayama C, Kimoto T, et al. Computed tomography of mediastinal bronchogenic cysts. J Comput Assist Tomogr 1982;6:733–738.

20. Medelson DS, Rose JS, Efremidis SC, Kirschmner PA, Cohen BA. Bronchogenic cysts with high CT numbers. AJR Am J Roentgenol 1983;140:463–465.

21. Nakata H, Sato Y, Nakayama T, Yoshimatsu H, Kobayashi T. Bronchogenic cyst with high CT number: analysis of contents. J Comput Assist Tomogr 1986;10:360–362.

22. Salonen O. CT characteristics of expansions in the middle and posterior mediastinum. Comput Radiol 1987;11:95–100.

23. Lupetin AR, Dash N. MRI appearance of esophageal duplication cyst. Gastrointest Radiol 1987;12:7–9.

24. Rhee RS, Ray CG, Kravetz MH, et al. Cervical esophageal duplication cyst: MR imaging. J Comput Assist Tomogr 1988;12:693–695.

Part 3

Therapeutic Bronchoscopy

18 | Flexible Bronchoscopy and the Use of Lasers

Atul C. Mehta, Francis Y. W. Lee, and Glen E. DeBoer

The concept of laser originated in 1917 when Albert Einstein proposed his theory on radiant energy (1). He postulated that "particles of light with energy of a particular frequency could stimulate atomic electrons to emit radiant energy as a light of the same frequency." The groundwork for the true theory of lasers was, however, not laid until 1958 by Charles Townes and Arthur Schawlow (2). The first working laser was developed by Theodor Maiman in 1961 using a ruby crystal as a lasing medium (3). In the same year, Javan and colleagues produced the first helium-neon (He-Ne) laser (4). Year 1964 saw the introduction of three new lasers. Geusic and coworkers from Germany succeeded in constructing the neodymium:yttrium-aluminum-garnet (Nd:YAG) laser (5). Patel (6) developed the first carbon dioxide (CO_2) laser and Bridges (7) the first argon (Ar) laser. Lasers have since been applied commercially in compact disc players, laser discs, CD-ROMs in computers, and even in supermarket checkout counters! The military has found it effective as aiming beams on weapons and guidance systems in "smart" bombs. The Strategic Defense Initiative (SDI) will perhaps be the ultimate military expression of laser technology.

The first clinical application of the CO_2 laser in the endobronchial tree was carried out in 1974 by Strong and associates (8). Godard and colleagues were the first to use the Nd:YAG laser clinically in 1979 (9).

Subsequently, work by Toty, Dumon, and Personne demonstrated the safety and effectiveness of the Nd:YAG laser in the management of symptomatic endobronchial lesions (10–12). Their technique soon caught the attention of pulmonologists and has led to the establishment of endobronchial laser surgery as an important clinical tool in many key centers in the United States (13–23) as well as in the rest of the world. Even so, Prakash and colleagues noted in a North American mail survey that only 11.3% of respondents (98 of 871) performed laser bronchoscopy; pulmonologists formed the majority of respondents (98.2%), whereas intensive care specialists and thoracic surgeons made up the rest (24,25). One of the key reasons given was the lack of available training facilities. Of all types of lasers used, the Nd:YAG laser was the one most often cited (83.7%). The flexible fiberoptic bronchoscope was used by 81.6% of respondents and exclusively so by 38.8%. For this reason and because it is the technique we use in practice, we concentrate our discussion on the use of the Nd:YAG laser through the flexible bronchoscope. We will discus this in a "cookbook" fashion just like our earlier chapter on basic techniques in bronchoscopy. We hope to make up for some of the deficiencies in training opportunities by providing a step-by-step guide. The latter portion of this chapter is devoted to the use of photodynamic therapy in lung diseases.

Laser Physics

The acronym *laser* stands for light amplification by stimulated emission of radiation. Laser light differs from ordinary light in three unique ways.

Coherence: This is the principle feature of laser light that distinguishes it from ordinary white light. Ordinary light waves do not travel in a fixed relationship even though they may be parallel to one another. Laser light waves, however, travel in phase with each other in relation to both time and space, constantly being parallel to one another.

Collimation: Laser light travels in a single direction with minimal divergence. Ordinary light, however, diverges rapidly from its source and tends to phase out at a short distance. Collimation or directionality allows laser light to project to a great distance without losing a significant amount of its original energy.

Monochromaticity: Sunlight or other forms of white light, such as that from an electric light bulb, is actually a combination of all the colors in the visible portion of the electromagnetic spectrum. The range of wavelengths of visible light varies from 390 to 800 nm. Laser light, however, represents a single wavelength, which if it came in the visible portion of the spectrum would emit the purest form of that color.

The medium that produces laser light is the cornerstone of any laser machine. Just about any medium can be excited to form a laser beam and can include gases like He-Ne, CO_2, Ar, and krypton (Kr), or solids like Nd:YAG, holmium:YAG, and potassium titanyl phosphate (KTP). Even semisolids like "Jello" have been used to generate laser light (26)! Laser medium with two or more components usually has one element that is more active than the other. For example, nitrogen is the active matrix in CO_2 lasers and neodymium in Nd:YAG lasers. The stimulus that excites a laser medium can be another laser (e.g., an argon-pumped dye laser, a flash lamp [Nd:YAG laser], or an intense electric current [He-Ne laser]). Regardless of the stimulus used, the energy applied to a lasing medium excites the electrons in the atom to a higher but less stable energy level. The electrons fall back to their usual energy level giving off spontaneous emission of packets of light called photons with a unique wavelength and frequency depending on the constitution of the lasing medium. As more energy is pumped into the medium, the majority of electrons are pushed into a higher energy level, a phenomenon known as population inversion.

The lasing medium is placed in a cavity with mirrors at either end, one completely reflective and the other only partially so, allowing some laser light to escape. The initial photons reflect off these mirrors and repeatedly strike the inverted population of electrons within the lasing medium. This produces more photons of the same wavelength and frequency (stimulated emission). The percentage of coherent light allowed to escape in form of a laser beam depends on the intrinsic refractility of the partial mirror and varies between systems. Up to 80% of energy is emitted from a Nd:YAG laser, whereas only 1% of light escapes from the much weaker He-Ne laser. The lasing medium ultimately determines the wavelength of light produced. The physical properties of the laser are in turn dependent on its wavelength. It can be in the visible spectrum or extend beyond it into the infrared or ultraviolet regions.

Laser light produces three main effects on living cells. These are thermal, photodynamic, and electromagnetic (27). We will discuss only the thermal and photodynamic mechanisms because electromagnetic effects are still being researched. The applications of lasers in pulmonary medicine based on their tissue effects are listed in Table 18.1.

The Use of Nd:YAG Laser in the Treatment of Airway Obstruction

The Nd:YAG laser operates at a wavelength of 1.064 μm (invisible near infrared spectrum), which allows it to be transmitted via flexible quartz optical fibers and can thus be introduced to the deeper recesses of the endobronchial tree either through the flexible fiberoptic bronchoscope or rigid bronchoscope. Besides, in comparison with the CO_2 as well as Ar laser, Nd:YAG laser light is poorly absorbed by both water as well as hemoglobin content of the tissue and has greater depth of tissue penetration, up to 4 to 5 mm. Thus, it affects a larger volume of tissue, creating the most appropriate power density for the best possible coagulation of the endobronchial lesion.

Table 18.1. The Application of Lasers in Pulmonary Medicine

Thermal Effects

Photoresection of airway lesions
  Malignant: Bronchogenic carcinoma, metastatic lesions
  Benign: Tracheal stenosis, broncholith, suture granuloma, carcinoid, amyloidosis
Photocoagulation
  Management of epistaxis
  Bleeding cavitary lesions

Photochemical Effects

Diagnostic usage (Kr laser)
  Carcinoma in situ
  Superficial bronchogenic carcinoma
Therapeutic usage (rhodamine B dye laser)
  Palliative resection of malignant airway lesions
  Curative therapy for carcinoma in situ, superficial bronchogenic carcinoma, and juvenile laryngotracheobronchial papillomatosis

---

Malignant Airway Obstruction

Indications and Contraindications

The ideal patient for Nd:YAG laser photoresection (LPR) has an unresectable, symptomatic, exophytic large airway lesion that is either recurrent or resistant to radiotherapy or chemotherapy (Plate 42). Symptoms associated with such lesions include shortness of breath, hemoptysis, intractable cough, asphyxiation, or those associated with postobstructive pneumonia. The goal of Nd:YAG LPR here is effective and safe palliation and not cure. Identifying the factors that make the outcome favorable or unfavorable from LPR is the next important step in patient selection (Table 18.2).

Lesions located in the trachea or main stem bronchi are ideally situated for Nd:YAG LPR, whereas lobar or segmental bronchi are not. The procedure in distal airways is difficult, associated with a high complication rate and often with less rewarding results. An exophytic or pedunculated tumor can obviously be treated more effectively than a submucosal and extrinsically compressing lesion. In fact, a lesion extrinsically compressing the airway without an endobronchial component is a contraindication to Nd:YAG surgery, and an alternative form of palliation such as stent placement or external beam radiation therapy should be sought. Treatment of lesions rising from one wall of the involved airway (localized) is much more rewarding as compared to a lesion arising from all the walls of the airway (extensive) (18). The length of the lesion should be no more than 4 cm with a readily visualized distal lumen (18). If the lesion extends more than 4 cm in length, the chances of finding viable lung parenchyma beyond the site of obstruction are reduced and the procedure itself is more time consuming and difficult. If the lumen is totally occluded, it would be difficult to determine the axis of the bronchus beyond the obstruction and could lead to the creation of a false track, perforation

Table 18.2. Factors that Influence Outcome of Nd:YAG Laser Photoresection

Factors	Favorable	Unfavorable
Type of lesion	Endobronchial, exophytic	Extrinsic compression of the airway
Appearance	Polypoid	Submucosal lesion
Extent*	Localized	Extensive
Length*	< 4 cm	> 4 cm
Distal lumen	Visible	Totally obstructed
Duration of lung collapse	Short, < 4–6 wk	Long standing, > 4–6 wk
Vascularity	Less vascular	Hemorrhagic
Clinical status	Hemodynamically stable	Hemodynamically unstable
Pulmonary vascular supply*	Intact	Compromised

See text for details.

of the bronchus (pneumothorax or pneumomediastinum), or an extrapulmonary vessel. When the distal lumen cannot be visualized, one of the ways to assess the airway axis is to pass a Fogarty's catheter (5 to 7 F) beyond the obstruction and then withdraw it after inflating the balloon with 1 to 2 cc of air for better visualization (19). An alternative is to insert a large bore transbronchial needle beyond the site of obstruction to inject dilute Dionisil to identify the distal tract under fluoroscopy (28). The duration of the airway obstruction and the corresponding collapse of the lung should be less than 4 to 6 weeks. A longer period of obstruction usually means the tumor has infiltrated sufficient lung parenchyma to make Nd:YAG LPR a futile and possibly dangerous exercise. Besides, the likelihood of restoring lung function following collapse of such a long duration is slim. Certainly, a less vascular lesion is easier to resect because visibility is less frequently impaired and less time is spent in securing hemostasis. A massive bleed from a highly vascular lesion can also lead to hypoxemia and cardiovascular compromise. A patient who is hemodynamically stable to begin with is likely to do better than one who is symptomatic and debilitated.

Involvement or compression of the corresponding segment of pulmonary artery by tumor is a contraindication to photoresection because recanalizing the airway will only lead to increased dead space ventilation and consequently worsening dyspnea and hypoxemia in the patient. Computed tomography (CT) of the chest may be useful in assessing such vascular involvement (Figure 18.1). Compression apart, CT of the chest also allows mapping of any distortion in the regular anatomy of the thoracic vasculature that might have occurred from the tumor process, radiation, or prior surgery (29,30). Extra care is then taken during surgery to avoid LPR on the endobronchial wall in close proximity to the large intrathoracic blood vessels as much as possible. When available, CT also allows assessment of the patency and axis of the distal lumen and the likelihood of viable lung parenchyma beyond the point of obstruction.

In cases of carcinoma of the esophagus or bronchus, CT evidence of contiguous involvement between these two structures is a contraindication to LPR because there is a great risk of producing a tracheoesophageal fistula. Other contraindications for the procedure include an abnormal coagulation profile,

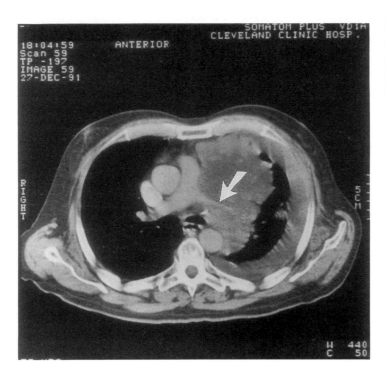

Figure 18.1. Contraindication for Nd:YAG LPR. CT scan of the chest reveals (*arrow*) encasement of the left pulmonary artery by the primary tumor.

raised intracranial pressure, acute bronchospasm, or marked hypoxemia requiring high supplemental fraction of inspired oxygen (FIO_2) to maintain an acceptable baseline oxygen saturation. High oxygen requirement increases the risk of ignition, and low baseline oxygen saturation leaves a narrow margin for error should hemorrhage or a pneumothorax occur.

Methodology

VENTILATORY MANAGEMENT: The most challenging part of performing Nd:YAG LPR is maintaining adequate ventilation throughout the procedure. This can be carried out in a variety of different fashions (Table 18.3). Nd:YAG LPR can be executed either through the rigid or the flexible bronchoscope. Photoresection through the rigid scope can be performed under neuroleptic analgesia or general anesthesia with either conventional or jet ventilation. In our experience, optimal neuroleptic analgesia is difficult to achieve. The patient is often too alert with an active cough reflex or too deep in anesthesia to maintain

spontaneous ventilation. Nd:YAG LPR can be achieved readily through the flexible scope. Although it can be done under local anesthesia, we prefer general anesthesia especially through the largest possible endotracheal tube (ETT) that allows a closed anesthetic circuit favored by our anesthesiologist. The ETT cuff is placed just distal to the vocal cords to allow maximum distance between the distal end of the inflammable polyvinyl chloride (PVC) ETT and the treatment site. For midtracheal lesions, we prepare several ETTs of different sizes, cutting the Murphy's eye just distal to the cuff (Figure 18.2). As the cuff inflation channel extends beyond the cuff to the tip of the ETT, cuff leakage is thus created. The distal opening of the channel is sealed with silicone cement and allowed to set for at least 24 hours (19). This once again provides a safe distance between the ETT and the midtracheal lesion. To secure the ETT in the patient's mouth, use only a single tape because in the event of ignition it can be readily removed and extinguished (31,32). We favor clear PVC ETTs over red rubber ones for several reasons (33,34). The latter tend to have a smaller

Table 18.3. Options for Ventilatory Management during Nd:YAG Laser Photoresection

Rigid Bronchoscope

Neuroleptic analgesia
 Spontaneous ventilation

General anesthesia
 Conventional ventilation
 Jet ventilation

Flexible Fiberoptic Bronchoscope

Local anesthesia
 Without endotracheal tube
  Transoral
  Transnasal
 With endotracheal tube

General anesthesia
 Conventional ventilation
 Jet ventilation

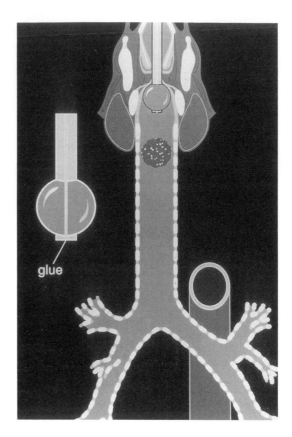

glue

Figure 18.2. Modification of ETT for midtracheal lesions with Murphy's eye cut off. Shown in vivo in cross section of trachea.

lumen for a comparable tube size. Red rubber tubes also tend to kink because of relatively poorer lateral support. Although PVC ETTs are supposedly more flammable, choosing one with fewer black markings will minimize absorption of laser energy (33–35). When it does ignite, however, it does so with a "blowtorch" effect and can lead to distal airway burns (32). The fumes from a PVC ignition produce hydrochloric acid and other toxic chemicals (36). Red rubber tubes do not burn as easily but produce large amounts of black acrid smoke. Another precaution that we take is to fill the ETT cuff with saline instead of air. The saline would act first as a heat sink, and should ignition occur, will spill out and douse at least the initial flames.

We reserve the use of jet ventilation through an experimental triple-lumen, inverted J-shaped steel jet injection cannula (JIC) for patients with high tracheal lesions that do not allow the placement of a regular ETT (Figure 18.3). The JIC has a total diameter of less than 4 mm. Two of the JIC channels are for ventilation and the third (most distal) for measuring airway pressure. The frequency of jet

ventilation is usually set at 70 to 150 cycles/min (19,37).

We have also developed a metal arch to hold the ETT in place during surgery (Figure 18.4). This obviates the need for an assistant to hold the ETT for the duration of Nd:YAG LPR. A detailed discussion of anesthetic agents is beyond the scope of this chapter and we refer the reader to a selection of articles pertaining to this subject (38–46). However, flammable anesthetic agents such as nitrous oxide should not be used during these procedures (34).

SELECTION OF APPROPRIATE ENDOSCOPE: The key deciding factor in choosing between the rigid scope and the flexible scope is the technical expertise of the operator (Table 18.4). Nd:YAG LPR was first developed by Toty and associates and Dumon and coworkers who

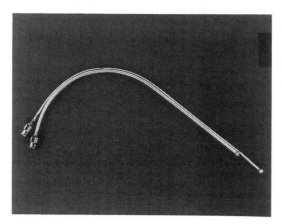

Figure 18.3. Jet injection cannula used during Nd:YAG LPR of high tracheal and subglottic lesions.

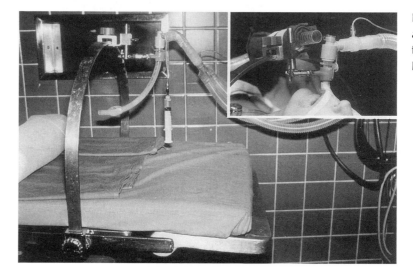

Figure 18.4. Metal arch and adjustable arm (*inset*) to hold ETT in place during Nd:YAG LPR.

Table 18.4. Rigid versus Flexible Bronchoscope for Nd:YAG Laser Therapy

Factor	Rigid	Fiberoptic
Expertise	Thoracic surgeon, otolaryngologist	Pulmonologist
Time commitment	Short	Long
Anesthesia	General only	General or local
Management of bleeding	Easier	Could be difficult*
Lesion		
Location	Trachea, major bronchi	Also lobar bronchi
Epistaxis	No	Yes
Bleeding cavity	No	Yes
Cervical spine, abnormalities	No	Yes
Endobronchial ignition	Less likely	Possible

*See text for details.

had a strong background in rigid bronchoscopy (10–12,47). It was not surprising then that physicians with similar training would elect to use the rigid scope in their own practice (48). With the advent of the flexible fiberoptic bronchoscope (49) and the declining numbers of pulmonologists being formally trained or practicing rigid bronchoscopy (24,25), use of the flexible scope has become a popular and practical choice in many practices including our own (13–20,50–52).

Because removal of debris and debulking of tumor tissue takes longer with the flexible forceps, Nd:YAG LPR is more time consuming when performed through the flexible scope. In our practice, however, we use the Fogarty catheter, flexible scissors, and polypectomy snare to a great advantage in reducing the time needed for debulking (52).

Debilitated patients with poor underlying cardiopulmonary function may not be able to undergo general anesthesia. For them rigid bronchoscopy under local anesthesia would be hazardous. Under the circumstances, it would be safer to perform the procedure with the flexible scope under local anesthesia.

Hemorrhagic lesions are probably dealt with better using the rigid scope because photocoagulation, suctioning, and direct tamponade of the bleeding site with the body of the scope can all be carried out simultaneously. A safe airway can also be established more rapidly with the rigid scope in cases of massive hemorrhage. In our experience with the flexible scope, we have required the use of the rigid bronchoscope for this purpose on three occasions during 330 procedures of Nd:YAG LPR. In the instance of perforation of a major intrathoracic vessel, neither the rigid scope nor the flexible fiberoptic scope will be effective in stopping the bleed or altering the outcome; these patients are usually poor candidates for open thoracic surgery due to their poor pulmonary reserve and the stage of their disease (14).

Although lesions in the trachea or main stem bronchi are ideally suited for Nd:YAG LPR, on occasion recannulating the lobar bronchus is necessary. In this setting, we use the flexible scope simply because it is easier to direct the tip of the laser fiber accurately toward the tumor compared to the rigid scope. Accuracy is of paramount importance given the proximity of major thoracic vessels to lobar bronchi.

Unusual indications for photocoagulation in our practice include epistaxis from polyps and arteriovenous malformations and bleeding pulmonary cavities (53,54). These procedures can only be performed with the flexible scope. Rheumatoid arthritis patients with atlanto-occipital joint involvement and patients with ankylosing spondylitis are obviously not candidates for rigid bronchoscopy.

Chances of the complication of an endobronchial fire are lower with the rigid scope because it is made of metal. The risk of the flexible scope, ETT, or laser fiber catching fire is higher because these are made of flammable materials.

The flexible bronchoscope is more economical because one instrument serves all diagnostic and therapeutic purposes including lasers. On the other hand, there are many different types of rigid scopes (Wolf, Karl Storz, Pilling, and Bryant). Each has its own distinct advantages and disadvantages and may prompt the user to purchase several costly systems to make up a comprehensive set of instruments. Endobronchial stenting and dilatation are, however, procedures best suited to the rigid bronchoscope.

Our practice model is to use the flexible scope with expertise and for ease and keep the rigid bronchoscope as a backup in the event significant bleeding occurs. Both instruments complement each other. Knowledge of the use of rigid bronchoscopy is desirable but not always mandatory especially if thoracic surgery backup is readily available.

Over the past 9 years, we have evolved an algorithm "Rule of Four" (Table 18.5) pertaining to limiting the risks of a fire hazard. The distal tip of the ETT should be kept at least 4 cm from the tumor. The laser fiber should extend approximately 4 mm beyond the tip of the bronchoscope and should be kept at least 4 mm away from the tumor (noncontact). The FIO_2 used during laser surgery should be kept to below 40%; a higher FIO_2 increases the risk of ignition. If a noncontact technique is used, we usually start with 40 W and adjust it according to the desired tissue effects. Synthetic sapphire crystal contact probes require much less power, and we usually start with 4 W during their usage. We use a single pulse mode with a duration of 0.4 seconds and pause every 40 pulses to remove the fiber to clean it of any blood or debris. This step is important because the presence of blood on the fiber will enhance the absorption of laser light and may lead to ignition or loss of the laser fiber tip (55). For the same reason the scope should be removed to clean the tip

periodically to prevent deposition of carbon particles or debris that may ignite if hit by the backscatter from the Nd:YAG laser beam. The single pulse mode is favored over the continuous mode. In addition, we limit the time spent in surgery to no more than 4 hours for the comfort of the laser team and to minimize mistakes resulting from fatigue. Finally, we try to keep the composition of the team constant with the same anesthetist and nurse at every surgery. This fosters familiarity with equipment and standard procedures, which leads to safer practice.

TISSUE EFFECTS: The Nd:YAG laser procedure can be carried out in either a contact or noncontact fashion, the latter using either sapphire probe or sculptured bare fiber. The following discussion mainly pertains to the noncontact method, which we predominantly use at our institution.

Laser tissue interaction is a dynamic process that depends on both the laser and the tissue characteristics. If the laser beam is directed perpendicularly to the tissue there is obviously greater penetration than with tangential entry (56). Varying the power (watts) and duration of the pulse will also enhance or diminish the tissue effect. The beam output divergence is 10° with a working focal length of 5 to 10 mm and a corresponding spot size of 1 to 2 mm (11,14). If both power and pulse duration are kept constant, then increasing the spot size by defocusing the beam will reduce the power density and tissue effect by spreading the area over which the power is distributed. By the same token, the patient's respiratory movements can also change the distance of the tumor and alter power density. How much energy is required to produce coagulation (pale discoloration) or carbonization (black discoloration) also depends on the "heat sink" effect in living tissue, which is determined by the local blood flow through the tumor (19,57). If the lesion is highly vascular-

Table 18.5. Rule of Four*

Duration of collapse	< 4 wk
Length of lesion	< 4 cm
Distance	
Endotracheal tube to lesion	> 4 cm
Fibertip to lesion†	4 mm
Bronchoscope to fibertip	4 mm
FIO_2	< 40%
Power (watts)	
Noncontact	40 W
Contact	4 W
Pulse duration	0.4 sec
Number of pulses between cleaning	40
Operating room time	< 4 h
Laser team	4

*See text for details.
†Noncontact method

ized, then a large fraction of the laser energy will simply be carried away from the tumor site with the blood flow. By increasing the length of each pulse or the power setting, this effect can be overcome. Also, by firing the laser at short intervals between the pulses, the heat built up in the tumor will increase accordingly. Finally, the color of the tumor will affect how much laser light is absorbed or scattered. Pale tissue will absorb less light and allow less penetration (forward scatter) while producing greater backscatter (20% to 40%) (58). Because unwanted transmural tissue damage can occur with forward scatter and deeper penetration, we keep the laser beam as parallel to the airway wall as possible. On occasion, we also biopsy the surface of a pale lesion in an attempt to produce contact bleeding, which will enhance surface absorption of laser light. As the tumor tissue darkens, absorption increases rapidly and carbonization and vaporization occur. If persistent sparks are seen, lower the FIO_2 if possible. If not, we suggest reducing the power or pulse duration and increasing the interval between pulses before continuing. Although not clinically significant, one may observe a sudden "popping" of the superficial layer of the tumor (known as the "popcorn" effect); it is due to concentration of the laser energy just below the tumor surface leading to a sudden rise in temperature and conversion of cellular water to steam (57).

For *hemorrhagic* lesions, where the goal is only hemostasis, we concentrate on coagulation (pale discoloration) without mechanical debulking (54). Firing the beam in a rosette formation (Plate 43) around the bleeding point effectively coagulates the feeder vessels and causes effective hemostasis (59). Unfortunately, if the bleeding vessel is hit end on, it will merely rupture the vessel wall causing further bleeding.

For relatively less vascular *mass* lesions we combine photocoagulation with mechanical excision to reduce the procedure time (Figure 18.5A). The laser is used primarily to control hemostasis in this setting with the bulk of the work being completed by mechanical excision. If the lesion is polypoid with a narrow base, we coagulate the base of the tumor a third of the way up from the endobronchial wall and then remove it with a polypectomy snare (Plate 44), flexible scissors, or large "crocodile" biopsy forceps.

For *hemorrhagic mass* lesions we vaporize from the luminal side of the tumor down to its base without mechanical excision, which could exacerbate the bleeding (Figure 18.5B). Metastatic renal cell carcinoma is an excellent example of this type of lesion and should be approached with caution. Familiarity with procedures to control a significant endobronchial bleed is essential in these cases (see Chapter 6).

Results and Survival Characteristics

In the management of unresectable malignant tracheobronchial lesions, Nd:YAG LPR is used mainly for palliation (19). In the experience of many authors, Nd:YAG LPR is able to achieve immediate palliation in over 80% of cases treated (10–12,17,19,20). Dumon and coworkers (11) and Unger (16) were able to achieve good or excellent results in 87% and 79% of their patients, respectively. Using similar classification, we were able to obtain excellent or good results following 94% of 211 procedures. Of 162 patients (Table 18.6), 6% who experienced no benefit (poor results) from the procedure either had extensive disease or total occlusion of the involved airway. Grouping immediate results into excellent, good, or poor categories, total resolution of symptoms of hemoptysis, asphyxiation, or intractable cough following Nd:YAG LPR was considered an excellent result. Evidence of improvement in the flow rate on flow volume loop of more than 20% or more than 20% improvement in quantitative ventilation or perfusion lung scan counts in the involved lung

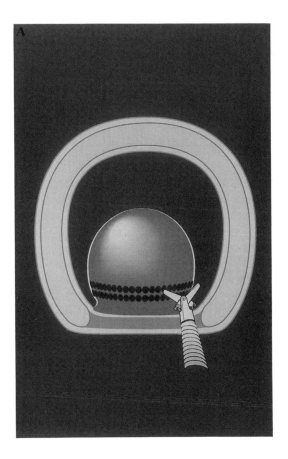
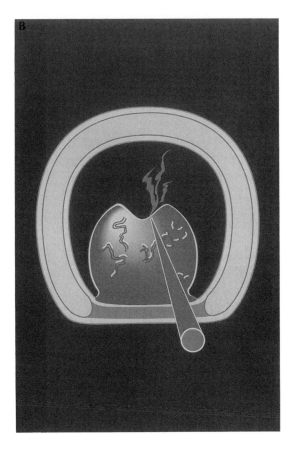

Figure 18.5. *A,* Mass lesion. A combination of photocoagulation (*arrow*) and subsequent mechanical excision with the scissors is used to remove this lesion. *B,* Hemorrhagic mass lesion. Start vaporization from the luminal aspect of the tumor, using a noncontact technique.

18.6. Immediate Palliation of Endobronchial Obstruction by Nd:YAG Laser Photoresection

Lesions	No. of Patients	Procedures	Results		
			Excellent	Good	Poor
Malignant	162	211	85 (40%)	118 (56%)	8 (4%)
Benign	55	89	50 (56%)	29 (33%)	10 (11%)
Total	217	300	135 (45%)	147 (49%)	18 (6%)

following the procedure was also considered as an excellent result. Radiologic evidence of reexpansion of a previously collapsed lung or lobe and clinicoradiologic resolution of postobstructive pneumonia were other objective criteria for an excellent result. A good result was significant symptomatic improvement without significant objective changes on radiography or spirometry. The absence of either symptomatic or objective benefit was considered a poor result.

In our review of the literature, we found few publications studying survival in patients with bronchogenic carcinoma after Nd:YAG LPR (20,60–62). Furthermore, no randomized trials have examined the effect of survival with Nd:YAG LPR followed by radiation therapy versus radiation therapy alone. Although studies done to date only included historical controls, early results were encouraging. Eichenhorn and colleagues (60) treated 19 patients with unresectable non–small-cell lung carcinoma by Nd:YAG LPR with sub-sequent external beam radiation therapy. Patients in whom satisfactory recanalization was achieved were found on rank testing to have significantly greater ($P < 0.006$) survival (median 340 days) versus those with poor Nd:YAG LPR results (median 39 days). In our initial study we found no significant improvement in the survival of 35 patients who were treated with both Nd:YAG LPR and radiation therapy over the historical controls who received palliative radiotherapy alone (61). However, comparing survival following Nd:YAG LPR as an emergency therapeutic intervention with historical controls who received emergent radiotherapy there was significant improvement in the laser group ($P = 0.04$). Although Nd:YAG LPR does not always produce an improvement over radiation therapy in all patient subgroups, those with critical endobronchial obstruction generally do worse with radiation therapy alone.

Ross and associates (62) treated 69 patients with palliative Nd:YAG LPR. They were successful in recanalizing the obstructed airway by at least 75% in 55 patients. They found that survival in their successful group as a whole was not significantly different from the unsuccessful group. However, a subset of patients with inoperable squamous cell carcinoma with successful Nd:YAG LPR survived significantly longer than those with unsuccessful Nd:YAG LPR or non-squamous cell carcinoma with successful LPR. They believe the reason to be the natural locally recurrent history of squamous cell carcinoma of the lung. The Radiation Therapy Oncology Group (RTOG) reports that intrathoracic recurrence occurs more frequently in patients with squamous cell carcinoma of the lung (80%) than other cell types (63). Therefore, control of local recurrence and its attendant complications, such as hypoxemia, hemoptysis, and postobstructive pneumonia/abscess formation appears to prolong survival for the squamous cell carcinoma subgroup (63,64). In a group of our patients who received a combination of endobronchial radiotherapy after Nd:YAG LPR and radiation therapy (17 of 300 patients) showed a significant increase in survival ($P = 0.022$) over historical controls receiving only radiotherapy (47 patients) (Figure 18.6, unpublished data). However, no demonstrable difference was seen between patients treated with radiation therapy and Nd:YAG LPR (66 of 300 patients) and those with radiotherapy alone. We believe the improvement in survival in the radiotherapy, Nd:YAG and endobronchial radiation group is related more to the endobronchial nature of the disease, which is suited to these therapeutic modalities, than the therapy itself. Nevertheless, the patients who do qualify for combined laser and endobronchial radiation therapy seem to survive longer with local control of the tumor process.

Overall survival, excluding a selected subset from unresectable non–small-cell carcinoma of the lung, has not been shown to improve with Nd:YAG LPR (61). We agree with previous authors (28,60) that randomized trials studying these therapeutic modalities are needed.

Complications

Perforation of a major vessel: This is a major complication of Nd:YAG LPR. A detailed knowledge of the anatomy of the airways in relation to major thoracic vessels is important before such surgery is undertaken. However, distortion of the normal anatomy can occur as a result of the tumor, radiation, or prior surgery (65), and contrast-enhanced CT or transverse magnetic resonance imaging (MRI) before LPR may be helpful in defining relationships with the endobronchial tumor. In selected patients, coronal MRI is able to visualize the main stem bronchi and trachea. Surface coil technology offers the best resolution of tumors in the proximal trachea (29). In

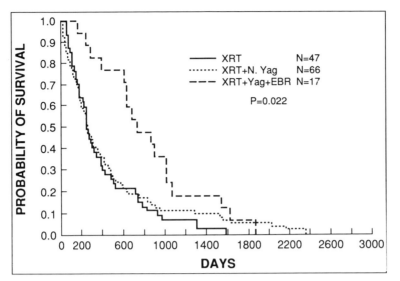

Figure 18.6. Cleveland Clinic Foundation 1992 survival estimates comparing historical controls (XRT), XRT + Nd:YAG, and XRT + Nd:YAG + EBR. XRT, external beam radiation; Nd:YAG, photoresection by Nd:YAG laser; EBR, endobronchial radiation therapy.

fact the first principle of endobronchial laser surgery is to fire the beam *parallel* to the bronchial wall; otherwise, it may perforate the airway. Careful planning prior to surgery to prevent perforation is the best course to take because little can be done once it occurs (14).

Endobronchial ignition: This is another dreaded complication of Nd:YAG LPR (31,32). On occasion, however, endobronchial ignition is minor and self-limiting (17). Fire can damage the plastic catheter of the laser fiber, resulting in loss of the metal nozzle that may or may not be recoverable (55). This can be prevented by keeping the fiber tip as clean as possible using hydrogen peroxide solution. We avoid using alcohol for this purpose because it is potentially flammable. The laser fiber should be frequently examined for wear and tear because the use of a damaged fiber could easily result in ignition of the flexible bronchoscope (Figure 18.7).

Major endobronchial ignition can result in serious injury to the patient's airways and damage the equipment. Best management of endobronchial ignition is its prevention. The choice of anesthesia, ETT, and bronchoscope have been discussed in our methodology section. An endobronchial fire is first suspected when black smoke (32) is seen emanating from the ETT or when a sustained yellow flare is seen through the scope optics (31). The first step is to stop ventilation. Then disconnect the oxygen source, remove the scope and ETT immediately and reintubate with a new ETT to reestablish ventilation. Apply mask ventilation in the interim if the new ETT is not immediately available. Reinsert the bronchoscope to assess the degree and extent of mucosal injury. The most serious immediate complication that can arise is airway obstruction from reactivebronchospasm, edematous mucosa, loss of mucosal ciliary clearance, and charred mucosal slough. Once the patient is in the recovery room, maintain an euvolemic state with intravenous normal saline infusion and start *humidified* oxygen supplementation. Follow through with aerosolized acetylcysteine and albuterol and four hourly chest physiotherapy and postural drainage. Call for a chest x-ray to exclude a pneumothorax or pneumomedia-stinum. Extended mechanical ventilation with or without positive end-expiratory pressure (PEEP) support may be needed in the event of significant thermal damage or inhalation of smoke (66). The indication for tracheostomy has to be individualized to the patient's clinical course. If the patient becomes dyspneic or hypoxic in the subsequent postoperative days, emergency bronchoscopy is required to ex-clude the development of mucus

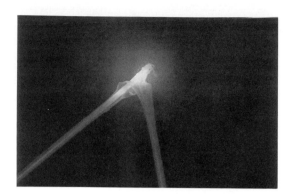

Figure 18.7. This laser fiber was fractured from regular wear and tear. Laser light can be seen emanating through its damaged end.

plugs. In our experience, these plugs appear to comprise tenacious mucoid secretions and charred mucosa on gross visual inspection. The use of empirical steroids and antibiotics has been advocated by Schramm and colleagues (66) and Casey and associates (31) but has not been favored by Herndon and coworkers (67). We also suggest clinicoradiographic assessment and follow-up bronchoscopy to assess the severity and progression of long-term airway damage that may lead to bronchial stenosis or endobronchial granuloma formation. Pulmonary function tests and ventilation perfusion scans are helpful adjuncts in diagnosing upper airway obstruction.

Hemorrhage from a vascular tumor: This complication can pose problems during surgery. Although minor bleeds will merely temporarily obscure the field of vision, a major and rapid bleed (250 to 500 mL) will necessitate inserting a rigid bronchoscope to tamponade the lesion, remove clot, and establish ventilation. Nd:YAG LPR is then used to cauterize the surface of the tumor to achieve hemostasis (19). Hemodynamic instability may ensue and blood products should be on hand if required.

Pneumothorax or pneumomediastinum: Either of these can occur as a result of laser surgery itself or as a complication of mechanical ventilation. This seems to occur more frequently while using jet ventilation. We recommend continuous peak airway pressure measurement throughout the procedure and keeping the laser beam parallel to the airway wall as far as possible to prevent inadvertent perforation.

Cerebral air embolism: This is an uncommon yet serious complication that may be secondary to a pneumothorax or pneumomediastinum. The air may also originate from the coaxial flow that cools sheathed fibers. Highly vascular lesions also add to the risk of air embolism. Using CO_2 instead of air for coaxial cooling may help to reduce the consequence of air embolism because CO_2 is more rapidly absorbed in the bloodstream.

Retinal damage: If Nd:YAG laser light is accidently reflected on the eyes of those present in the operating room, it would pass through the cornea, anterior chamber, lens and vitreous humor and produce retinal damage. Protective goggles should always be used by the laser team to prevent such complications (36,68,69).

Laser plume: Although no definite detrimental effects have been attributed to laser plume, we wish to draw attention to the presence of human immunodeficiency virus (HIV) DNA detected by Baggish and colleagues (70). This study was an in vitro experiment using the CO_2 laser to vaporize HIV-infected tissue pellets. Although they were unable to culture the virus, polymerase chain reaction analysis revealed proviral HIV DNA in particulate debris from laser smoke. Therefore, we suggest that masks be worn and an effective smoke evacuator be used during laser surgery until further studies are done to confirm or refute risks of viral infection to the laser team.

Table 18.7 compares key patient-related complications in major Nd:YAG LPR series reported in the world literature (12,17, 20,47,71). Of 5771 treatments, there has been an overall complication rate of only 0.85% and an acceptably low mortality rate of

Table 18.7. Comparison of Major Patient-Related Complications as a Direct Consequence of Laser Use

Author	No. of Treatments	Vessel Perforation	Ignition	Pneumothorax	Pneumomediastinum	Death	% of Complications
Personne	2284	3	0	21	3	18	1.18
Dumon	1503	1	0	3	1	1	0.34
Cavaliere	1396	0	0	4	2	0	0.43
Mehta	330	1	1	4	1	4	2.12
Brutinel	176	3(?)	0	1	0	3	2.27
Kvale	82	0	0	0	0	0	0.0
Total	5771	8	1	33	7	26	0.85

0.45%. One should be fully aware of all reported complications of the procedure before undertaking the endeavor. If due precautions are taken, these complications are to a great extent preventable.

Benign and Low-Grade Malignant Airway Obstruction

Tracheal Stenosis

Tracheal strictures are among the most common benign indications for Nd:YAG LPR. The underlying etiology is usually prolonged or traumatic intubation or prior tracheostomies. In 1986, Personne and colleagues performed 389 resections with the laser for this condition (12). The practical point from this series is that tracheal strictures that involve damage to or loss of cartilage are not suitable for Nd:YAG LPR because of the attendant tracheomalacia after surgery. In the following year, Shapshay and coworkers modified the technique using a combination of radial incisions with Nd:YAG laser and gentle dilatation with the rigid bronchoscope (72). In our study of 18 patients with tracheal stenosis (in press), 12 were successfully treated using this technique (Plates 45–47). The most suitable lesions to treat were single thin concentric weblike stenoses less than one cm in length with intact tracheal cartilage rings. Factors that led to failure of treatment included lesions of more than one cm in length and tracheomalacia. Total ablation of the scar using laser invariably results in recurrence and should be avoided. The technique of laser dissection followed by gentle dilatation is an excellent initial therapeutic option because surgical resection and end-to-end anastomosis had reported failure rates of up to 27% and total mortality rates of up to 19% (73).

Endobronchial Granulomas

Granulomas can form as a result of the presence of a foreign body, tracheostomy tube, transtracheal oxygen catheter, and suture material from previous surgery to the endobronchial tree (11,12,15,52,71). Such granulomas when symptomatic can be easily removed with Nd:YAG LPR. The procedure also offers a closed surgical approach to fracture the broncholith obstructing the airway for easy removal without thoracotomy (74–76).

Carcinoid Tumor

Carcinoid tumors are low-grade malignant tumors and we emphasize that Nd:YAG LPR is *not* indicated as primary therapy. Historically, endoscopic resection was successful initially but recurrences were documented up to 12 years after the initial surgery (77). Nd:YAG LPR should thus be used to palliate unresectable disease (11,12,14,20,71) or limit the extent of lung resection (78). Although the definitive surgical treatment was sleeve resection of the involved bronchus in Okike's series of 203 patients with typical bronchial carcinoid tumor, the most common indication for pneumonectomy was suppuration distal to the obstruction. Provided the tumor is in a suitable location, relief of the obstruction with Nd:YAG LPR and treatment of the suppuration with appropriate antibiotics will enable the surgeon to limit the margins of resection and conserve as much lung tissue as possible. Use of laser resection prevents excessive bleeding that can follow simple forceps biopsy. Acute carcinoid syndrome can also occur during Nd:YAG LPR, which we have successfully prevented by pretreating with ciproheptadine in a single case (unpublished data).

Other benign tumors

Although uncommon, a variety of histologically benign endobronchial lesions can be treated with Nd:YAG LPR. Reported cases include hemangiomas, lipomas, myoblastomas, chondromas, leiomyomas, histiocytomas (11–13), and hamartomas (79). Total patency can often be achieved with excellent results and prognosis given the benign nature of these conditions.

Contact Probes

Contact probes for Nd:YAG laser surgery were originally intended for open surgery to use as a scalpel and also where tactile appreciation of underlying tissue is essential. These probes are made of synthetic sapphire crystal that couples low thermal conductivity and mechanical strength. These probes also possess a high melting point in excess of 2000°C. They are placed at the distal end of the fiber using a special type of metal nozzle. The geometry of the probe (unless frosted) allows the laser beam to focus as desired—rounded geometry for vaporization, a conical probe for fine incisions, and flat probe for coagulation. Frosted tips are for simultaneous cutting and coagula-

tion and interstitial hyperthermia. The advantages of contact probes include low wattage requirements (10 to 15 W) better precision, less forward as well as backward scatter, less smoke production, tactile feedback, easy cleaning, and use in interstitial hyperthermia. Limited forward scatter limits penetration of the laser light and thus damage to important deeper structures. Contact probes also allow safe application of laser in lobar or segmental bronchi where the noncontact technique would be unsafe. The relative power density for a contact versus noncontact probe is 1:4, that is, 20 W will produce the same tissue effect as 80 W by noncontact Nd:YAG LPR. The disadvantage of the contact probe is that it blocks the view of the surface being treated and may create a track through the lesion and its attendant complications. Tissue sticking is another problem with use of the probes. If the probe is left embedded in the tumor following the laser pulse and allowed to cool before attempting withdraw it, the probe will adhere to the lesion. By withdrawing the probe before the end of the laser pulse, this effect can be avoided. Certain precautions have to be observed when using a contact probe. Start with a low wattage of 5 to 10 W. It is almost never necessary to exceed 25 W with contact probes. To prevent the major catastrophe of endobronchial ignition, avoid placing inflammable instruments distal to the treatment site. Stray laser light may then inadvertently cause ignition (32). Keep the probes as clean as possible. Use the probe for indications it is meant for and replace it if it appears misshapen (80,81). In our own practice, we have found few situations that specifically indicate usage of the contact probe. Our preference is to be able to see what we are treating while we treat it, a privilege not offered by the contact probe.

Another option of carrying out Nd:YAG LPR in a contact fashion is applying the tip of the quartz fiber (sculptured or polished) directly on the tumor tissue, which offers similar advantages and disadvantages of a sapphire probe. However, unlike sapphire probes, quartz fibers are vulnerable to damage and melting because of their lower melting point and mechanical strength and may require frequent polishing or resculpturing. In our opinion, safety of the unsheathed quartz fiber through the flexible fiberoptic broncho-scope needs to be established (31). Nevertheless, use of contact versus noncontact techniques remains operator as well as institution specific.

Summary

Given its low morbidity and mortality, Nd:YAG LPR is a safe procedure. We believe that most of these complications are related to the initial learning curve each operator has with the modality. We also suggest that safety would improve with actual "hands-on" experience under the supervision of a qualified laser bronchoscopist for at least the first 10 cases (24,25). We also agree with the recommendations of the American Society for Laser Medicine and Surgery that the following criteria are fulfilled before laser privileges are granted (82):

1. A review of the literature and a laser bronchoscopy course with a "hands-on" laser workshop that occupies a total of at least 8 to 10 hours
2. A minimum of at least 6 to 8 hours of observation and practice in the presence of an experienced operator

We believe that these guidelines offer a fair and balanced appraisal of the individual physician who wishes to perform laser surgery without being overly restrictive on hospital privileges.

Photochemical Effects

Intracellular activation of photosensitizers by light of a specified wavelength that leads to either tissue necrosis or fluorescence at a different wavelength or both is known as photochemical effect. Because some photosensitizers are preferentially retained by the majority of malignant and some premalignant lesions, they can be used in both treatment as well as early diagnosis of endobronchial tumors.

The use of photochemical effect of laser dates back to the turn of the century. In 1900, Raab noted that ordinary light and acridine orange proved fatal to paramecia (83). Three years later, eosin and white light was used by von Tappenier to treat skin tumors (84). In 1924, Policard discovered that both human and animal malignant tumors accumulated endogenous porphyrins and exhibited a red fluorescence, which was attributed to hemolytic bacteria (85). In the 1960s Lipson's work with hematoporphyrin derivative (Hpd) led to the first therapeutic use in a patient with recurrent carcinoma of the breast (86–89). In 1981, Dougherty was able to purify the active component of HpD subsequently known as dihematoporphyrin ethers (DHE), which for the same tumoricidal dose had the benefit of far less cutaneous photosensitization (90). DHE is the most widely studied photosensitizer today. Once DHE has been administered intravenously it is initially distributed to all body tissues. However, after 6 hours DHE is cleared from most normal tissues. The lungs retain it for about 12 hours, and the reticuloendothelial system for 24 hours in a ratio initially higher than tumor tissue. This ratio, however, reverses by 48 hours (91) with tumor tissue holding a DHE concentration of 2 to 3:1 (except for intracranial tumors where the ratio can rise as high as 28:1) for the next few days (92). Skin cells still hold small amounts of DHE for 30 to 80 days, enough to be responsible for photosensitivity reactions to direct light. Hence, patients must cover their entire body (Figure 18.8) and avoid direct exposure especially to sunlight for at least one month. If there is extravasation of porphyrin and inadvertent exposure to direct light, marked photosensitivity followed by ulceration and sloughing of the skin will follow. Great care has to be taken to prevent this during injection of DHE.

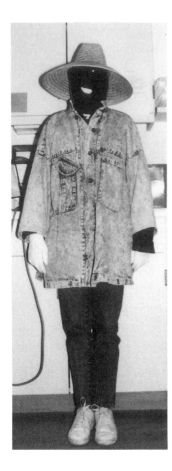

Figure 18.8. Patient for photodynamic therapy is dressed up in light-protective gear.

Diagnostic Application

Endobronchial carcinoma in situ and superficial tumors that cannot be distinguished from normal mucosa can be made to fluoresce at 630 to 690 nm 48 hours after HpD/DHE injection by illumination with violet light (405 nm) from a Kr ion laser (Figure 18.9). The amount of porphyrin retained by these diminutive tumors is very small and hence fluorescence is difficult to detect with the naked eye (93–95). Several image intensifiers have been developed to enhance the fluorescence signal that can be translated into audio signals, digital outputs, or amplified visual images (93–100). Tumor localization is followed by multiple biopsies for histologic confirmation because HpD fluorescence is nonspecific and moderate to marked metaplasia will also fluoresce (94,

101). Clinical studies from Mayo Clinic and Tokyo Medical College have shown the great potential of photosensitizers in early diagnosis of lung cancer. However, because there can be false negatives or false positives on fluorescence alone, histology must be reviewed in all cases before a clinical decision is made (101).

Therapeutic Application

The role of photodynamic therapy (PDT) in both malignant and benign lesions is currently the subject of intense research (Figure 18.10) (102–114). PDT has the potential to cure carcinoma in situ or unresectable yet early stage lung carcinoma where infiltration is limited to the bronchial mucosa without lymphatic or hematogenous spread (102–106). In the series of Hayata and colleagues, 8 of 13 patients who were treated solely with PDT were free of disease 13 to 41 months after therapy (103). Cortese and Kinsey achieved complete remission with PDT in 6 of 19 patients with early stage carcinoma over a follow-up period of 8 to 31 months (105). Balchum and Doiron were successful in treating 5 of 6 patients with early stage lung cancer although the period of follow-up was not specified (106). Kato reported data on a 59-year-old woman with stage Ia disease he treated exclusively with PDT who remained disease free for 5 years following a single treatment (104). For resectable lesions, Hayata has demonstrated anecdotally that PDT before surgery can on occasion limit the extent of lung excised by reducing the margin of resection necessary to achieve tumor clearance (102). By doing so lung function is better preserved postoperatively. Unresectable airway lesions have also been shown to be effectively palliated by PDT (102,103, 105–107,109).

Criteria used to determine success or failure in lung carcinoma have included Karnofsky's performance status (KPS) (106,107), loss of weight (106), relief of symptoms such as cough and hemoptysis (107), improvement on chest

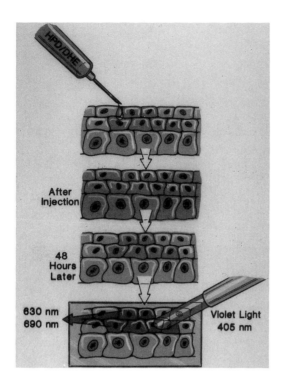

Figure 18.9. Schematic diagram shows diagnostic application of photodynamic technique.

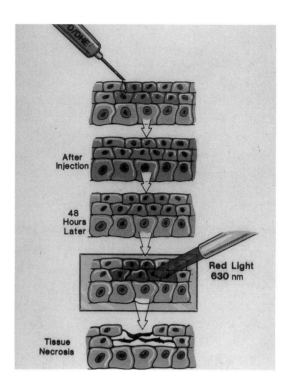

Figure 18.10. Schematic diagram represents principle of photodynamic therapy.

x-ray (107,109), and endobronchial appearance of the tumor (102,109).

Earlier work by Hayata failed to demonstrate significant improvement in survival in 14 patients, which was attributed to the advanced stages of lung cancer the patients were in (102). Balchum and Doiron, however, demonstrated in a group of patients that KPS of 70 to 100 was significantly associated with better survival than KPS of 40 to 60 ($P < 0.002$), independent of weight loss (106). McCaughan later noted that KPS taken on its own was not completely reliable. It is also important to distinguish if the poor KPS is associated more with potentially treatable pulmonary symptoms or metastatic disease (109).

The factors associated with treatment failure include remote physical location of tumor, incorrect assessment of depth of penetration of tumor, difficulty in calculating light dosage or lack of specialized equipment to measure dosimetry (107), and technical difficulties with

argon-pumped dye laser equipment (102,107). Toilet bronchoscopy 2 to 4 days after PDT was also cited by several authors as being critical in achieving good results (102,103,105–107,109). Removal of post-PDT necrotic tumor debris reduced significantly the complication rate following therapy including acute respiratory distress secondary to tumor swelling adding to airway obstruction. This emphasizes the fact that effects of PDT are delayed and may contribute to significant morbidity.

The side effect most commonly associated with PDT is photosensitivity, which manifests itself as sunburn or periorbital edema (102, 103,105,107,109). Cortese and coworkers also cited significant cough productive of blood-tinged sputum and necrotic material (105,109). They also described early airway obstruction attributed to post-PDT bronchial edema. Eleven patients died of delayed pulmonary hemorrhage after PDT in series by

Balchum, Cortese, and McCaughan (105,106, 109,110). Possible contributing factors include tumor that had eroded into the wall of the bronchus and extensive disease extending beyond the bronchus visible on chest x-ray. These authors believe that PDT was contributory in extending tumor necrosis with subsequent fatal hemoptysis although many of these patients had symptomatic hemoptysis before treatment. It is interesting to note that in Balchum and Doiron's (106) and Cortese and Kinsey's (105) series, of seven patients who died from delayed pulmonary hemorrhage, five had squamous cell carcinoma. It is also noteworthy that massive hemoptysis is not an uncommon sequela of cavitating squamous cell carcinoma regardless of prior radiation therapy or PDT (115).

Photodynamic therapy is hence effective and potentially curative for superficial or intramural tumors (103). The main limitation is the depth of penetration of red light, which extends 5 to 15 mm below the tumor surface (103,107). Once the lesion has extended deeper into the muscle or cartilage of the bronchial wall, PDT is solely palliative and other therapeutic modalities should be included in the patient's management. Interstitial PDT with implantable quartz fibers has been used in an attempt to overcome the problem of depth of penetration but dosimetry is difficult at best (105,107,109). Cortese and associates advocate selecting patients with radiologically occult tumors with an estimated surface area of less than 3 cm^2 and a superficial appearance on bronchoscopy (105,109). They also suggest that patients with large obstructing tumors should not be treated because of the inherent risk of delayed massive hemoptysis. Balchum and Doiron (106) and McCaughan and colleagues (107) advocate using the KPS to select relatively fit patients for PDT. Unfit patients whose poor KPS can be attributable to local disease may also benefit from PDT. McCaughan and coworkers also suggested

performing Nd:YAG LPR and a debulking procedure in patients with erosive lesions presenting with hemoptysis prior to PDT in an effort to reduce the risk of delayed massive pulmonary hemorrhage (107).

Most of the clinical literature in the treatment of benign lesions with PDT has centered on recurrent juvenile laryngotracheobronchial papillomatosis (JLTBP) due to human papilloma virus (HPV) types 6 and 11. Although juvenile laryngeal papillomas are the most common benign lesions to involve the larynx, tracheobronchial extension is seen in 5% to 20% of patients (116,117). Although the incidence of parenchymal involvement by JLTBP is less than 1%, it can potentially lead to progressive deterioration in lung function and repeated pneumonias (118–120). The natural history of JLTBP may involve episodes of hemoptysis, airway obstruction, and even progression to malignancy. Airway obstruction can occasionally necessitate tracheostomy with its attendant morbidity. Patients who receive radiotherapy have a 14% incidence of malignant change, whereas those without prior irradiation have a 2% incidence (121–123). Therapeutic options for JLTBP have been largely ineffective. Radiation therapy, ultrasound, cryotherapy, autologous tumor tissue vaccines, sex hormones, steroids, and tetracyclines have been unsuccessful in the long term (124). Although the Papilloma Study Group has recently reported a median remission of 550 days in 22 of 60 patients with a complete response to lymphoblastoid interferon alfa-n1, they also noted 25 with only partial remission and 13 with no response at all (125). Continuous therapy was also required to maintain control of the disease.

Abramson and colleagues have documented in 33 patients that PDT can reduce the average growth rate of JLTBP by about 50% (126). Patients with more severe disease appeared to achieve a better response based on Kashima's scoring system (127). Three of 33 patients remain disease free over a 2-year follow-up period, a response reflected in a case report by Kavuru and associates (128). At present, parenchymal disease may not be amenable to treatment with PDT given its inaccessibility to laser light (129).

We believe that PDT will play a key role in the management of JLTBP prior to involvement of the parenchyma for the following reasons. Although no other current treatment modalities have been successful, PDT has been curative in selected cases of endobronchial disease. PDT may also treat adjacent areas infected by HPV but having a macroscopically normal-looking appearance on bronchoscopy. If treated early enough, malignant change may also be avoided. Finally, apart from photosensitivity there are almost no other complications of PDT (101).

Summary

The application of photosensitizers in the diagnosis and treatment of early lung cancer, palliation of unresectable endobronchial carcinoma, and control of JLTBP with potential for cure, has brought its use to the brink of regular clinical practice. In patients with resectable disease, pretreatment with PDT may allow a more conservative margin of resection. Lung carcinoma in situ may potentially be cured with PDT. New photosensitizers currently under investigation such as benzoporphyrin derivative analogues have more favorable tumor-skin ratios and faster systemic clearance than DHE (130). In the future these advantages may lead to better patient acceptance and wider usage among physicians. Further studies have to be made into improving the depth of penetration that still has a cytocidal effect, attaining uniform dosimetry, and methods of reducing the incidence and severity of photosensitization reactions. The potential synergy between PDT and other therapeutic modalities such as Nd:YAG laser photoresection, brachytherapy, and hyperthermia should be the subject of future studies (101).

Laser-induced Autofluorescent Detection of Early Lung Cancer

This last section focuses on laser-induced autofluorescent detection of early lung cancer with the lung imaging fluorescence endoscope or LIFE diagnostic imaging system.

Early lung cancers are difficult to detect with conventional white light bronchoscopy. Woolner and colleagues noted that only 30% of all centrally located squamous cell carcinoma in situ were visible to an experienced bronchologist (131). Dysplasias and carcinoma in situ lesions are hard to diagnose even with bronchoscopy because they are only a few millimeters in radius and less than a millimeter in depth. Precancerous lesions and early cancers are also usually asymptomatic. Only 25% of all patients with lung cancer present early enough for curative surgical resection (132). Survival becomes significantly hampered by the time the patient becomes symptomatic or a lesion appears on the chest x-ray (133). Thomas and associates reported a local recurrence and second primary rate of 3.6% per annum in patients with resected T1N0M0 lung carcinomas (134). Pastorino and coworkers noted that 17% of completely resected stage I lung cancers developed a second primary over a 3-year follow-up period (135). Cortese and colleagues reported the development of a second primary lung carcinoma at a rate of 5% per annum in patients with radiologically occult, sputum cytology-positive tumors who underwent surgical resection (136) Efforts in the past to diagnose early cancer have been hampered by the need to use photosensitizers such as HpD or DHE that are preferentially retained by tumor (94,100,137,138). HpD has an affinity for tumor tissue that emits a fluorescent signal in the red portion of visible light peaking at 630 and 690 nm when excited by a Kr laser or short-arc mercury lamp with a narrow band pass optical interference filter (405 nm) via a thin 400 μm flexible quartz filament. Forty-eight hours following intravenous injection of HpD, bronchoscopy is performed and the bronchial tree screened for fluorescence. It is of interest to note that a number of distinct techniques have been developed to identify the fluorescence induced by the photosensitizer. Tokyo Medical College and the University of California (Santa Barbara) used image intensifiers and cathode ray tube displays to locate the green fluorescence from these lesions. The Mayo Clinic system, however, used a frequency modulator to produce an audio signal that was directly proportional to the intensity of the fluorescence detected. Using this system, Kato and Cortcse studied 11 patients with true occult lung carcinoma who had central airway squamous cell carcinomas not visible on chest x-ray (94). They were able to make the diagnosis in 10 of these patients. Unfortunately, the use of these drugs, which required relatively high doses (2 to 3 mg/kg intravenously), put fluorescence bronchoscopy at a disadvantage because of their dermatologic photosensitivity (139). Recently, Lam and coworkers developed a real-time diagnostic imaging system based on natural autofluorescence of early bronchogenic carcinoma and precancerous lesions (LIFE) (140). Two image-intensifying charged couple device (CCD) cameras were used to capture the weak, low-intensity fluorescence. This system is coupled to the eyepiece of the flexible bronchoscope (Olympus BF20D). The CCD cameras capture simultaneous red (more than 630 nm) and green (480 to 520 nm) images in real time. A helium-cadmium laser, which emits blue light at 442 nm, is delivered through the illumination fiberoptic bundle of the scope. This blue laser light acts as the excitation light source, which induces autofluorescence of the bronchial mucosa without the use of photosensitizers (141). Precancerous and early carcinomas have an autofluorescent spectrum distinct from normal mucosa when excited by light at 442 nm (142). A computer-controlled image processor creates a real-time color pseudoimage using the unique fluorescent signals induced by the laser and captured by the CCD camera. Normal mucosa is arbitrarily assigned a green color while red or brownish red identifies precancerous or early cancer lesions for biopsy on an RGB monitor. The physician is able to determine the area for biopsy more accurately with the diagnosis always based on histopathology. Preliminary work was reported in 94 subjects (mean age 63 years) of whom 41 were volunteers who did not have a history of lung cancer and 53 who had suspected or known carcinoma. Altogether, 328 histology specimens revealed 62 dysplasias (14 mild, 33 moderate, 15 severe), 29 carcinoma in situ, 64 invasive cancers, and 173 normals. Interestingly, ex-smokers (stopped for more than 10 years) in the volunteer group had 13% carcinoma in situ and 31% moderate or severe dysplasias. Of 64 patients known to have lung carcinoma, 15% had one or more areas of carcinoma in situ in addition to the grossly visible invasive cancer. Overall, the LIFE diagnostic imaging system had a 72.5% sensitivity and 94% specificity, representing a 50% improvement over white light bronchoscopy in detecting carcinoma in situ or dysplasia (140). Its main limitation is the range of the bronchoscope, which cannot access the outer third of the lung and identify early peripheral lesions. A multicenter trial is presently underway to establish the value and place this procedure has within the context of current accepted practice.

Conclusion

Although the use of Nd:YAG laser in treatment of benign and malignant conditions remains the best established in clinical practice, PDT appears to be gaining wider acceptance in specific areas, particularly for early lung cancer and JLTBP.

The LIFE diagnostic system should not be viewed as a mass screening tool for early detection of lung cancer. However, it offers selected high-risk patients and patients with surgically resected disease a greater chance for early detection of lung cancer within the range of the bronchoscope. Combined with newer photodynamic agents with shorter periods of cutaneous photosensitivity, this could provide a rational basis for a new multicenter prospective randomized survival studies in the early diagnosis and treatment of lung cancer.

REFERENCES

1. Einstein A. Zur quantientheoric der strahlung. Physikalishe Zeitschrift 1917;18: 121–128.
2. Schawlow AL, Townes CH. Infrared and optical masers. Phys Rev 1958;112:1940–1949.
3. Maiman TH. Optical and microwave-optical experiment in ruby. Phys Rev Lett 1960; 4:564–566.
4. Javan A, Bennett WR Jr, Herriot DR. Population inversion and continuous optical laser oscillation in gas discharge containing helium-neon mixture. Phys Rev Lett 1961; 6:106.
5. Geusic JE, Marcos HW, Van Uitert LG. Laser oscillation and Nd:doped yttrium aluminum, ytrrium gallium and gadolinium garnets. Appl Physics Lett 1964;4:182.
6. Patel CKN. Selective excitation through vibrational energy transfer and optical laser action in N_2-CO_2. Phys Rev Lett 1964; 13:617.
7. Bridges WB. Laser oscillation in singly ionized argon in the visible spectrum. Appl Physics Lett 1964;4:128.
8. Strong MS, Vaughan CW, Polanyi T, Wallace R. Bronchoscopic carbon dioxide laser surgery. Ann Otol 1974;83:769–776.
9. Godard P, Draussin M, Lopez FM, et al. Utilisation du rayonnement laser en bronchologie. Resection de deux tumeurs tracheobronchiques. Poumon Coeur 1979; 35:147–150.
10. Toty L, Personne C, Colchen A, Vourc'h G. Bronchoscopic management of tracheal lesions using Nd:YAG laser. Thorax 1981; 36:175–178.
11. Dumon JF, Reboud E, Garbe L, Aucomte F, Meric B. Treatment of tracheobronchial lesions by laser photoresection. Chest 1982; 3:278–284.
12. Personne C, Colchen A, Leroy M, Vourc'h G, Toty L. Indications and technique for endoscopic laser resections in bronchology. A critical analysis based on 2284 resections. J Thorac Cardiovasc Surg 1986;91: 710–715.
13. Unger M, Atkinson GW. Nd:YAG laser application in pulmonary and endobronchial lesions. In: Joffe SN, ed. Neodymium:YAG lasers in medicine and surgery. New York: Elsevier, 1983:71–81.
14. McDougall JC, Cortese DA. Neodymium-YAG laser therapy of malignant airway obstruction. Mayo Clin Proc 1983;58:35–39.
15. Parr GVS, Unger M, Trout RG, Atkinson WG. One hundred Nd-YAG laser ablation of obstructing tracheal neoplasms. Ann Thorac Surg 1984;38:374–379.
16. Unger M. Bronchoscopic utilization of the Nd:YAG laser for obstructing lesions of the trachea and bronchi. In: Kirschner RA, Unger M, eds. Surgical clinics of North America. Philadelphia: WB Saunders, 1984; 64:931–938.
17. Kvale PA, Eichenhorn MS, Radke JR, Miks V. YAG laser photoresection of lesions obstructing the central airways. Chest 1985; 87:283–288.
18. Mehta AC, Golish JA, Ahmad M, Zurick A, Padua NS, O'Donnell J. Palliative treatment of malignant airway obstruction by Nd:YAG laser. Cleve Clin Q 1985;52:513–524.
19. Livingston DR, Mehta AC, Golish JA, Ahmad M, DeBoer G, Tomaszewski MZ. Palliation of malignant tracheobronchial obstruction by Nd:YAG laser: an update of experience at the Cleveland Clinic Foundation. Journal of the American Osteopathic Association 1987;87:226–233.
20. Brutinel WM, Cortese DA, McDougall JC, Gillio RG, Bergstralh EJ. A two year experience with the neodymium-YAG laser in endobronchial obstruction. Chest 1987;91: 159–165.
21. Gelb AF, Epstein JD. Neodymium-yttrium-aluminum-garnet laser in lung cancer. Ann Thorac Surg 1987;43:164–167.

22. Goldberg M. Endoscopic laser treatment for bronchogenic carcinoma. In: Farrell EM, Keon WJ, eds. Surgical clinics of North America. Philadelphia: WB Saunders, 1988; 68:635–644.

23. Chan AL, Tharratt RS, Siefkin AD, Albertson TE, Volz EG, Allen RP. Nd:YAG laser bronchoscopy. Rigid or fibreoptic mode? Chest 1990;98:271–275.

24. Prakash UBS, Stubbs SE. The bronchoscopy survey. Chest 1991;100:1660–1667.

25. Prakash UBS, Offord KP, Stubbs SE. Bronchoscopy in North America: The ACCP survey. Chest 1991;100:1668–1675.

26. Enderby E. Medical laser fundamentals. In: Fleisher D, Jensen D, Bright-Asare P, eds. Therapeutic laser endoscopy in gastrointestinal disease. Dudrecht, Netherlands: Martinus Nijhoff, 1983:1–8.

27. Mehta AC, Golish JA, Ahmad M. Lasers in medicine: a clinician's guide to the physics. J Respir Dis 1987;8:37–44.

28. Joyner LR Jr, Maran AG, Sarama R, Yakaboski A. Neodymium-YAG laser treatment via the flexible fiberoptic bronchoscope. Chest 1985;87:418–427.

29. Ross JS, O'Donovan PB, Mehta A, Golish J, Paushter DM. Magnetic resonance and computed tomography evaluation of tracheobronchial lesions prior to laser photoresection. Cleve Clin Q 1986;53:335–344.

30. Pearlberg JL, Sandler MA, Kvale P, Beute GH, Madrazo BL. Computed tomographic and conventional linear tomographic evaluation of tracheobronchial lesions for laser photoresection. Radiology 1985;154:759–762.

31. Casey KR, Fairfax WR, Smith SJ, Dixon JA. Intratracheal fire ignited by the Nd:YAG laser during treatment of tracheal stenosis. Chest 1983;84:295–296.

32. Krawtz S, Mehta AC, Wiedemann HP, De Boer G, Schoepf KD, Tomaszewski MZ. Nd:YAG laser-induced endobronchial burn. Management and long term followup. Chest 1989;95:916–918.

33. Geffin B, Shapshay SM, Bellack GS, Hobin K, Setzer SE. Flammability of endotracheal tubes during Nd:YAG laser application in the airway. Anesthesiology 1986;65:511–515.

34. Wolf GL, Simpson JI. Flammability of endotracheal tubes in oxygen and nitrous oxide enriched atmosphere. Anesthesiology 1987;67:236–239.

35. Andrews AH, Goldenberg RA, Moss HW, Shaker MH. Carbon dioxide laser for laryngeal laser surgery. Surg Annu 1974; 6:459–476.

36. Healy GB. Complications of laser surgery. In: Simpson GT, Shapshay SM, eds. Otolaryngology clinics of North America. Philadelphia: WB Saunders, 1983;16:815–820.

37. Mehta AC, Livingston DR, Levine HL, et al. Ventilatory management during neodymium:yttrium aluminum garnet photoresection of subglottic and higher tracheal lesions. Presented at the meeting of the American Broncho-esophagological Association, Palm Beach, Florida, May 5–6, 1986. In: Transactions of the American Broncho-esophagological Association 1986:148–153.

38. George PJM, Garrett CPO, Nixon C, Hetzel MR, Nanson EM, Millard FJC. Laser treatment for tracheobronchial tumors: local or general anesthesia? Thorax 1987;42: 656–660.

39. Hanowell LH, Martin WR, Savelle JE, Foppiano LE. Complications of general anesthesia for Nd:YAG laser resection of endobronchial tumors. Chest 1991;99:72–76.

40. McCaughan JS, Barabash RD, Penn GM, Glavan BJ. Nd:YAG laser and photodynamic therapy for esophageal and endobronchial tumors under general and local anesthesia. Effect on arterial blood gases. Chest 1990;98:1374–1378.

41. Warner ME, Warner MA, Leonard PF. Anesthesia for neodymium-YAG (Nd-YAG) laser resection of major airway obstructing tumors. Anesthesiology 1984;60:230–232.

42. Vourc'h G, Tannieres ML, Toty L, Personne C. Anesthetic management of tracheal surgery using the neodymium-yttrium-aluminum-garnet laser. Br J Anaesth 1980; 52:993–997.

43. Donlon JV. Anesthesia for airway surgery. Seminars in Anesthesia 1987;6:17–26.

44. George PJM, Clarke G, Tolfree S, Garrett CPO, Hetzel MR. Changes in regional ventilation and perfusion of the lung after endoscopic laser treatment. Thorax 1990;45: 248–253.

45. Rouby JJ, Simonneau G, Benhamou D, et al. Factors influencing pulmonary volumes and CO_2 elimination during high-frequency jet ventilation. Anesthesiology 1985;63:473–482.

46. Jakobsen CJ, Ahlburg P, Holdgard HO, Olsen KH, Thomsen A. Comparison of intravenous and topical lidocaine as a suppressant of coughing after bronchoscopy during general anesthesia. Acta Anaesthesiol Scand 1991;35:238–241.

47. Dumon JF, Shapshay SM, Bourcereau J, et al. Principles for safety in application of neodymium-YAG laser in bronchology. Chest 1984;86:163–168.

48. Beamis JF, Shapshay SM. More about the YAG. Chest 1985;87:277–278.

49. Ikeda S, Yanai N, Ishikawa S. Flexible bronchofiberscope. Keio J Med 1968;17:16–18.

50. Parr GVS, Unger M, Trout RG, Atkinson WG. One hundred neodymium-YAG laser ablations of obstructing tracheal neoplasms. Ann Thorac Surg 1984;38:374–379.

51. Arabian A, Spagnolo SV. Laser therapy in patients with primary cancer. Chest 1984;86:519–523.

52. Mehta AC. Laser applications in respiratory care. In: Kacmarek RM, Stoller JK, eds. Current respiratory care. Toronto: BC Decker, 1988:100–106.

53. Mehta AC, Livingston DR, Crisostomo A, Golish JA, Ahmad M. Radiation necrosis of bronchus and its palliative management using Nd:YAG laser. Am Rev Respir Dis 1987;135:A243.

54. Mehta AC, Livingston DR, Levine HL. Fiberoptic bronchoscope and Nd:YAG laser in the treatment of severe epistaxis from nasal hereditary hemorrhagic telangiectasia and hemangioma. Chest 1987;91:791–792.

55. Mehta AC, Golish JA, Livingston DR. Loss of fiberoptic laser tip. Chest 1985;88:796.

56. Unger M. Neodymium:YAG laser therapy for malignant and benign endobronchial obstructions. In: Unger M, ed. Clinics in chest medicine. Philadelphia: WB Saunders, 1985;6:277–290.

57. Polanyi TG. Physics of surgery with lasers. In: Unger M, ed. Clinics in chest medicine. Philadelphia: WB Saunders, 1985;6:179–202.

58. Polanyi TG. Laser physics. In: Simpson GT, Shapshay SM, eds. Otolaryngology clinics of North America. Philadelphia: WB Saunders, 1983;16:753–774.

59. Gorisch W, Boergen KP. Heat induced contraction of blood vessels. Lasers Surg Med 1982;2:1–13.

60. Eichenhorn MS, Kvale PA, Miks UM, Seydel HG, Horowitz B, Radke JR. Initial combination therapy with YAG laser photoresection and irradiation for inoperable non-small cell carcinoma of the lung. A preliminary report. Chest 1986;89:782–785.

61. Desai SJ, Mehta AC, Medendorp SV, Golish JA, Ahmad M. Survival experience following Nd:YAG laser photoresection for primary bronchogenic carcinoma. Chest 1988;94:939–944.

62. Ross DJ, Mohsenifar Z, Koerner SK. Survival characteristics after neodymium:YAG laser photoresection in advanced stage lung cancer. Chest 1990;98:581–585.

63. Perez CA, Pajak TF, Rubin P, et al. Long term observations of the patterns of failure in patients with unresectable non-oat cell carcinoma of the lung treated with definitive radiotherapy: report by the Radiation Therapy Oncology Group (RTOG). Cancer 1987;59:1874–1881.

64. Petrovich Z, Stanley K, Cox JD, Paig C. Radiotherapy in the management of locally advanced lung cancer of all cell types: final report of randomized trial. Cancer 1981;48:1335–1340.

65. Cordasco EM Jr, Rice T, De Boer G, Mehta AC. Fatal mistaken identity. Am Rev Respir Dis 1991;144:469–470.

66. Schramm VL, Mattox DE, Stool SE. Acute management of laser ignited intratracheal explosion. Laryngoscope 1981;91:1417–1426.

67. Herndon DN, Thompson PB, Traber DL. Pulmonary injury in burned patients. Crit Care Clin 1985;1:79–96.

68. Duncavage JA, Ossoff RH. Laser application in the tracheobronchial tree. In: Parkin JL, ed. Otoloaryngology clinics of North America. Philadelphia: WB Saunders, 1990;23:67–75.

69. Dedhia HV, Lapp NL, Jain PR, Thompson AB, Withers A. Endoscopic laser therapy for respiratory distress due to obstructive airway tumors. Crit Care Med 1985;13:464–467.

70. Baggish MS, Poiesz BJ, Joret D, Williamson P, Refai A. Presence of human immunodeficiency virus DNA in laser smoke. Lasers Surg Med 1991;11:197–203.

71. Cavaliere S, Foccoli P, Farini PL. Nd:YAG laser bronchoscopy. A five year experience

with 1396 applications in 1000 patients. Chest 1988;94:15–21.

72. Shapshay SM, Hybels RL, Beamis JF, Bohigian RK. Endoscopic treatment of subglottic and tracheal stenosis by radial laser incision and dilation. Ann Otol Rhinol Laryngol 1987;96:661–664.

73. Maassen W, Greschuchna D, Vogt-Moykopf I, Toomes H, Lullig H. Tracheal resection—state of the art. Thorac Cardiovasc Surg 1985;33:2–7.

74. Miks VM, Kvale PA, Riddle JM, Lewis JW. Broncholith removal using the YAG laser. Chest 1986;90:295–297.

75. Cahill BC, Harmon KR, Shumway SJ, Mickman JK, Hertz MI. Tracheobronchial obstruction due to silicosis. Am Rev Respir Dis 1992;145:719–721.

76. Faber LP, Jensik RJ, Chawla SK, Kittle CF. The surgical implication of broncholithiasis. J Thorac Cardiovasc Surg 1975;70:779–789.

77. Okike N, Bernatz PE, Woolner LB. Carcinoid tumors of the lung. Ann Thorac Surg 1976;22:270–275.

78. Desai SJ, Mehta AC, Rice TW, Ahmad M. Role of Nd:YAG laser photoresection in limiting the extent of pulmonary resection in obstructive carcinoid tumor. Am Rev Respir Dis 1988;137:467S.

79. Aboussouan LS, Mehta AC, Ahmad M, DeBoer G. Definitive treatment of endobronchial hamartomas using Nd:YAG laser photoresection. Am Rev Respir Dis 1991;143:A65.

80. Mehta AC, Livingston DR, Golish JA. Artificial sapphire contact endoprobe with Nd:YAG laser in the treatment of subglottic stenosis. Chest 1987;91:473–474.

81. Mehta AC, Grimm M. Breakage of Nd:YAG laser sapphire contact probe inside the endobronchial tree. Chest 1988;93:1119.

82. American Society for Laser Medicine and Surgery. Standards of practice for the use of lasers in medicine and surgery. Clin Laser Monthly 1984;2:59.

83. Raab C. Uber die wirkung fluresziender stoffe auf infusoren. Z. Biol 1900;39:524–526.

84. Von Tappenier H, Jesioneck A. Therapeutische versuche mit flureszierenden stoffen. Muench Med Wochschr 1903;1:2042.

85. Policard A. Etudes sur les aspects offerts par des tumeur experimentales examinee a la lumiere de woods. C R Soc Biol 1924;91:1423–1424.

86. Lipson RL, Baldes EJ, Olsen AM. Hematoporphyrin derivative. A new aid of endoscopic detection of malignant disease. J Thorac Cardiovasc Surg 1961;42:623–629.

87. Lipson RL, Baldes EJ, Olsen AM. A further evaluation of the use of hematoporphyrin derivative as a new aid for the endoscopic detection of malignant disease. Dis Chest 1964;46:676–679.

88. Lipson RL, Gray MJ, Olsen AM. Hpd for detection and management of cancer. Proc: IX. Internat Cancer Congr 1966:393.

89. Lipson RL, Pratt JH, Baldes EJ, et al. Hematoporphyrin derivative for the detection of lung cancer. Obstet Gynecol 1964;24:78.

90. Dougherty TJ, Boyle DG, Wieshaupt KR, et al. Photoradiation therapy—clinical and drug advances. In: Kessel D, Dougherty TJ, eds. Porphyrin photosensitization. New York: Plenum Press, 1983.

91. Dougherty TJ, Kaufman JE, Goldfarb A, et al. Photoradiation therapy for the treatment of malignant tumors. Cancer Res 1978;38:2628–2635.

92. Brown SG. The future of lasers in cancer therapy. Br J Hosp Med 1988;40:161.

93. Profio AE, Doiron DR, King EG. Laser fluorescence bronchoscope for localization of occult lung tumors. Med Phys 1979;6:523–525.

94. Kato H, Cortese DA. Early detection of lung cancer by means of hematoporphyrin derivative fluorescence and laser photoradiation. In: Unger M, ed. Clinics in chest medicine. Philadelphia: WB Saunders, 1985;6:237–253.

95. Kato H, Konaka C, Ono J, et al. Cancer localization by detection of fluorescence by means of HpD administration and krypton ion laser photoradiation in canine lung cancer. Lung Cancer 1981;21:439–445.

96. Profio AE, Doiron DR, Sarnaik J. Fluorometer for endoscopic diagnosis of tumors. Med Phys 1984;11:516–520.

97. Hirano T, Ishizuka M, Suzuki K, et al. Photodynamic cancer diagnosis and treatment system consisting of pulsed lasers and endoscopic spectro-image analyzer. Laser Life Sci 1989;3:1–18.

98. Wagnieres G, Depeursinge CH, Monnier PH, et al. Photodetection of early cancer by laser induced fluorescence of a tumor-selective dye: apparatus design and realization. SPIE 1990;1203:43–52.

99. Montan S, Svanberg K, Svanberg S. Multicolor imaging and contrast enhancement in cancer-tumor localization using laser-induced fluorescence in hematoporphyrin-derivative-bearing tissue. Optic Lett 1985;10:56–58.

100. Cortese DA, Kinsey JH, Woolner LB, Payne WS, Sanderson DR, Fontana RS. Clinical application of a new endoscopic technique for detection of in situ bronchial carcinoma. Mayo Clin Proc 1979;54:635–642.

101. Mehta AC, Golish JA, Ahmad M. Photosensitizers as diagnostic and therapeutic tools in oncology. In: Goldson AL, ed. Cancer management in man. Detection, diagnosis, surgery, radiology, chronobiology, endo-crine therapy. Boston: Kluwer Academic Publishers, 1989;9:220–226.

102. Hayata Y, Kato H, Konaka C, Ono J, Takizawa N. Hematoporphyrin derivative and laser photoradiation in the treatment of lung cancer. Chest 1982;81:269–277.

103. Hayata Y, Kato H, Konaka C, et al. Photoradiation therapy with hematoporphyrin derivative in early and stage I lung cancer. Chest 1984;86:169–177.

104. Kato H, Konaka C, Kawate N, et al. Five year disease-free survival of a lung cancer patient treated only by photodynamic therapy. Chest 1986;90:768–770.

105. Cortese DA, Kinsey JH. Hematoporphyrin derivative phototherapy in the treatment of bronchogenic carcinoma. Chest 1984;86:8–15.

106. Balchum OJ, Doiron DR. Photoradiation therapy of endobronchial lung cancer. In: Unger M, ed. Clinics in chest medicine. Philadelphia: WB Saunders, 1985;6:255–275.

107. McCaughan JS, Williams TE, Bethel BH. Photodynamic therapy of endobronchial tumors. Lasers Surg Med 1986;6:336–345.

108. Lam S, Muller NL, Miller RR, et al. Predicting the response of obstructive endobronchial tumors to photodynamic therapy. Cancer 1986;58:2298–2306.

109. Edell ES, Cortese DA. Bronchoscopic phototherapy with hematoporphyrin derivative for treatment of localized bronchogenic carcinoma; a 5-year experience. Mayo Clin Proc 1987;62:8–14.

110. McCaughan JS, Hawley PC, Walker J. Management of endobronchial tumor: a comparative study. Semin Surg Oncol 1989; 5:38–47.

111. Kavuru MS, Mehta AC, Eliachar I. Effect of photodynamic therapy and external beam radiation therapy on juvenile laryngotracheobronchial papillomatosis. Am Rev Respir Dis 1990;141:509–510.

112. Basheda SG, Mehta AC, DeBoer G, Orlowski JP. Endobronchial and parenchymal juvenile laryngotracheobronchial papillomatosis. Chest 1991;100:1458–1461.

113. Mullooly VM, Abramson AL, Shikowitz MJ. Dihematoporphyrin ether-induced photosensitivity in laryngeal papilloma patients. Lasers Surg Med 1990;10:349–356.

114. Abramson AL, Shikowitz MJ, Mullooly VM, Steinberg BM, Amella CA, Rothstein HR. Clinical effects of photodynamic therapy on recurrent laryngeal papillomas. Ann Otol Head Neck Surg 1992;118:25–29.

115. Miller RR, McGregor DH. Hemorrhage from carcinoma of the lung. Cancer 1980; 46:200–205.

116. Majoros M, Parkhill EM, Devine KD. Papilloma of the larynx in children: a clinicopathologic study. Am J Surg 1964;108: 470–475.

117. Strong MS, Vaughn CW, Healey GB, Cooperband SR, Clemente MA. Recurrent respiratory papillomatosis: management with the CO_2 laser. Ann Otol Rhinol Laryngol 1976;85:508–516.

118. Kramer SS, Wehunt WD, Stocker JT, Kashima H. Pulmonary manifestations of juvenile laryngotracheal papillomatosis. AJR Am J Roentgenol 1985;144:687–694.

119. Rosenbaum HD, Alari SM, Bryant LR. Pulmonary parenchymal spread of juvenile laryngeal papillomatosis. Radiology 1968; 90:654–660.

120. Smith L, Gooding CA. Pulmonary involvement in laryngeal papillomatosis. Pediatr Radiol 1974;2:161–166.

121. Matsuba HM, Thawley SE, Spector GJ, Mauney M, Pikul FJ. Laryngeal epidermoid carcinoma associated with juvenile laryngeal papillomatosis. Laryngoscope 1985;95: 1264–1266.

122. Siegel SE, Cohen SR, Isaacs H, Stanley P. Malignant transformation of tracheobronchial juvenile papillomatosis without prior radiotherapy. Ann Otol Rhinol Laryngol 1979;88:192–197.

123. Zehnder PR, Lyons GD. Carcinoma and juvenile papillomatosis. Ann Otol Rhinol Laryngol 1975;84:614–618.

124. Robbins KT, Woodson GE. Current concepts in the management of laryngeal papillomatosis. Head Neck Surg 1984;6:861–866.

125. Leventhal BG, Kashima HK, Mounts P, et al., and the Papilloma Study Group. Long term response of recurrent respiratory papillomatosis to treatment with lymphoblastoid interferon alfa-n1. N Engl J Med 1991; 325:613–617.

126. Abramson AL, Shikowitz MJ, Mullooly VM, Steinberg BM, Amella CA, Rothstein HR. Clinical effects of photodynamic therapy on recurrent laryngeal papillomas. Ann Otol Head Neck Surg 1992;118:25–29.

127. Kashima H, Leventhal B, Mounts P, and the Papilloma Study Group. Scoring system to assess severity and course in recurrent respiratory papillomatosis. In: Howley PM, Broker TR, eds. Papillomavirus: molecular and clinical aspects. Proceedings of the Burroughs-Wellcome-UCLA Symposium held in Steamboat Springs, Colorado. New York: Alan R Liss, 1985:125–135.

128. Kavuru MS, Mehta AC, Eliachar I. Effect of photodynamic therapy and external beam radiation therapy on juvenile laryngotracheobronchial papillomatosis. Am Rev Respir Dis 1990;141:509–510.

129. Basheda SG, Mehta AC, De Boer G, Orlowski JP. Endobronchial and parenchymal juvenile laryngotracheobronchial papillomatosis—effect of photodynamic therapy. Chest 1991;100:1458–1461.

130. Allison B, Richter A, Jiang F, Jiang S, Liu D, Levy JG. Approach to improved delivery of photosensitizers. SPIE 1990;IS6:167–176.

131. Woolner LB, Fontana RS, Cortese DA, et al. Roentgenographically occult lung cancer: pathologic findings and frequency of multicentricity during a ten year period. Mayo Clin Proc 1984;59:453–466.

132. Shields TW. Surgical therapy for carcinoma of the lung. Clin Chest Med 1982;3:369–387.

133. Fontana RS, Sanderson DR, Taylor WF, et al. Early lung cancer detection: results of the initial (prevalence) radiologic and cytologic screening in the Mayo Clinic study. Am Rev Respir Dis 1984;130:561–565.

134. Thomas P, Rubinstein L, and the Lung Cancer Study Group. Cancer recurrence after resection of T1N0 non small cell lung cancer. Ann Thorac Surg 1990;48:242–247.

135. Pastorino U, Infante M, Maiol M. A randomized chemoprevention trial in stage I lung cancer with high dose retinol palmitate. Lung Cancer 1991;7:11. Abstract.

136. Cortese DA, Pairolero PC, Bergstralh EJ, et al. Roentgenographically occult lung cancer. A ten year experience. J Thorac Cardiovasc Surg 1983;86:373–380.

137. Hayata Y, Kato H, Konaka C. Fiberoptic bronchoscopic laser photoradiation for tumor localization in lung cancer. Chest 1982;82:10–14.

138. Profio AE, Doiron DR, King EG. Laser fluorescence bronchoscope for localization of occult lung tumors. Med Phys 1979;6: 523–525.

139. Dougherty TJ, Cooper M, Mang TS. Cutaneous photoxic occurrences in patients receiving photofrin. Lasers Surg Med 1990; 10:485–488.

140. Lam S, MacAulay C, Hung J, Le Riche J, Profio AE, Palcic B. Detection of dysplasia and carcinoma in situ with a lung imaging fluorescence endoscope device. J Thorac Cardiovasc Surg 1993;105:1035–1040.

141. Palcic B, Lam S, Hung J, MacAulay C. Detection and localization of early lung carcinoma by imaging techniques. Chest 1991;99:742–743.

142. Hung J, Lam S, LeRiche JC, Palcic B. Autofluorescence of normal and malignant bronchial tissue. Lasers Surg Med 1991; 11:99–105.

19 | Endobronchial Radiation Therapy

Basil S. Hilaris, Michael S. Porrazzo, and Chitti R. Moorthy

The incidence of bronchogenic carcinoma continues to rise. The American Cancer Society estimates that there will be 172,000 new cases in 1994, and that 153,000 patients will die of their disease. Lung cancer ranks among the most lethal of human malignancies (1). Surgery is the treatment of choice, but most cases present at an advanced stage. Only 25% of cases are considered operable, and only one third of these actually undergo curative resection (2).

Therapeutic alternatives for patients with locally advanced or otherwise nonresectable tumors include chemotherapy and radiation. For patients without pulmonary symptoms, chemotherapy is appropriate as the initial treatment. It offers some measure of systemic coverage and may produce local tumor shrinkage. However, a complete response is rarely achieved and many patients may experience disease progression despite treatment. Radiation therapy produces a superior level of local control and is indicated in any patient with significant pulmonary symptoms.

shown to be dose dependent (3). The Radiation Therapy Oncology Group (RTOG) is currently recommending doses greater than 6000 cGy to maximize local control (4). To safely deliver large doses, computed tomography (CT)-guided treatment planning should be used. Shrinking fields delivered from multiple directions are usually necessary. The tolerance of surrounding organs, such as the spinal cord, heart, esophagus, bone, and normal lung, must be respected.

High-dose external beam therapy requires many weeks of daily treatment and often results in significant morbidity, such as pneumonitis, esophagitis, and generalized fatigue (5). Recurrence following radiation therapy is not uncommon. Disease progression within the treated field has been reported to occur in approximately one third of patients within 18 months (6–8). Autopsy studies have shown that local regional disease is responsible for nearly 50% of deaths (9). Local recurrence is a cause of significant morbidity, including hemoptysis, dyspnea, cough, and chest pain.

Radiation Therapy

External beam therapy is the most frequently used radiation technique for lung cancer. High-energy linear accelerators are most appropriate for treatment of the lung. The lesion itself, any suspicious lymph nodes, and the surrounding areas at risk are included in the treatment field. Local control has been

Brachytherapy

Brachytherapy is a localized form of radiation. When applicable, it offers distinct advantages over external beam therapy in terms of reduction in the integral dose. Large doses can be delivered to accessible tumors while sparing the surrounding structures because of the inverse square law (10). It has been postulated that brachytherapy is less affected by low oxygen tension than external beam radiotherapy (11). Endobronchial brachytherapy (EBBT) can be used in combination with external beam therapy, usually to boost the lesion itself (12). Occasionally, treatment with EBBT alone may be appropriate. In patients with recurrent disease after prior high-dose radiotherapy, EBBT is usually a treatment option. Whether used alone or in combination with either limited field external beam radiation or laser resection, it has been shown to produce prolonged palliation of symptoms (13–15).

The concept of EBBT is not new. In 1922, Yankauer reported data on two patients with lung cancer in whom encapsulated radium sources were placed via the bronchoscope (16). In 1933, Kernan reported on several cases of lung cancer treated with diathermy and the bronchoscopic implantation of radon seeds (17). The largest experience with radon im-plantation came from Memorial Hospital by Pool in 1961 (18). Hilaris later updated the Memorial experience with radon, and he introduced ^{125}iodine a new radioisotope suitable for implantation (19). All of these reports involved the permanent implantation of radioactive sources via the bronchoscope.

This technique has largely been replaced by temporary implantation using afterloading catheters (20–23). Bronchoscopy is still necessary to locate the lesion and place the catheter. However, the procedure differs from permanent implantation in that once the catheter is in place, the bronchoscope is removed. The radioactive material, usually ^{192}iridium is then afterloaded in the catheter. The radioactive material remains in place for a specified period of time, and then along with the catheter, is removed from the patient. Treatments may be repeated several times. At present, several literature reports have assessed the efficacy and safety of temporary EBBT (Table 19.1).

Indications and Contraindications

Endobronchial brachytherapy is applicable in certain clinical situations. Patients should have biopsy-proven disease involving the trachea or accessible bronchi. Patients who have received large doses of external beam therapy can still receive additional treatment with brachytherapy provided that the treatment catheter can be placed in proximity to the lesion (Figure 19.1). Symptoms such as hemoptysis, dyspnea, and cough are usually due to endobronchial

Table 19.1. Endobronchial Radiation Therapy—Literature Review

First Author	Technique	Dose	Depth	Response	Complications
Schray (24)	LDR	3000 cGy	5–10 mm	60%	18%
Roach (10)	LDR	3000 cGy	5 mm	67%	6%
Cotter (12)	LDR	3000 cGy	10 mm	90%	10%
Mehta (34)	LDR	2500 cGy	20 mm	83%	10%
Allen (14)	LDR	3000 cGy	5 mm	100%	N/A
Speiser (27)	LDR	2000 cGy	5 mm	69%	3%
Seagren (22)	HDR*	1000 cGy	10 mm	>90%	25%
Nori (23)	HDR	2000 cGy†	10 mm	80%	<5%
Stout (26)	HDR	1500 cGy	10 mm	71%	<5%
Miller (25)	HDR	1000 cGy	10 mm	78%	<5%

*Cobalt 60
†Multiple fractions
HDR, high-dose rate; LDR, low-dose rate

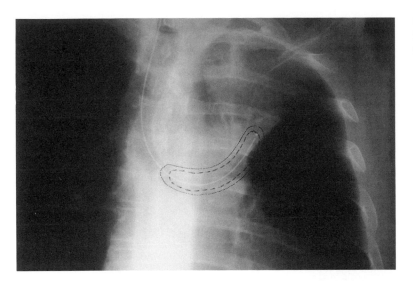

Figure 19.1. Chest x-ray identifying the position of the treatment catheter.

lesions, and these can be effectively palliated with high-dose localized radiation. Lesions causing complete airway obstruction can be debulked with laser therapy, and this should be followed with EBBT to prolong the palliation (24,25). Selected extrabronchial lesions can be adequately treated using a multicatheter technique (Figure 19.2).

Peripheral parenchymal lesions, bulky disease, and the presence of a fistula arc contraindications to the use of EBBT. Patients with poor performance status, advanced age, or without biopsy-proven disease are not eligible for treatment. The presence of metastatic disease is not a contraindication to therapy in patients who are symptomatic from their endobronchial disease.

Technique

General
The placement of an afterloading catheter is done under direct visualization using the flexible bronchoscope (Figure 19.3). The patient is given a mild sedative and the procedure is carried out with local anesthetics. The lesion is first located via bronchoscopy. The afterloading catheter is then inserted transnasally, although some investigators prefer to do this transorally. The catheter is positioned adjacent to the lesion with its tip placed a few

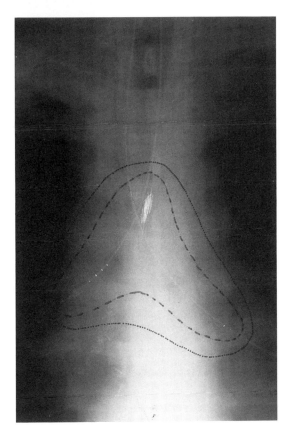

Figure 19.2. Chest x-ray with composite isodose distribution of two treatment catheters. Selected extrabronchial lesions can be adequately covered using a multicatheter technique.

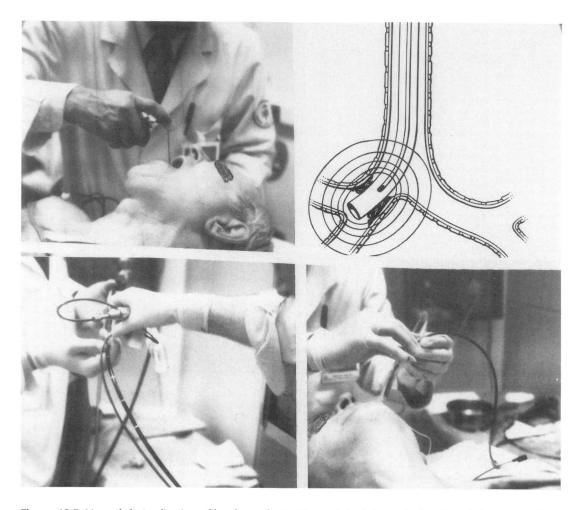

Figure 19.3. *Upper left,* Application of local anesthetic. *Upper right,* Schematic drawing of placement of treatment catheter in proximity to lesion. *Lower left,* Preparation of the bronchoscope and treatment catheter. *Lower right,* Treatment catheter is placed under direct visual guidance.

centimeters beyond the distal end of the tumor to allow for some movement.

Once the afterloading catheter is in place, the bronchoscope is removed, and the catheter is secured. Marker seeds are inserted into the catheter and a chest x-ray in anteroposterior and lateral views is obtained. This documents the treatment and can be compared with other films when multiple applications are used. An isodose distribution is overlaid on the films and the dosimetry should be reviewed before the actual treatment begins (Figures 19.4, 19.5).

Low-Dose Rate

The conventional technique of EBBT involves the afterloading of ^{192}Ir sources into polyethyl-ene catheters. This can be done either manually or mechanically. Dose rates in the range of 50 to 75 cGy/h at 10 mm are achieved. Applications that deliver 1500 to 4500 cGy require 24 to 72 hours of exposure. Patients require hospitalization in private rooms for the duration of the treatment. They are not confined to bed, but should be behind lead shields when others are in the room. Patients tend to tolerate this therapy fairly well. The greatest concern during a low-dose rate (LDR) endo-bronchial application is displacement of the catheter. The exposed portion of the tube is securely taped in place. If the patient has a patent tracheostomy, this can be used to insert the afterloading catheter. This technique may

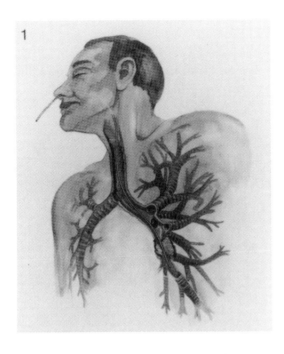

Figure 19.4. Anatomic drawing depicts placement of treatment catheter.

Courtesy of Nucletron Corporation, Columbia, Maryland.

be more comfortable for the patient and may reduce the risk of catheter displacement.

High-Dose Rate

The growing popularity and availability of high-dose rate (HDR) afterloading devices has provided an alternative technique for EBBT (Figure 19.6). The major advantages of this approach include the convenience of outpatient treatments and reduced exposure to personnel. Dose rates in the range of 50 to 100 cGy at 10 mm/min can be delivered. The afterloading catheter is positioned under bronchoscopic guidance. It is secured in place and connected to the HDR device. A high-activity ^{192}Ir source, connected to a cable, is driven through the catheter. The ^{192}Ir source stops at a number of predetermined positions for various lengths of time. In this way, a composite isodose distribution is produced, which should encompass the target volume. A unique feature of the HDR system is that by varying the dwell

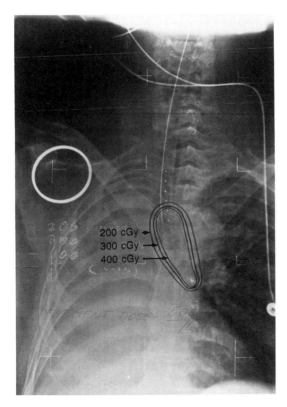

Figure 19.5. Chest x-ray confirms placement of treatment catheter with isodose distribution.

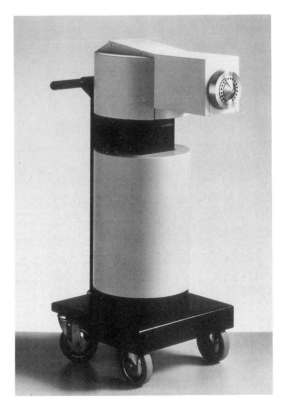

Figure 19.6. Micro–Selectron high-dose rate afterloader by Nucletron Corporation.

times at the various resting stations, the iso-dose distribution can be customized. Because of the rapid rate of dose delivery, no more than 1000 cGy to 10 mm depth should be given in one sitting. The actual application requires a matter of minutes depending on the activity of the source and the prescribed dose. Procedures are done on an outpatient basis and are performed within the radiation department. Multiple applications are usually performed except in cases where only a single bronchoscopy is advisable (26).

Comparison of Low-Dose with High-Dose Rate

No available randomized data compare LDR with HDR for bronchial lesions. Both are effective in prolonging palliation and neither can claim to improve survival. The advantages of HDR therapy include:

1. Treatments are done on an outpatient basis and so hospitalization is avoided.
2. Treatment lasts only a few minutes, so there is less chance for applicator movement.
3. Radiation exposure to the patient and staff is reduced.

Disadvantages of HDR therapy include:

1. Because more than one application is generally prescribed, multiple bronchoscopies must be performed for catheter placement.
2. A high dose is given in a short period of time, some of which reaches normal tissue, and this may result in a greater incidence of acute and late effects.
3. HDR afterloaders require dedicated shielded rooms.

Low-dose rate EBBT is generally delivered in a single sitting, and so only one bronchoscopy is necessary. When careful technique is used, there should be minimal exposure to the staff because the sources are afterloaded. The major disadvantages of LDR therapy are:

1. There is a risk of catheter movement during the 1 to 3 days that an application requires.
2. The patient is hospitalized and confined to a private room for the duration of the application.
3. Close observation is required throughout the duration of treatment to assess the patient's status.

We and others have also used intermediate-dose rate (IDR) technique that requires a high-activity single ^{192}Ir ribbon (27). The catheter remains in place for several hours. Patients need to be behind shields but do not require overnight hospitalization. Dose rates range from 250 to 500 cGy/h, and 1500 to 2000 cGy can be given in a single sitting. Multiple applications are generally required and this necessitates several bronchoscopies for catheter placement. High-activity iridium ribbons are readily available, saving the patient the cost of a hospital admission, but there is the potential for increased exposure to the staff.

Treatment Planning

Several critical aspects of EBBT must be considered. Proper positioning of the afterloading catheter is obviously of prime importance. For LDR and IDR therapy, a technique to secure the catheter in place to allow only minimal movement during treatment is necessary. Of equal importance is the dose per fraction and the prescription point. For instance, when 1000 cGy is prescribed to a point 10 mm from the source, there is certain to be some normal tissue less than 10 mm from the source, and this can receive significantly more than the 1000 cGy prescribed dose (Figure 19.7). In addition, if there is curvature of the catheter, hot and cold spots can be produced. For HDR EBBT, it is particularly important to have an

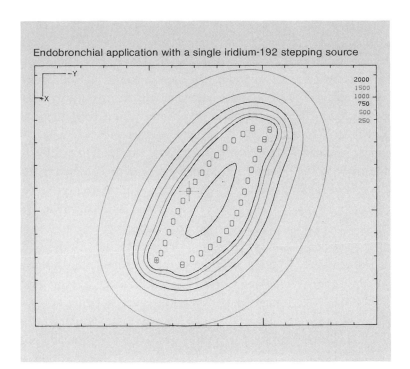

Endobronchial application with a single iridium-192 stepping source

Figure 19.7. Isodose distribution reveals rapid fall off of dose with increasing distance from the source.

Courtesy of Nucletron Corporation

Table 19.2. New York Medical College Treatment Guidelines: Group I*

Technique	Dose/Fraction	Depth	No. of Fractions	Total Dose
LDR	4500 cGy	5 mm	1	4500 cGy
IDR	2000 cGy	5 mm	2	4000 cGy
HDR	1000 cGy	5 mm	3	3000 cGy

Prior radiation therapy < 5000 cGy, Karnofsky ≥ 90, no symptomatic distant metastases.
HDR, high-dose rate; IDR, intermediate-dose rate; LDR, low-dose rate

Table 19.3. New York Medical College Treatment Guidelines: Group II*

Technique	Dose/Fraction	Depth	No. of Fractions	Total Dose
LDR	3000 cGy	5 mm	1	3000 cGy
IDR	1250 cGy	5 mm	2	2500 cGy
HDR	500 cGy	5 mm	3	1500 cGy

Prior radiation therapy > 5000 cGy, Karnofsky < 90, symptomatic distant metastases.
HDR, high-dose rate; IDR, intermediate-dose rate; LDR, low-dose rate

accurate determination of the surface dose and any hot spots to avoid acute and late effects.

At New York Medical College, we place candidates for EBBT into two categories. Group I consists of patients who have received no more than 5000 cGy external radiation, have a Karnofsky performance status of 90 or greater, and have no symptomatic distant metastases. Group II consists of patients who have received more than 5000 cGy external radiation, have a Karnofsky performance status less than 90, and are symptomatic from distant metastasis. Our treatment policies according to group are shown in Tables 19.2 and 19.3. For tracheal lesions, we prescribe to 10 mm depth.

Treatment needs to be planned in advance. The length and depth of the lesion must be known so that a target volume can be determined and a proper isodose can be generated. Pretreatment bronchoscopy and CT scan are helpful in this regard. Recently, we have begun to investigate advantages of pretreatment three-dimensional brachytherapy treatment planning based on three-dimensional reconstruction of the tumor and surrounding anatomy (Figure 19.8). This requires the patient to undergo either magnetic resonance imaging or CT scan of the target area using 2-mm slices. A three-dimensional view of the region can be reconstructed. We are currently investigating ways to link the three-dimensional isodose distribution to the reconstructed anatomy to assess the adequacy of coverage prior to the actual procedure. When used together with modern HDR treatment planning systems, we will be able to vary the depth of the prescription point throughout the tumor to ensure proper coverage.

Placement of the catheter should always be done under bronchoscopic guidance to ensure proper placement and reduce the risk of perforation. In addition, the condition of the affected airway should be periodically reevaluated. Impending fistula formation is a contraindication to therapy. The physician should keep in mind that a fistula, although not originally present, can develop during the course of therapy as a tumor regresses. When the bronchoscope is removed, a chest x-ray is obtained to document placement of the catheter and demonstrate an isodose distribution.

Evaluation during Treatment

The LDR and IDR therapies require several hours to days of exposure. Patients need to be in private rooms with lead shields available when either staff or visitors enter the room. Patients should be checked frequently to guard against movement of the catheter. In the case of HDR therapy, patients remain within the treatment room for the several minutes required to deliver the prescribed dose. They are observed on camera for the duration of the treatment. Catheter movement is not a major concern. When treatment is complete, the catheter is removed. The patient is observed for a period of several hours. A repeat chest x-ray should be obtained after any LDR or IDR treatment. (Figure 19.9)

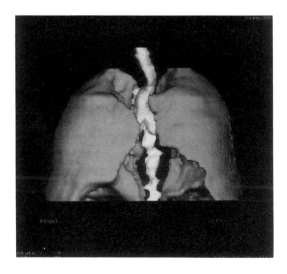

Figure 19.8. Three-dimensional reconstruction of the chest used for treatment planning. *Courtesy of Nucletron Corporation.*

Laser Therapy

The neodymium:yttrium-aluminum-garnet (Nd:YAG) laser has been of value for palliating

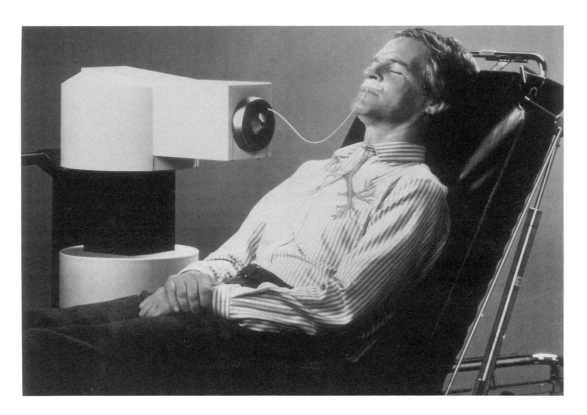

Figure 19.9. Patient receiving endobronchial brachytherapy treatment using the high-dose rate afterloader. *Courtesy of Nucletron Corporation.*

proximal intraluminal tumors. Since its introduction in the 1980s, this technique has become popular because of its ability to produce rapid relief of airway obstruction (28–31). The Nd:YAG laser has also been effective in controlling hemoptysis. The procedure is now generally considered safe, but it is not without risks. Massive hemorrhage is the most feared complication. Fistula formation is also potentially life threatening. The perioperative mortality rate for the procedure has been reported to be as high as 10% (30,32,33).

There are several limitations to the use of laser debulking. The treatment of distal obstructions or extrinsic disease is technically difficult and carries with it a higher risk of perforation. The palliative effect of laser debulking alone is usually short lived. Repeated treatment tends to be less effective and is associated with a higher incidence of complications.

It should be kept in mind that laser therapy is not tumoricidal and that the palliation it produces generally lasts an average of 3 months. Several reports have documented the efficacy of the combination of laser and endobronchial radiation. It has been reported by Schray and colleagues that brachytherapy appears to prolong the duration of palliation obtained by laser by a factor of two to three (24). Others have suggested that no difference exists in the duration of palliation when comparing laser plus EBBT versus EBBT alone. With this in mind many institutions reserve the use of laser to cases where the obstruction is severe enough that the afterloading catheter cannot be passed (14). A totally occluded bronchus should be lasered until a channel is produced to pass the treatment catheter. Endobronchial radiation can then be effectively delivered. Thus, in many cases, the two techniques are considered complementary.

Table 19.4. Endobronchial Carcinoma—Survival Data

First Author	No. of Patients	Median Survival (mo)
Cotter (12)	30	10.0
Seagren (22)	18	9.0
Roach (10)	17	6.5
Stout (26)	100	5.5
Fish (35)	15	5.1
Mehta (34)	38	5.0
Schray (24)	65	4.0
Overall	283	5.8

Results

The patient population for which EBBT has found its greatest applicability are those cases with central recurrence. Neither EBBT, nor laser therapy, nor the combination of both modalities has had a significant impact on survival. The median survival of patients who present with malignant bronchial obstruction is less than 6 months (Table 19.4). This is not surprising because most patients who develop central recurrence will also manifest distant metastases. Occasionally, central recurrence in the absence of distant metastases may be detected, and such patients are potentially long-term survivors with proper endobronchial treatment.

Central recurrence is associated with significant morbidity, including hemoptysis, cough, and shortness of breath. Improvement in these symptoms can be measured, and, at present, this offers the best method to assess the success of treatment. These symptoms have been consistently and effectively palliated with the use of EBBT. Overall response rates have been in the range of 80% to 90%, with most cases considered a complete response. Hemoptysis appears to be particularly responsive to endobronchial therapy. Cough and shortness of breath can be palliated in more than 50% of cases.

The effectiveness of treatment depends on a number of factors, with dose being the most important; 1000 cGy to 5 mm using HDR appears to be as effective as 4500 cGy using LDR. Doses higher than this may give slightly better response rates but at the cost of increased morbidity. Other factors affecting the success of treatment include proper positioning of the catheter and the duration of symptoms. Gelb and Epstein found that the degree of bronchial occlusion was inversely correlated with the response to therapy (32). They suggested initial laser debulking of a totally occluded bronchus to allow for effective EBBT. Schray and associates reported that a prior response to irradiation lasting greater than one year was associated with a higher response to subsequent therapy (24).

Complications

Endobronchial brachytherapy involves both bronchoscopy and radiation therapy, each with its attendant risks. The potential morbidity of bronchoscopy includes hemoptysis, pneumothorax, and perforation. The incidence of these complications is acceptably low, and the reader is referred to other chapters in this book for a more complete discussion.

The major complications of EBRT include hemorrhage and fistula formation. In some initial reports of EBBT, the incidence of these problems was reported to be greater than 20%, although it is impossible to distinguish disease progression from radiation reaction (Table 19.5). Follow-up studies and more recent reports have suggested a much lower incidence of complications. Some of the early HDR afterloading devices used cobalt sources and this may be associated with a greater incidence of tissue damage. Currently, most HDR units use ^{192}Ir sources.

Follow-up bronchoscopic examinations of treated patients have identified a surprisingly high incidence of mucosal necrosis and slough-

Table 19.5. Endobronchial Radiation Therapy Treatment-related Complications

First Author	No. of Patients	Complications*		
		Hemorrhage	Fistula	Necrosis
Mehta (34)	38	–	2	2
Schray (24)	65	–	11	1
Seagren (22)	18	5	–	–
Stout (26)	100	1	–	–
Cotter (12)	30	1	1	1
Total	218	7	14	4
	(100%)	(3.2%)	(6.4%)	(1.5%)

May represent disease progression.

ing. Patient condition, tumor extent, and aggressiveness of therapy have obvious effects on the incidence of morbidity. No more than 1000 cGy prescribed to 10 mm depth should be given in a single application using the HDR technique. At New York Medical College, our policy for all bronchial lesions is to prescribe to 5 mm depth. In patients who are debilitated or who have received large doses of external beam therapy, 500 cGy to 5 mm depth is preferred. For patients treated with LDR therapy, 4500 cGy to 5 mm depth given in a single sitting represents a safe limit. This may need to be reduced in debilitated or previously treated patients.

Conclusions

The efficacy and safety of EBBT is becoming well established. Numerous studies have shown that this method can provide significant palliation of recurrent endobronchial disease. The technique is becoming more commonly used as part of the initial curative therapy for applicable patients. Regardless of the dose rate technique used, similar response and toxicity can be expected. We feel that when HDR is available, it is the preferred method of treatment because of advantages in patient com-

fort, convenience, and safety. At present, however, there is no consensus as to proper fraction size, prescription point, or dose rate. Until more is known about mucosal tolerance, we choose to be conservative with fraction size and prescription point. Ran-domized studies are clearly needed to answer these questions.

REFERENCES

1. Garfinkle L, Silverberg E. Lung cancer and smoking trends in the United States over the past 25 years. CA Cancer J Clin 1991;41: 137–145.
2. Holmes EC. Combined modality therapy for non-small cell lung cancer. Cancer 1988;4: 12–21.
3. Perez CA, Stanley K, Grundy G, et al. Impact of radiation technique and tumor extent in tumor control and survival of patients with unresectable non-oat cell carcinoma of the lung. Cancer 1982;50:1091–1099.
4. Enami B, Perez CA, Hershovic A, et al. Phase I/II study of treatment of locally advanced (T3 T4) non-oat cell lung cancer with high dose radiotherapy (rapid fractionation). Radiation Therapy Oncology Group Study. Int J Radiat Oncol Biol Phys 1988;15:1021–1025.
5. Collins TM, Ash DV, Close HJ, Thorogood J. An evaluation of the palliative role of brachytherapy in inoperable carcinoma of the bronchus. Clin Radiol 1988;39:284–286.

6. Eisert DR, Cox JD, Komaki R. Irradiation for bronchial carcinoma: reasons for failure. Cancer 1976;37:2665–2670.

7. Salazar OM, Rubin P, Brown JC, et al. Predictors of radiation response in lung cancer. Cancer 1976;37:333–336.

8. Perez CA, Stanley K, Rubin P, et al. Patterns of tumor recurrence after definitive irradiation for inoperable non-oat cell carcinoma of the lung. Int J Radiat Oncol Biol Phys 1980; 6:987–994.

9. Luomanen R, Watson W. Autopsy findings. In: Watson W, ed. Lung cancer: a study of five thousand Memorial Hospital cases. St. Louis: CV Mosby, 1968:504–510.

10. Roach M, Leidholdt EM, Tatera BS, Joseph J. Endobronchial radiation therapy (EBRT) in the management of lung cancer. Int J Radiat Oncol Biol Phys 1990;18:1449–1454.

11. Hall EJ. Radiotherapy for the radiologist. Philadelphia: Harper & Row, 1978:1505–161.

12. Cotter GW, Herbert DE, Ellingwood KE. Inoperable endobronchial obstructing lung carcinoma treated with combined endobronchial and external beam irradiation. Southern Med J 1991:84;562–565.

13. Schray MF, McDougall JC, Martinez A, et al. Management of malignant airway obstruction using an iridium-192 afterloading technique in conjunction with the neodymium-YAG laser. Int J Radiat Biol Phys 1985;11:403–409.

14. Allen MD, Baldwin JC, Fish VJ, et al. Combined laser therapy and endobronchial radiotherapy for unresectable lung carcinoma with bronchial obstruction. Am J Surg 1985;150:71–77.

15. Lang N, Maners A, Broadwater J, et al. Management of airway problems in lung cancer patients using the neodymium-YAG laser and endobronchial radiotherapy. Am J Surg 1988;156:463–465.

16. Yankauer S. Two cases of lung tumor treated bronchoscopically. N Y Med J 1922; 115:741–742.

17. Kernan JD. Carcinoma of the lung and bronchus treated with radon implantation and diathermy. Arch Otolaryngol 1933;17: 457–475.

18. Pool JL. Bronchoscopy in the treatment of lung cancer. Ann Oto Rhinol Laryngol 1961; 70:1172–1178.

19. Hilaris BS, Martini N, Luomanen RK. Endobronchial interstitial implantation. Clin Bull 1979;9:17–20.

20. Mendiondo OA, Dillon M, Beach LJ. Endobronchial brachytherapy in the treatment of recurrent bronchogenic carcinoma. Int J Radiat Biol Phys 1983;9:579–582.

21. Schray MF, Martinez A, McDougall JC, et al. Malignant airway obstruction: management with temporary intraluminal brachytherapy and laser treatment. Endocurie Hypertherm Oncol 1985;1:237–245.

22. Seagren SL, Harrell JH, Horn RA. High dose rate intraluminal irradiation in recurrent endobronchial carcinoma. Chest 1985;86:810–814.

23. Nori D, Hilaris BS, Martini N. Intraluminal irradiation in bronchogenic carcinoma. Surg Clin North Am 1987;67:1093–1102.

24. Schray MD, McDougall JC, Martinez A, et al. Management of malignant airway compromise with laser and low dose rate brachytherapy, the Mayo Clinic experience. Chest 1988;93: 264–269.

25. Miller JI, Phillips TW. Neodymium-YAG laser and brachytherapy in the management of inoperable bronchogenic carcinoma. Activity Selectron Brachytherapy Journal Suppl 1990; 1:23–29.

26. Stout R, Burt PA, Barber PV, et al. HDR brachytherapy for palliation and cure in bronchial carcinoma: the Manchester experience using a single dose technique. Activity Selectron Brachytherapy Journal Suppl 1990;1:48–50.

27. Speiser B, Spratling L. Intermediate dose rate remote afterloading brachytherapy for intraluminal control of bronchogenic carcinoma. Int J Radiat Biol Phys 1990;18:1443–1448.

28. Dumon JF, Reboud E, Garbe A, et al. Treatment of tracheobronchial lesions by laser photoresection. Chest 1982;81:278–284.

29. Toty L, Personne C, Colchen A, et al. Bronchoscopic management of tracheal lesions using the neodymium yttrium aluminum-garnet laser. Thorax 1981;36:175–178.

30. McDougall JC, Cortese DA. Neodymium-YAG laser therapy of malignant airway obstruction. A preliminary report. Mayo Clinic Proc 1983; 58:35–39.

31. Unger M, Atkinson GW. Nd-YAG endobronchial photoradiation therapy. Am Rev Respir Dis 1983;127:83–90.

32. Gelb AF, Epstein JP. Laser in treatment of lung cancer. Chest 1984;86:662–666.

33. Arabian A, Spagnolo SV. Laser therapy in

patients with primary lung cancer. Chest 1984;86:519–523.

34. Mehta MP, Shahabi S, Jarjour NN, et al. Endobronchial irradiation for malignant airway obstruction. Int J Radiat Biol Phys 1989;17:847–851.

35. Fish VJ, Cannon WB, Ray GH, et al. Treatment of malignant tumor causing obstruction of major airways using intrabronchial brachytherapy. Endocurie Hypertherm Oncol 1985;1: 177–183.

Bronchoscopy in Foreign Body Removal

David P. Meeker and Atul C. Mehta

20

Foreign body (FB) aspiration remains a common worldwide problem (1-6). Most cases occur in children less than 3 years of age, but a significant number of cases occur in older children and adults. Originally associated with a high mortality rate particularly in children, FB aspiration-associated mortality has fallen with the advent of bronchoscopy. Gustav Killian has been credited with performing the first bronchoscopic removal of a FB in 1887 (6). Improved bronchoscopic and anesthetic techniques have resulted in a current mortality rate of less than one percent.

This chapter reviews the clinical and radiographic presentation of FB aspiration, associated complications, and the available techniques for FB removal. Specific attention will be paid to the relative advantages of flexible fiberoptic bronchoscopy (FOB) and rigid bronchoscopy.

Clinical Presentation

Foreign body aspiration remains predominantly a problem of childhood. As outlined in Table 20.1, the majority of patients in most large series are less than age 3. The tendency of young children to place objects in their mouth, their inability to masticate well, their incomplete control of deglutition, as well as a propensity toward laughing, talking, crying, or playing with food or objects in their mouth predisposes to FB aspiration. A careful history will elicit the diagnosis in 40% to 50% or

more of the patients (3,5,7). Although the classic triad of coughing, choking, and wheezing is present in only a small percentage of patients, 80% or more will have at least one feature of the triad (5,8,9).

Many patients present after a significant delay despite having a witnessed choking event. In several large series 34% to 60% of patients presented within 24 hours of aspiration (1,8,10); 20% to 50% may present after a delay of days to weeks and most series included some patients with a delay of months to years (4,8,11). In patients presenting after a significant delay, the coughing episode usually subsides and the presenting manifestations may include fever (3,8,11,12), phlegm production (1,3,8,10), and hemoptysis (12).

Patients with laryngotracheal obstruction may present with stridor, severe dyspnea, cyanosis, and rarely full cardiopulmonary arrest (8). Esclamado and coworkers (13) reviewed 20 cases of laryngotracheal FB aspiration in children. Ninety percent presented with a history of choking or aspiration. Eleven of 20 (55%) presented within 24 hours and 19 (95%) were correctly diagnosed within one week. Nine of the patients were initially misdiagnosed as croup (5 patients), pneumonia/bronchiolitis (3 patients), and asthma (11 patients). The complication rate was significantly higher, 6 of 9 (67%) versus 3 of 11 (27%), in those patients with a delay in diagnosis of greater than 24 hours. Early complications included 2 cases of cardiopulmonary

Table 20.1. Foreign Body Aspiration

First Author	No. of Patients	Age	Delay in Diagnosis	Organic Material (%)
Banerjee (8)	223	63% < 3 y	52% < 24 h	66
Puhakka (10)	83	55% < 2 y	60% < 24 h	59
Weissberg (11)	66	40% < 2 y	53% < 24 h	67
Elhassani (1)	1822	"Majority" 1–2 y	34% < 24 h	81
McGuirt (2)	88	61% < 3 y	NA	66
Steen (3)	94	77% 1–3 y	70% < 72 h	89
Daniilidis (4)	90	65% < 2	29% < 24 h	78
Wiseman (5)	157	80% < 3 y	46% < 24 h	65
Kosloske (18)	41	50% < 16 mo	50% < 48 h	71
Black (9)	262	81% < 3 y	61% < 48 d	74
Abdulmajid (7)	250	42% < 2 y	NA	85

NA, Not available

arrest, one of whom died. Late complications consisted of subglottic edema, aspiration pneumonia, respiratory failure, and bilateral pneumothorax. Their review underscores the greater morbidity associated with laryngotracheal FBs and the increased incidence of associated complications when the diagnosis is delayed whether the FB is proximally or distally located.

Radiographic Presentation

The chest radiograph is of only limited help in the diagnosis of FB aspiration. A definitive diagnosis can be made in the small percentage of patients with an opaque aspirated FB. Subtle signs such as air trapping may be present in 40% to 50% of patients (8,9), with atelectasis and pulmonary infiltrates present in a smaller percentage (8,9). Fluoroscopy may identify a mediastinal shift during active respiration confirming air trapping in the patient with a normal film (2,5).

Unusual radiographic presentations such as pneumomediastinum in a child less than 2 years of age should suggest FB aspiration (14).

Lateral neck films revealing a subglottic density or swelling may be suggestive in the patient with a laryngotracheal FB (13). However, initial localization of the FB by chest radiograph does not negate the need to perform a complete endobronchial examination because the object can change position between the time of the initial radiographic examination and FB removal (11). Furthermore, other FBs in addition to the one suggested by the chest radiograph may be present in the airway (2).

Type of Foreign Body

The majority of aspirated FBs consist of organic material. Cultural differences account for the diversity in the most commonly aspirated materials. Peanuts universally head the list of series originating from the United States and northern Europe with an incidence of 30% to 50% (2,3,5,8,10). Pumpkin seeds accounted for 22 of 90 (24%) of cases reported from Greece with peanuts the second most commonly aspirated substance at 12 of 90 (13%) (4). Melon seeds are commonly aspirated in Middle Eastern countries (1,7). Watermelon seeds accounted for 1208 of 1822 (66%) of cases of

FB aspiration in a series from Iraq where watermelon is eaten frequently and young children are often given fruit without the seeds removed (1). Prayer beads and worry beads are common in Islamic countries and explain their prominence in 42 of 188 (22%) cases among the nonorganic types of foreign body (1).

Lifestyle may predispose to unusual types of aspiration. Nussbaum and colleagues (15) reported 9 cases of hypodermic needle aspiration in drug addicts who held the needle between their lips while drawing heroin into the syringe. Similarly, activities such as the use of a blow gun may result in aspiration of the dart (16). Finally, in rare cases, FBs may migrate from other parts of the body into the endobronchial tree as in the case of a intracervical Steinmann pin that migrated through the posterior tracheal wall and lodged in the left bronchus (17).

Different objects pose different challenges to the bronchoscopist attempting their removal. As discussed below, identification of the type of FB enables the bronchoscopist to choose the appropriate instruments and approach as well as to anticipate complications.

Location of the Foreign Body

A greater percentage of FBs tend to lodge in the right bronchus, most likely related to the less acute angle between trachea and bronchus. Reported right versus left bronchus aspirations range from 30% to 40% on the left to 40% to 70% on the right with a smaller percentage, 10% to 20%, lodging in the laryngotracheal area (2,7,8,10,18). Aspirated material may be located bilaterally in a small percentage of cases (5).

Foreign Body Aspiration in Adults

Foreign body aspiration in the adult is much less common than in children and has received proportionately less attention in the medical literature. However, most series not limited to children include some adults, and several authors have specifically examined the issue of adult FB aspiration (19–21). Limper and coworkers (19) reviewed data on 60 adults with FB aspiration presenting to the Mayo Clinic between 1956 and 1989. The median age was 60 with a range of 18 to 88 and a predominance of cases in the seventh decade.

As in children, vegetable matter was most commonly aspirated, 24 of 60 (40%). Most aspirations occurred in patients with a normal sensorium. Dental equipment or prostheses, tracheostomy tube segments, and endotracheal tube appliances inadvertently lost in the airway comprised the second largest group, 19 of 60 (31%). A miscellaneous assortment of nonorganic items such as pins, coins, and a beverage can top accounted for the remaining 17. Eleven of 60 (18%) patients had primary neurologic disorders such as seizures, mental retardation, or a prior cerebral vascular accident. Trauma with cervical facial injury and loss of consciousness was a factor in 6 and alcohol or sedative use contributed to aspiration in 5 patients. The supine position and local anesthesia contributed to the high frequency of aspirated dental-related equipment. Forty-seven of 48 conscious patients were symptomatic with cough being most commonly reported; the remaining 12 patients were comatose at the time of FB aspiration.

As previously noted, cultural (1), occupational (22), or lifestyle (15) preferences may predispose to specific types of aspiration. For example, aspiration of small animal bones is common in an area where small game is cooked in the form of a soup or stew (20). Needle aspiration occurs more frequently in the drug addict population (15).

The median delay between symptom onset and bronchoscopy was 10 days with a range of 1 hour to 13 years. Delay often occurred because patients ignored their symptoms or were misdiagnosed and initially received alternate treatment. Interestingly, Lan and associates (21) in a series from Taiwan also reported a significant delay between symptom onset and bronchoscopy with 21 of 33 patients presenting more than one week after the onset of symptoms. The delay in diagnosis in both series underscores a decreased awareness of the possibility of FB aspiration in the adult on the part of the patient and physician. Conceivably, the aspirated FB may be less likely to cause severe respiratory distress in the larger adult airways; a picture of obstruction or postobstructive pneumonia may be slower to develop, again leading to a delay in diagnosis.

Aspirated FBs in the adult airway may be misdiagnosed as more commonly occurring endobronchial lesions such as tumors. Figure 20.1 reveals an aspirated tooth cap removed from the right bronchus in a patient referred with a diagnosis of cancer. The off-white color of the dental cap along with the surrounding granulation tissue contributed to the misdiagnosis.

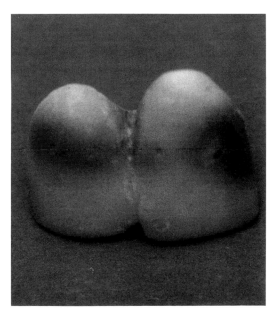

Figure 20.1. Aspirated tooth cap.

Management of Foreign Body Aspiration

The patient with suspected FB aspiration should remain under medical observation until the diagnosis can be confirmed or excluded and an appropriate management plan for its removal is devised; sudden, proximal migration of the FB to the trachea may lead to asphyxiation and cardiopulmonary arrest, particularly in the small child (18,23). Once an FB is identified, it should be removed promptly. The likelihood and extent of tissue reaction increases the longer an FB remains in the airway (3,5,24). Wiseman (5) noted absent or mild endobronchial inflammation in 96% of 72 patients presenting less than 24 hours after aspiration. Severe bronchial inflammation defined by the presence of erythema, edema, granulation tissue, and purulent secretions was noted in 36% of 85 patients presenting more than 24 hours after the event. However, in the absence of acute respiratory distress a delay of several hours to ensure an organized coordinated approach to removal is appropriate.

Rigid bronchoscopy, FOB, and chest physical therapy have been proposed as possible management strategies. Thoracotomy has been required in a small number of cases where the above strategies fail or resection of a bronchiectatic segment is required (1,10). Nonremoval of a nonobstructing inert FB may be appropriate in selected cases, avoiding the morbidity associated with thoracotomy. The relative advantages and disadvantages of each therapeutic option will be discussed.

Postural Drainage

Cotton and coworkers (25) in 1973 reported their experience with bronchodilator inhalation and postural drainage in FB removal in 24 children aged 10 months to 16 years. Twenty-two of 24 patients successfully coughed up the FB; the other 2 patients experienced cardiopulmonary arrest following proximal migration of the object. In a report from the same institution, Campbell and colleagues (26) proposed a dual approach to FB removal. Centrally located FBs, 29 of 57 (51%), were removed directly by rigid bronchoscopy. Children with peripherally located FBs, 28 of 57 (49%), received 48 hours of postural drainage. The object was successfully coughed out in 18 (64%) with 8 of 10 remaining FBs removed via rigid bronchoscopy. No major complications were encountered. Hospital stay was slightly longer (4.2 versus 3.4 days) in the chest physical therapy group. Law and Kosloske (24) subsequently compared postural drainage and bronchoscopy. The FB was successfully cleared in 12 of 49 (25%) of children treated with postural drainage as compared to 56 of 63 (89%) FBs successfully removed with rigid bronchoscopy. Complications were higher and hospital stay was longer in those patients requiring bronchoscopy after a failed course of chest physical therapy. Respiratory arrest was not reported in that series, but the same authors subsequently reported a cardiopulmonary arrest after postural drainage using the same protocol at their institution (27).

In summary, bronchodilator inhalation and postural drainage are not recommended in the initial management of FB aspiration; proximal migration of the FB may lead to cardiopulmonary arrest in a small percentage of patients. A delay in proceeding to bronchoscopy increases the risk of complications such as pneumonia and atelectasis while decreasing the likelihood of successful bronchoscopic removal. Recent advances in bronchoscopic technology make bronchoscopy a safe, reliable, and superior method of FB removal. Furthermore, bronchoscopy permits direct visualization of the bronchial tree to ensure complete removal of the FB.

Rigid Bronchoscopy

Rigid bronchoscopy has been extensively used in FB removal and is currently recommended as the procedure of choice by many authors. The development of the Hopkins rod-lense magnification system has significantly improved airway visualization over that afforded by the open tube bronchoscope. The success rate using rigid bronchoscopy exceeds 95% to 99% in several large reported series (1,3,4,7,9, 10,18,19). Rigid bronchoscopy in the pediatric population is performed under general anesthesia. Ventilation may be achieved via the bronchoscope and complete control of the airway is ensured. A variety of bronchoscopic sizes are available, increasing in size from a 4-mm outer diameter sheath for use in infants.

In addition to improved airway visualization, the development of more sophisticated extraction instruments has contributed to the improved success rate for bronchoscopic FB removal. Available instruments include the optical forceps that permit complete visualization of both the FB and the grasping jaws during use of the instrument (9). Alligator forceps, four-prong flexible grasping hooks, the Dormier basket, and the Fogarty balloon are also available (Figure 20.2) (23).

The type of FB should dictate the choice of extraction instrument. Depending on the location of the FB, more than one instrument is frequently used. Forceps are used in the removal of the flat nonorganic FB (Plate 48). However, forceps may fracture the round organic FB during attempted removal (18). The basket (28) or the Fogarty balloon technique described by Kosloske (29) are more appropriate in this instance. Figure 20.3 reveals a pea embedded in the bronchus and its subsequent intact removal with a Dormier basket. The pea readily fractured as it was removed from the basket. The Fogarty balloon technique consists of passing the balloon distal to the FB. The inner sheath and telescope are then withdrawn 8 to 10 mm within the outer sheath, creating a hollow space in the tip of the bronchoscope. The balloon is inflated and the FB is retracted into the tip of the bronchoscope. Once secured, the entire

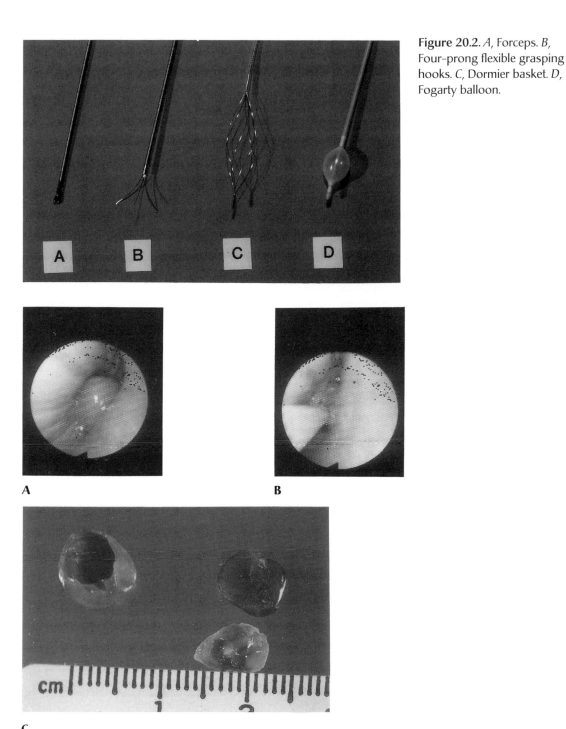

Figure 20.2. *A*, Forceps. *B*, Four-prong flexible grasping hooks. *C*, Dormier basket. *D*, Fogarty balloon.

A

B

C

Figure 20.3. Clockwise from upper left: *A*, Pea imbedded in main stem bronchus. *B*, Pea encircled by Dormier basket. *C*, Pea was removed in one piece, but fragmented with removal from the basket.

assembly is removed. Complications with this technique are rare although separation of a catheter tip in the bronchial tree has been reported related to excessive traction on the Fogarty balloon catheter (30).

More unusual presentations have mandated an equally creative approach to FB removal. Robinson (31) described a toothpick device used to manipulate an FB in the airway, thereby permitting its removal with the forceps, and a specially designed corkscrew to remove a plastic bullet with a central hole.

The sharp FB poses its own unique set of challenges. For example, the sharp end of an aspirated needle may imbed in the airway mucosa. Bending the needle in the middle may disengage the needle tip allowing its safe removal. If possible, sharp objects should be removed along with the bronchoscope with the pointed end shielded within the bronchoscope to minimize trauma to the airway mucosa and lessen the likelihood the object will be lost passing through the glottis (15). Rigid bronchoscopy is preferable in this setting because it affords better control of the sharp object.

Inflammation and the development of surrounding granulation tissue may impede or prevent removal of some FBs. Neodymium:yttrium-aluminum-garnet (Nd:YAG) laser has been used to vaporize the granulation tissue freeing the FB (32,33). Nd:YAG laser poses additional risks and should be used only by those endoscopists skilled in its use. In occasional instances, it may avoid the need for a thoracotomy when more traditional extraction methods have failed.

Flexible Fiberoptic Bronchoscopy

The development of flexible FOB has revolutionized the practice of pulmonary medicine. Increased experience with FOB has broadened the indication for its use to areas such as laser therapy, endobronchial radiation, and not surprisingly FB removal. In addition to increased experience with FOB, the development of more sophisticated instruments has increased the safety and viability of FOB as a therapeutic alternative to rigid bronchoscopy. Zavala and Rhodes (28,34) described using a variety of different extraction instruments in an artificial and animal model using the flexible bronchoscope. As listed in Table 20.2, FOB offers a number of advantages over rigid bronchoscopy. The procedure may be safely performed with the use of mild sedation and topical anesthesia eliminating the risk of general anesthesia. The flexible scope permits a more thorough airway examination and removal of the distally located FB out of reach of the rigid bronchoscope (15,35,36). The procedure may be performed through an endotracheal tube, guaranteeing continued control of the airway in the mechanically ventilated patient. However, objects too large to be removed through the scope and the endotracheal tube may require removal of the FB, scope, and endotracheal tube simultaneously with immediate reintubation (37). Loss of the FB as the assembly is pulled through the cords is a major concern with this maneuver. Skilled personnel and appropriate equipment for resuscitation should be immediately available. Flexible FOB may also be performed in the patient with a neck injury without further risk to the spine.

Limitations associated with the use of FOB in FB removal are listed in Table 20.3. Many FBs are too large to be retracted through the narrow channel of the flexible scope. Successful removal in this case necessitates removal of the scope along with the FB with the risk of losing the unshielded object in the subglottic area. The narrow channel also limits the size of the extraction instruments available for use with the flexible scope. Lost objects may fall to a more distal location, further complicating their attempted removal. Small extraction instruments may result in

Table 20.2. Advantages of Flexible Fiberoptic Bronchoscopy

Increased experience

Improved instruments

Small objects/peripheral airways

Use of local anesthesia and preservation of cough reflex

May be performed via endotracheal tube

Use in patients with cervical facial injury

Table 20.3. Disadvantages of Flexible Fiberoptic Bronchoscopy

Narrow channel

Small extraction instruments

Potential for distal displacement of the foreign body

Loss of objects in subglottic area

Fracture of organic objects

Limited use in pediatric patients

fracture of organic material with incomplete removal from the airway.

Each of the above limitations is magnified in the smaller airway of the pediatric patient. Although FOB is safely performed in the pediatric population, most authors agree FB removal in a child should only be attempted with a rigid bronchoscope (38,39). Rigid bronchoscopy ensures better control of the airway and decreases the risk of sudden asphyxiation due to loss of the FB during attempted removal in a large airway.

Wood and Gauderer (38) have advocated the diagnostic use of the flexible scope in pediatric patients with a questionable diagnosis of FB aspiration. FBs were identified in 10 of 52 (19%) of cases in their series. Patients with a definite diagnosis of FB aspiration went directly for open tube bronchoscopy; FBs identified by FOB were also removed by open tube bronchoscopy. Twelve patients underwent FOB following FB removal to ensure complete removal of the FB. Increased awareness of FOB as a diagnostic option by the referring physician should permit earlier diagnosis of the retained FB.

Most reported cases of FB removal by FOB are in adults (5,15,19,21,27,36,37,40–43). Cunanan (27) successfully used FOB in 89% of 300 cases of FB aspiration. His patients were 10 years or older with most being mentally delayed and physically handicapped. The remaining 11% required rigid bronchoscopy or a combination of the two. Lan and colleagues (21) reported their experience with FOB in 33 adults aged 19 to 78 years. Seventy percent of the patients presented with a FB of one to 19 months duration. The FB was successfully removed at the first bronchoscopy in 9 of 12 patients with minimal surrounding granulation tissue. Two patients required a second bronchoscopy; a third patient subsequently coughed up three broncholiths after three unsuccessful flexible bronchoscopies and one attempted rigid bronchoscopy. FOB successfully identified 18 of 21 (85%) of the chronically impacted FBs. Fifteen of 18 (71%) were successfully removed with one attempt, wheras the remainder required additional bronchoscopies. Endobronchial resection of sur-rounding granulation tissue facilitated FB removal and did not result in significant bleeding.

Foreign body removal using flexible FOB was less successful in a series of 60 adult patients reported from the Mayo Clinic (19). FOB was performed at the discretion of the bronchoscopist. FOB was successful in 14 of 23 (60%) of attempted cases as compared to 43 of 44 (98%) of successful attempts using rigid bronchoscopy, including 6 of 7 cases where FOB had failed. FOB was specifically useful in 2 cases of distally located FBs and one case of severe cervical facial trauma precluding the neck extension required for rigid bronchoscopy. No significant complications were encountered in this series.

Several specific technical aspects related to FB removal via flexible FOB should be considered. FOB should be performed via the oral route as opposed to the nasal route if an FB is suspected. Intubation of the patient over the flexible scope should be considered; the FB that is too large to be extracted through the scope may be shielded by the endotracheal tube again minimizing the risk of losing the FB in the subglottic area. Larger FBs as noted may require simultaneous removal of the endotracheal tube. Movement of an FB to a more proximal airway and then asking the patient to cough is an option in the cooperative adult patient.

Fluoroscopy may be a useful adjunct when the FB is not visible endoscopically. Ali (22) described using a cytology brush to localize a peripherally aspirated nail under fluoroscopy. Forceps were then advanced into the identified subsegment and the nail was successfully removed with fluoroscopic guidance. Saito and colleagues (42) retrieved a broken biopsy forceps using a magnetic extractor, again under fluoroscopic guidance.

Summary

Foreign body aspiration is common in children but may occur in any age group. Organic material is most commonly aspirated. Transient symptoms or lack of suspicion may lead to a delay in diagnosis. Organic material may swell as it absorbs moisture, but it does not dissolve, leading to late complications such as postobstructive pneumonia and bronchiectasis. Radiography may be useful in individual cases, but bronchoscopy remains the diagnostic procedure of choice. Rigid bronchoscopy should be used in the pediatric population, although flexible FOB is a useful diagnostic procedure in questionable cases. Rigid bronchoscopy offers the advantages of airway control, larger extraction instruments, and an increased ability to manipulate the FB. Most cases are performed under general anesthesia although it may be performed with topical anesthesia and sedation alone (19). Flexible FOB has been used increasingly in the adult population. Increased experience, improved instrumentation, and the ability to remove distally located FBs has made it a viable therapeutic alternative in specific cases. Furthermore, the combined use of the rigid bronchoscope and the flexible bronchoscope may be preferable in other cases. FB removal should be attempted by those skilled in this procedure and fully aware of the possible complications.

REFERENCES

1. Elhassani NB. Tracheobronchial foreign bodies in the Middle East: a Baghdad study. J Thorac Cardiovasc Surg 1988;96:621–625.
2. McGuirt WF, Holmes KD, Feehs R, Browne JD. Tracheobronchial foreign bodies. Laryngoscope 1988;98:615–618.
3. Steen KH, Zimmerman T. Tracheobronchial aspiration of foreign bodies in children: a study of 94 cases. Laryngoscope 1990;100:525–530.
4. Daniilidis J, Symeonidis B, Triaridis K, Kouloulas A. Foreign body in the airways: a review of 90 cases. Arch Otolaryngol 1977;103:570–573.
5. Wiseman NE. The diagnosis of foreign body aspiration in childhood. J Pediat Surg 1984;19:531–535.
6. Aytac A, Yurdakul Y, Ikizler C, Olga R, Saylam A. Inhalation of foreign bodies in children: report of 500 cases. J Thorac Cardiovasc Surg 1977;74:145–151.
7. Abdulmajid OA, Ebeid AM, Motaweh MM, Kleibo IS. Aspirated foreign bodies in the tracheobronchial tree: report of 250 cases. Thorax 1976;31:635–640.
8. Banerjee A, Subba Rao KSVK, Khanna SK, et al. Laryngo-tracheo-bronchial foreign bodies in children. J Laryngol Otol 1988;102:1029–1032.
9. Black RE, Choi KJ, Syme WC, Johnson DG, Matlak ME. Bronchoscopic removal of aspirated foreign bodies in children. Am J Surg 1984;148:778–781.
10. Puhakka H, Svedstrom E, Kero P, Valli P, Iisao E. Tracheobronchial foreign bodies: a persistent problem in pediatric patients. Am J Dis Child 1989;143:543–545.
11. Weissberg D, Schwartz I. Foreign bodies in the tracheobronchial tree. Chest 1987;91:730–733.
12. Pattison CW, Leaming AJ, Townsend ER. Hidden foreign body as a cause of recurrent hemoptysis in a teenage girl. Ann Thorac Surg 1988;45:330–331.
13. Esclamado RM, Richardson MA. Laryngotracheal foreign bodies in children. Am J Dis Child 1987;141:259–262.
14. Burton EM, Riggs W Jr, Kaufman RA, Houston CS. Pneumomediastinum caused by foreign body aspiration in children. Pediatr Radiol 1989;20:45–47.

15. Nussbaum M, Nash M, Cho H, Cohen J, Pincus R. Hypodermic needles: an unusual tracheobronchial foreign body. Ann Otol Rhinol Laryngol 1987;96:698–700.

16. Salm TJV, Ellis N. Blowgun dart aspiration. J Thorac Cardiovasc Surg 1986;91:930–932.

17. Richardson M, Gomes M, Tsou E. Trans-tracheal migration of an intravertebral Steinmann pin to the left bronchus. J Cardiovasc Surg 1987;93:939–941.

18. Kosloske AM. Bronchoscopic extraction of aspirated foreign bodies in children. Am J Dis Child 1982;136:924–927.

19. Limper AH, Prakash UBS. Tracheobronchial foreign bodies in adults. Ann Intern Med 1990;112:604–609.

20. Casson AG, Guy JRF. Foreign-body aspiration in adults. Can J Surg 1987;30:193–194.

21. Lan RS, Lee CH, Chiang YC, Wang WJ. Use of fiberoptic bronchoscopy to retrieve bronchial foreign bodies in adults. Am Rev Respir Dis 1989;140:1734–1737.

22. Ali MM. Retrieval of a construction nail from a peripheral airway. Chest 1988;94:224.

23. Kosloske AM. Tracheobronchial foreign bodies in children: back to the bronchoscope and a balloon. Pediatrics 1980;66:321–323.

24. Law D, Kosloske AM. Management of tracheobronchial foreign bodies in children: a reevaluation of postural drainage and bronchoscopy. Pediatrics 1976;58:361–367.

25. Cotton EK, Abrams G, Vanhoutte J, Burrington J. Removal of aspirated foreign bodies by inhalation and postural drainage. Clin Pediat 1973;12:270–276.

26. Campbell DN, Cotton EK, Lilly JR. A dual approach to tracheobronchial foreign bodies in children. Surgery 1982;91:178–182.

27. Cunanan OS. The flexible fiberoptic bronchoscope in foreign body removal: experience in 300 cases. Chest 1978;73:725–726.

28. Zavala DC, Rhodes ML. Foreign body removal: a new role for the fiberoptic bronchoscope. Ann Otol 1975;84:650–656.

29. Kosloske AM. The Fogarty balloon technique for the removal of foreign bodies from the tracheobronchial tree. Surg Gynecol Obstet 1982;155:72–73.

30. Carpenter RJ III, Snyder GG III. A complication in the use of a Fogarty catheter for foreign body removal during bronchoscopic management. Otolaryngol Head Neck Surg 1981;89:998–1000.

31. Robinson CLN. New bronchoscopic instruments: a toothpick and a corkscrew. Can J Surg 1991;34:13–14.

32. Hayashi AH, Gillis DA, Bethune D, Hughes D, O'Neil M. Management of foreign-body bronchial obstruction using endoscopic laser therapy. J Pediat Surg 1990;25:1174–1176.

33. Unger M. Neodymium YAG laser therapy for malignant and benign endobronchial obstructions. Clin Chest Med 1985;6:277–290.

34. Zavala DC, Rhodes ML. Experimental removal of foreign bodies by fiberoptic bronchoscopy. Am Rev Respir Dis 1974;110:357–360.

35. Lillington GA, Ruhl RA, Peirce TH, Gorin AB. Removal of endobronchial foreign body by fiberoptic bronchoscopy. Am Rev Respir Dis 1976;113:387–391.

36. Smith LJ, Khan MA. Role of fiberoptic bronchoscopy in removal of a foreign body. Chest 1977;72:264.

37. Verea-Hernando H, Garcia-Quijada RC, Ruiz De Galarreta AA. Extraction of foreign bodies with fiberoptic bronchoscopy in mechanically ventilated patients. Am Rev Respir Dis 1990;142:258.

38. Wood RE, Gauderer MWL. Flexible fiberoptic bronchoscopy in the management of tracheobronchial foreign bodies in children: the value of a combined approach with open tube bronchoscopy. J Pediat Surg 1984;19:693–698.

39. Nussbaum E. Flexible fiberoptic bronchoscopy and laryngoscopy in infants and children. Laryngoscope 1983;93:1073–1075.

40. Clark PT, Williams TJ, Teichtahl H, Bowes G, Tuxen DV. Removal of proximal and peripheral endobronchial foreign bodies with the flexible fiberoptic bronchoscope. Anaesth Intensive Care 1989;17:205–208.

41. Wager GC, Williams JH Jr. Flexible bronchoscopic removal of radioccult polyurethane foam, with pneumonitis in a hyperventilated lobe. Am Rev Respir Dis 1990;142:1222–1224.

42. Saito H, Saka H, Sakai S, Shimokata K. Removal of broken fragment of biopsy forceps with magnetic extractor. Chest 1989;95:700–701.

43. Klayton RJ, Donlan CJ, O'Neil TJ, Foreman DR. Foreign body removal via fiberoptic bronchoscopy. JAMA 1975;234:806.

The Role of Bronchoscopy in Hemoptysis

21

Sunit R. Patel and James K. Stoller

Hemoptysis is the coughing up of blood from a source below the glottis (1). It is a common clinical symptom (2) that has been reported to be responsible for 6.8% of outpatient chest clinic visits (3), 11% of admissions to the hospital chest service (4), 38% of patients referred to a chest surgical practice (5), and up to 15% of all pulmonary consultations (6). Hemoptysis poses a great diagnostic challenge because it has been described in many cardiopulmonary diseases and some hematologic disorders (7–11). Most episodes of hemoptysis are reportedly associated with chronic bronchitis, bronchiectasis, bronchogenic carcinoma, or tuberculosis (4,7,8,12–15). However, over the years the spectrum of leading causes of hemoptysis has been changing, perhaps contributing to the diagnostic dilemma (4,7,16,17).

The four major concerns in evaluating hemoptysis are to rule out bronchogenic cancer, determine whether the underlying cause is treatable, localize the site of bleeding in case further therapeutic intervention is needed (6), and decide which treatment to implement if the bleeding persists, recurs, or is massive and when to treat. In this regard, bronchoscopy (particularly flexible fiberoptic bronchoscopy [FOB]) has assumed a central role in diagnosis and localization of bleeding and also in performing different therapeutic interventions to control bleeding (18). Indeed, hemoptysis is one of the most frequent indications for bronchoscopy, accounting for 10% to 30% of bronchoscopic procedures in major medical centers (7,15,19,20). For example, a 1989 survey of 871 bronchoscopists in North America, conducted by the American College of Chest Physicians (ACCP), reported that 81.1% of respondents listed hemoptysis as one of five most common indications for bronchoscopy. Overall, hemoptysis was the second most commonly cited indication for bronchoscopy (21).

With this background, this chapter reviews the definitions, pathogenesis, and differential diagnosis of hemoptysis and provides a systematic diagnostic approach to patients with hemoptysis, emphasizing the role of bronchoscopy in both diagnosis and therapy.

Definitions and Characterization of Hemoptysis in Available Literature

Defining by Severity: Massive and Nonmassive Hemoptysis

Hemoptysis may range from a small amount of blood-streaked sputum to a massive amount of bleeding that causes asphyxiation and exsanguination. Because the overall management of hemoptysis depends on the severity of bleeding, most authors distinguish between massive (e.g., potentially life-threatening) and nonmassive hemoptysis (1,11,22,23). Although no clear-cut definitions of nonmassive hemoptysis are available, hemoptysis has been arbitrarily graded as small or mild when the amount ranges from blood-tinged sputum to less than 15 to 30 mL over 24 hours (1,23,24). The term "gross" or "frank"

298

hemoptysis is sometimes used to refer to a quantity of bleeding that is smaller than massive but greater than blood streaking (11).

Table 21.1 summarizes different available definitions of massive hemoptysis, which subsume definitions based on the volume of expectorated blood (e.g., at least 600 mL/24 h) and those based on the magnitude of the clinical effect associated with hemoptysis (e.g., hemoptysis threatening asphyxia) (2,25–30). The most lenient volume definition of massive hemoptysis has been proposed by Amirana and colleagues (25) and Bobrowitz and coworkers (26) (expectorating 100 mL or more of blood a day at least once). At the other extreme of volume definitions are those proposed by Crocco and associates (27) (more than 600 mL of expectorated blood in 48 hours) and Corey and Hla (28) (1000 mL or more of expectorated blood in 24 hours).

As an alternative to volume definitions, other authors have defined massive hemoptysis by the magnitude of the clinical consequences. For example, based on the fact that

Table 21.1. Definitions of Massive Hemoptysis

Massive hemoptysis
   Spectrum of "volume" definitions
      ≥ 100 mL/24 h (25,26)
      > 600 mL/48 h (27)
      Major (≥ 200 mL/24 h) versus massive
      (≥ 1000 mL/24 h) (28)
"Magnitude of effect" definitions (29)
   Presents risk of large aspiration
   Life-threatening by virtue of airway
      obstruction, hypotension, or anemia
Exsanguinating hemoptysis (30)
   Hemoptysis that threatens because of actual
      volume of blood lost
   Loss of ≥ 1000 mL total at rate of ≥ 150 mL/h
Commonly accepted definition (31–36)
   ≥ 600 mL over 24 h

Modified and reproduced with permission from Stoller JK. Diagnosis and management of massive hemoptysis: a review. Respir Care 1992;32:564–581.

the anatomic dead space of the measured airways is 100 to 200 mL in most individuals, massive hemoptysis has been defined as the volume of expectorated blood that poses risk for lung aspiration or that is life-threatening by virtue of airway obstruction, hypotension, or blood loss. Finally, an operational definition of massive hemoptysis has been proposed by Holsclaw and colleagues (29), who offer three criteria for massive hemoptysis as pulmonary bleeding that causes death or requires hospitalization, is large enough to give laboratory or clinical evidence of systemic blood loss, or requires blood or plasma transfusion.

Garzon and coworkers (30) distinguished "exsanguinating" hemoptysis as pulmonary bleeding that is brisk enough to threaten life not only by asphyxiation, but also by blood loss itself, that is, a volume of 1000 mL or greater at a rate of at least 150 mL/h.

Although varying definitions have been proposed, a commonly accepted definition of massive hemoptysis is the expectoration of at least 600 mL over 24 hours (31–36). The practical difficulty of measuring the volume of expectorated blood under usual clinical circumstances limits the value of finer distinctions in defining massive hemoptysis (2). Also, beyond the actual quantity of expectorated blood, the rate of bleeding appears to be clinically important (36,37). In a study of 67 patients with at least 600 mL expectorated blood in 48 hours, Crocco and coworkers (27) showed that mortality was strikingly related to bleeding rate regardless of treatment. Specifically, patients expectorating 600 mL of blood over 4 hours had a combined mortality of 71%, those with more than 600 mL in 4 to 6 hours had a 45% mortality, and those with more than 600 mL in 16 to 48 hours had a 5% mortality.

Defining by Cause: Idiopathic Hemoptysis

Despite a careful work-up that includes FOB, the cause of hemoptysis cannot be determined in some patients. This so-called "idiopathic," "essential," or "cryptogenic" hemoptysis has been reported in 2% to 18% of patients with hemoptysis (4,8–10,13,15). The typical presentation and course of idiopathic hemoptysis is a single bout of bleeding with minimal or no respiratory symptoms, a normal chest radiograph, normal bronchoscopic findings, and bronchial washings without evidence of infection or malignancy (7,38). Fortunately, the usual prognosis in "idiopathic hemoptysis" is favorable with resolution of bleeding within 6 months of evaluation (38).

Defining by Cause: Pseudohemoptysis

Pseudohemoptysis is the expectoration of blood from a source other than the lower respiratory tract, causing diagnostic confusion, especially in patients who cannot clearly describe the source of the bleeding (11). In addition to upper gastrointestinal bleeding (hematemesis), which can sometimes mimic true hemoptysis (when the blood is aspirated into the lungs), pseudohemoptysis may occur when blood from the oral cavity (39) or nasopharynx (39,40) drains to the back of the throat and initiates the cough reflex (8). Pseudohemoptysis has also been described in patients with pneumonia from *Serratia marcescens*, when the red-pigment-producing bacteria imparts a red color to the phlegm (41), and in patients with rifampin overdose, when the drug imparts a reddish color to sputum (42).

Defining by Frequency: Recurrent Hemoptysis

Recurrent hemoptysis is usually defined as bleeding episodes that recur at an interval of less than one year (43).

Differential Diagnosis of Hemoptysis and Massive Hemoptysis

Table 21.2 presents the differential diagnosis of hemoptysis, which has been amply described in several reviews (8–11,44).

Changing rates of disease occurrence (e.g., declining rates of new-onset bronchiectasis) and diagnostic advances (e.g., the advent of flexible FOB in the 1970s) likely account for a changing spectrum of the common causes of hemoptysis (2). For centuries, hemoptysis was considered pathognomonic of pulmonary tuberculosis, an association highlighted by the Hippocratic aphorism: "Spitting of pus follows the spitting of blood, consumption follows the spitting of this and death follows consumption" (4). Studies done in the 1940s and 1950s reported tuberculosis, bronchiectasis, and bronchogenic carcinoma as the most common causes of hemoptysis (5,12–15). However, more recent series indicate that hemoptysis is now most commonly caused by bronchitis and less commonly by tuberculosis and bronchiectasis (16,17).

Massive hemoptysis accounts for a minority of patients with hemoptysis (4.8% to 6.7% of hospitalized patients with hemoptysis) (4,28) and the spectrum of causes of massive hemoptysis is narrower (Table 21.3). The most common causes of massive hemoptysis are bronchiectasis, TB (active and inactive), bronchogenic carcinoma, lung abscess, and mycetoma (2,27,30,32,33,45–47), and unlike lesser hemoptysis (for which tuberculosis and bronchiectasis have become less frequent causes) (16,17), the spectrum of causes of massive hemoptysis has changed little among series that span three decades.

Pathophysiology of Hemoptysis

A rational approach to managing hemoptysis requires knowledge of the vascular anatomy of the lungs, which is summarized below. Sources of pulmonary bleeding include the pulmonary circulation, a low pressure circuit (with normal pulmonary artery pressures of 15 to 20 mm Hg systolic and 5 to 10 mm Hg diastolic), and the bronchial circulation, consisting of the bronchial arteries (which branch from the aorta and have systemic arterial pressures),

Table 21.2. Differential Diagnosis of Hemoptysis

Pulmonary Disorders

Infections

Lung abscess

Pneumonia (bacterial or nonbacterial)*

Mycetoma (e.g., aspergilloma)*

Tuberculosis (active or inactive)*

Parenchymal fungal infections
(coccidioidomycosis, mucormycosis,
histoplasmosis, cryptococcosis, etc.)

Parasitic infections (amebiasis, ascariasis,
clonorchiasis, echinococcosis, hookworm
infestations, paragonimiasis,
schistosomiasis, etc.)

Others (actinomycosis, nocardiosis, viral, etc.)

Neoplasms

Bronchogenic carcinoma*

Pulmonary metastasis from extrapulmonary
primary

Bronchial adenoma (including carcinoid
tumors)

Others (sarcoma, hamartoma, hydatidiform
mole, etc.)

Tracheobronchial disease

Acute tracheobronchitis*

Chronic bronchitis*

Aspirated foreign body

Tracheoesophageal or tracheovascular fistula

Mucoid impaction of the bronchus

Bronchiecstasis (including cystic fibrosis)*

Broncholithiasis

Suture granuloma or airway dehiscence at
airway anastomotic site (e.g., in lung
transplant patients)

Bronchial telangiectasia

Congenital disease

Bronchopulmonary sequestration

Bronchogenic cysts

Pulmonary vascular disease

Pulmonary thromboembolism/infarction

Pulmonary venous varix

Pulmonary artery aneurysms

Fat/tumor embolism

Arteriovenous malformation (including
Osler–Weber–Rendu syndrome)

Pulmonary hemorrhage syndromes
(Goodpasture's syndrome, idiopathic
pulmonary hemosiderosis, Wegener's
granulomatosis, etc.)

Vasculitis (Behcet's syndrome, Churg–Strauss
syndrome, Henoch–Schonlein purpura,
systemic lupus erythematosus, rheumatoid
arthritis, scleroderma, mixed cryoglobu-
linemia, mixed connective tissue disease,
IgA nephropathy)

Bronchial artery rupture

Drug/toxin related

Toxic/smoke inhalations

Aspirin

Anticoagulants

Solvents

Penicillamine

Trimellitic anhydride

Inhaled isocyanides

Traumatic

Blunt chest trauma (contusion, hematoma)

Penetrating lung injury

Fractured bronchus

Miscellaneous

Amyloidosis

Endometriosis (catamenial hemoptysis)

Pneumoconiosis

Extrinsic allergic alveolitis

Aspiration of gastric contents

Cardiovascular Diseases

Left ventricular failure*

Mitral stenosis*

Superior vena cava syndrome

Subclavian artery aneurysm

Postmyocardial infarction syndrome

Congenital heart disease

Aortic aneurysm

Cardiac catheterization

Coronary artery bypass grafting

Hematologic Disorders

Coagulopathy

Thrombocytopenia

Disseminated intravascular coagulation

Leukemia

Iatrogenic

Bronchoscopy including laser therapy

Lung biopsy and surgery

Cardiac catheterization

Intubation

Idiopathic

*Common causes

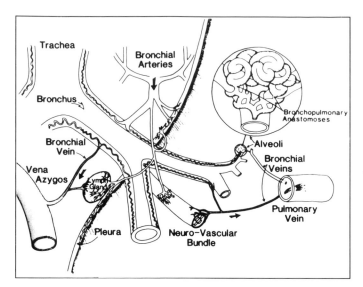

Figure 21.1. Schematic of the systemic blood supply to the lung. Note that flow from the extrapulmonary airways and supporting structures returns to the right heart, whereas intra-pulmonary flow drains into the pulmonary veins and returns to the left heart.

Reproduced by permission from Deffebach ME, Charau NB, Lakshminarayan S. State of the art: the bronchial circulation–small but vital attribute of the lung. Am Rev Respir Dis 1987;135:467.

and the bronchial veins (which drain via systemic veins into the right heart) (2). The bronchial arteries are the main vascular supply to the airways (from the main stem bronchi to terminal bronchioles), and the supporting framework of the lung (i.e., the pleura, intra-pulmonary lymphoid tissue, large branches of the pulmonary vessels, and nerves) (11,48). The pulmonary arteries supply the pulmonary parenchymal tissue including the respiratory bronchioles (11,48). As depicted in Figure 21.1, the bronchial and pulmonary circulations are normally connected; bronchial arterial blood feeding the proximal airways drains into the bronchial veins and empties into the right heart, whereas bronchial arterial blood perfusing the intrapulmonary airways and lung tissue drains through bronchopulmonary anastomoses into the pulmonary veins and left heart (2,49). Anastomoses between bronchial arteries and tributaries of the pulmonary veins have been demonstrated in normal lungs at autopsy and may be a major source of massive hemoptysis (49). Arteriographic studies in patients with active hemoptysis have demonstrated that the usual source of bleeding (92% of cases) is the systemic circulation (50).

Pathogenesis

The pathogenesis of hemoptysis depends on the type and location of the underlying disease

(13). Because a detailed discussion of the pathogenesis of hemoptysis in individual diseases is beyond the scope of this chapter, only the pathogenesis of some of the common causes of hemoptysis is discussed. The reader should refer to other published reviews for further information (10,11,13,36).

In tuberculosis, bleeding may result from several mechanisms (51). First, an acute exudative pneumonia can cause necrosis of adjacent bronchial vessels or local mucosal ulceration (13). In endobronchial tuberculosis, hemoptysis may result from ulceration of the bronchial mucosa or bronchiectasis (11). In healed and fibrotic parenchymal disease, bleeding may arise from irritation of granulation tissue in the walls of bronchiectatic airways in the same areas (11). A healed calcified lymph node may impinge on the bronchial wall and erode into a bronchial lumen; if a blood vessel lies in the path of a broncholith, hemoptysis may result, occasionally associated with coughing up gravel (lithoptysis) (52). Chronic inactive fibrocaseous tuberculosis is a common setting for massive hemoptysis in tuberculosis. Although some controversy surrounds the precise source of the hemoptysis, it is commonly believed that the mechanism of this bleeding is rupture of Rasmussen's aneurysms (51–55), which are ectatic portions of the pulmonary artery traversing the thick-walled cavities caused by tuberculous involvement of the adventitia and media vessels.

In bronchogenic carcinoma, pathologic studies have shown an increase in bronchial arterial supply to the region of the tumor (56). Hemoptysis in cancer results from necrosis, mucosal invasion, or direct local invasion of a blood vessel (10,11,13). About 10% of patients with bronchogenic cancer experience massive hemoptysis during the course of their disease (57). More than 80% of cases of massive hemoptysis in lung cancer are associated with squamous cell carcinoma, which are generally located in the central airways and may cavitate in half the cases (36).

Bronchiectasis is a frequent cause of massive hemoptysis (see Table 21.3). In autopsy specimens from patients with bronchiectasis, Liebow and colleagues (58) reported striking bronchial artery enlargement with tortuosity, marked by increased anastomoses with pulmonary arteries. These investigators postulated that budding capillaries in the granulation tissue of areas with organizing pneumonitis increased the capillary bed supplied by the bronchial arteries, leading to increased load and hypertrophy. In addition, the destruction of the pulmonary arterial capillary bed and local spasm in the pulmonary circulation from hypoxemia and inflammation may cause opening of bronchial-to-pulmonary artery communications and penetration of the high pressure blood flow from the bronchial to the pulmonary circulation (36,59). The enlarged vessels that lie in the wall of the bronchiectatic sacs are susceptible to further injury from the products of local inflammation and infection (36).

Mycetomas result from saprophytic colonization of preexisting cavities from tuberculosis, sarcoidosis, lung abscess, infarction, or bronchiectasis. Putative causes of hemoptysis in this setting include mechanical trauma of the highly vascular granular tissue of the cavity wall (from movement of a fungus ball), release of anticoagulant and trypsin-like pro-teolytic enzymes, aspergillus-associated endotoxin causing vascular injury, or a type III hypersensitivity reaction causing vascular damage (60,61).

In acute left ventricular failure and mitral stenosis, blood-streaked sputum is caused by rupture of pulmonary veins or capillaries or anastomoses between bronchial and pulmonary arteries distended by elevated intravascular pressure or pulmonary venous hypertension (10,56,62).

In both acute and chronic bronchitis, bleeding results from irritation of friable and inflamed mucosa (10,13).

Finally, the pathogenesis of bleeding from a lung abscess is not entirely clear, but may be due to progression of local inflammatory processes causing necrosis of branches of the pulmonary artery (63).

Diagnostic Approach to the Patient with Hemoptysis

All instances of hemoptysis require careful evaluation to determine the cause and to localize the bleeding source. Bronchoscopy is helpful for both of these goals.

Routine Prebronchoscopy Evaluation

The routine evaluation before bronchoscopy is outlined in Table 21.4. In patients with massive hemoptysis, localizing the site of bleeding and specific therapy (including airway maintenance, transfusion, and therapeutic interventions) should proceed simultaneously with diagnostic studies to determine the cause of bleeding (10).

A detailed history and physical examination should be performed to rule out hematemesis and other causes of pseudohemoptysis and to provide clues to the site and cause of hemoptysis. As outlined by Lyons (8), features of blood from the lung that may distinguish between hemoptysis and hematemesis are that blood from the lung is coughed versus vomited, partly frothy, alkaline versus acid (unless

Table 21.3. Causes of Massive Hemoptysis in Selected Series

First Author	Definition	Patient Total	Active	Inactive	Lung Cancer	Bronchiectasis	Abscess	Mitral	Fungoma	Unknown	Other
						Cause of Massive Hemoptysis, % (No.)					
Crocco, 1968 (27)	> 600 mL/48 h	67	49% (33)	24% (16)	8% (5)	10% (7)	9% (6)	–	–	–	–
Garzon, 1974 (32)	≥ 600 mL/24 h	62	26% (16)	47% (29)	3.2% (2)	11.3% (7)	6.5% (4)	–	–	–	6.5% (4)
McCollum, 1975 (46)	Asphyxia threat	15	33% (5)	33% (5)	6.7% (1)*	20% (3)	–	–	13.3% (2)	6.7% (1)	20% (3)
Yang 1978 (47)	> 200 mL/24 h	20	25% (5)	25% (5)	15% (3)	15% (3)	–	5% (1)	5% (1)	10% (2)	–
Garzon, 1982 (30)	> 1000 mL/6 h	24	29% (7)	17% (4)	13% (3)	17% (4)	8% (2)	–	–	8% (2)	8% (2)
Conlan, 1983 (33)	NS	123	38% (47)	–	4.9% (6)	30% (37)	4.9% (6)	–	3.3% (4)	–	18.7% (23)
Ullacker, 1985 (45)	NS	75	76% (57)	–	–	1.3% (1)	2.6% (2)	–	16% (12)	–	3.9% (3)

*Metastatic
NS, not specified
Modified and reproduced with permission from Stoller JK. Diagnosis and management of massive hemoptysis: a review. Respir Care 1992;32:564–581.

Table 21.4. Routine Prebronchoscopic Evaluation*

History and physical examination ± nasopharyngeal evaluation

Complete blood count, urinalysis, coagulation profile (e.g., prothrombin time, partial thromboplastin time)

Chest radiographs (posteroanterior and lateral)

Sputum examination (cytology, acid-fast smear, and culture)

Electrocardiogram

Arterial blood gases (in moderate to massive hemoptysis)

Evaluation can be individualized to each patient.

hematemesis is so massive that stomach acid is neutralized by blood), and mixed with pus, organisms, and macrophages versus sometimes mixed with food. Also, patients with hemoptysis sometimes report gurgling in the chest and may even localize a bleeding site in the thorax versus experiencing nausea and vomiting, as is more typical in upper gastrointestinal bleeding (4). Additional historical clues that may help establish true hemoptysis are reviewed in Table 21.5 (7,10,11,23,44,64).

Physical findings may also offer diagnostic clues (Table 21.6) (10,11,43,64). Finally, routine laboratory studies may help identify the cause of hemoptysis (10,11,43). The complete blood count may suggest the presence of an infection, chronic blood loss (e.g., idiopathic pulmonary hemosiderosis), or a hematologic disorder. Coagulation studies may suggest an underlying hematologic disorder. The electrocardiogram may suggest pulmonary hypertension, mitral stenosis, or ischemic heart disease as a marker of left ventricular dysfunction. The urinalysis may suggest a systemic disease or pulmonary-renal syndrome (e.g., Goodpasture's syndrome, Wegener's granulomatosis). Finally, collection of all expectorated sputum will allow both qualitative examination of the sputum (cytology, smear for acid-fast bacilli, and cultures for tuberculosis, fungi, and bac-

teria) and measurement of the quantity of expectorated blood, although because sputum collection is often unappealing and cumbersome, it is not undertaken.

The chest radiograph can be useful to diagnose the site and cause of bleeding (7), and both standard posteroanterior and lateral chest radiographs should be obtained routinely before bronchoscopy (10,64). As reviewed elsewhere (11,43,64,65), both the characteristics of the infiltrate and the side and location of the infiltrate can suggest the cause of bleeding and its site. Unilateral infiltrates usually indicate the side from which bleeding emanates (4), but chest radiographs showing bilateral infiltrates understandably offer little help in lateralization. Whenever abnormalities are found, obtaining older radiographs for comparison is advisable (43). For example, abnormal findings can be obscured by aspirated blood or the changes may be chronic and unrelated to the recent hemoptysis (43). Up to 30% of patients with hemoptysis will have normal chest radiographs (11), which should not discourage further investigation (10). Conditions that may cause hemoptysis with a normal (or minimally abnormal) chest radiograph include bronchitis, bronchiectasis, small areas of infection, angiomas, infarction, or any endobronchial lesion that is not large enough to cause occlusion of the bronchus (64).

Besides bronchoscopy, ancillary tests may also be useful. Examples include echocardiography when mitral stenosis or congenital heart disease is suspected, a ventilation/perfusion lung scan or even pulmonary angiography when pulmonary embolism is suspected, antiglomerular basement membrane antibody, antineutrophilic cytoplasmic antibody, or renal biopsy in suspected pulmonary-renal syndromes.

Localizing the Bleeding: The Role of Bronchoscopy

Once the lung has been established as the cause of bleeding, attention turns to localizing

Table 21.5. Some Historical Clues That May Help to Establish Cause of Hemoptysis

Clues	Diagnostic Possibility
Young age	Adenoma, bronchiectasis, mitral stenosis, sequestration arteriovenous malformation
Age > 40, smoking, abnormal chest x-ray, small amounts of hemoptysis occurring daily for weeks	Bronchogenic carcinoma
Recurrence over months to years	Adenoma, bronchiectasis
Hematuria	Goodpasture's syndrome, Wegener's granulomatosis, polyarteritis nodosa
Occurrence during menses	Endometriosis (catamenial hemoptysis)
Fever, weight loss, night sweats, cough	Tuberculosis, fungal disease
Chronic phlegm	Chronic bronchitis, bronchiectasis
Dyspnea, acute pleuritic chest pain	Pulmonary embolism with infarct or pneumonia
Associated with exertion, orthopnea or paroxysmal nocturnal dyspnea	Congestive heart failure, mitral stenosis
History of rheumatic fever	Mitral stenosis
History of anticoagulation	Coagulopathy from large dose or pulmonary embolism from too small a dose
History of deep venous thrombosis	Pulmonary embolism
Infertility, diabetes mellitus, malabsorption	Cystic fibrosis
Recent procedure	Iatrogenic (bronchoscopy, Swan–Ganz catheterization, etc.)
Sputum appearance	
Mixed with gritty white material	Broncholithiasis
Pink frothy	Left ventricular failure
Rusty brown	Pneumonia
Mixed with pus	Lung abscess, bronchiectasis
Travel history	
Southwest USA	Coccidioidomycosis
Midwest river valleys in USA	Histoplasmosis
Far East	Paragonimiasis
South America, Africa, Far East	Schistosomiasis

the bleeding, particularly in recurrent or large-volume hemoptysis, because optimal treatment requires accurate knowledge of the bleeding site (2). Localizing the bleeding source will also help guide further diagnostic techniques such as washings, biopsies, etc. Using all available methods, overall success rates for specifically localizing bleeding have been 75% to 93% (66). Lateralizing the bleeding source without more specific lobar localization has been reportedly accomplished in 95% of instances (67). The yield of individual strategies for localizing the bleeding site has been assessed by Pursel and Lindskog (4) in a series of 105 patients with hemoptysis. Patients' self-assessment was least useful, offered by only 10% of patients and inaccurate in 30% of these. Clinical examination correctly localized the bleeding source in 43% of patients but was inaccurate 2% of the time. Chest radiographs were correct in 60% of patients and no instance of inaccuracy was found. Finally, bronchoscopy during active bleeding was most accurate (86% of

Table 21.6. Physical Findings That May Help to Establish the Cause of Hemoptysis

Physical Findings	Diagnostic Possibility
Telangiectasia on lips, skin, and buccal mucosa	Osler–Weber–Rendu disease
Ecchymoses, petechiae	Hematologic disorder
Clubbing	Non–small-cell bronchogenic carcinoma, bronchiectasis, lung abscess
Tachypnea, phlebitis, pleural rub	Pulmonary embolism with infarct
Ulceration of nasal septum	Wegener's granulomatosis
Diastolic rumble, opening snap, loud S_1, loud P_2	Mitral stenosis
Loud P_2, holosystolic murmur tricuspid area	Pulmonary hypertension
Unilateral wheeze	Bronchial adenoma, carcinoma
Palpable cervical scalene	Bronchogenic carcinoma
Supraclavicular lymph node	Lymphoma
Localized wheezes, rhonchi, crackles	Area of hemorrhage, consolidation, bronchiectasis, or airway narrowed by blood clots
Flow murmur over the chest	Arteriovenous malformation

evaluations), but was possible in only a minority (20%) of all patients in that series.

Because bronchoscopy is widely considered the preferred initial procedure for localizing bleeding in hemoptysis (whether massive or nonmassive) (11,44), an optimal diagnostic approach requires understanding the role of bronchoscopy.

Indications for Bronchoscopy

Although firm guidelines regarding bronchoscopy for hemoptysis are not available, it is generally agreed that bronchoscopy is indicated for patients with hemoptysis and parenchymal infiltrates on the chest radiograph (e.g., mass, infiltrate, cavity, or lobar atelectasis). In this setting, the diagnostic yield of bronchoscopy has been reported to be approximately 80% (20,68–74), with carcinoma comprising one third of cases (68).

The indications for bronchoscopy in patients with hemoptysis and either a normal or nonlocalizing chest radiograph are more controversial. The yield of bronchoscopy may be increased in the presence of several clinical features (especially when cancer is suspected), including age over 40 years, bleeding duration exceeding one week, volume of expectorated blood greater than 30 mL, a smoking history over 40 pack-years, and male gender (67–69,75,76). Whether to perform bronchoscopy in patients without these features remains a matter of individual discretion. Although some studies recommend that such patients may be observed following a negative sputum cytology and otolaryngologic examination (68–70, 75–77), others have recommended bronchoscopy in all patients, because bronchogenic carcinoma has been reported in 5% to 22% of patients with hemoptysis and normal or nonlocalizing chest radiographs (20,71,78–80). Specifically, Lederle and coworkers found bronchogenic carcinoma in 4.7% of 106 bronchoscopies performed in men older than 40 years with normal and nonlocalizing chest radiographs (81). Features associated with bronchogenic cancer in this series included smoking history greater than 20 pack-years and a centrally obscuring abnormality, but not a large volume of coughed blood. Although uncommon, bronchogenic cancer has been described in patients younger than 40 years and bronchoscopy should be considered in these patients as well. For example, Snider reported that 5% of 955 patients with bronchogenic carcinoma were less than 45 years of age (70). Similarly, Cortese and colleagues reported that 5.5% of patients with radiographically occult lung cancer were younger than 50 years (82). Based on these considerations, the authors' view is that bronchoscopy should be performed to evaluate hemoptysis unless a clear cause is already established. For example, it would seem prudent to defer bronchoscopy if a small volume of expectorated blood develops in the setting of acute bronchitis. On the other hand, persistent or new-onset bleeding as the infection is resolving should be investigated.

Having performed bronchoscopy once for "cryptogenic hemoptysis," a controversial question is whether and when to repeat bronchoscopic examination if bleeding recurs. Adelman and coworkers (38) reviewed the clinical outcome of 67 patients with hemoptysis and a normal or nonlocalizing chest radiograph with a prior nondiagnostic fiberoptic bronchoscopic examination. During a follow-up period up to 6 years, 85% of patients remained well without evidence of active tuberculosis or overlooked bronchogenic carcinoma, and 9 patients died of nonpulmonary conditions. Only one patient developed bronchogenic carcinoma 20 months after bronchoscopy and resolution of symptoms. Hemoptysis had resolved by one week in 57% of patients, and within 6 months in 90%. Only 4.5% of patients experienced recurrence of bleeding. The authors concluded that the prognosis for these patients is generally very good. In agreement with previous studies using rigid bronchoscopy (9,83), most of these studies have assessed the role of a single bronchoscopy in patients with recurrent hemoptysis. In contrast, the diagnostic role of multiple bronchoscopies in patients with recurrent hemoptysis

was reviewed by Gong (84) in 14 patients over a 6-year period. Ten patients had two procedures, 3 patients underwent three procedures, and one patient had five bronchoscopies at various intervals. Definitive diagnosis was available in 17.6% of all bronchoscopies, all in patients with bronchogenic carcinoma. Although the optimal number of bronchoscopies and the optimal time between these procedures was not definitely identified in this series, a second diagnostic bronchoscopy did increase diagnostic yield and caused subsequent changes in management compared to the first bronchoscopy. Based on these findings and the report by Adelman and associates that bleeding stops by 6 months in 90% of patients with cryptogenic hemoptysis (38), it seems justifiable to repeat bronchoscopy in 6 months if hemoptysis recurs after an initial nondiagnostic examination. Although bronchoscopy is generally indicated for any significant or new hemo-ptysis, it may not be needed in some clinical situations. Examples include patients with known chronic bronchitis with mild occasional blood streaking, particularly if associated with an exacerbation of acute tracheobronchitis (11,18); patients with acute lower respiratory infections (11); patients who have recent documentation of the site of bleeding by bronchoscopic examination (11); and patients with obvious cardiac or pulmonary vascular disease such as congestive heart failure and pulmonary embolism (11). Despite these broad indications, the decision to perform bronchoscopy should be individualized and depends on the degree of confidence assigned to the presumed cause of hemoptysis.

Timing of Bronchoscopy

Whether to perform bronchoscopy early (i.e., within 48 hours of acute bleeding) or remotely remains controversial. Table 21.7 presents the three available studies comparing early versus delayed bronchoscopy (4,20,85), all of which show a higher rate of successful localization with early bronchoscopy. However,

Table 21.7. A Summary of Available Studies of Delayed versus Immediate Bronchoscopy for Hemoptysis

First Author	No.	Bronchoscopy	Yield of Locating Bleeding	
			Delayed	Early
Pursel, 1961 (4)	105	Rigid	52%	86%
Smiddy, 1973 (66)	71 (active)	Flexible	NS	93%
Gong, 1981 (20)	129	Flexible	11%	34%
Bobrowitz, 1983 (26)	25	Flexible	NS	86%
Rath, 1973 (73)	31	Flexible	NS	68%
Corey, 1987 (28)	59	NS	NS	39%
Saumench, 1989 (85)	36	Flexible	50%	91%

NS, not stated
Modified and reproduced by permission from Stoller JK. Diagnosis and management of massive hemoptysis: a review. Respir Care 1992;32:564–581.

careful analysis of the diagnostic impact of bronchoscopy has shown that although active bleeding and the site of bleeding are visualized more commonly with early versus delayed bronchoscopy (34% versus 11%, respectively), the timing of bronchoscopy rarely alters the suspected cause of bleeding or overall patient management (20). Despite this controversy, we recommend early bronchoscopy because localizing the source can be critical if massive hemoptysis develops later and because early bronchoscopy also lessens the chance that an old clot will become redistributed by coughing or that gravitational pooling from the true bleeding site will occur (44).

Choice of Instruments

The flexible bronchoscope is the instrument of choice for nonmassive hemoptysis because flexible FOB can be performed in an outpatient setting or at the bedside under local anesthesia, is well tolerated by most patients, and provides an extended visual range into subsegmental bronchi including upper lobe orifices (7,44,72).

Whether to use a rigid or flexible bronchoscope in massive hemoptysis is debated, but in the absence of a head-to-head comparison, no firm conclusion can be offered. Currently, the choice reflects the user's experience. Many surgeons advocate using a rigid instrument, whereas most pulmonologists favor a flexible bronchoscope. The important advantages of rigid bronchoscopy include improved suctioning capacity and a larger lumen to introduce tamponading materials, perform lavage, and allow continuous airway control (6).

However, the rigid bronchoscope is limited by reduced visual range and the need for general anesthesia and an operating room. As summarized by Neff, "In cases of massive hemoptysis, the use of a rigid bronchoscope for emergency examinations seems more advantageous than using a fiberoptic bronchoscope. The selection of which scope to use for hemoptysis seems less important, however, than the close communication between the experienced pulmonary physician and skilled thoracic surgeon" (86).

If the flexible bronchoscope is used and there has been recent massive bleeding, airway control should be maintained by inserting a large-caliber oral endotracheal tube, through which the bronchoscope can be passed (36). Intubation also allows repeated easy removal and reinsertion in case the viewing lens needs to be cleaned after the lens is clouded by blood (36,87). Besides providing airway control, a large-bore suction catheter can also be passed through the endotracheal tube to suction larger clots (87). The flexible bronchoscope can be used to wash each segmental lobe orifice carefully for specimens, followed by close observation for the appearance of fresh blood (36). The larger channel flexible bronchoscope with a 2.6-mm aspiration channel diameter is recommended when a flexible instrument is used (87). At times when the rate of hemorrhage exceeds the suction capacity of the flexible bronchoscope, the flexible instrument can be passed via the rigid scope, thus combining safety (airway control and suctioning capacity) and maneuverability (36,44). This practice is also used in laser treatment for tracheobronchial tumors (18,88,89).

In situations when uninterrupted ventilation is required, high-frequency jet ventilation can be used with either rigid or flexible bronchoscopy. The open system used in jet ventilation allows simultaneous bronchoscopy, ventilation, suctioning, and localization.

Route of Passing the Fiberoptic Bronchoscope

If the source of bleeding is known to be subglottic, either the transnasal or transoral approach can be used. However, if doubt exists regarding the source of bleeding, the upper airways should be examined along with the standard evaluation of the tracheobronchial tree. Selecky (7) states that the transoral approach provides a unique view of the posterior nasopharynx and recommends flexing the tip of the bronchoscope cephalad 180° to view the posterior aspect of the nasal passages and turbinates. If an upper airway source is suspected and the transnasal approach is selected, both sides of the nose should be examined.

Bronchoscopic Findings

Although bronchoscopy remains the best diagnostic and localizing modality in hemoptysis,

it may not identify the bleeding to a specific site. For example, Smiddy and Elliot (66) performed FOB in 71 patients with active hemoptysis and identified a single bleeding point in 46.5%. Bleeding was localized to a bronchopulmonary segment in 38% of patients, multiple bleeding sites were identified in 8.45%, and the bleeding site could not be localized in 7%. To optimize the bronchoscopic yield, each bronchial orifice should be examined to its furthest extent, preferably to a subsegmental bronchus (18). At times, using a small caliber or pediatric bronchoscope may enhance the diagnostic yield by allowing examination of the more distal bronchial tree (89). Segmental lavage with sterile saline solution may also help identify the source of bleeding, as discussed earlier (36). All abnormalities must be appropriately biopsied, brushed, or lavaged for adequate specimens, depending on the underlying clinical situation (7). The bronchoscopist should pay special attention to the mucosa and visible vessels. Obvious vascular capillaries, bronchial inflammation, and subtle mucosal abnormalities are all considered valuable findings (18). In the ACCP survey on hemoptysis (31), clinicians were asked to grade the clinical value of bronchoscopic findings and their impact on management in patients with normal or nonlocalizing chest radiographs. A specific diagnosis (e.g., lung cancer) was perceived to be more useful than a nonspecific result, but more than 80% of respondents considered nonspecific findings (objective bronchitis, normal airways, or either localized or diffuse tracheobronchial blood) valuable in clinical decision-making.

Diagnostic Techniques Other than Bronchoscopy

When bronchoscopy does not indicate the source of bleeding, other diagnostic tests may be required, including bronchial arteriography, chest computed tomography (CT), and bronchography.

The comparative value of bronchial arteriography versus bronchoscopy has been examined in two studies. Saumench and associates (85) assessed the value of FOB versus angiography for diagnosing the bleeding site in 36 patients with hemoptysis. Bronchial arteriography was performed in all 36 patients and the bleeding site was identified in 55.5%. Bronchoscopy was performed in 25 patients and the bleeding site was identified in 68%. Arteriography identified the bleeding site in only 2 of the 8 patients with nondiagnostic bronchoscopies. In keeping with other studies, these authors concluded that the main advantage of arteriography was to plan bronchial artery embolization. In the second study, Katoh and coworkers (90) compared bronchoscopic findings with bronchial arteriography in 7 patients with hemoptysis. The lesions were located in the second to fifth order bronchi and were either bulge lesions or mass lesions. Intrabronchial bulge was discovered by bronchoscopy in 5 patients. In one of these, the bulge corresponded to the site of an aneurysm in the bronchial arteriogram, while in the other 4, the bulge corresponded to the site of hypervascularity on the bronchial arteriogram. An intrabronchial mass in 2 patients corresponded to obstruction with focal dilatation on one arteriogram and hypervascularity on the other. These intrabronchial lesions disappeared or diminished in size after bronchial artery embolization. However, some case reports suggest that some bronchial arterial lesions may resemble the bronchoscopic appearance of a tumor and thus predispose to serious hemorrhage if biopsy is attempted (91,92).

Three studies have compared the diagnostic impact of chest CT to bronchoscopy in patients with hemoptysis. Haponik and associates (93) performed plain chest radiographs, chest CT scans, and flexible FOB in 32 patients with hemoptysis of various causes. Chest CT scans provided unique imaging information in 47% of patients (15 of 32), including 10 patients whose plain films were normal. However, in only 2 patients did CT provide diagnostic information not available after bronchoscopy, leading to alternative treatment in only one patient (3%). The authors concluded that although CT markedly enhances radiographic diagnostic yield, the management impact of CT is more meager and does not support its routine use in evaluating patients with hemoptysis (93). Naidich and coworkers (94) retrospectively correlated chest CT and chest radiographic findings with those found at FOB in 58 patients presenting with hemoptysis. Chest CT depicted focal abnormalities involving the central airways in 18 (31%) and bronchiectasis in 10 (17%). Focal abnormalities were seen at bronchoscopy in 18 cases (31%) and all were apparent with CT. Malignancy was diagnosed in 24 patients and CT was abnormal in all 24. Bronchoscopic examination was normal in 3 of these 24 patients (12.5%), but malignant cells were identified on transbronchial biopsy. In 11 of 21 patients (52%) with non–small-cell lung cancer, CT allowed definitive staging by documenting either direct mediastinal invasion or metastatic disease. Bronchoscopy allowed definitive staging in only 3 patients by documenting tumor within 2 cm of the carina. In only 6 of 24 patients (25%) with malignancy did the CT fail to disclose new information compared to the plain chest radiograph and bronchoscopy. Because chest CT provided no false negative results, the authors concluded that CT was effective in evaluating patients with hemoptysis. Only 10 patients in the series were evaluated using a specific high-resolution protocol, but results of this protocol or comparison with conventional techniques were not given. Finally, Millar and colleagues (95) performed chest CT in 40 patients with a history of hemoptysis and normal findings on both chest radiograph and bronchoscopy. Previously unsuspected abnormalities were detected in 20 patients (50%), 7 of whom had evidence of bronchiectasis (18%). Using the contralateral lung of 93 patients undergoing CT for preoperative assessment of bronchogenic carcinoma as controls, the relative risk of having an abnormality on CT in the study group was 7.75. The authors concluded that chest CT scan was valuable in patients with unexplained hemoptysis and suggested that in patients with normal chest radiographs, CT should precede bronchoscopy to direct bronchoscopic techniques to areas of abnormality and to detect peripheral neoplasms and bronchiectasis not visible at bronchoscopy.

Based on the available evidence, the current authors' view is to reserve chest CT for evaluating hemoptysis when the cause of bleeding remains unclear after bronchoscopy and plain chest radiography.

Finally, bronchography (i.e., instilling lipophilic dye into the bronchi) can be performed to localize bleeding, but recent developments have led to decreased dependence on bronchography (96). High-resolution CT has a high degree of sensitivity for diagnosing bronchiectasis and has essentially replaced bronchography where CT is available (96). Some of the dyes traditionally used for bronchography (e.g., Dionosil) are no longer commercially available.

Overall, bronchoscopy and plain film radiography remain the mainstays for evaluating patients with hemoptysis. Chest CT is reserved to evaluate some patients with lung cancer or whose source of hemoptysis is elusive after initial work-up.

Therapeutic Role of Bronchoscopy in Hemoptysis

The development of several endobronchial topical treatments has revolutionized the role of bronchoscopy in managing hemoptysis (97). These measures are used mainly to control massive or life-threatening hemoptysis and can be combined with surgical treatment. As adjunct maneuvers, they help to "buy time" to restore clinical stability and to perform essential diagnostic and definitive management procedures such as embolotherapy or surgery. Treatments using the bronchoscope include lung isolation and airway control techniques, endobronchial balloon or direct bronchoscopic tamponade, cold saline lavage, laser therapy, electrocautery, brachytherapy, and application of topical vasoconstrictors or coagulants. Several of these techniques are discussed below. Others, such as laser and brachytherapy, are discussed elsewhere (see Chapters 18 and 19).

Lung Isolation and Airway Control

When there is active bleeding, the airway can be maintained during bronchoscopic localization by rigid bronchoscopy alone or by use of a fiberoptic bronchoscope through a large-caliber endotracheal tube (ETT). The flexible fiberoptic bronchoscope can also be used to facilitate intubation, change ETTs, and extubate over the bronchoscope when edema or closure of upper airway structures is a concern (98). For airway management, the 5-mm outer diameter (OD) fiberoptic bronchoscope is optimal; to use this bronchoscope, an ETT with at least 8-mm internal diameter (ID) has been recommended in adults (98). This will allow the remaining endotracheal ring size to approximate a 7-mm ID ETT even with the bronchoscope in place. The 6-mm OD fiberoptic bronchoscope is not recommended for use with an ETT (98), except possibly when bleeding is controlled and bronchoscopy is being done only for intubation.

Double-Lumen Endotracheal Tube

Urgent management of massive hemoptysis must protect the uninvolved lung from aspiration of blood. One method of isolating the lungs is to place a double-lumen ETT, which can be guided over a flexible bronchoscope (99,100). Available double-lumen ETTs include the Carlen's tube (introduced in 1949 and less popular now because of the small caliber of the individual lumens), the Robertshaw rubber tube (102) (right and left-sided models), and disposable polyvinyl chloride variations of the Robertshaw tube, including the Mallinckrodt Broncho-Cath, the Rusch endobronchial tube, and the Sheridian Broncho-Trach (99). Some recent double-lumen tube models now have diaphragms on the ventilation adaptors to allow bronchoscopy without loss of airway pressure in patients undergoing mechanical ventilation (99). Double-lumen tubes are currently available in five sizes (28 F, 35 F, 37 F, 39 F, and 41 F) and size selection depends on the size of the patient. The largest possible tube through the glottis is preferred because it will have little chance of advancing too far down the left main stem bronchus and creates a better air seal. On the other hand, using a smaller tube requires more endobronchial cuff pressure, increasing the chance of cuff herniation across the carina with resultant airway occlusion (99). In general, most adult men can accommodate a 41 F double-lumen tube, whereas women more commonly accommodate a 39 F double-lumen tube (103). The fiberoptic bronchoscope has two roles with double-lumen tubes: first, to facilitate difficult intubations, and second, to confirm correct tube placement and position. Diagnostic bronchoscopy through double-lumen tubes is difficult because of the small caliber of each lumen.

Intubation over the bronchoscope usually requires shortening the double-lumen tube by 7 cm from the proximal end to allow an adequate working length for the bronchoscope (104). A pediatric bronchoscope is recommended for use with double-lumen tubes smaller than 39 F (98,99) because the outside diameter of the smallest adult bronchoscope (4.9 mm) interferes with passage of the instrument through the smaller tubes (99).

The technique of double-lumen tube placement using a bronchoscope has been well described by Dellinger (98). The tube is first inserted into the trachea, either with a bronchoscope or by using direct laryngoscopy, and the tracheal cuff is inflated and mechanical ventilation begun or resumed. The bronchoscope is then advanced through the endobronchial lumen of the double-lumen tube and for left-sided tube placement, advanced into the left main stem bronchus (Figure 21.2). In general, left-sided double-lumen tubes are preferred because adequate cuff seal is difficult to achieve on the right; the short distance between the main carina and the takeoff of the right main stem bronchus prevents easy placement of right-sided tubes or assurance of an adequate seal. After the bronchoscope is fixed in the left main stem bronchus, the endobronchial tube is advanced into the left main stem bronchus using the bronchoscope as an obturator. The bronchoscope is then withdrawn and passed through the tracheal lumen. Once the bronchoscope passes out of the tracheal lumen, the left endobronchial tube can be visualized. The bronchial cuff is positioned and inflated in proper position. For correct double-lumen tube placement, the blue endobronchial cuff should be easily seen just beyond the carina, the cuff should not be

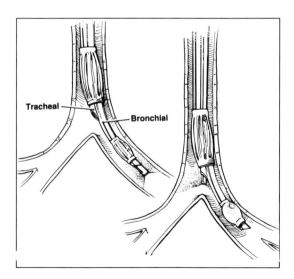

Figure 21.2. Fiberoptic bronchoscopic insertion of the double–lumen endobronchial tube (left bronchial type). See text for details of technique.

Reproduced by permission from Dellinger RP. Fiberoptic bronchoscopy in adult airway management. Crit Care Med 1990;18:884.

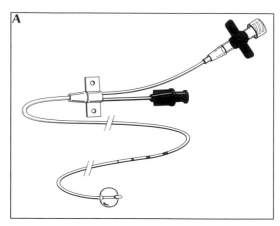

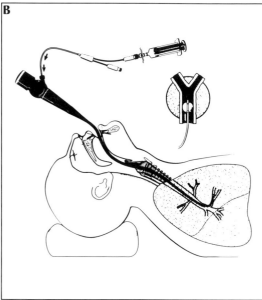

Figure 21.3. *A,* Fogarty balloon embolectomy catheter with balloon inflated. *B,* Fogarty balloon embolectomy catheter inserted through the channel of the fiberoptic bronchoscope with balloon inflated after insertion.

herniating, and the double-lumen tube should not be too distal in the main stem bronchus (99).

Endobronchial Balloon Tamponade

Another catheter that can be placed using the bronchoscope is for endobronchial balloon tamponade, which has been used to control life-threatening hemoptysis in nonintubated patients (105–109). Balloon tamponade involves occluding the bleeding airway by

inflating a Fogarty embolectomy catheter (4 F for segmental bronchi and up to 14 F for the left main stem bronchus), which is passed either through a fiberoptic or rigid broncho-scope, followed by removal of the broncho-scope over the catheter (Figure 21.3) (2). The balloon is deflated after 24 to 48 hours and then removed. An alternative approach is to pass the Fogarty catheter alongside the flexible bronchoscope (110).

In 1974, Hiebert (105) reported data on a patient with such brisk hemoptysis that visu-alization with a rigid bronchoscope could not be maintained. In desperation, a Fogarty catheter was passed into the right main stem bronchus and inflated with successful tam-ponade of the bleeding, thus saving the patient's life. Thereafter, several others have reported successful use of this technique (106–109). Saw and coworkers (107) reported data on 10 patients in whom balloon tamponade successfully controlled acute bleeding. None of the patients died from hemoptysis or experi-enced recurrent bleeding (without surgical resection) for up to 9 months of follow-up. In 4 patients with cystic fibrosis and massive hemoptysis, Swersky and associates (109) achieved acute control of bleeding with bal-loon tamponade, although bleeding recurred in 3 of 4 patients. No complications of endo-bronchial tamponade were reported in either of these series.

Overall, although the reported experience is limited, the universal reported success with controlling acute bleeding and the lack of reported complications have caused endo-bronchial balloon tamponade to be widely used (2). Balloon occlusion is a rapid method to isolate the bleeding from the good lung, allowing stabilization before more definitive treatment can be undertaken (36).

Selective Bronchial Intubation

If the bleeding site can be localized only to the involved lung rather than to a specific lobe, Gourin and Garzon have recommended a

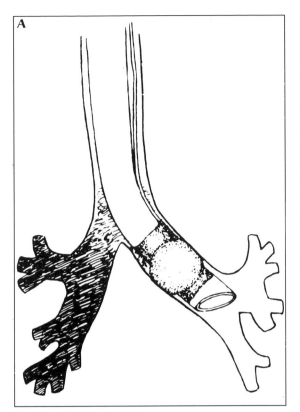
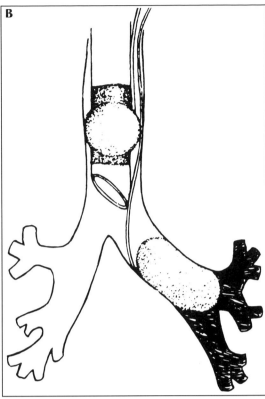

Figure 21.4. *A,* During right-sided bleeding, a cuffed ETT in the left main bronchus protects the left lung from spillover. *B,* During left-sided bleeding, a balloon occlusion catheter inflated below the carina in the left main stem isolates the left lung while an ETT in the trachea ventilates the right lung.

Reproduced by permission from Gourin A, Garzon A. Control of hemorrhage in emergency pulmonary resection for massive hemoptysis. Chest 1975;68:120–121.

technique of selective bronchial intubation or balloon catheter blockage of the bleeding bronchus (111,112). During right-sided bleeding the endotracheal tube can be advanced into the left main stem bronchus under bronchoscopic guidance to allow unilateral lung ventilation while simultaneously blocking spillover of blood to the left side (Figure 21.4*A*). Because of normal anatomic asymmetry, selective intubation of the right lung carries a risk of occluding the right upper lobe bronchus, which generally rises just below the main carina (36). Thus, a different approach is recommended for left-sided bleeding. An occluding Fogarty catheter can be placed into the left main stem bronchus and the endotracheal tube is left in place in the trachea to ventilate the right side (Figure 21.4*B*). Of 25 patients in Gourin and Garzon's series (111) in whom single-lung

anesthesia was used, 18 patients underwent bronchial intubation or balloon catheter blockage. Only 3 patients showed contralateral aspiration on postoperative chest radiographs and only one died (of respiratory and renal failure). The effectiveness of selective bronchial intubation allows pulmonary resection or embolization therapy to be performed safely (97). If medical therapy is indicated, supportive therapy can be maintained (97). This technique can be combined with iced saline lavage to the bleeding site while aeration is maintained to the other lung and is also considered a first-line technique for managing of major bronchovascular fistula (97).

Direct Tamponade with a Bronchoscope

In the event of overwhelming hemoptysis that occurs during the bronchoscopic evaluation, the fiberoptic bronchoscope can be advanced into the appropriate segmental or subsegmental bronchus under direct vision to act as an occlusive wedge (36,43). This is a temporizing measure that will allow the bleeding site to clot off while preventing spillage to normal areas. If the source of hemoptysis is proximal and a rigid bronchoscopy is being performed, the rigid instrument can also be used to directly tamponade the bleeding site using the side of the bronchoscope while maintaining the airway (18).

Use of Topical Vasoconstrictors and Coagulants

Instillation of epinephrine (1:20,000) through the bronchoscope is commonly used with the aim of achieving topical vasoconstriction with diminution of blood flow and thrombotic obstruction of the distal vessels (18,113). Topical epinephrine is effective to control endobronchial hemorrhage after biopsy of a vascular tumor or severe bleeding from the mucosa (97,113). Following balloon tamponade, regular endobronchial instillation of epinephrine through an irrigation catheter has also been proposed (109). However, the benefits of topical epinephrine in controlling massive hemoptysis are uncertain.

Vasopressin is another topical vasoconstrictor that has been used for controlling hemoptysis. Worth and colleagues (114) compared endobronchial versus intravenous vasopressin in lung bleeding during bronchoscopy. Eleven patients were treated with one mg intravenous vasopressin and 16 patients received the same dose endobronchially at the site of bleeding. Endobronchial administration was equally efficacious to intravenous treatment, but lacked hemodynamic effects.

Instillation of topical coagulants through the bronchoscope has been reportedly useful to control hemoptysis and several coagulants like bosmin (115), reptilase (116), thrombin (117,118), fibrinogen-thrombin (118,119), and fibrin precursors (120) have been des-

cribed. Tsukamoto and coworkers (118) treated 19 patients with thrombin (5 to 10 mL of 1000 units/mL solution), and noted substantial efficacy (i.e., no recurrence within 14 days) in 14 (74%), partial efficacy (i.e., hemoptysis recurred between 24 hours and 14 days after treatment) in one patient, and failure to control bleeding in 4 patients (21%). In another 14 patients treated with fibrinogen-thrombin (5 to 10 mL of 2% fibrinogen solution), substantial efficacy was noted in 11 (79%) and partial efficacy in 3 (21%). A topical coagulant consisting of fibrin precursors (fibrinogen, fibronectin, factor XIII, and aprotinin), which are activated by adding calcium chloride and thrombin, has been described by Bense (120). With this approach, a four-channel catheter (OD 2 mm) is introduced into the bleeding bronchus with a flexible bronchoscope and the two main components, which together form a fibrin sealant, are mixed, heated to 37°C, and injected simultaneously but separately into two channels of the four-channel catheter. Using this technique, Bense safety arrested four episodes of hemoptysis that were resistant to other therapy (120). Despite enthusiasm for using topical coagulants for even massive hemoptysis, lack of any controlled comparison and the paucity of available studies advise the reader to reserve judgment currently. A further concern is that the continuous stream of blood in massive hemoptysis may flush away the fibrin glue before a stable clot forms (18).

Cold Saline Lavage through the Bronchoscope

In keeping with a time-honored treatment of upper gastrointestinal bleeding, cold saline lavage has been used to stop bleeding in massive hemoptysis. For example, Conlan and Hurwitz (121) reported that bronchial irrigation with 50-mL aliquots of cold (4°C) normal saline administered through a rigid bronchoscope successfully arrested bleeding in 12 patients with massive hemoptysis. The average volume of saline required was 500 mL (range 300 to 750 mL).

The mechanism by which lavage arrests bleeding is presumably hypothermic vasoconstriction with diminution of blood flow and thrombotic obstruction of the distal vessels.

Bronchoscopic Laser Therapy and Electrocautery

As discussed in Chapter 18, the neodymium: yttrium-aluminum-garnet laser (Nd:YAG), applied through either the flexible or rigid bronchoscope, has been used to achieve hemostasis in patients with hemoptysis from airway neoplasms.

Electrocautery is an alternative bronchoscopic treatment for hemoptysis. For example, Gerasin and Shafirovsky (122) performed endobronchial electrosurgery with the aid of a flexible bronchoscope and a diathermic snare in 14 patients with tracheal and bronchial tumors. Total tumor eradication was achieved in 9 patients with benign tumors and airway patency was effectively established in 3 of 5 patients with malignant tumors. In one patient, emergent endobronchial electrosurgery successfully controlled massive hemorrhage caused by an endobronchial metastasis from thyroid carcinoma. Compared with laser, advantages of electrocautery for treating hemoptysis through the bronchoscope include lower cost and availability, more rapid removal of tumor by diathermic snare, and the capability for excising tumors with cartilaginous and ostial components resistant to laser coagulation. A limitation of electrocautery with a diathermic snare is the inability to surround the tumor when the base is broad, when the bronchial lumen is tightly obstructed, or when the tumor is inaccessible (e.g., in a segmental bronchus) (122). Two practical precautions about electrocautery should be noted: 1) contact of the diathermic snare with the tip of the bronchoscope should be avoided because the bronchoscope is not electrically grounded, and 2) excessive current or pressure while closing the snare may lead to rapid cutting without cauterization of the vessel, resulting in further bleeding. Given the paucity of data, the precise role of electrocautery in managing hemoptysis remains to be defined.

In summary, although many endobronchial treatments for hemoptysis are available, the paucity of comparative studies precludes a clear recommendation about which treatment to use first. For nonmassive hemoptysis, our practice is to instill epinephrine topically, followed by bronchial balloon tamponade. For massive hemoptysis, immediate treatments would include intravenous vasopressin, placing the bleeding lung in the dependent position, and possibly selective bronchial intubation to stabilize the patient while bronchial embolization or surgery is planned.

REFERENCES

1. Marini JJ. Hemoptysis. In: Respiratory medicine for the house officer, 2nd ed. Baltimore: Williams and Wilkins, 1987;29:223–225.
2. Stoller JK. Diagnosis and management of massive hemoptysis: a review. Respir Care 1992;32:564–581.
3. Chaves AD. Hemoptysis in chest clinic patients. Am Rev Tuberc 1951;63:144–201.
4. Pursel SE, Lindskog GE. Hemoptysis: a clinical evaluation of 105 patients examined consecutively on a thoracic surgical service. Am Rev Respir Dis 1961;84:329–336.
5. Abbott OA. The clinical significance of pulmonary hemorrhage: a study of 1316 patients with chest disease. Dis Chest 1948;14:824–842.
6. Johnston RN, Lockhart W, Ritchie RT, Smith DM. Hemoptysis. Br Med J 1960;1:592–595.
7. Selecky PA. Evaluation of hemoptysis through the bronchoscope. Chest 1978;73:741–745.
8. Lyons HA. Differential diagnosis of hemoptysis and its treatment. ATS News 1976;26–30.
9. Barrett RJ, Tuttle WM. A study of essential hemoptysis. J Thorac Cardiovasc Surg 1960;40:468–474.

10. Wolfe JD, Simmons DH. Hemoptysis: diagnosis and management. West J Med 1977; 127:383–390.

11. Irwin RS, Curley FJ. Hemoptysis. In: Rippe JM, Irwin RS, Alpert JS, et al., eds. Intensive care medicine, 2nd ed. Boston: Little Brown, 1991;48:513–524.

12. Jackson CL, Diamond S. Hemorrhage from the trachea, bronchi, and lungs of nontuberculosis origin. Am Rev Tuberc 1942; 46:126–138.

13. Souders CR, Smith AT. The clinical significance of hemoptysis. N Engl J Med 1952;247:790–793.

14. Heller R. The significance of hemoptysis tubercule. 1946;26:70–74.

15. Moersch HJ. Clinical significance of hemoptysis. JAMA 1952;148:1461–1465.

16. Johnston H, Reisz G. Changing spectrum of hemoptysis: underlying causes in 148 patients undergoing diagnostic flexible bronchoscopy. Arch Intern Med 1989;149:1666–1668.

17. Santiago S, Tobias J, William AJ. A reappraisal of the causes of hemoptysis. Arch Intern Med 1991;151:2449–2451.

18. Prakash UBS. Bronchoscopy. In: Bone RC, Dantzker DR, George RB, Matthay RA, Reynolds HY, eds. Pulmonary and critical care medicine, vol 1. St. Louis: Mosby-Year Book, 1993;F(5):1–18.

19. Kahn MP, Whitcomb ME, Snider GL. Flexible fiberoptic bronchoscopy. Am J Med 1976;61:151–155.

20. Gong H, Salvatierra C. Clinical efficacy of early and delayed fiberoptic bronchoscopy in patients with hemoptysis. Am Rev Respir Dis 1981;124:221–225.

21. Prakash UBS, Offord KP, Stubbs SE. Bronchoscopy in North America: the ACCP survey. Chest 1991;100:1668–1675.

22. Howard WJ, Rosario EJ, Calhoon SL. Hemoptysis: causes and practical management approach. Postgrad Med 1985;77:53–57.

23. Karlinsky JB, Lau J, Goldstein RH. Hemoptysis. In: Decision making in pulmonary medicine. Philadelphia: BC Decker, 1991:10–11.

24. Clausen JL. Hemoptysis. In: Bordew RA, Moser KM, eds. Manual of clinical problems in pulmonary medicine. Boston: Little, Brown, 1991;14:67–71.

25. Amirana M, Frater R, Tirschwell P, Janis M, Bloomberg A, State D. An aggressive surgical approach to significant hemoptysis in patients with pulmonary tuberculosis. Am Rev Respir Dis 1968;97:187–192.

26. Bobrowitz ID, Ramkrishna S, Shim YS. Comparison of medical vs. surgical treatment of major hemoptysis. Arch Intern Med 1983;143:1343–1346.

27. Crocco JA, Rooney JJ, Fankushen DS, DiBenedetto RJ, Lyons HA. Massive hemoptysis. Arch Intern Med 1968;121: 495–498.

28. Corey R, Hla RM. Major and massive hemoptysis: reassessment of conservative management. Am J Med Sci 1987;294: 301–309.

29. Holsclaw DS, Grand RJ, Shuachman H. Massive hemoptysis in cystic fibrosis. J Pediatr 1970;76:829–838.

30. Garzon AA, Cerruti MM, Golding ME. Exsanguinating hemoptysis. J Thorac Cardiovasc Surg 1982;84:829–833.

31. Haponik EF, Chin R. Hemoptysis: clinician's perspective. Chest 1990;97:469–475.

32. Gourin A, Garzon AA. Operative treatment of massive hemoptysis. Ann Thorac Surg 1974;18:52–60.

33. Conlan AA, Hurwitz SS, Krige L, Nicolau N, Pool R. Massive hemoptysis: a review of 123 cases. J Thorac Cardiovasc Surg 1983;85: 120–124.

34. Bone RC. Massive hemoptysis. In: Sahn S, ed. Pulmonary emergencies. New York: Churchill Livingston, 1982:225–236.

35. Rogers RM (Moderator). The management of massive hemoptysis in a patient with pulmonary tuberculosis. Chest 1976;70: 519–526.

36. Winter SM, Ingbar DH. Massive hemoptysis: pathogenesis and management. J Intensive Care Med 1988;3:171–188.

37. Wedzicha JA, Pearson MC. Management of massive hemoptysis. Respir Med 1990; 84:9–12.

38. Adelman M, Haponik EF, Bleecker ER, Britt EJ. Cryptogenic hemoptysis. Ann Intern Med 1985;102:829–834.

39. Stiernberg C. Hemoptysis of undetermined etiology. Tex State J Med 1964;60:630–633.

40. Thomson SC. Hemoptysis from the throat (hemoptysis not of pulmonary origin). Ann Otol Rhinol Laryngol 1928;37:209–212.

41. Gale D. Overgrowth of *Serratia marcescens* in respiratory tract simulating hemoptysis. JAMA 1957;164:1328–1330.

42. Newton RW, Forest ARW. Rifampicin overdosage—"the red man syndrome." South Med J 1975;20:55–57.

43. Israel RH, Poe RH. Hemoptysis. Clin Chest Med 1987;8:197–205.

44. Ingbar D. A systematic workup for hemoptysis. Contemporary Int Med July/August 1989: 60–70.

45. Uflacker R, Kaemmerer A, Picon PD, et al. Bronchial artery embolization in the management of hemoptysis: technical aspects and longterm results. Radiology 1985;157:637–644.

46. McCollum WB, Mattox KL, Guinn GA, Beall AC. Immediate operative treatment for massive hemoptysis. Chest 1975;67:152–155.

47. Yang CT, Berger HW. Conservative management of life-threatening hemoptysis. Mt. Sinai J Med 1978;45:329–333.

48. Remy J, Arnaud A, Fardou H, et al. Treatment of hemoptysis by embolisation of bronchial arteries. Radiology 1977;122: 33–39.

49. Deffebach ME, Charau NB, Lakshminarayan S. State of the art: the bronchial circulation—small but a vital attribute of the lung. Am Rev Respir Dis 1987;135:463–481.

50. Rabkin JE, Astafjer VI, Gothman LN, et al. Transcatheter embolization in the management of pulmonary hemorrhage. Radiology 1987;163:361–365.

51. Thompson JR. Mechanisms of fatal pulmonary hemorrhage in tuberculosis. Dis Chest 1954;25:193–205.

52. Dixon GF, Donnerberg RL, Schonfeld SA, Whitcomb MI. Advances in the diagnosis and treatment of broncholithiasis. Am Rev Respir Dis 1984;129:1028–1030.

53. Auerbach O. Pathology and pathogenesis of pulmonary arterial aneurysm in tuberculosis cavities. Am Rev Tuberc 1939;39:99–115.

54. Plessinger VA, Jolly PN. Rasmussen's aneurysms and fatal hemorrhage in pulmonary tuberculosis. Am Rev Tuberc 1949;60:589–603.

55. Rasmussen V. Hemoptysis, especially when fatal, in its anatomical and clinical aspects (translated by WD Moore). Edinburgh Med J 1868;14:385–486.

56. Wood DA, Miller M. Role of dual pulmonary circulation in various pathologic conditions of the lungs. J Thorac Surg 1938;7:649–654.

57. Miller RR, McGregor DH. Hemorrhage from carcinoma of the lung. Cancer 1980; 46:200–205.

58. Liebow AA, Hales MR, Lindskog GE. Enlargement of the bronchial arteries and their anastomoses with the pulmonary arteries in bronchiectasis. Am J Pathol 1949;25: 211–220.

59. Tadavarthy SM, Klugman J, Casjaneda-Zuinga WR, et al. Systemic pulmonary collaterals in pathological states. Radiology 1982;144:55–59.

60. Joynson DHM. Pulmonary aspergilloma. Br J Clin Pract 1977;31:207–221.

61. Varkey B, Rose HD. Pulmonary aspergilloma —a rational approach to treatment. Am J Med 1976;61:626–631.

62. Ferguson FC, Kobilak RE, Deitrick JE. Varices of bronchial veins as a source of hemoptysis in mitral stenosis. Am Heart J 1944;28:445–449.

63. Thoms NW, Wilson RF, Puro HE, Arbula A. Life-threatening hemoptysis in primary lung abscess. Ann Thorac Surg 1972;14:347–357.

64. Strickland B. Investigating hemoptysis. Br J Dis Chest 1986;245–251.

65. Soll B, Selecky PA, Chang R, et al. The use of the fiberoptic bronchoscope in the evaluation of hemoptysis. Am Rev Respir Dis 1977; 115:165–168.

66. Smiddy JR, Elliot RC. The evaluation of hemoptysis with fiberoptic bronchoscopy. Chest 1973;64:158–162.

67. Shamji FM, Vallieres E, Todd ER, Sach HJ. Massive or life-threatening hemoptysis. Chest 1991;100:78S.

68. O'Neil KM, Lazarus AA. Indications for bronchoscopy. Arch Intern Med 1991;151: 171–174.

69. Weaver LJ, Solliday N, Cugell DW. Selection of patients for fiberoptic bronchoscopy. Chest 1979;76:7–10.

70. Snider GL. When not to use the bronchoscope for hemoptysis. Chest 1979;76:1–2.

71. Zavala DC. Diagnostic fiberoptic bronchoscopy. Chest 1975;68:12–19.

72. Mitchell DM, Emerson CJ, Collyer J, Collins JV. Fiberoptic bronchoscopy: ten years on. Br Med J 1980;281:360–363.

73. Rath GS, Schaff JT, Snider GL. Flexible fiberoptic bronchoscopy: techniques and review of 100 bronchoscopies. Chest 1973;63: 689–693.

74. Peters J, McClung H, Teague R. Evaluation of hemoptysis in patients with a normal chest roentgenogram. West J Med 1984; 141:624–626.

75. Jackson CV, Savage PJ, Quinn DL. Role of fiberoptic bronchoscopy in patients with hemoptysis and a normal chest roentgenogram. Chest 1985;87:142–144.

76. Poe RH, Israel RH, Marin MG, et al. Utility of fiberoptic bronchoscopy in patients with hemoptysis and a nonlocalizing chest roentgenogram. Chest 1988;92:70–75.

77. Heimer D, Bar-Ziv J, Scharf SM. Fiberoptic bronchoscopy in patients with hemoptysis and nonlocalizing chest roentgenographs. Arch Intern Med 1985;145:1427–1428.

78. Kallenbach J, Song E, Zwi S. Hemoptysis with no radiologic evidence of tumors: the value of early bronchoscopy. S Afr Med J 1981;59:556–558.

79. Richardson RH, Zavala DC, Mukerjee PK, Bedell GN. The use of fiberoptic bronchoscopy and brush biopsy in the diagnosis of suspected pulmonary malignancy. Am Rev Respir Dis 1974;109:63–66.

80. Heaton RW. Should patient with hemoptysis and normal chest x-ray be bronchoscoped? Postgrad Med J 1987;63:947–949.

81. Lederle FA, Nichol KL, Parenti CM. Bronchoscopy to evaluate hemoptysis in older men with nonsuspicious chest roentgenograms. Chest 1989;10:43–47.

82. Cortese DA, Parvolero PC, Bergstrach EJ, et al. Roentgenographically occult lung cancer: a ten year experience. J Thorac Cardiovasc Surg 1983;86:373–380.

83. Douglas DE, Carr DT. Prognosis in idiopathic hemoptysis. JAMA 1952;150:764–765.

84. Gong J Jr. Repeat fiberoptic bronchoscopy in patients with recurrent unexplained hemoptysis. Respiration 1983;44:225–233.

85. Saumench J, Escarrabil J, Padro L, Montana J, Clariana A, Canto A. Value of fiberoptic bronchoscopy and angiography for diagnosis of the bleeding site in hemoptysis. Ann Thorac Surg 1989;48:272–274.

86. Neff JA. Hemoptysis. West J Med 1977; 127:411–412.

87. Imgrund SP, Goldberg SK, Walkenstein MD, Fischer R, Lippmann ML. Clinical diagnosis of massive hemoptysis using the fiberoptic bronchoscope. Crit Care Med 1985; 13:438–443.

88. George PJM, Garrett CPO, Nixon C, et al. Laser treatment for tracheobronchial tumors: Local or general anesthesia? Thorax 1987; 42:656–660.

89. Prakash UBS. The use of the pediatric fiberoptic bronchoscope in adults. Am Rev Respir Dis 1985;132:715–717.

90. Katoh O, Yamada H, Hiura K, Nakanishi Y, Kishikawa T. Bronchoscopic and angiographic comparison of bronchial arterial lesions in patients with hemoptysis. Chest 1987;91:486–489.

91. Takeuchi Y, Namikawa S, Kusagawa M, Higashi K, Sakai T, Hashizume T. Bronchofiberscopic findings of bronchial artery lesions: a report of two cases. J Jpn Soc Bronchology 1985;7:71–76.

92. Flick MK, Wasson K, Dunn LJ, Block AJ. Fatal pulmonary hemorrhage after transbronchial lung biopsy through the fiberoptic bronchoscope. Am Rev Respir Dis 1975;111:853–856.

93. Haponik EF, Britt EJ, Smith PL, Bleecker ER. Computed chest tomography in the evaluation of hemoptysis: impact on diagnosis and treatment. Chest 1987;91:80–85.

94. Naidich DP, Funt S, Ettenger NA, Arranda C. Hemoptysis: CT-bronchoscopic correlations in 58 cases. Radiology 1990;177:357–362.

95. Millar AB, Boothroyd AE, Edwards D, Hetzel M. The role of computed tomography (CT) in the investigation of unexplained hemoptysis. Respir Med 1992;86:39–44.

96. Shephard JO, McLoud TC. Imaging the aneurysm: computed tomography and magnetic resonance imaging. Clin Chest Med 1991;12:151–168.

97. Conlan AA. Massive hemoptysis: diagnostic and therapeutic implications. Surg Ann 1985;17:337–355.

98. Dellinger RP. Fiberoptic bronchoscopy in adult airway management. Crit Care Med 1990;18:882–887.

99. Strange C. Double-lumen endotracheal tubes. Clin Chest Med 1991;12:497–506.

100. Shivaram U, Finch P, Nowak P. Plastic endobronchial tubes in the management of life-threatening hemoptysis. Chest 1987; 92:1108–1110.

101. Bjork VO, Carlens E. The prevention of spread during pulmonary resection by the use of a double lumen catheter. J Thorac Surg 1951;20:151–154.

102. Robertshaw FL. Low resistance double-lumen endobronchial tubes. Brit J Anaesth 1962;34:576–579.

103. Brodsky JB. Isolation of the lungs. Probl Anesth 1990;4:264–269.

104. Shulman MS, Brodsky JB, Levesque PR. Fiberoptic bronchoscopy for tracheal and endobronchial intubation with a double lumen tube. Can J Anaesth 1987;34: 172–175.

105. Hiebert CA. Balloon catheter control of life-threatening hemoptysis. Chest 1974; 66:308–309.

106. Gottlieb LS, Hillberg R. Endobronchial tamponade therapy for intractable hemoptysis. Chest 1975;67:482–483.

107. Saw EC, Gottlieb LS, Yokoyama T, Lee BC. Flexible fiberoptic bronchoscopy and endobronchial hemoptysis. Chest 1976;70: 589–591.

108. Faloney JP, Balchum OJ. Repeated massive hemoptysis. Successful control using multiple balloon-tipped catheters for endobronchial tamponade. Chest 1978;74:683–685.

109. Swersky RB, Chang JB, Wisoff BG, Gorvoy J. Endobronchial balloon tamponade of hemoptysis in patients with cystic fibrosis. Ann Thorac Surg 1979;27:262–264.

110. Thompson AB, Teschler H, Rennard SI. Pathogenesis, evaluation and therapy for massive hemoptysis. Clin Chest Med 1992; 13:69–82.

111. Garzon AA, Gourin A. Surgical management of massive hemoptysis: a ten year experience. Ann Surg 1978;187:267–271.

112. Gourin A, Garzon AA. Control of hemorrhage in emergency pulmonary resection for massive hemoptysis. Chest 1975;68:120–121.

113. Zavala DC. Pulmonary hemorrhage in fiberoptic transbronchial biopsy. Chest 1976;70:584–588.

114. Worth H, Breuer HWM, Charchut S, Trampisch HJ, Glanzer K. Endobronchial versus intravenous application of Glypressin for the therapy and prevention of lung bleeding during bronchoscopy. Am Rev Respir Dis 1987;135:A108.

115. Kaneko M, Ono R, Yoneyama T, Ikada S. A case of aortitis syndrome with massive hemorrhage following a transbronchial biopsy. J Jpn Soc Bronchology 1980;3:73–80.

116. Nakano S. Use of Reptilase with an endoscope against bronchial hemorrhage. Chin Rep 1986;20:229–235.

117. Kinoshita M, Shiraki R, Wagai F, Watanabe H, Kitamura S. Thrombin instillation therapy through the fiberoptic bronchoscope in cases of hemoptysis. Jpn J Thorac Dis 1982;20:251–254.

118. Tsukamoto T, Sasaki H, Nakamura H. Treatment of hemoptysis patients by thrombin and fibrinogen-thrombin infusion therapy using a fiberoptic bronchoscope. Chest 1989; 96:473–476.

119. Takagi O, Kohda Y, Yamazaki K, et al. Effect on bronchial bleeding by local infusion of fibrinogen and thrombin solution. J Jpn Soc Bronchology 1983;5:455–464.

120. Bense L. Intrabronchial selective coagulative treatment of hemoptysis. Chest 1990;97: 990–996.

121. Conlan AA, Hurwitz SS. Management of massive hemoptysis with the rigid bronchoscope and cold saline lavage. Thorax 1980; 35:901–904.

122. Gerasin VA, Shafirovsky BB. Endobronchial electrosurgery. Chest 1988;93:270–274.

Endoscopic Management of Subglottic and Tracheal Stenosis

22

Randall J. Harris, Glen E. DeBoer, and Atul C. Mehta

The presentation of airway stenosis varies from asymptomatic to life-threatening situations, depending on the degree of stenosis and the patient's pulmonary reserve. Subglottic and tracheal stenosis has become a significant clinical problem because both the number of endotracheal intubations and emergency medical procedures have increased (1). Previous therapies such as electrocautery, cryotherapy, and bougie dilation resulted in unpredictable healing and significant failure rates. No single conservative modality has yet been found uniformly effective. Moreover, some patients do not desire open tracheotomy for aesthetic reasons. Curative laryngotracheal resection or reconstruction is frequently successful, but may result in vocal cord and recurrent laryngeal nerve damage (2). For these reasons, endoscopic management has become the preferred therapy for many types of airway stenosis.

Recent improvements in laser technology afford more precise and less traumatic airway management, in addition to better hemostasis. The goals for endoscopic management of airway stenosis are to treat inoperable lesions, decannulate tracheotomies, return the patient to near-normal voice, and provide good exercise capacity.

Current endoscopic procedures are directed toward preserving the epithelium and minimizing thermal and mechanical mucosal injury. Multimodality approaches used include carbon dioxide (CO_2), argon, and neodymium:yttrium-aluminum-garnet (Nd:YAG) laser photodissections, gentler dilations, and indwelling stents. These conservative modalities are used to avoid the morbidity of an open operation or permanent tracheotomy. All conservative avenues should be exhausted before committing to open reconstruction. Aggressive endoscopic management does not preclude future open procedures if necessary.

The key to successful endoscopic management is careful patient selection, atraumatic dissection and dilation, meticulous postoperative care, and the use of serial procedures. Questions remain, however, as to the best combination of techniques, the use of adjuvant therapies, the number of required treatments, and the timing of surgical options. This chapter addresses these issues and is an update to our previous discussion on the endoscopic management of benign airway stenosis (3).

Anatomic Classification of Airway Stenosis

Stenosis management depends on both the location and degree of involvement. Stenosis may occur at the level of the larynx, subglottis, or the trachea (Table 22.1). It is important to anatomically distinguish these as separate entities because the treatment regimens differ. Because this book is mainly directed toward the pulmonologist, the discussion will be restricted to benign subglottic and tracheal stenosis. Discussion of laryngeal stenosis can be found elsewhere (4,5).

Table 22.1. Anatomic Classification and Causes of Airway Stenosis

Laryngeal	Subglottic	Tracheal
Supraglottic	Membranous web	Membranous web
Posterior glottic	Tracheomalacia	Tracheomalacia
Anterior glottic	Closed first ring	Vascular anomaly
	Trauma-related	Trauma-related
	Systemic disease	Systemic disease

Subglottic Stenosis

Subglottic stenosis is defined as a narrowing of the immediate airway below the glottis. It can be divided into congenital and acquired types (1). Congenital types may be membranous webs or cartilaginous in nature and usually present within the first few weeks of life. Intrinsic narrowing resulting from completed cartilaginous rings can also produce congenital obstruction. Audible biphasic stidor and prolonged "croup" are two common presenting symptoms. In 1976, Holinger and colleagues (6) stated that congenital subglottic stenosis was the third most common congenital upper airway malformation, and 44% of his patients required tracheotomy.

Acquired subglottic stenosis usually occurs secondary to trauma. External trauma includes anterior neck injury from motor vehicle accidents; internal trauma includes endotracheal intubations, emergency tracheotomies, burn inhalational injuries, and prior endoscopic treatment attempts. Acquired stenosis can also be a manifestation of systemic disease, namely amyloidosis, papillomatosis, tuberculosis, and Wegener's granulomatosis. Of the reported 158 National Institutes of Health patients with Wegener's granulomatosis, 16% had subglottic stenosis (7). Positive pressure ventilation can also cause acquired subglottic stenosis (1). Positive pressure ventilation creates direct pressure at the site of the endotracheal tube cuff as well as shearing stress on the tracheal mucosa with each inspiratory and expiratory

exchange. The most common cause of internal trauma by far, however, is endotracheal intubation.

Factors responsible for the airway obstruction secondary to an endotracheal tube are intubation trauma, duration of intubation, the size of the endotracheal tube relative to the size of the larynx or trachea, chemical irritants on the tube, tube motion, cuff pressure and necrosis, superimposed tracheal infections, and the patient's general condition (8).

Tracheal Stenosis

Tracheal stenosis is secondary to scarring and stricture of the trachea, tracheomalacia, tumor, or systemic disease. Congenital tracheal stenosis may result from membraneous webs, ring anomalies, or tracheomalacia. Unfortunately, only 10% of patients with tracheal stenosis have simple weblike stenosis (5). The majority of patients have more complex stenosis or combinations of intrinsic scarring and malacia. In rare instances, vascular anomalies can cause external compression at the innominate artery or vascular ring level, resulting in airway compromise. Acquired tracheal stenosis is caused by internal or external injury. Internal injury is caused by endotracheal intubation or tracheotomy and is best characterized as acute or chronic benign scarring of the trachea, which can occur at any one or more of four predictable locations (9). Montgomery (10) described these four locations and related each of them to the various causal factors responsible for scar development. First, strictures that occurred above the tracheotomy site were caused by a high tracheotomy, trauma to the anterior tracheal wall during tracheotomy, or intubation trauma. Second, at the level of the tracheotomy itself, inflammatory changes caused by injury, infection, polyps, or granulation tissue resulted in a loss of cartilaginous support and scarring that led to airway stenosis. Third, just below the tracheotomy site, granuloma formation or ulceration secondary to excessive cuff pressure were present in the acute stage of injury, whereas the loss of cartilaginous support and circumferential stenosis were identified in the chronic stage. The fourth site of involvement was the area at the distal tip of the endotracheal tube. Here, excessive pressure and motion against the anterior tracheal wall led to granuloma formation and the loss of cartilaginous support.

Definitive treatment options for tracheal stenosis include tracheal reconstruction, tracheoplasty, endoscopic incision or excision of scar tissue, dilation, and airway stenting. Total occlusion of the airway or the inability to visualize the distal lumen mandates a tracheotomy. Otherwise, the presence or absence of tracheomalacia, the characterization of the stenosis, and the presence of skeletal deformity significantly influence selection of the therapeutic procedure.

Diagnosis and Evaluation of Airway Stenosis

Signs and Symptoms

Patients with airway stenosis may present with acute or chronic complaints. Signs and symptoms related to subglottic and tracheal stenosis depend on the anatomic location of the obstruction and its severity. Major signs and symptoms include hoarseness, stridor or wheezing, dyspnea, and respiratory failure. A difficult intubation is yet another sign that airway stenosis may be present. If stenosis is related to prior intubation, frequently the patient is extubated and able to breathe relatively comfortably until an upper respiratory infection causes additional airway narrowing and subsequent respiratory distress.

Noninvasive Testing

Noninvasive testing is usually the first step after physical examination in the evaluation of airway stenosis. Chest roentgenograms can be revealing for airway narrowing but are not sensitive. Tracheal tomograms are occasionally helpful (Figure 22.1). Flow-volume loops obtained with spirometry can indicate dynamic or fixed upper airway obstruction. Enhanced noninvasive imaging, namely, magnetic resonance and computed tomography, have gained prominence as diagnostic tools for airway obstruction (11). These techniques can characterize the length of the stenotic segment, identify the external length of the stenotic segment, identify external compression causes, and quantify the degree of anatomic severity.

Invasive Imaging

The gold standard for assessing airway obstruction is direct visualization through flexible fiberoptic bronchoscopy (FOB). Direct visualization allows for the proper anatomic classification of the stenosis. It also permits assessment of the cause and degree of obstruction (Plate 49). Moreover, the information provided by FOB can help physicians formulate strategies for future treatment.

Available Endoscopic Options

Intraluminal Stenting

Intraluminal stenting has been used for many years in select patients with variable success. It is used most often in patients in whom endoscopic management is incomplete or in patients who present with tracheomalacia. At this time, what type of a stent is optimal and for how

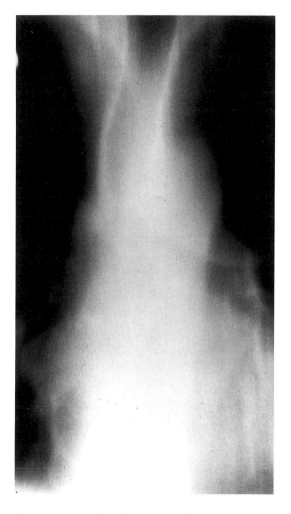

Figure 22.1. Tracheal tomogram demonstrates stenosis.

long it should be left in place are unknown. Because many cases of subglottic stenosis are caused by rigid indwelling endotracheal tubes (which act as stents), it seems logical that a therapeutic stent should be soft enough to avoid further pressure necrosis and elastic enough to prevent the formation of exuberant granulation tissue (12). Internal pressure should be light enough to allow epithelial migration beneath the stent. Stents should also be inert and elicit little or no tissue reaction. A commonly used stent is the Montgomery T-tube Silastic stent, which is described in detail elsewhere (10). Indwelling times of 2 weeks to 6 months have been arbitrarily used (5,12).

The disadvantages of stents include required maintenance of a tracheotomy, stomal infections, stent migration, and respiratory distress because of obstruction by dried secretions (2).

Simpson and colleagues (13) reported a large experience with intraluminal stenting as part of a multimodality protocol. Thirty-nine of 60 (65%) patients with subglottic or tracheal stenosis had stents placed for internal support. Silastic stents were deemed useful (or at least not harmful) because they were used in 84% of the successful subglottic cases.

Recently, Colt and coworkers (2) described the technique of percutaneous external fixation of bronchoscopically placed subglottic stents. Under direct videobronchoscopic control, a 14-gauge angiocatheter is inserted through the skin, subcutaneous tissues, anterior tracheal wall, and anterior silicone stent. A second catheter is inserted about one cm distal to the first. A suture is placed through the catheter ports. Once secure, the catheters are removed and the suture pulled taut. A polypropylene button is tied snugly to the anterior neck for external stabilization. This technique can be considered in carefully selected patients with severe malacia and subglottic stenosis who have failed indwelling stent placement because of stent migration.

Dilation

Currently, endoscopic intervention is a multimodality approach, with dilation relegated to a minor role. Historically, subglottic stenosis had been managed with dilation alone using Jackson dilators and rigid bronchoscopes. Success in these cases was measured by the ability to wean these patients from their tracheotomy tubes. Hawkins (8) managed eight patients in this manner. However, the process was laborious and required an average of six dilations over an 8-week period. Other workers have suggested that acquired subglottic stenosis is commonly refractory to dilation alone and that dilation can cause stenosis (14).

Rigid versus Flexible Bronchoscopy

Rigid bronchoscopes have been specialized for simultaneous laser fiber introduction, the use of flexible suction catheters, and an application of a rigid telescope with either an open or a closed ventilating system. The advantages of a rigid bronchoscope are that it allows for secure ventilation, rapid evacuation of blood clots, the ability to tamponade bleeding, and a less flammable system during photocoagulation. The disadvantages of the rigid bronchoscope compared to the flexible bronchoscope are limited access to the proximal bronchi and the need for general anesthesia (15).

The advantages of a flexible bronchoscopic system include the ability to perform operations under local anesthesia and better access to more distal lesions. The disadvantages of FOB include its minimal suction capability, the inability to compress bleeding, and the risk of igniting the plastic covering of the bronchoscope (15).

Laser Systems

The CO_2 and the Nd:YAG lasers are the most common systems used. It is unclear which laser is optimal for stenosis therapy. The CO_2 laser is a more precise cutting instrument. The Nd:YAG laser has a greater coagulation than cutting effect and may provide better hemostasis (16). The Nd:YAG has the ability to pass readily through flexible quartz fibers, allowing application through the flexible scope. Nd:YAG lasers also have greater penetration (5 mm) but unfortunately less predictable soft tissue effects. Hence, it should at all times be directed parallel to the tracheal wall, skimming the surface of the target tissue to avoid damaging the underlying cartilaginous rings and deeper structures (14).

"Mucosal-Sparing" Techniques

Techniques that minimize mucosal trauma should be used at all times. Procedures (such as dilation by using progressively larger bougies or rigid bronchoscopes) in which treatment can destroy normal airway mucosa at the stenotic site may predispose a patient to disorganized healing by second intention, excessive fibrous tissue proliferation, and scar recurrence (14). Avoiding both excessive laser energy and mechanical trauma to normal mucosa is paramount to overall success. Three reported series that used mucosal-sparing techniques will be reviewed.

In 1983, Dedo and Sooy (17) presented an innovative approach to the difficult problem of subglottic and tracheal stenosis. A "micro-trapdoor" flap was made in the trachea for tracheal stenosis and in the posterior glottic region for posterior glottic stenosis. A thin, superiorly based flap of epithelium was elevated using the CO_2 laser. The laser was then used to remove the underlying scar tissue by vaporization. This biologic flap was then put back into position to reepithelialize the wound area. Success was reported in 8 of 9 (89%) patients treated with this technique for posterior glottic stenosis. Nine of 10 (90%) patients with subglottic or tracheal stenosis less than one cm thick were also successfully treated. Resolution of dyspnea on exertion and decannulation were the criteria for success. The average thickness of the tracheal and subglottic stenosis was 6 mm. Success was attributed to reepithelialization that prevented scar formation.

In 1987, Shapshay and colleagues (18), in hopes of developing a less traumatic technique, used the Nd:YAG or CO_2 laser through the rigid bronchoscope to introduce radial incisions coupled with dilation. The radial incisions were made through the epithelium and underlying fibrous tissue using intermittent exposures of laser energy just sufficient to vaporize, not to coagulate, the soft tissue. The rationale behind this technique was that islands of epithelium between the radial laser incisions could be preserved and rapidly reepithelialize the tracheal wall. Initially performed in five patients, durable success was noted in three patients at the end of a one-year follow-up period after the application of one to five treatments. A modification of this technique adding the use of 12- to 14-mm silicone T-tube airway stents to the previous application of multiple radial incisions and increasing rigid bronchoscope dilations, was later successful in 8 of 12 (67%) tracheotomy patients with total cervical stenosis (15). The average duration of initial T-tube placement in this series was 6 months. However, six of these eight (75%) successful patients required additional laser treatment over a follow-up period of one to 6 years. One patient died of an acute myocardial infarction at decannulation. Of the other three with poor results, two underwent sleeve resection of the trachea with a good final result.

In 1993, Mehta and coworkers (14) used a mucosal-sparing technique that included Nd:YAG photodissection, radial incisions, and gentle dilation (without stenting) and reported a 67% (12 of 18) success rate for select patients with benign concentric stenosis. Of the 12 successful patients, 8 required a single treatment, whereas only 4 required two or more treatments. No patients required new tracheostomy to carry out the procedure. Follow-up periods ranged from 2 to 85 months (mean 32 months). Lengthy scars (greater than one cm) and tracheomalacia were the clinical features common to those patients in whom the treatment was unsuccessful. The number of procedures needed to achieve success in this series, even without using increasing dilation or stenting, was less than that of Simpson and associates (1.5 vs. 2.4 per patient) (13).

Procedure Description

The operative procedure and protocol for endoscopic management of airway stenosis is both operator and institution dependent. This following discussion is restricted primarily to our mucosal-sparing technique performed at the Cleveland Clinic Foundation.

Anesthesia

General anesthesia is used in the majority of cases. It ensures airway control, provides full cooperation from the patient, and eliminates some psychological trauma. Our preference is to use the Nd:YAG laser. Ventilation during the Nd:YAG laser photodissection (LPD) is provided by a jet ventilator using an experimental stainless steel jet injection cannula (JIC) (Figure 22.2). This ventilation technique is used to overcome hypoventilation caused by an air leak that can occur while performing Nd:YAG LPD through the beveled distal end of a rigid bronchoscope, especially if the patient has subglottic stenosis. The methods and equipment used during this procedure have been described previously (14,19). A stainless steel, triple-lumen cannula delivers jet

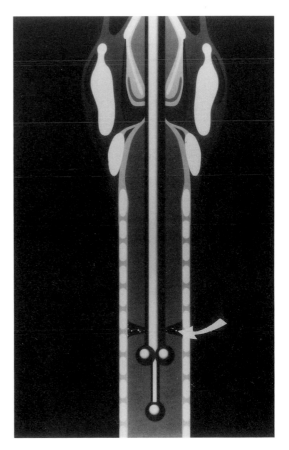

Figure 22.2. Schematic of stainless steel jet injection cannula (JIC). Note that the three ports (see text) are distal to the obstructing lesion (see arrow).

ventilation. Two proximal lumina of this cannula deliver jet ventilation while the third one simultaneously measures airway pressure. This cannula, approximately 3 mm in total diameter and of variable length, is introduced under laryngoscopic guidance, and its ventilation port is placed distal to the lesion. Thus, preoperative tracheostomy is avoided. The jet ventilation frequency used is between 70 and 120, and the driving pressure is adjusted for each patient.

Technical Aspect

Patients with short-segment concentric subglottic or tracheal stenosis who are selected on the basis of bronchoscopic findings usually undergo Nd:YAG LPD of the stenotic area with flexible bronchoscopy, in addition to a single gentle dilation using a rigid bronchoscope. Nd:YAG LPD is used to produce radial incisions through the entire vertical length of the stenotic lesion, usually at the 9, 12, and 3 o'clock positions (18) (Plate 50). Islands of epithelium that remain between these laser incisions facilitate rapid generation of epithelial cover. To avoid thermal trauma to surrounding tissues, minimal laser energy is used. Average power settings of 30 to 40 W with a 0.4-second pulse duration are used for most cases. To prevent endotracheal combustion, the fractional inspired oxygen is kept below 40% during the actual use of the laser beam. Although extremely rare, an endobronchial fire can occur. The immediate response is prompt removal of all flammable materials, especially the flexible bronchoscope.

In our protocol, Nd:YAG LPD is followed by a gentle dilation using a size 7.0-, 8.0-, or 9.0-mm rigid bronchoscope while still providing ventilation with the JIC system. The rigid bronchoscope is used under telescopic guidance, for only the purpose of gentle dilation. Unlike routine dilation with increasing sizes of bougies or rigid bronchoscopes, gentle dilation consists of only a single insertion of the largest possible rigid bronchoscope that the patient's trachea can accommodate after the laser dissection. This single insertion minimizes the mechanical trauma of repeated insertions to the treatment site and spares as much normal mucosa as possible. It is imperative to avoid exposure of the perichondrium to prevent chondritis and inflammation.

Postoperative Care

If significant endobronchial mucopurulent material is noted during the procedure, patients are placed on a 7- to 10-day course of empirical antibiotics. Patients with a history of reactive chronic obstructive pulmonary disease or bronchial asthma receive a 2- to 3-week course of oral corticosteroids after the procedure. Cortico-steroids are also prescribed for patients in whom it is suspected that laryngeal trauma from the procedure may lead to laryngeal edema. We do not empirically use systemic or intralesional corticosteroids to reduce operative inflammation. Most patients undergo Nd:YAG LPD and gentle dilation treatment on an outpatient basis. Patients are observed for several hours in the recovery room or the short-stay unit. Reevaluation is at 6 weeks, unless symptoms arise earlier.

The operative strategy sometimes commands a stepwise procedure. Nonetheless, the majority of patients undergo a repeat procedure only as dictated by recurrence of symptoms or if significant stenosis is identified during follow-up bronchoscopic surveillance. The number of repeat treatments is usually limited to three in our practice. If stenosis recurs following the third endoscopic treatment, the patient is referred to either an otolaryngologist or a thoracic surgeon for definitive surgical intervention.

Endoscopic laser management is judged as successful if postoperative, bronchoscopically verified patency or near normalization of the flow-volume loop are confirmed, and symptomatic improvement is noted.

Review of Published Series

Other major reported series are summarized in Table 22.2. Each series is discussed in chronologic order.

In 1979, Strong and colleagues (12) reported the initial experience with endoscopic management for airway stenosis. They used the original 50-W CO_2 laser coupled to the Ziess surgical microscope in 23 patients, with an age range of 10 months to 72 years. The patient population consisted of 5 patients with supraglottic stenosis, 7 with glottic stenosis, and 11 with subglottic stenosis. Sixteen (70%) presented with existing tracheotomies. Eight (35%) patients received an indwelling stent for a variable period of time. Endoscopic management using vaporization was successful in 18 (78%) of their 23 patients.

In 1981, Koufman and associates (20) reported 13 cases of subglottic stenosis that were managed endoscopically with the CO_2 laser. The stenoses ranged in severity from 50% to 90% occlusion (average 77%). Six (46%) of these patients previously had undergone repeated dilations. In 10 (77%) of 13 patients, a satisfactory airway was reestablished within a one-year period. Patients in this study underwent one to five laser procedures (average 2.7 per patient). However, their experience with laser excision followed by stenting (3 cases) was discouraging. In each of these cases, copious granulation tissue filled the subglottic region after stent removal. In 2 cases, the stenoses appeared worse after the stent was removed. None of the 3 patients treated with stents were decannulated.

In 1982, Simpson and coworkers (13) retrospectively analyzed the outcome in 49 patients with laryngeal stenosis (31 subglottic), 6 with tracheal stenosis, and 5 with combined laryngeal and tracheal stenoses (total 60 patients) who had been treated with first-generation 25- to 50-W CO_2 laser instrumentation. Dilation was not required in any patient in this series. Silastic stents were used in 39 (65%) patients. Follow-up ranged from one to 8 years. Multiple procedures (average 2.2 per patient) were required in 35 (73%) of 49 laryngeal patients. Thirty-nine (80%) of 49 patients with laryngeal stenosis had successful outcomes. Of 31 patients with subglottic stenosis, 25 (81%) were managed successfully (average 2.4 procedures per patient). Of 11 patients with combined laryngeal and tracheal procedures, only 3 (27%) were successfully managed endoscopically. Overall, 41 (68%) of 60 patients were successfully managed by endoscopic techniques. Thirteen (22%) patients who failed endoscopic management underwent

Table 22.2. Reported Series of Endoscopic Management of Airway Stenosis

First Author	Date	Technique	Success Rate No./No. (%)
Strong (12)	1979	CO_2 laser; stents (most)	18/23 (78)
Koufman (20)	1981	CO_2 laser	10/13 (77)
Simpson (13)	1982	CO_2 laser; stents	41/60 (68)
Dedo (17)	1983	CO_2 laser; microtrapdoor technique	17/19 (89)
Ossoff (9)	1985	CO_2 laser; intralesional steroids; stents	8/14 (57)
Shapshay (18)	1987	Nd:YAG or CO_2 laser; radial incisions; dilation; stents	8/12 (67)
Mehta (14)	1993	Nd:YAG laser; gentle dilation	12/18 (67)

open surgery. This landmark study justifies a trial of endoscopic management, at all levels of stenosis, if certain anatomic features are absent.

Ossoff and colleagues (9) in 1985 examined their endoscopic experience among 14 patients using the rigid, ventilating bronchoscope and the CO_2 laser. Twelve (86%) of 14 patients had tracheotomies at the time of their referral. Neither intralesional steroid injections nor Silastic stents were used in this series. Eight (57%) of 14 patients with tracheal stenosis were successfully managed by bronchoscopic laser technique, but each required multiple procedures. In the 6 cases that were unsuccessful, circumferential scarring greater than one cm in width was present on examination. Open procedures were subsequently performed in 5 of the 6 failed cases and were successful in 3. These investigators concluded that patients with narrow, noncircumferential strictures should first be treated with the CO_2 laser, with successful results achievable in the majority.

Anatomic Features Predictive of Outcome

Given that the location, extent, and severity of stenoses are highly variable, corrective measures need to be selected to suit the individual problem. Invasive endoscopists need to be aware of these prognostic features and select patients with favorable features. It is clear that successful endoscopic outcome depends on proper patient selection.

Favorable Features

The presence of certain anatomic features that account for the reported variable short and long-term success rates are presented in Table 22.3. Favorable features in our experience include a thin weblike concentric stenosis of less than one cm in vertical length and the absence of tracheomalacia (14).

Table 22.3. Unfavorable Predictive Features of Outcome of Endoscopic Management

Circumferential scarring with cicatricial contracture (9,13)

Scarring longer than 1 cm in vertical dimension (9,13,14)

Tracheomalacia (13,14)

History of bacterial infection associated with tracheotomy (13)

Carinal involvement of stenosis (9)

Combined laryngeal and tracheal stenoses (13)

Unfavorable Features

Patients with collapsing cartilage (tracheomalacia) or the so-called hourglass or bottleneck stenosis should not be selected (14–16). Simpson and colleagues (13) identified anatomic features that connote poor response rates or failure: circumferential scarring with cicatricial contracture, scarring greater than one cm in vertical dimension, tracheomalacia with loss of cartilage support, and a history of severe bacterial infections with tracheotomy. Ossoff and coworkers (9) retrospectively add carinal involvement as predictive of an unfavorable outcome. In these circumstances, multiple procedures, more extensive alternative surgeries, or maintenance of tracheotomy were usually necessary.

Perioperative Adjuvant Therapies

Corticosteroids and Antibiotics

Each reported series used different perioperative adjuvant therapies such as corticosteroids (systemic or intralesional) and antibiotics. However, these adjuncts have not been adequately studied. Controlled studies are not available that substantiate or refute their efficacies in the endoscopic management of airway stenosis.

Koufman and coworkers (20) gave each of their 13 patients who underwent CO_2 laser surgery for subglottic stenosis a single intraoperative dose of intravenous dexamethasone (0.5 to 1.0 mg/kg) in hopes of reducing postoperative edema. Early in the series, patients were treated postoperatively with a 2-week course of oral prednisone (0.5 mg/kg daily). This practice of systemic steroids was abandoned and replaced by the use of intralesional corticosteroids. Depomedrol (20 to 40 mg) was injected with a 22-gauge needle into the scar, granulation tissue, or both, before laser use.

There is concern that systemic corticosteroids delay epithelialization and inhibit effective healing (16). Shapshay and coworkers (15) avoided corticosteroids in their series of 12 patients with total cervical tracheal stenosis for fear of delayed epithelial migration and the potential prolongation of susceptibility to infection. To date, there is no consensus on the proper use of corticosteroids or their effect on outcome. Randomized, controlled studies are necessary. Pending further data, we use corticosteroids only if procedure-induced laryngeal edema is suspected or bronchospastic disease exists.

The possibility of infection and its potential sequelae prompt some endoscopists to use prophylactic antibiotics (13). Sasaki (21) has shown in an animal model that infection predisposes the host to scar tissue formation and airway stenosis. The amount of scar tissue produced was directly related to the length of time required for wound healing and to the presence or absence of localized infection. Based upon this work, both Simpson (13) and Friedman (1) suggested the prophylactic use of antibiotics. Moreover, Koufman and associates (20) used parenteral antibiotic therapy selected on the basis of perioperative stomal and subglottic cultures. Shapshay and colleagues (15,18) gave each patient a broad-spectrum antibiotic for 10 days. Infection rates and the antibiotics' effect on procedure success are not adequately analyzed in any of these investigations. Pending further data, we do not believe empirical antibiotics are necessary for every case. In our protocol, we use antibiotics only if mucopurulent secretions are identified in the operating room. Randomized, controlled studies are needed to investigate the role of antibiotics and their effect on outcome.

Complications

Endoscopic management of benign airway stenosis is a safe procedure. Complications are infrequent. Technical improvements in the laser instrumentation, jet ventilation, and flexible bronchoscopes have reduced the potential for serious complications. Trends toward minimizing thermal and mechanical trauma have had an impact and have reduced the risk for mishaps, such as bleeding or perforation. Jet ventilation with a steel cannula can provide uninterrupted instrument access in addition to adequate ventilation because of the cannula's small diameter and mobility. The nonflammable nature of the steel cannula also reduces the threat of endobronchial ignition. More-over, jet ventilation can minimize the need for tracheostomy before the procedure.

No significant complications occurred among 23 patients reported by Strong's group (12). In 2 patients, minor infection developed adjacent to the exit of the stent transfixation wire; both infections were readily controlled by antibiotic therapy. Shapshay and colleagues (15,18) reported no laser complications among their 12 patients. No tracheal perforations occurred despite using rigid dilations. Persistent granulation tissue and a minor degree of fibrosis were the only complications (8 of 12 patients). In the largest collection of patients to date, Simpson and associates (13) did not report any significant complications among their 60 patients. Similarly, respiratory complications (infections, airway perforation, and hemorrhage) were not recorded for any patient during the treatment and follow-up by Mehta's group (14). A small laceration of the upper lip during insertion of the rigid bronchoscope in one patient was the only complication in this series.

Special Endoscopic Modalities

Photodynamic Therapy

Juvenile laryngotracheobronchial papillomatosis (JLTBP) is the most common benign tumor of the larynx (22). It can present as upper airway stenosis (Plates 51 and 52). Extension into the trachea and proximal bronchi occurs with a reported incidence of 5% to 20% (23). It is well established that human papillomavirus (subtypes HPV 1, 6) is the causative agent (23). Papillomas are not neoplastic but are benign squamous lesions that tend to occur in clusters and are composed of a vascular connective tissue core covered by stratified squamous epithelium, with little tendency to invade submucosal tissue. They are usually multiple and sessile, but may pedunculate. Although variable, these epithelial tumors have the tendency to aggressively recur. The clinical course may be complicated by airway stenosis, hemoptysis, or malignant transformation of the papillomas. Current management is symptomatic and involves frequent and repeated endoscopic removal of papillomas with cup forceps and laser surgery. Numerous therapies including radiation, cryotherapy, local podophyllum, human leukocyte interferon, hormones, and chemotherapy have little long-term success. Endoscopic management using photodynamic therapy (PDT) is a promising alternative.

Currently, PDT uses the combination of dihematoporphyrin ether (DHE), a photosensitive compound characterized by its ability to localize in dividing tissues, and red light to destroy dividing cells (HPV or tumor). The proposed mechanism for therapy is cellular destruction via the production of toxic oxygen radicals after the direct excitation of DHE by a laser beam of appropriate wavelength. The oxygen radicals disrupt cell membranes by lipid and protein sulfydrol oxidation and also affect the microcirculation of rapidly dividing tissue. Current experimental protocols use DHE intravenously (22). Forty-eight hours later, PDT is carried out using red light (630 nm) obtained from an argon-pumped dye laser. Another repeat FOB for clean-up at 96 hours demonstrates significant necrosis of laryngeal and endobronchial papillomas. DNA hybridization techniques have confirmed the disappearance after DHE of the HPV genome from the endobronchial mucosa (22).

Photodynamic therapy has potential as therapy for JLTBP. Precautions must be taken to have the patient avoid direct sunlight or fluorescent light for approximately 30 days postoperatively because of the risk of serious skin photosensitization and sunburn. PDT has been successful for treating this disease in isolated cases (22,23). However, confirmatory studies are necessary.

Open Surgical Options for Airway Stenosis

Open procedures are indicated when unfavorable findings preclude endoscopic intervention or conservative approaches have been unsuccessful. However, open surgical procedures involve certain potential risks not associated with endoscopic techniques, including increased anesthesia time, longer hospitalizations, blood loss, pneumothorax, and increased risk of infection (9). Open surgical repair consists of *resecting* the stenotic segment or *restoring* circular architecture over which respiratory epithelium can regenerate (24).

Resection

Resection of the stenotic portion of trachea with primary end-to-end anastomosis has been the preferred method of tracheal reconstruction for lesions up to 3 cm in length (9). Grillo and Mathisen (25) had a failure rate of only 4% and a mortality rate of 1.8% in 279 patients with tracheal stenosis. Maggi and colleagues (26) reported a failure rate of 17.8% (5 patients) in 28 cases of benign tracheal stenosis. They reported dehiscence in 3.6% (one case), restenosis in 7.1% (2 patients), and death in 7.1% (2 patients). Maassen and associates (27), however, reported an alarming failure rate of 27% and a total mortality of 19%. This disparity in results for open reconstruction is probably related to surgical technique and patient selection.

The tracheal sleeve procedure is another resection option. Bisson and coworkers (28) performed 200 sleeve resections for iatrogenic subglottic and tracheal stenosis. Preoperative Nd:YAG laser use was of paramount help in opening the stenosis and stabilizing the patient before the operation. In this group, 175 (87.5%) patients were definitively cured, but 16 patients required a Montgomery T-tube for 6 months to one year. Three (1.5%) patients required an emergency operation for rupture of the innominate artery. Nine (4.5%) patients died postoperatively. Five (2.5%) patients experienced a disabling recurrent laryngeal nerve palsy. Mediastinal sepsis occurred in one (0.5%) patient. Sixteen (8%) had recurrent stenosis. Two patients needed a second tracheal sleeve resection. Thus, successful sleeve resection is not without attendant risk.

Restoration

The restoration techniques require ensuring adequate cartilaginous or bony structure for support of the airway. Restoration techniques involve either splitting of the cricoid ring and stepladdering the cartilage, or inserting a graft of bone or cartilage (20) to create internal support.

Children

Although spontaneous resolution of congenital subglottic stenosis has been reported (29), usually mandating tracheotomy until resolution, most patients require definitive intervention. Maddalozzo and Holinger (30) reported their experience with laryngotracheal reconstruction (LTR) in 20 children using autologous costal cartilage grafts. Eight (40%) patients had both anterior and posterior costal grafts, plus stent insertion (typically for 6 to 10 weeks). Sixteen (80%) of the 20 children were successfully decannulated. Most patients had an endoscopic procedure between LTR and decannulation, however. The authors reported a failure rate of 20% and a complication rate of 30%, with a total mortality of 5%. The complication rate was high, but the majority of complications were minor. Two patients did have a pneumothorax as a result of harvesting the costal cartilage. One child died within 24 hours of the LTR, possibly of apnea or obstruction of the tracheotomy tube. In this series, LTR was undertaken only if conservative therapy was unsuccessful, and the child was tracheotomy dependent. It is possible some children may have benefited from earlier open procedures.

Adults

In the adult population, McCaffrey (24) surgically treated, by restoration, 21 patients with severe subglottic stenosis refractory to endoscopic treatment. Patients were treated with anterior or anterior plus posterior cricoid division with costal cartilage grafting. Sixteen (77%) of the patients were successfully decannulated and able to perform normal daily activities without restriction. There was significantly better outcome in patients with isolated subglottic stenosis compared to those with combined glottic and subglottic stenoses.

Controversies Regarding Endoscopic Management

In a short time, endoscopic management using laser technology has become the cornerstone of management for benign airway stenosis. Despite encouraging results, many questions remain unanswered. The exact timing of laser therapy is controversial. It is unknown if the progression of disease can be halted in the acute stage by using early excision or if excision is most effective in the chronic stage after mature scar tissue has formed. Laser can cause thermal injury that possibly results in further scarring.

The precise roles of adjuvant perioperative corticosteroids and antibiotics need to be addressed in prospective studies. Which patient populations these drugs benefit or harm remains to be determined. If indeed useful, the optimal timing is not known.

It appears that "gentle dilation" as proposed by Mehta and colleagues (14) is as efficacious as repeated enlarging rigid dilations. This observation awaits confirmation. Moreover, the additional benefit provided by any dilation has not yet been quantified.

It is also unknown in which patient population indwelling stents are beneficial. The optimal time that stents should be left in place is not known. Finding answers to these questions should be the goals of future prospective, randomized studies.

Summary

Tracheotomy and open repair of airway stenosis have significant associated morbidity. The application of laser technology has advanced the success rate of endoscopic management. Successful outcome occurs in the majority of patients when patients are properly selected. Predictive anatomic features have been identified that aid proper patient selection. Additionally, we recommend that mucosal-sparing techniques be used at all times. Given its clinical effectiveness and low complication rate, endoscopic management should remain the first option for subglottic and tracheal stenosis. Importantly, endoscopic management does not preclude the use of open surgical procedures if necessary. Further studies are necessary to refine and optimize the endoscopic operative technique.

REFERENCES

1. Friedman EM, Healy GB, McGill TJ. Carbon dioxide laser management of subglottic and tracheal stenosis. Otolaryngol Clin North Am 1983;16:871.
2. Colt HG, Harrell J, Neuman TR, et al. External fixation of subglottic tracheal stents. Chest 1994;105:1653.
3. Mehta AC, Harris RJ, DeBoer GE. Endoscopic management of benign airway stenosis. In: Clinics in chest medicine. Philadelphia: WB Saunders, 1994 (in press).
4. Duncavage JA, Ossoff RH. Laser surgery for benign laryngeal lesions. In: Davis RK, ed. Lasers in otolaryngology—head and neck surgery. Philadelphia: WB Saunders, 1990: 26–32.
5. Shapshay SM. Laser bronchoscopy. In: Davis RK, ed. Lasers in otolaryngology—head and neck surgery. Philadelphia: WB Saunders, 1990:85–105.
6. Holinger PH, Kutnick SL, Schild JA, et al. Subglottic stenosis in infants and children. Ann Otol 1976;85:591-599.
7. Hoffman GS, Kerr GS, Leavitt RY, et al. Wegener granulomatosis: an analysis of 158 patients. Ann Intern Med 1992;116:488.
8. Hawkins DB. Glottic and subglottic stenosis from endotracheal intubation. Laryngoscope 1977;87:339-346.
9. Ossoff RH, Tucker GF Jr, Duncacage JA, et al. Efficacy of bronchoscopic carbon dioxide laser surgery for benign strictures of the trachea. Laryngoscope 1985;95:1220-1223.
10. Montgomery WW. Current modifications of the salivary bypass tube and tracheal T-tube. Ann Otol Rhinol Laryngol 1986;95:121.
11. Fletcher BD, Dearborn DG, Mulopulos GP. MR imaging in infants with airway obstruction:

preliminary observations. Radiology 1986; 160:245.

12. Strong MS, Healy GB, Vaughan CW, et al. Endoscopic management of laryngeal stenosis. Otolaryngol Clin North Am 1979;12:797–805.

13. Simpson GT, Strong MS, Healy GB, et al. Predictive factors of success or failure in the endoscopic management of laryngeal and tracheal stenosis. Ann Otol Rhinol Laryngol 1982;91:384–388.

14. Mehta AC, Lee FY, Cordasco EM, et al. Concentric tracheal and subglottic stenosis. Chest 1993;104:673–677.

15. Shapshay SM, Beamis JF, Dumon JF. Total cervical tracheal stenosis: treatment by laser, dilation, and stenting. Ann Otol Rhinol Laryngol 1989;98:890-895.

16. Shapshay SM, Beamis JF Jr. Use of CO_2 laser. Chest 1989;95:449–456.

17. Dedo HH, Sooy CD. Endoscopic laser repair of posterior glottic, subglottic, and tracheal stenosis by division or micro-trapdoor flap. Laryngoscope 1984;94:445–450.

18. Shapshay SM, Beamis JF, Hybels RL, et al. Endoscopic treatment of subglottic and tracheal stenosis by radial laser incision and dilation. Ann Otol Rhinol Laryngol 1987; 96:661–664.

19. Mehta AC, Livingston DR, Levine HL, et al. Ventilatory management during neodymium: yttrium aluminum garnet photoresection of subglottic and higher tracheal lesions. Trans Am Broncho-esophagological Association, 1986:148–153.

20. Koufman JA, Thompson JN, Kohut RI. Endoscopic management of subglottic stenosis with the CO_2 surgical laser. Otolaryngol Head Neck Surg 1981;89:215–220.

21. Sakasi CT, Horiuchi M, Koss N. Tracheostomy-related subglottic stenosis: bacteriologic pathogenesis. Laryngoscope 1979;89: 857–865.

22. Basheda SG, Mehta AC, DeBoer GE, et al. Endobronchial and parenchymal juvenile laryngotracheobronchial papillomatosis: the effect of photodynamic therapy. Chest 1991;100:1458–1461.

23. Kavuru MS, Mehta AC, Eliachar I. Effect of photodynamic therapy and external beam radiation therapy on juvenile laryngotracheobronchial papillomatosis. Am Rev Respir Dis 1990;141:509.

24. McCaffrey TV. Management of subglottic stenosis in the adult. Ann Otol Rhinol Laryngol 1991;100:90–94.

25. Grillo HC, Mathisen DJ. Surgical management of tracheal strictures, vol 68. In: Farrell EM, Keon WJ, eds. Philadelphia: WB Saunders, 1988:511–524.

26. Maggi G, Ardissone F, Cavallo A, et al. Tracheal stenosis: a study of 100 cases. Int Surg 1990;75:225–230.

27. Maassen W, Greschuchna D, Vogt-Moykopf K, et al. Tracheal resection—state of the art. Thorac Cardiovasc Surg 1985;33:2.

28. Bisson A, Bonnette P, El Kadi B, et al. Tracheal sleeve resection for iatrogenic stenoses (subglottic, laryngeal, and tracheal). J Thorac Cardiovasc Surg 1992;104:882–887.

29. Rosenfeld RM, Bluestone CD. Does early expansion surgery have a role in the management of congenital subglottic stenosis? Laryngoscope 1993;103:286–290.

30. Maddalozzo J, Holinger LD. Laryngotracheal reconstruction for subglottic stenosis in children. Ann Otol Rhinol Laryngol 1987;96:665–669.

Part 4

Special Considerations

23 | Pediatric Flexible Fiberoptic Bronchoscopy for the Adult Bronchoscopist

Marc S. Rovner and Paul C. Stillwell

Although flexible bronchoscopy was first introduced in the United States in 1969, it was not until 1978 that the first reports of flexible fiberoptic bronchoscopy (FOB) in infants and young children appeared (1). In 1991, the American College of Chest Physicians published the results of a survey of bronchoscopy in North America revealing that 13% to 20% of adult pulmonologists performed bronchoscopy in pediatric patients despite having limited exposure to pediatric bronchoscopy during their training (2,3).

This chapter delineates for the adult bronchoscopist the indications and limitations of bronchoscopy in pediatric patients. General considerations and the relevant anatomy are introduced. Technical aspects of the equipment and important methods of patient preparation and sedation are then addressed. Further, medical situations in which the adult pulmonologist should be able to comfortably perform pediatric bronchoscopy, bronchoscopy in the pediatric critical care setting, special diagnostic techniques, and the use of the pediatric bronchoscope in adult patients are discussed. Finally, attention is turned toward the contraindications and complications of bronchoscopy in children.

General Considerations

One of the issues in a discussion of pediatric bronchoscopy, in the context of adult pulmonology, is defining the population in question. A simplistic definition would be to define the pediatric pulmonary patient as that patient who otherwise would be seen and evaluated by a pediatric pulmonologist. In reality, no single characteristic determines what constitutes a pediatric pulmonary patient but a constellation of chronological age, emotional development, physiology, anticipated disease process, and if the primary care physician is a pediatrician or other pediatric health care specialist.

The number of pediatric pulmonologists is still insufficient to satisfy projected needs (4) and because infants, children, adolescents, and young adults can present with a range of complex respiratory disorders (Table 23.1), the adult pulmonologist may be the only person

Table 23.1. Pediatric Pulmonary Diseases Likely to be Encountered by the Adult Bronchoscopist

Bronchopulmonary dysplasia

Cystic fibrosis

Lower respiratory tract infections

Pulmonary intensive care of infants and children

Airway appliances and chronic ventilatory assistance

Aspiration syndromes (tracheoesophageal fistulas, gastroesophageal reflux disease)

Congenital anomalies of the respiratory system

Chronic suppurative lung disease

Evaluation of pulmonary problems in the compromised patient

capable of adequately evaluating and performing bronchoscopy on this group of patients (5).

The comfort (or discomfort) felt by adult pulmonologists with pediatric patients should not be based solely on the age of the patient, but on how comfortable they are with the diseases, physiology, and anatomy of younger patients, the psychosocial stage of the patient, and the acuity of the need for bronchoscopy. Each of these factors must be carefully considered before adult pulmonologists accept pediatric patients for evaluation (6).

Bronchoscopy in pediatric patients has many similarities to those procedures performed in adult patients. Driving the bronchoscope is the same except for the smaller field of view, the shorter distances traversed, and less distal reach. However, significant differences between adult and pediatric bronchoscopy do exist and it is important for adult pulmonologists to objectively decide whether the relative urgency of the procedure justifies avoiding delay and referral to a more experienced, preferably pediatric, bronchoscopist.

In general, differences with equipment, sample collections, medications, and patient-physician interaction are greatest for newborns and infants (Table 23.2).

The bronchoscopy equipment is smaller and the light fibers are more easily broken, a working channel may not be present, and the viewing image is smaller. Therefore, less of the anatomy is visible at any given time. Further, because dynamic airway collapse occurs more often in pediatric patients, the viewing area is often in motion and a videotape of the procedure with playback review is often necessary before specific diagnoses can be made.

Special procedures and invasive techniques such as transbronchial biopsies are infrequently performed and fluoroscopy is not usually necessary. However, if fluoroscopy is used, full lead protection for the patient takes on greater significance.

Specimens from brushings or bronchoalve-

olar lavage (BAL) are of smaller volume and hospital laboratories need to be organized to process these smaller samples.

The total procedure time may be shorter when compared to adult procedures. In the infant, in whom the bronchoscope may be only marginally smaller than the airway, procedures can be done in several repeated insertions each of no longer than 30 to 40 seconds with recovery with bagging and hyperoxygenation between views (7–9).

Attention to medication dosing is crucial, with dosage amounts based on weight (versus fixed dosing in adults).

Patient preparation and explanations in terms commensurate with age have heightened importance in this group of patients and family involvement is often greater than with adult patients.

Pediatric pulmonary diseases can be quite different from adults and to the uninitiated obvious or important pathologic findings

Table 23.2. Differences between Adult and Pediatric Flexible Bronchoscopy

Age-appropriate explanations are vital.

Family involvement with decisions is greater.

Equipment and specimens are smaller.

Suction channel is absent on the smallest bronchoscopes.

Transbronchial biopsies and fluoroscopy are used less frequently.

Bronchoscopy is almost exclusively performed via the nasal route.

Dynamic airway collapse is a more common finding.

Synchronous abnormalities are more common.

Medications are more often dosed by weight and given in titrated fractions.

Lower medication doses are required.

Total procedure time is shorter.

Potential exists for less patient cooperation.

Specific monitoring personnel are necessary.

could be missed or, at best, misinterpreted. The adult pulmonologist needs to be mindful that pediatric patients, particularly infants, toddlers and preteens, are not small adults and that experience with bronchoscopy in adults cannot always be transposed directly to these patients.

Anatomic Considerations

A full discussion of the pediatric airway anatomy is beyond the scope of this chapter. However, a basic understanding of the age-related differences between adult and pediatric airway anatomy can help the bronchoscopist better anticipate equipment and procedure needs. Although vascular and parenchymal development are important in several congenital diseases (vascular rings, pulmonary sequestration, etc.), for the purposes of pediatric bronchoscopy, these sites are less important and will not be discussed.

The immature larynx matures proportionally from infant to adult, with the larynx of children less than age 15 years showing many distinct differences from the adult larynx. The first major difference is the shape and position of the epiglottis. In the newborn and young child the epiglottis is elongated, more rounded (omega or U shaped) and appears much softer than in the adult, as shown in Plate 53 (10). The epiglottis can prove difficult to navigate in children when attempting to enter the larynx with the bronchoscope. The larynx itself is positioned more cephalad than in the adult. Further, whereas the glottis is the most narrow portion of the adult airway, the subglottic space or that portion within the cricoid ring is most narrowed in infants and young children. Therefore, the selection of the bronchoscope or endotracheal tube for infants and young children must take into consideration that the area beneath the vocal cords is the area of limitation, not the space between the vocal cords as in adults (11).

Finally, the immature larynx and glottis consist primarily of cartilaginous tissue. In the adult, they are composed mostly of muscle and soft tissue. The immature airway is more collapsible than in the adult, especially in the dynamic sense (malacia) and such collapse is often localized to anatomic sites (*laryngo*malacia, *tracheo*malacia, *broncho*malacia).

Although there is some debate, the bronchial tree appears to grow in proportion to the size of the patient after the first year. The neonatal tracheal diameter is on average 3.5 to 4.0 mm with a tripling of the diameter by adulthood (11 to 13 mm) (12–15). Therefore, the large airway anatomy and branching pattern of the normal pediatric patient will look quite similar to that of the adult patient except for the relatively smaller size. In fact, it has been suggested that the bronchial tree of the infant and young child are a miniature of the adult (12). The airway epithelium of the infant and young child has a higher ratio of mucous glands than that of the adult and tracheal mucociliary clearance is decreased in children when compared to adults (13). Therefore, increased normal secretions relative to the adult may be encountered at bronchoscopy. Finally, the airway of pediatric patients, even the very young, shows the expected physiologic and pharmacologic responses to commonly used medications (i.e., bronchodilators, topical anesthetics, vasoconstrictors, etc.) (16,17).

Equipment and Instrument Selection

Advances in fiberoptic and digital imaging technology have made available a number of high quality instruments with variable geometries. Table 23.3 lists the operating characteristics of the available pediatric bronchoscopes (arbitrarily defined as those scopes with outside diameters of less than 5.5 mm) from two large endoscopy manufacturers (Olympus America, Inc., Lake Success, New York, and Pentax Precision Instrument Corporation, Orangeburg, New York). Although adult-proportioned bronchoscopes are of limited use

Table 23.3. Operating Characteristics and Geometries of Pediatric Flexible Bronchoscopes

	Model*	Outside Diameter (mm)	Suction Channel (mm)	Smallest Endotracheal Tube (mm)	Age for Use	Comments
Ultrathin	BFN20	2.2	None	2.5–3.0	Premature infants	Smallest available scope
Pediatric	BF3C10	3.5	1.2	4.0–4.5 older	Term infants and no longer available	BF3C10 and BF3C20 are
	BF3C20	3.5	1.2	4.0–4.5		
	FI10P	3.5	1.2	4.0–4.5		
	FB10X	3.5	1.2	4.0–4.5		
	BF3C30	3.6	1.2	4.0–4.5		
Small adult	BFP10	4.9	2.2	5.5–6.0	Age 7 or older†	BFP10 and BFP20D are no longer available
	BFP20D	4.9	2.2	5.5–6.0		
	BFP30	4.9	2.2	5.5–6.0		
	FB15X	4.9	2.2	5.5–6.0		
	BFP200	5.3	2.0	6.0–6.5	Age 10 or older	

*BFN, BF3C, BFP series are manufactured by Olympus. FB10X, FB15X and FI-10P are manufactured by Pentax.
†Younger patients can be safely (albeit carefully) instrumented with selected larger bronchoscopes if biopsies, brushings, or aggressive suctioning is necessary.

in children because they have large outside diameters (6.0 mm or greater), they are sometimes used for their larger instrument channel. Adult bronchoscopes must be used with great care in pediatric patients to avoid unnecessary trauma and are generally not indicated in children aged 10 or younger (8). Obviously any pediatric-sized bronchoscope can be used in larger or older patients.

The proper selection of which instrument is best suited for use in a given patient is based on the size of the airway and the indication for bronchoscopy.

One method to assist in the selection of the appropriate-sized bronchoscope for a given age of the patient is to estimate the expected endotracheal tube size the patient would be able to accept (18,19). Then, based on the inside diameter of the endotracheal tube one can estimate which bronchoscope can safely pass through the glottis or subglottic space. Table 23.4 shows the expected endotracheal tube (ETT) size for age and the recommended

bronchoscope. A useful caveat is that the size of the patient's fifth digit is often a reasonable estimation of the outside diameter of the appropriate ETT (19).

Technique of Bronchoscopy in Pediatric Patients

Once the need for bronchoscopy has been established, the proper steps for performing a successful procedure are not too dissimilar from adult requirements.

Equipment and Personnel

In general, the equipment available should include the appropriate pediatric-sized flexible fiberoptic bronchoscope and a high-intensity light source. The availability of a still camera for photographic documentation is useful. A video camera and video recording system (preferably VHS) is also desirable not only for teaching and archiving purposes, but also to allow playback to the family and

Table 23.4. Endotracheal Tube Size-for-Age and Suggested Bronchoscope

Age	Endotracheal Tube* (Inside Diameter, mm)	Outside Diameter (mm)	Bronchoscope
Premature	2.5	3.6	
	3.0	4.3	
Newborn (< 30 d)	3.0	4.3	BFN20
	3.5	4.9	
Infant (1–12 mo)	3.5	4.9	
	4.0	5.6	
1 y	4.0	5.6	
	4.5	6.2	BF3C10
			BF3C20
3 y	4.5	6.2	BF3C30
	5.0	6.9	FB10X
			FI–10P
6 y	5.0	6.9	
	5.5	7.5	
10 y	6.0	8.2	
	6.5	8.9	BFP10
			BFP20D
Adolescent	7.0	9.6	BFP30
	7.5	10.3	FB15X

*The appropriate endotracheal tube size can be estimated by the formula: ETT (mm) $= \dfrac{Age\ (in\ y) + 16}{4} \pm 0.5\ mm$

patient for discussion of the findings. Pediatric-sized equipment for the bronchoscope should be readily available as well as a list of calculated medication doses based on the weight of the patient. Two suction setups should be simultaneously maintained, one for use through the bronchoscope and one for control and care of oral secretions. A dual system for humidified oxygen delivery with the appropriate connectors and with pediatric high-flow capabilities should also be readily available.

As in adult procedures, specimen collection devices (protected brushes, cytology brushes, cytology slides, fixatives, BAL syringes, and the appropriate collection media) need to be available in quantity. Resuscitation equipment with bag, mask, laryngoscope blades, and endotracheal tubes sized appropriately for infants and children must be present at the bedside as well as a fully stocked pediatric "crash" cart. A resuscitation dosage card should be created before every procedure, as illustrated in Figure 23.1. Fluoroscopy is not necessary for most pediatric bronchoscopy cases. However, if transbronchial biopsy is anticipated with fluoroscopic guidance, the procedure requires the same expertise and precautions as in adults. Covering *the patient* below the chest with lead shielding if fluoroscopy is needed and using no more than 5 minutes' total exposure time for any given procedure are recommended. Finally, oxygen can be delivered with the nasal prongs placed directly in the mouth of infants or insufflated via the suction channel at 1 to 3 L/min.

**PEDIATRIC
CARDIOPULMONARY RESUSCITATION DRUGS**

Name_____
Age_____
Weight_____

Epinephrine (first dose) 1:10,000 (0.01 mg/Kg)   = _____ mg = _____ cc @ 0.1 mg/ml
Epinephrine (subsequent doses) 1:1000 (0.1 mg/Kg)   = _____ mg = _____ cc @ 1.0 mg/ml
Adenosine (0.1-0.2 mg/Kg)   = _____ mg = _____ cc @ 3.0 mg/ml
Atropine (0.02 mg/Kg)   = _____ mg = _____ cc @ 1.0 mg/ml
Lidocaine (1.0 mg/Kg)   = _____ mg = _____ cc @ 10 mg/ml
Naloxone (0.01-0.2 mg/Kg)   = _____ mg = _____ cc @ 0.4 mg/ml

Defibrillation (2-3 joules/Kg) = _____ joules (watt-sec)

ET Tube Size = $\dfrac{16 + \text{age in years}}{4}$ = _____ mm

Dopamine or Dobutamine Drip (2-20 mcg/Kg/min) = 6 x weight in Kg = mg added to diluent to make 100 ml; then 1.0 ml/hr = 1.0 mcg/Kg/min - titrate to effect

Epinephrine Drip (0.1-1.0 mcg/Kg/min) = 0.6 x weight in Kg = mg added to diluent to make 100 ml; then 1.0 ml/hr = 0.1 mcg/Kg/min - titrate to effect

Lidocaine Drip (20-50 mcg/Kg/min) = 120 mg of 40 mg/ml solution added to 97 ml D_5W; then infuse 1.0 ml x Kg/hr = 20 mcg/Kg/min

Physician_____
Date_____

Figure 23.1. Pediatric resuscitation dosage card.

Monitoring Equipment

Monitoring pediatric patients during bronchoscopy (20) is similar to monitoring any patient undergoing conscious sedation for an invasive procedure. The first rule of monitoring is that trained eyes are often the best monitors. The bronchoscopist needs to avoid paying too much attention to the technical aspects of the procedure and not enough to the young patient. Frequent assessment of color, respirations, head position, and apparent comfort are important. Mechanical monitoring of the patient should include vital signs, continuous electrocardiography (ECG), and continuous pulse oximetry. However, mechanical monitoring of the child should be used only to alert the bronchoscopy team to look at the child more closely. Special attention to the patient should be made after the procedure is complete, remembering that patients are still sedated. A sedated patient should never be left alone or unobserved. Monitoring should continue for the pediatric patient until the child is awake. Supplemental oxygen should be continued after the procedure until oxygenation is adequate (i.e., greater than 92%) on room air. The patient should be tolerating oral intake prior to discharge.

Personnel

In addition to the bronchoscopist, two or three trained assistants who are comfortable both with normal and abnormal children are necessary for the success and safety of the procedure. All personnel should be trained in at least basic life support and pediatric advanced life support certification is encouraged. The bronchoscopy team usually consists of a bronchoscopy nurse who assists with medications, specimen collection, equipment care, and with the specific technical needs of the procedure and two to three nurses or assistants. One person should be primarily responsible for monitoring the patient, which is often done while holding and comforting the child. All members of the team function as "human monitors" and need always to be on guard for changes in the patient.

Patient Preparation

It cannot be emphasized enough how important the approach and setting for bronchoscopy is for pediatric patients. Establishing a firm, caring rapport with the patient and parents is necessary to gain trust and cooperation before and during the procedure. Bronchoscopy performed in the anxious adolescent can be just as difficult as that performed in a 2-year old.

If the procedure is relatively elective, the child (and family) should have the procedure explained to them in terms that are appropriate for the age and level of education of the patient. Parents play an important role by helping to facilitate the understanding of the procedure. Using positive, nonthreatening words can minimize anxiety. Once in the bronchoscopy area, maintenance of a quiet reassuring atmosphere will not only help calm the patient and allow for a better examination, but can greatly minimize the need for additional intravenous sedation. Even young children can be calmed by the proper atmosphere.

Children are very alert to changes in their surroundings, being particularly sensitive to negativity, unexpected movement, or unfamiliar faces. Conversations within the procedure area should be made with awareness of their effect on the patient and family; extraneous conversation should be kept to a minimum (21). The scene should remain calm and consistent and, when possible, the lights should be dimmed. Having the parents or a familiar person remain in the room during the procedure or at least until the child is sufficiently sedated is encouraged.

Additional preparation before the use of sedation includes maintenance of an empty stomach at least 4 hours prior to bronchoscopy for all children greater than 5 years old. For infants and young toddlers, clear liquids up to 2 hours before the procedure are permissible.

Sedation

The sedation of pediatric patients undergoing diagnostic and therapeutic procedures has received considerable attention in recent years. Sedation protocols for bronchoscopy vary from the use of general anesthesia to topical lidocaine alone (20,22,23).

The form of sedation used most commonly for bronchoscopy in North America is known as "conscious sedation" and is defined as a medically controlled state of depressed consciousness that: 1) allows protective reflexes to be maintained, 2) preserves the patient's ability to maintain a patent airway independently and continuously unless intubated, and 3) permits response by the patient to physical stimulation or verbal command (23).

Pharmacologic sedation is dosed by weight and titrated to effect starting with half the lower end of the dose range. It can be useful to calculate the dose for all the medications expected to be used and to have this reference readily available. Table 23.5 is a list of the most frequently used medications for pediatric sedation and the relevant pharmacologic properties (18,24–26).

Intravenous access can be difficult to obtain in children and should be placed *before* the start of the procedure. Not only does this provide the necessary access route for sedation, it also avoids having to place the line in a child who acutely needs resuscitation or reversal of medications. Once the intravenous line, monitoring equipment, and personnel are in place and the atmosphere sufficiently calm, pharmacologic sedation can be initiated.

Because of the difficulty with absorption and onset of action, only rarely are medications delivered intramuscularly and this route is discouraged.

A sedation protocol for bronchoscopy in pediatric patients can be found in Table 23.6 (9). Intravenous sedation combined with topical anesthesia is successfully accomplished in

Table 23.5. Intravenous Sedating Agents for Pediatric Flexible Bronchoscopy*

Class	Name	Starting Dose (IV)	Maximum Dose	Onset	Duration	Comments
Narcotics	Meperidine (Demerol)	0.5–2 mg/kg	50–100 mg	4 min	3–5 h	
	Fentanyl (Sublimaze)	1–2 µg/kg	3 µg/kg/h	1–2 min	1–2 h	Fentanyl can be used as a continuous drip starting at 1 µg/kg/h
Benzodiazepines	Midazolam (Versed)	0.05–0.1 mg/kg	0.2 mg/kg	3–5 min	2–6 h	All have amnestic effects
	Lorazepam (Ativan)	0.1 mg/kg	4.0 mg	15–20 min	6–8 h	
	Diazepam (Valium)	0.1 mg/kg	0.6 mg/kg	10–15 min	6–20 h	Can have rebound sedation with diazepam at 6–8 h
Barbiturates, sedatives, and anesthetics	Methohexital (Brevital)	1–1.5 mg/kg	50–100 mg	< 1 min	5–10 min	Short-acting agents
	Pentobarbital (Nembutal)	1–3 mg/kg	100 mg	1 min	Variable (< 1 h)	
	Propofol (Diprivan)	1–2 mg/kg	Titrated to effect	< 1 min	Variable (< 5 min)	Propofol requires a continuous drip starting at 100 µg/kg/min
	Ketamine (Ketalar)	0.5–2 mg/kg	4.5 mg/kg	< 1 min	10–30 min	Lower doses and fewer side effects when used with benzodiazepine
Reversing agents	Flumazenil (Romazicon)	2 mg	1–3 mg	3 min	10–60 min	
	Naloxone (Narcan)	0.01–0.1 mg/kg	None	2 min	1–4 h	May repeat Narcan every 3–5 min until achieve effect

*See references 18, 24, 25, and 26 for more details.

almost every case. General anesthesia should rarely, if ever, be required (8,9).

Some authors prefer to begin with aerosolized lidocaine in the dose of 20 to 40 mg delivered via face mask nebulizer prior to intravenous sedation. After this step, intravenous benzodiazepine or a narcotic is titrated to achieve adequate sedation and analgesia. It is important that sufficient time be given for fractional doses to take effect. Oversedation should be avoided because dynamic evaluation of the pediatric airway is of particular importance.

After initial sedation is achieved, additional doses of benzodiazepines or narcotic can be given alternately depending on the duration of the procedure. It is important to recognize that synergistic effects are possible when narcotics and benzodiazepines are used together

that may lower the effective individual dose of each for a given patient. The advantages of midazolam are that it is short acting and has amnestic properties affording better patient recovery. Both meperidine and fentanyl are relatively short-acting narcotics. Fentanyl has the added advantage of antitussive effects.

Topical Anesthesia

Topical anesthesia of the upper airway applied after intravenous sedation greatly facilitates the examination. Even with adequate intravenous sedation, topical anesthesia can minimize laryngospasm and vagal stimulation as well as minimize the cough reflex. Lidocaine solution is used at 0.5% to 1.0% concentrations for patients less than one year of age and in 1% to 2% concentrations for patients one year or older (8,9). Viscous lidocaine in concentrations

Table 23.6. Sedation for Bronchoscopy in Pediatric Patients

Before Procedure

NPO for at least 4 h in older children; clear liquids for infants and toddlers

Age-appropriate discussion with patients and family to create a level of trust and comfort

Introduction of bronchoscopy team to patient and family

Assemble or check bronchoscopy and resuscitation equipment

Calculation of medication doses and maximum limits per patient weight

Establish intravenous access

In Bronchoscopy Room

Confirm IV line and ease of flush

Initiate monitoring with continuous pulse oximeter, ECG, and blood pressure cuff

Prepare video equipment for recording (rewind or reset tape, note counter number, set to record)

Dim lights, avoid loud noises, minimize stimulation, create positive atmosphere with quiet reassuring suggestions, maintain environment of relaxation with calming, quiet words.

Administration of Intravenous Sedation

   Note: All medications are titrated to effect starting with half the lower end of the dose range with careful observation of the patient and monitors.

   IV midazolam 0.05–0.1 mg/kg over 2–5 min

and   IV meperidine 0.5–2.0 mg/kg over 2–5 min

or   IV fentanyl 1–2 µg/kg (max: 3 µg/kg) over 2–5 min

or   IV ketamine 0.5–2.0 mg/kg (max: 4.5 mg/kg) over 2–5 min

   (Atropine 0.02 mg/kg IV can be used for vasoconstriction and secretion control)

    Note: Propofol 0.5 mg/kg IV given over 1-2 min (max: 3.0 mg/kg) may be used for sedation instead of midazolam, but requires a continuous infusion of 0.2 mg/kg/min.

Administration of Topical Anesthesia

   Lidocaine 1% or 2% solution 0.5–1.0 mL

   Instill into selected nostril with cotton-tipped applicator and repeat as necessary

   (Some bronchoscopists use 1–3 mL lidocaine 1% or 2% aerosol for initial topical anesthesia)

then   Instill 1–3 mL lidocaine 1% viscous gel with a cotton-tipped applicator through the same nostril and ask patient to sniff in if possible.

   (When using the smallest bronchoscopes, this step may be omitted.)

    Note: The maximum dose of lidocaine is 7 mg/kg

If Additional Sedation Is Required

   Titrate midazolam, meperidine, fentanyl, ketamine or propofol to maximum doses:

   Midazolam 0.05 mg/kg boluses up to 0.2 mg/kg

   Meperidine 0.5 mg/kg boluses up to 3.0 mg/kg

   Fentanyl 1.0 µg/kg boluses up to 3.0 µg/kg

   Propofol 0.5 mg/kg boluses up to 2.0 mg/kg

   Ketamine 0.5 mg/kg boluses up to 4.5 mg/kg

or   Use IV methohexital 1.0 mg/kg (may repeat once)

   (Provides 1–2 min of anesthesia with rapid recovery and facilitates effect of other sedatives)

    Note: Larger doses of sedative medications are permissible but will prolong recovery and may interfere with dynamic evaluations.

Postprocedure

Continue monitoring until patient is awake, talking, and able to swallow liquids (to ensure topical anesthesia has worn off).

Continue to provide nasal cannula oxygen until well-saturated on room air.

Continue to provide positive feedback and maintain calm atmosphere.

Discuss procedure and findings with the patient and family and view the videotape if appropriate.

of 1% to 2% can be used for nasal anesthesia and lubrication. However, viscous lidocaine can plug the suction channel and obscure the field of view in smaller bronchoscopes if not used sparingly. The total cumulative dose of lidocaine should be recorded and, in general, should not exceed 7 to 10 mg/kg.

Prior to the insertion of the bronchoscope, 1 to 2 mL lidocaine solution on a cotton-tip applicator is applied to the nostril and then gently passed posteriorly to the nasal pharynx. This is followed by passing another cotton-tip applicator saturated with 1% viscous lidocaine jelly through the nostril to provide further topical anesthesia and lubrication. This procedure has several important effects:

1. Provides anesthesia of the nares and nasopharynx
2. Establishes the size and patency of the nasal passage for placement of the bronchoscope
3. Provides assessment of the adequacy of intravenous sedation
4. Provides nasal lubrication and dilatation for easy passage of the bronchoscope
5. Allows for the removal of excess nasal secretions

If a suction channel is present on the bronchoscope, additional lidocaine can be applied to the larynx, glottis, and tracheobronchial tree (with the suction temporarily off) under direct vision to minimize discomfort and cough. Intravenous atropine or other agents to control secretions are not usually used in young children but may be helpful in the young adult.

Insertion of the Bronchoscope

Once adequate sedation and topical anesthesia are achieved, the flexible bronchoscope can be passed through the nose, rather than through the mouth, in virtually all cases (8). Obvious exceptions are patients who are intubated and those with nasal anomalies. The nasal approach is the preferred route because of its stability, relative comfort to the patient, and ease of approach to the larynx; most importantly, it allows inspection of the nasopharynx. It is stated that there is almost no child whose nose is too small to accommodate the 2.2-mm (BFN20) or 3.5-mm (BF3C series) bronchoscopes (8). If the oral route is indicated, and for those children intubated in the intensive care unit (ICU), a bite block can help prevent damage to the relatively fragile smaller instruments.

Indications for Bronchoscopy in Pediatric Patients

Bronchoscopy in pediatric patients, performed in the appropriate setting by experienced personnel, is just as safe and useful as in the adult patient. Table 23.7 lists the indications for flexible FOB in pediatric patients as outlined by the American Thoracic Society (27). The adult pulmonologist can be falsely reassured to find that many of these indications overlap with those for adult flexible FOB. Unlike adults, there is frequently more than one finding and that not necessarily related to the primary indication for the procedure (8,28). In one large series of flexible bronchoscopic procedures in patients less than age 16, seven categories accounted for over 85% of the indications for bronchoscopy (Figure 23.2) (8,28). These indications included stridor (24%), atelectasis (18%), tracheostomy evaluation (15%), suspected upper airway abnormalities (8%), recurrent or persistent pneumonia (7%), wheezing (6%), and lower airway abnormalities (i.e., ETT management, aid to intubation, positioning; 5% to 10%). The diagnostic yield for bronchoscopy in this series was 76%, but it has been reported as high as 88% in other series (29).

Stridor

Stridor is one of the most common indications for flexible FOB in pediatric patients. Stridor is acute or chronic with the acute form most

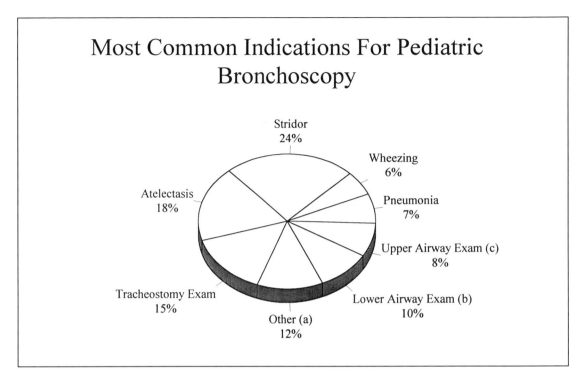

Most Common Indications For Pediatric Bronchoscopy

Stridor 24%
Wheezing 6%
Pneumonia 7%
Upper Airway Exam (c) 8%
Lower Airway Exam (b) 10%
Other (a) 12%
Tracheostomy Exam 15%
Atelectasis 18%

Figure 23.2. *A*, Includes airway compression, nonspecific x-ray findings, suspected foreign body, hemoptysis, cough. *B*, Includes endotracheal tube management, follow-up foreign body, parenchymal mass lesion, presurgical evaluation, immotile cilia syndrome, hemosiderosis, tuberculosis. *C*, Includes abnormal vocalization apnea, aspiration, prolonged intubation, upper airway obstruction, vocal cord paralysis.

commonly associated with infections. The chronic causes of stridor are listed in Table 23.8.

Acute stridor does not warrant endoscopy particularly when the diagnosis of epiglottitis is being considered. Endoscopy in this setting is performed in the operating room prepared for emergent tracheostomy if necessary (30). Acute stridor is usually the manifestation of infectious laryngotracheobronchitis (croup), epiglottis, or laryngeal foreign body (FB) (9,31,32). It is sometimes difficult to make the important distinction between stridor caused by croup from epiglottis and there is a great temptation to visualize the airway. The primary reason not to perform bronchoscopy or laryngoscopy in this setting is the high likelihood of causing total upper airway obstruction (30–32). Because the clinical information needed can be obtained safely in other ways, routine endoscopy for acute stridor is contraindicated.

Chronic stridor is most often due to dynamic airway collapse, fixed upper airway lesions, or both. The majority of patients are less than one year of age with 85% less than age 6 (8,33). The most common form of dynamic collapse is laryngomalacia (Plate 54), but frequently multiple regions of collapse can be observed. Stridor due to laryngomalacia is caused by involution of the supraglottic structures on inspiration. Tracheomalacia (Plate 55), although occasionally a cause of stridor, more often causes wheezing. In a recent study, both laryngomalacia and tracheomalacia were found to coexist in 20% of pediatric patients evaluated for stridor and in 40% of cases all airway segments (i.e., bronchomalacia as well) were involved (8,33).

The degree of dynamic collapse observed is subjectively characterized as normal, mild, moderate, or severe on the basis of the proximity of the opposing bronchial walls during

Table 23.7. Indications for Bronchoscopy in Pediatric Patients

Chronic stridor
Persistent atelectasis
Persistent wheezing (unresponsive to appropriate therapy)
Recurrent or persistent pulmonary infiltrates
Lung lesions of unknown etiology (i.e., radiographic abnormality)
Persistent or chronic cough
Hemoptysis
Suspected bronchial or tracheal foreign body
Assessment of damage from toxic inhalation or aspiration
Evaluation of upper airway trauma (i.e., accidental or prolonged intubation)
Vocalization abnormalities or vocal cord dysfunction
Assessment of the position, patency, or airway damage related to endotracheal or tracheostomy tubes
Samples of lower airway secretions and/or cells by bronchoalveolar lavage
Brush biopsies or transbronchial biopsies for pathology
Aid to difficult intubations
Therapeutic bronchoalveolar lavage
Removal of airway secretions and mucous plugs

Table 23.8. Causes of Chronic Stridor in Children

Dynamic collapse 40%–60%
    Laryngomalacia 5%–40%*
    Tracheomalacia 2%–4%
    Both 20%
    All airways (including bronchomalacia) 30%–40%

Fixed lesion 21%–50%
    Subglottic stenosis or edema 25%*
    Adenoid hypertrophy 5%
    Vocal cord paresis 2%–9%
    Tracheal stenosis 1%–8%
    Hemangioma 2%–6%
    Tracheal compression (i.e., vascular ring, etc.) 2%–5%

Dynamic collapse and fixed lesion 14%

Normal examination 2%–3%

Other 1%–2%
    Laryngeal papillomatosis
    Nasal obstruction
    Laryngeal sarcoma

*Percentages in the subgroups are percents of the total in that group (8,33).

respiration. Fixed lesions are less common causes of stridor most often in the subglottic space (i.e., stenosis or edema), but adenoidal hypertrophy, vocal cord paresis, tracheostenosis, hemangiomas, vascular rings, and cysts can be observed.

Some authors advocate the empirical diagnosis of laryngomalacia (i.e., without diagnostic bronchoscopy) in the child who is in no respiratory distress and is eating and growing normally. However, recent studies suggest that this may not be optimal because a surgically correctable lesion can be found in up to 24% of cases (33). Therefore, it is recommended that all children with chronic stridor be evaluated by bronchoscopy. Further, because children who present with stridor have more than one lesion in approximately 15% of cases, it is important to examine the airway at least to the carina in every case (8).

Atelectasis

Atelectasis in pediatric patients, unlike adult patients, is a common indication for bronchoscopy. In adults, good chest physiotherapy is usually sufficient to resolve atelectasis. This is not always the case for children partly because of the inability to use incentive spirometry. In fact, if atelectasis is persistent or recurrent in children in the face of good physical therapy, bronchoscopy is necessary to rule out other causes (such as FB aspiration) as well as to obtain specimens for culture or to clear tenacious secretions (Figure 23.3).

In one study of 201 pediatric patients undergoing bronchoscopy for atelectasis, a treatable cause was found in approximately two thirds of patients, the most common being central mucous plugging (8). Unsuspected FB was found in approximately 5% of cases. A

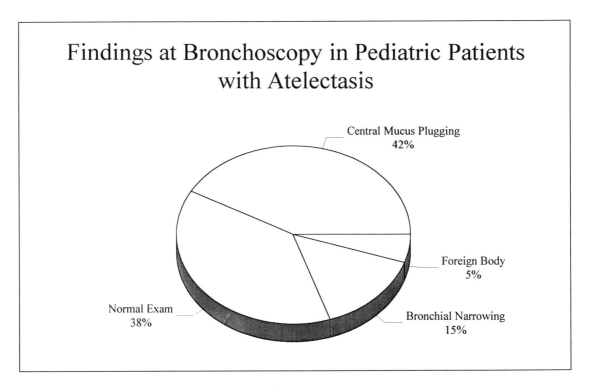

Figure 23.3. Common causes of atelectasis in pediatric patients.

completely normal examination was present in less than 10% of cases in this series. It is important to note that most children (60% to 70%) with atelectasis are infants, often intubated and in the pediatric or neonatal ICU (8,34). It is only infrequently that the adult pulmonologist may be called on to evaluate these patients. In the ICU setting, bronchoscopy for the removal of mucous plugging results in radiographic and clinical improvement in over 80% of cases (34,35).

The ultrathin bronchoscopes (outside diameter 2.2 mm, suction channel 0.9 mm) have also been used in neonates for pulmonary toilet with good success (35), but these instruments are not routinely available to the adult pulmonologist. For some older children with a history of bronchopulmonary dysplasia who present with atelectasis secondary to mucous plugging, bronchoscopy may be helpful (36). Otherwise, for the older child, bronchoscopy is effective in relieving atelectasis in only 60% of cases and chest physiotherapy with incentive spirometry and suctioning are preferred (7,34).

Tracheostomy Evaluation

Bronchoscopic evaluation of pediatric patients with tracheostomies is common and similar to the evaluation in adult patients. The usual indications include obstructing granulation tissue, subglottic edema or stenosis (Plate 56), assessment of tracheostomy positioning, trauma, mucous plugging, and general secretions management (8,37).

Granulation tissue can be extensive and warrants removal by forceps to decrease the risk of occluding the tracheostomy tube. Also in any pediatric patient with a tracheostomy requiring bronchoscopy for any indication, the procedure is often accomplished more easily than in the patient without tracheostomy primarily because topical anesthesia of the glottis is not necessary.

Careful attention to the inside diameter of the tracheostomy tube or stoma is necessary for proper instrument selection. The endotracheal tube diameters in Table 23.4 can serve as guidelines in selecting the appropriate instrument. As in the patient without a tracheostomy tube, adequate topical anesthesia of the carina will greatly facilitate the procedure and decrease cough. Finally, a view of the glottis is easily obtained via retroflection of the endoscope and can often reveal unsuspected pathology.

In general, the evaluation of tracheostomies in children is elective and performed by an otolaryngologist or pediatric pulmonologist (37).

Foreign Bodies

One of the most important indications for flexible FOB in the young patient is to make the diagnosis of FB aspiration (Plate 57). There is an urgency to making the diagnosis because the complication rate is higher and the outcomes are worse if the diagnosis is delayed (38). In the absence of bronchoscopy, the diagnosis can be elusive. In one series of 76 patients with proven FBs, the diagnosis was delayed by up to 8 weeks in approximately 12% of patients (39). Persistent or new-onset wheezing, stridor, or cough may be the only clues to the diagnosis but are nonspecific. The chest film is of limited value in the diagnosis of FB aspiration and several large series of pediatric patients with proven FB aspiration have shown a low yield, finding a normal chest radiograph in up to 25% (38,40,41).

When less obvious by history, physical examination, or chest radiograph, FBs are found in only 19% to 25% of cases. Therefore, flexible FOB has its greatest utility in excluding FB aspirations in the 75% to 80% of cases in which the clinical findings are equivocal (39,42).

Although the diagnosis of FBs in the airway of a child is an appropriate indication for flexible FOB, removal of airway FBs is usually done via the rigid bronchoscope (42,43). In cases of high clinical suspicion, rigid bronchoscopy should be considered for both diagnosis and removal without an initial flexible procedure. In one series of 29 patients in whom the history, physical examination, or chest roentgenogram suggested a high likelihood of an FB, 27 (93%) patients actually had an FB requiring removal at the time of bronchoscopy (42).

Successful removal of FBs in children via the flexible instrument has been reported (44–47). However, 85% of children who have an FB in the airway are less than 5 years old (46). Because the instruments used for FB removal cannot fit through the small flexible bronchoscopes in the majority of children with FBs, the rigid bronchoscope remains the instrument of choice for their removal.

Removal of an FB via the flexible instrument should be attempted only when the rigid bronchoscope has failed, there is inaccessibility to the rigid instrument, or when the flexible instrument appears to be more likely to succeed (as in the case of an FB in a distal bronchus) (43,45).

Several other important differences between adult and pediatric FB aspiration have been noted. Although the adult literature suggests that most FB aspirations occur to the right main stem bronchus, in children aspirations occur equally to both the left and right side (39). Fragmentation or multiple FBs are common and often occur distal to the rigid bronchoscope. Therefore, another important role of the flexible bronchoscope in FB aspiration is for careful airway inspection after FB removal (via the rigid bronchoscope if necessary) or in outpatient follow-up.

Vocal Cord Dysfunction

Vocal cord dysfunction or paradoxical vocal cord adduction as described in adults (48) is also an important cause of "factitious or functional" wheezing in children (49,50). The diagnosis can be made by flexible laryngoscopy or FOB during an acute spontaneous episode or by provocation. Videotape recordings of the endoscopy with postprocedure frame-by-frame playback can be useful to quantify the degree of adduction as well as an educational aid in the therapy of the patient. In the majority of cases, the patients are adolescent females and high achievers presenting as either recalcitrant asthma or with an inability to perform athletics at their previous competitive level. Failure to correctly diagnose vocal cord dysfunction may result in deleterious treatment including prolonged tracheostomies and excessive corticosteroid therapy.

Recurrent or Persistent Infiltrates

Recurrent or persistent infiltrates on chest radiography are frequent indications for bronchoscopy particularly if an adequate sputum sample cannot be obtained. Noninfectious as well as infectious etiologies need to be considered and bronchoscopy is often necessary for definitive evaluation or treatment. Persistent infiltrates due to infections are assessed using BAL and, for older patients, protected specimen brushes. Although the technique of BAL and protected specimen brush in children is somewhat different from that in adults and not standardized, the information obtained is as valuable.

The presence and quantification of lipid-laden macrophages in BAL fluid is highly suggestive of aspiration as a cause for recurrent pulmonary infiltrates (51,52). By assessing the amount of lipid within alveolar macrophages a "lipid-laden alveolar macrophage index" can be calculated. For adults, an index of greater than 100 has a sensitivity and negative predictive value each of 100%; an index of less than 100 makes the diagnosis of aspiration unlikely. In children the cut-off values are less well defined with an index greater than 86 suggesting aspiration and an index less than 72 making aspiration unlikely. If aspiration pneumonia is diagnosed in children, further evaluation is indicated.

Noninfectious causes for persistent infiltrates, such as compression from a vascular ring, need to be considered in children. Endobronchial tumors as a cause for persistent or postobstructive pneumonia are rare. It is also important to note that although FB is often suspected in children with persistent infiltrates, it is, in fact, a rare finding (less than 1%) (8).

Pneumonia in the Immunocompromised Host

The immunocompromised pediatric patient often requires early bronchoscopic evaluation. Bronchoscopy and BAL in immunocompromised children is effective for the diagnosis of infiltrates due to infection and has proven to be an alternative to open lung biopsy (53–61).

In pediatric patients of any age with acquired immunodeficiency syndrome (AIDS), the recovery of *Pneumocystis carinii* via BAL is as effective as in adults for making the diagnosis. The diagnostic sensitivity of BAL for pneumocystis in children with AIDS is approximately 90% (54). The overall diagnostic yield of BAL to detect any infectious pathogen in children with AIDS is also high (54–58). In bone marrow transplantation, BAL has a reported diagnostic sensitivity of 75% to 100% in pediatric patients (59).

Transbronchial biopsy does not add to the diagnostic utility of BAL for infection in immunocompromised pediatric patients and is not routinely recommended (54). The role of the protected specimen brush and quantitative cultures in children for the diagnosis of infectious diseases has not been determined. However, in pediatric patients old enough to accommodate the larger bronchoscopes, use of the protected specimen brush is likely to be of similar efficacy as in adults. Encouraging data for the use of protected specimen brush in neonates has recently been reported (62).

Persistent Wheezing

Persistent wheezing requiring rapid escalation of therapy or unresponsive to therapy is a common indication for bronchoscopic evaluation in children. In one large series of patients with chronic wheezing, an abnormality that explained that patient's symptoms was found in 87% (8). Of these patients, 91% had findings in the lower airway and 9% had findings in the upper airway. The most common lower airway causes were tracheomalacia, left main stem bronchus compression, extrinsic tracheal compression from vascular structures, and FBs. Common upper airway causes for wheezing included laryngomalacia, vocal cord dysfunction, and subglottic edema. Although treatment is often reassurance and careful follow-up, definitive diagnosis allows for the discontinuation of unnecessary therapy in those cases when an anatomic cause for the chronic wheezing is found.

Endotracheal Tube Management and Bronchoscopy in the Pediatric Intensive Care Unit

Bronchoscopy in the ICU (pediatric or neonatal) can be performed for any non-ICU indication previously described (63,64). However, a common ICU indication for bronchoscopy and a frequent indication for pediatric bronchoscopy in general is for artificial airway management. The fiberoptic bronchoscope is particularly useful as an aid to intubation and for nonradiographic assessment of ETT position.

Aid to Intubation

A small group of infants and children pose difficult challenges for endobronchial intubation with the usual techniques. This can occur during an elective procedure, in the operating room, as an acute respiratory emergency, or as an urgent need for reintubation after inadvertent extubation (65,66). The adult pulmonologist may be the only endoscopist available to assist with these intubations. Regardless of the etiology, patient age, or the urgency of the situation, intubation can be accomplished either through the mouth or the nose using the endoscope (64). The neonate can be safely intubated using the Olympus BFN20. For the term infant or older child, the Olympus BF3C30 or the Pentax FB10X can be used. In addition Pentax has a

specific bronchoscope designed for intubation (FI10P) that is more stiff with less angulation (see Table 23.3). After intubation a repeat bronchoscopy via the newly placed ETT can be performed to confirm appropriate positioning. With this technique, blind nasotracheal intubation of neonates or young children is unnecessary.

In most cases where bronchoscopy or laryngoscopy is needed to assist intubation, the procedure is easily accomplished. However, if the anatomy is of sufficient complexty (67,68) or if the initial attempts at bronchoscopic intubation fail, immediate surgical referral for possible tracheostomy is indicated. The use of ETT changers for extubation and reintubation is not recommended in pediatric patients. If a properly positioned ETT in a patient with a "difficult airway" needs replacement (i.e., cuff failure, mechanical failure), rapid extubation and reintubation over the bronchoscope are preferable and safer (69).

Positioning of Endotracheal Tubes

In the pediatric ICU, determination of appropriate ETT positioning after intubation is routine. This assessment is usually confirmed on the basis of symmetrical chest rise, bilateral auscultatory breath sounds, and the presence of "misting" or condensation within the ETT during exhalation. However, a portable anteroposterior chest x-ray is usually the final arbiter of the adequacy of ETT placement.

With the advent of the ultrathin bronchoscope, several studies have shown that the assessment of correct ETT position by flexible FOB is as safe and as effective as radiologic assessment and avoids unnecessary repeated exposure to radiation (70,71).

Further, the information obtained from flexible FOB is immediately available, whereas assessment by chest x-ray can be delayed depending on the availability of radiologic services (71).

Special Techniques

This section discusses the mechanics of performing common adjunct procedures in pediatric patients undergoing bronchoscopy.

Bronchoalveolar Lavage in Children

If the adult pulmonologist is asked to perform a bronchoscopy in a pediatric patient, BAL is often indicated. As alluded to earlier, BAL is used in children in a similar fashion to that in adults. The difference is in the actual performance of the technique as it applies to children. Even the smallest of channels can be used for successful BAL. If a specific site for lavage is chosen based on chest x-ray, physical examination, or endobronchial findings, the flexible bronchoscope is advanced to the selected site until it can advance no further with gentle pressure ("wedge position"). As for adults, if the process is diffuse, the lingula and the right middle lobe are the areas of choice when lavage is performed because of their favorable anatomic location, ease of obtaining a good wedge, and higher volume of return compared to other areas (72).

The volume of lavage fluid used in children depends on the size of the bronchoscope relative to the pediatric airway and to the size of the patient. Obviously, a smaller pediatric bronchoscope can be advanced further in an older child. Therefore, less volume is necessary to fill the lung segment distal to the wedged bronchoscope tip. Although no specific data quantify the diagnostic yield of BAL on the basis of the volume instilled, the actual volume of fluid used for BAL in children needs to be carefully considered.

Several methods have been used to estimate the maximum volume of BAL fluid that can be used safely in young patients. Some authors use 1 to 3 aliquots of 10 mL each for children over 3 kg in weight (8). Another method is to use an amount no more than 5% to 15% of the functional residual capacity (FRC). If the FRC has been measured by spirometry, the maximum volume can be determined directly. Otherwise, the FRC can be estimated from the patient's height using the equation:

$$FRC = 1.3 \text{ to } 1.5 \text{ mL} \times height$$
$$(or \text{ } length) \text{ in centimeters.}$$

For example, if a 3 year-old patient requires BAL and is 97 cm (50th percentile) in length, the estimated FRC would then be 126.1 to 145.5 mL and the maximum estimated BAL fluid volume would be 12.6 mL to 14.5 mL if 10% of the FRC is used (73). Once the maximum value has been calculated, the solution for BAL (sterile normal saline without preservatives) is then instilled via the suction port of the bronchoscope in aliquots of no more than 2 mL/kg of body weight up to a maximum of 10 mL/aliquot. The fluid can then be recovered by applying manual suction to a syringe attached to the port after instillation or by attaching a specimen trap in-line to the wall suction. The volume of return is usually between 50% and 75% of the total volume instilled.

Complications associated with BAL, apart from bronchoscopy itself, occur in less than 1% of procedures and include hypoxia, hemorrhage, pneumothorax, tachypnea, and arrhythmias. Fever occurs in up to 40% of patients following BAL. It is usually low grade, lasting 24 to 48 hours, and can be treated with acetaminophen 10 to 15 mg/kg per dose every 4 to 6 hours (72,74).

Transbronchial Biopsy

Transbronchial biopsy has been used infrequently in children. The reasons for this have been the relatively few indications for transbronchial biopsy in children and the small size of the suction channel on pediatric bronchoscopes. Currently, the smallest biopsy forceps is 2.0 mm in diameter and the smallest flexible bronchoscope through which this forceps can pass is the Olympus BFP30. For children unable to accommodate this bronchoscope, transbronchial biopsy via flexible FOB is not possible.

More recently, transbronchial biopsy in children has been used in patients following lung transplantation to assess rejection and opportunistic infection and the adult pulmonologist may be asked to perform transbronchial biopsy in these patients (75). In the older child and adolescent, the technique is the same as in the adult. In small children biopsy may require general anesthesia and intubation to pass a sufficiently large flexible bronchoscope to obtain the specimen via the forceps (76).

Brushings

Although ample data describe the use and benefits of both open and protected specimen brushes in adults, there is no such information for children and infants (77–79). Again, as for transbronchial biopsy, the use of brushings in children is limited by the size of the working channel. For older children and adolescents who can accommodate large enough bronchoscopes, open and protected specimen brushes are used similarly to that in adults. And, since the specimen size obtained is determined by the size of the brush not by the actual return (as in BAL), specimen processing for brushes in children is accomplished exactly as that for adults.

Recently, the technique of protected BAL has been described, combining the protected brush with BAL for microbiologic sampling of the lower respiratory tract (80). Unfortunately, these catheters are also too large to pass through the pediatric-sized bronchoscope. Until smaller brushes become available for widespread use, BAL will continue to be the most reliable technique for microbiologic assessment of the lower respiratory tract in infants and small children.

Instillation of Medications

Standard medications such as lidocaine and epinephrine are routinely instilled via the bron-
choscope with good therapeutic effect. Cautious instillation of N-acetyl cysteine (Mucomyst) solution into areas of mucous plugging has also been used as an adjunct to therapy during bronchoscopy.

Recent work in the field of recombinant DNA technology has resulted in the availability of new gene therapy strategies that may have a significant impact on children with hereditary pulmonary diseases (81,82). In the future, the delivery of these gene products such as the CFTR gene for the treatment of cystic fibrosis or the alpha1-antitrypsin gene for the treatment of hereditary emphysema may best be accomplished by direct, definitive instillation to the lower tract via flexible FOB (71). Further, studies using aerosolized alpha1-antitrypsin and aerosolized insulin suggest that the lung is a potential safe portal of delivery for a variety of therapeutic proteins. At least initially, these drugs may need to be delivered with the precision afforded by flexible FOB (83).

Use of Pediatric Bronchoscopes in Adult Patients

Even when considering all of the possible indications and uses for bronchoscopy in pediatric patients, it is still unlikely that the adult pulmonologist will have much opportunity to use these pediatric instruments in children. It is more likely that the adult pulmonologist will use the smaller pediatric bronchoscopes in adults. It was not until 1985 that the first reported use of pediatric bronchoscopes in adults appeared (84). Because their length is the same as the adult bronchoscope (550 mm), the smallest pediatric instruments with suction channels allow entry into an additional three to five distal generations of bronchi with good visualization. Because of their small size, the pediatric bronchoscope can be a useful diagnostic adjunct in certain adult patients (Table 23.9).

Table 23.9. Uses of Pediatric Bronchoscopes in Adult Patients

Entry through small nasal passage

Upper airway endoscopy

Entry through an area of airway stenosis

Entry alongside an endotracheal or tracheostomy tube

Cryptogenic hemoptysis

Chronic cough

Aid to intubation

Carlens tube placement and positioning

Exercise laryngoscopy

For the evaluations of cryptogenic hemoptysis and chronic cough in which the airway examination is negative with the adult bronchoscope, repeating the examination with a pediatric instrument for access to the more distal subsegments has been suggested as a method for increasing the diagnostic yield (84).

The smaller bronchoscopes may allow entry and examination into regions the larger bronchoscopes cannot safely traverse such as through areas of airway stenosis or narrowing. Carlens tube insertion and placement can be performed using the smaller instruments and the smallest bronchoscopes can be passed *alongside* an endotracheal tube, if indicated.

One other use of the pediatric bronchoscope is when entry via the nasal route is desired and partial obstruction or narrowing of the anatomy prevents safe passage of a larger bronchoscope. Similarly, comfortable resting and exercise laryngoscopy can be adequately performed using the pediatric bronchoscope in adults if a flexible laryngoscope is not available (50).

Contraindications and Complications

There are no absolute contraindications to flexible FOB in children. However, if the adult pulmonologist is inexperienced or uncomfortable with performing bronchoscopy in children and the situation is not emergent, referral is prudent. Table 23.10 lists situations that present a serious risk of complication during pediatric bronchoscopy (27). Patients with thrombocytopenia, serious bleeding disorders, or coagulopathies can almost always safely undergo diagnostic bronchoscopy and lavage, particularly if no biopsy is obtained. Serious upper airway obstruction or severe bronchospasm do warrant careful consideration because FOB can induce or exacerbate both conditions (8). Never should the endoscope be passed through an area of severe narrowing in the upper airway that could lead to total occlusion. If hypoxia is amenable to correction via bronchoscopy, such as in the removal of mucous plugging, then obviously the procedure should not be withheld.

Serious complications related to flexible FOB in children are uncommon (7,8,36,85). Table 23.11 lists the most common complications that may occur related to flexible FOB in pediatric patients. The complications can be divided into adverse effects of medication used before or during the procedure and adverse effects related to the bronchoscopic examination itself.

Over 50% of all reported complications are related to adverse reactions to medications (27). In one large series of pediatric bronchoscopies, reported complications included transient bradycardia (1%), epistaxis (0.7%), anesthetic complications (0.5%), laryngospasm (0.3%), and pneumothorax (0.2%) with an overall complication incidence of 2.9% (8). In another series of bronchoscopy procedures performed in children with bronchopulmonary dysplasia, the overall complication rate was 3.1%, none of which were severe (36). Minor complications such as transient bradycardia or transient hypoxemia often occur in infants or small children during any type of manipulation and can be avoided by careful attention to technique. Hypoxemia may require supplemental oxygen during the procedure. In one

Table 23.10. Situations That Present Serious Risk of Complications during Pediatric Bronchoscopy

Coaguloapathy

Bleeding diathesis (that cannot be corrected)

Massive hemoptysis

Severe airway obstruction

Severe refractory hypoxemia

Unstable hemodynamics

Arrhythmias

Inexperienced physicians

Inadequate training in pediatric life support

Table 23.11. Complications of Pediatric Flexible Bronchoscopy

Procedure Related

Transient bradycardia

Transient hypoxemia

Epistaxis

Laryngospasm

Pneumothorax

Hemoptysis

Nosocomial infection

Aspiration

Medication Related

Patient discomfort (undersedation)

Respiratory depression (oversedation)

Inadequate topical anesthesia

    Vagal stimulation

    Laryngospasm

    Excessive cough

    Bradycardia

Urticaria

Paradoxical agitation (i.e., benzodiazepines)

study of 36 children undergoing bronchoscopy for a variety of indications, 81% had a fall in the oxygen saturation of greater than 5% during the procedure, although the majority still maintained saturations above 90% (86). Patients less than 12 months of age had the greatest drop in saturation and those over 7 years of age, the smallest drop. All patients returned to their baseline values after the procedure. In general, if patients develop hypoxia during bronchoscopy that is correctable with supplemental oxygen, the procedure can be completed safely.

Hemoptysis as a result of bronchoscopy is most commonly associated with transbronchial biopsy and is therefore uncommon in pediatric patients (7,8). If hemoptysis occurs but is localized and does not obscure the field of view, wedge or Fogarty occlusion can sometimes control the bleeding segment.

Inadequate use of topical anesthesia (either too much or too little) can result in adverse reactions such as laryngospasm, bradycardia or other vagally mediated phenomena. Nosocomial infections should not occur with proper sterilization and maintenance of bronchoscopy equipment.

Recent evidence suggests that BAL induces a local influx of neutrophils into the lung with the release of cytokines (87,88). This effect may be responsible for the fever that is fre-

quently observed to occur after bronchoscopy with BAL. However, if persistent for more than 24 hours, another cause for the fever should be sought. Finally, there is only one reported death related to FOB in children, occuring in a 20-month-old patient 22 hours following flexible FOB (89). However, there are no reported cases of fatality during or as a direct result of the procedure itself in pediatric patients.

Summary

Flexible FOB is now a part of the routine diagnostic and therapeutic examination for neonates, infants, and children with selected pulmonary diseases and for children in the pediatric ICU. Pediatric pulmonologists continue to be trained to meet the volume demands of these patients. However, until supply meets demand, adult pulmonologists will need to be able to perform bronchoscopy in pediatric patients. Technically, there are many similarities between adult and pediatric bronchoscopy. However, unsuspected differences between the two procedures preclude automatic extrapolation from adults to children (21,90). The adult pulmonologist can feel comfortable and competent to perform bronchoscopy in pediatric patients if careful attention is paid to the limitations imposed on bronchoscopy when applied to children.

REFERENCES

1. Tucker JA, Silberman JM. Flexible fiberoptic pediatric bronchoscope: a new instrument. Ann Otorhinolaryngol 1978;87:558–559.
2. Prakash UBS, Offord KP, Stubbs SE. Bronchoscopy in North America: the ACCP survey. Chest 1991;100:1668–1675.
3. Prakash UBS, Stubbs SE. The bronchoscopy survey: some reflections. Chest 1991;100:1660–1667.
4. Pediatric Pulmonary 1985 Manpower Study. Long range planning committee for pediatric pulmonology. Pediatrics 1988;81:680–685.
5. Graduate Medical Education Directory 1993–1994. American Medical Association, 99–101;108–109.
6. Wood RE, Pick JR. Model systems for learning pediatric flexible bronchoscopy. Pediatr Pulmonol 1990;8:168–171.
7. Wood RE, Postma D. Endoscopy of the airway in infants and children. J Pediatr 1988;112:1–6.
8. Wood RE. Spelunking on the pediatric airways: explorations with the flexible fiberoptic bronchoscope. Pediatr Clin North Am 1984;31:785–799.
9. Wood RE. Bronchoscopy. In: Laughlin GM, Eigen H, eds. Respiratory disease in children: diagnosis and management. Baltimore: Williams & Wilkins, 1994:117–133.
10. Tucker HM. Embryology and developmental anatomy. In: The larynx. New York: Thieme Medical Publishers, 1993:19–22.
11. Eavey RD. The pediatric larynx. In: Fried MF. The larynx: a multidisciplinary approach. Boston: Little, Brown, 1988.
12. Hislip A, Muir DCF, Jacobsen M, Simon G, Reid L. Postnatal growth and function of the pre-acinar airways. Thorax 1972;27:265–274.
13. Wohl MEB, Mead J. Age as a factor in respiratory disease. In: Chernick V, ed. Disorders of the respiratory tract in children. Philadelphia: WB Saunders, 1990:175–182.
14. Murry JF. Postnatal growth and development of the lung. In: The normal lung, 2nd ed. Philadelphia: WB Saunders, 1986:23–25.
15. Motoyama EK, Brody JS, Colten NR, Warshaw JB. Postnatal lung development in health and disease. Am Rev Respir Dis 1988;137:742–746.
16. Hiatt P, Eigen H, Yu P, Tepper RS. Bronchodilator responsiveness in infants and young children with cystic fibrosis. Am Rev Respir Dis 1988;137:119–122.
17. Motoyama EK, Fort MD, Klesh KW, Mutich RL, Guthrie RD. Early onset of airway reactivity in premature infants with bronchopulmonary dysplasia. Am Rev Respir Dis 1987;136:50–57.
18. Johnson K, ed. The Harriet Lane handbook, 13th ed. St. Louis: Mosby-Yearbook, 1993:13–14.
19. Arnold J, Casto C. Endotracheal intubation. In: Blummer JL, ed. A practical guide to pediatric intensive care, 3rd ed. St. Louis: Mosby-Yearbook, 1990:926–927.
20. American Academy of Pediatrics, Committee on Drugs. Guidelines for monitoring and management of pediatric patients during and after sedation for diagnostic and therapeutic procedures. Pediatrics 1992;89:1110–1115.
21. Wood RE. Pitfalls in the use of the flexible bronchoscope in pediatric patients. Chest 1990;97:199–203.
22. Snodgrass WR, Dodge WF. Lytic/"DPT" cocktail: time for rational and safe alternatives. Pediatr Clin North Am 1989;36:1285–1291.
23. American Academy of Pediatrics, Committee on Drugs, Section of Anesthesiology. Guidelines for the elective use of conscious sedation, deep sedation and general anesthesia in pediatric patients. Pediatrics 1985;76:317–332.
24. Goodman-Gilman A, ed. The pharmacological basis of therapeutics, 8th ed. New York: Pergamon Press, 1990.

25. Physician's desk reference, 48th ed. Montvale, NJ: Medical Economic Data Production Company, 1994.

26. Drug facts and comparisons, 48th ed. St. Louis: Facts and Comparisons, 1994.

27. Green CG, Eisenberg J, Leong A, Nathanson I, Schnapf BM, Wood RE. Flexible endoscopy of the pediatric airway. Am Rev Respir Dis 1992;134:233–235.

28. Wood RE. The diagnostic effectiveness of the flexible bronchoscope in children. Pediatr Pulmonol 1985;1:188–192.

29. Fitzpatrick SB, Marsh B, Stokes D, Wang KP. Indications for flexible fiberoptic bronchoscopy in pediatric patients. Am J Dis Children 1983;137:595–597.

30. Vernon DD, Sarnaik AP. Acute epiglottitis in children: a conservative approach to diagnosis and management. Crit Care Med 1986; 14:23–25.

31. Levin DS, Springer MA. Croup and epiglottitis. In: Hilman B, ed. Pediatric respiratory disease: diagnosis and treatment. Philadelphia: WB Saunders, 1993:238–240.

32. Swan Y, Newth CJL. Acute upper airway obstruction. In: Laughlin GM, Eigen H, eds. Respiratory diseases in children: diagnosis and management. Baltimore: Williams & Wilkins, 1994:319–333.

33. Stillwell PC, Radford PJ. Should all children with stridor undergo fiberoptic bronchoscopy? J Bronchol 1994;13:276–280.

34. Nussbaum E. Pediatric flexible bronchoscopy and its application in infantile atelectasis. Clin Pediatr 1985;24:379–382.

35. Shinwell ES. Ultrathin fiberoptic bronchoscopy for airway toilet in neonatal pulmonary atelectasis. Pediatr Pulmonol 1992; 13:48–49.

36. Cohn RC, Kercsmar C, Dearborn D. Safety and efficacy of flexible endoscopy in children with bronchopulmonary dysplasia. Am J Dis Child 1988;142:1225–1228.

37. Benjamen B, Curley JW. Infant tracheostomy: endoscopy and decannulation. Int J Pediatr Otorhinolaryngol 1990;20:113–121.

38. Mu L, Sun D, He P. Radiological diagnosis of aspirated foreign bodies in children: review of 343 cases. J Laryngol Otol 1990;104:778–782.

39. Mantor PC, Tuggle DW, Tunell WP. An appropriate negative bronchoscopy rate in suspected foreign body aspiration. Am J Surg 1989;158:622–624.

40. Svedstrum E, Puhakka H, Kero P. How accurate is chest radiography in the diagnosis of tracheobronchial foreign bodies in children? Pediatr Radiol 1989;19:520–522.

41. Pasaoglu I, Dogan R, Demircin M, Hatipoglu A, Bozer AY. Bronchoscopic removal of foreign bodies in children: retrospective analysis of 822 cases. Thorac Cardiovasc Surg 1991;39:95–98.

42. Wood RE, Gauderer MWL. Flexible fiberoptic bronchoscopy in the management of tracheobronchial foreign bodies in children: the value of a combined approach with open tube bronchoscopy. J Pediatric Surg 1984;19:693–695.

43. Wood RE. Flexible bronchoscopy to remove foreign bodies in children—yes, maybe, but ... J Bronchol 1994;1:87.

44. Castro M, Midthun DE, Edell ES, Stelck MJ, Prakash UBS. Flexible bronchoscopic removal of foreign bodies from pediatric airways. J Bronchol 1994;1:92–98.

45. Rayet I, Navez M, Freycon MT, Prudes JM. Endoscopic extraction of a foreign body from the distal bronchus in the middle lobe, inaccessible by usual techniques, in a 3-year-old child. Pediatrics 1992;47:589–591.

46. Cohen SR, Levis GB, Herbert WI, Geller KA. Foreign bodies in the airway. Five-year retrospective study with special reference to management. Ann Otol 1980;89:437–444.

47. Cunanan OS. The flexible fiberoptic bronchoscope in foreign body removal: experience in 300 cases. Chest 1979;73:725–726.

48. Christopher KL, Wood RP, Eckert C, Blager FR, Raney RA, Souhrada MD. Vocal cord dysfunction presenting as asthma. N Engl J Med 1983;308:1566–1570.

49. Brugman SM, Howell JH, Rosenberg DM, Blager FB, Lack G. The spectrum of pediatric vocal cord dysfunction. Am J Resp Crit Care Med 1994;149:A353.

50. Rovner MS, Stillwell PC. Exercise-induced vocal cord dysfunction in pediatric athletes with exercise-induced asthma. Am J Resp Crit Care Med 1994;149:A354.

51. Colombo JF, Halberg TK. Recurrent aspiration in children: lipid-laden alveolar macrophage quantitation. Pediatr Pulmonol 1987;3:86–89.

52. Corwin RW, Irwin RS. The lipid-laden macrophage as a marker of aspiration in

parenchymal lung disease. Am Rev Respir Dis 1985;132:576–581.

53. Prober CG, Whyte H, Smith CR. Open lung biopsy in immunocompromised children with pulmonary infiltrates. Am J Dis Child 1984;138:60–63.

54. Griffiths MH, Kocjan G, Miller RF, Godfrey-Faussett P. Diagnosis of pulmonary disease in human immunodeficiency virus infection: role of transbronchial biopsy and bronchoalveolar lavage. Thorax 1989;44:554–558.

55. Abadco DL, Amaro-Galvez R, Rao M, Steiner P. Experience with flexible fiberoptic bronchoscopy with bronchoalveolar lavage as a diagnostic tool in children with AIDS. Am J Dis Child 1992;146:1056–1059.

56. Birriel JA, Adams JA, Saldana MA, et al. Role of flexible bronchoscopy and bronchoalveolar lavage in the diagnosis of pediatric acquired immunodeficiency syndrome-related pulmonary disease. Pediatrics 1991; 87:897–899.

57. Bye RM, Bernstein L, Shah K, Ellawie M, Rubinstein A. Diagnostic bronchoalveolar lavage in children with AIDS. Pediatric Pulmonol 1987;3:425–428.

58. deBlic J, Blanche S, Danel C, LeBourgeois M, Caniglia M, Scheinmann P. Bronchoalveolar lavage in HIV infected patients with interstitial pneumonitis. Arch Dis Child 1989;64: 1246–1250.

59. McCubbin MM, Trigg ME, Hendrickar CM, Wagener JS. Bronchoscopy with bronchoalveolar lavage in the evaluation of pulmonary complications of bone marrow transplantation in children. Pediatr Pulmonol 1992;12:43–47.

60. Pattishall EN, Noyes BE, Orenstein DM. Use of bronchoalveolar lavage in immunocompromised children with pneumonia. Pediatr Pulmonol 1988;5:1–5.

61. Stokes DC, Shenep JL, Perham D, Bozeman DM, Marienchek W, Mackert PW. Role of flexible bronchoscopy in the diagnosis of pulmonary infiltrates in pediatric patients with cancer. J Pediatr 1989;115:561–567.

62. Rigal E, Roze JC, Villers D, et al. Prospective evaluation of the protected specimen brush for the diagnosis of pulmonary infections in ventilated newborns. Pediatr Pulmonol 1990;8:268–272.

63. Fan LL, Sparks LM, Fix JE. Flexible fiberoptic endoscopy for airway problems in a pediatric intensive care unit. Chest 1988;93: 556–560.

64. Mallory GB, Stillwell PC. Flexible fiberoptic bronchoscopy in the critically ill infant and child. In: Dieckmann RA, Fiser DH, Selbst S. Illustrated textbook of pediatric emergency and critical care procedures. St. Louis: CV Mosby, in press.

65. Baines DB, Goodrick MA, Beckenham EJ, Overton JA. Fiberoptically guided endotracheal intubation in a child. Anesth Intensive Care 1989;17:354–356.

66. Finer NN, Muzyka D. Flexible endoscopic intubation of the neonate. Pediatr Pulmonol 1992;12:48–51.

67. Wilder RT, Belani KG. Fiberoptic intubation complicated by pulmonary edema in a 12-year-old child with Hurler's syndrome. Anesthesiology 1990;72:205–207.

68. Scheller JG, Schulman SR. Fiberoptic bronchoscopic guidance for intubating a neonate with Pierre-Robin syndrome. J Clin Anesth 1991;3:45–47.

69. deLina LA, Bishop MJ. Lung laceration after tracheal extubation over a plastic tube changer. Anesth Analg 1991;73:350–351.

70. Vigneswaran R, Whitfield JM. The use of a new ultrathin fiberoptic bronchoscope to determine endotracheal tube position in the sick newborn infant. Chest 1981;80:174–177.

71. Dietrich KA, Strauss RH, Cabalka AK, Zimmermann JJ, Scanlan KA. Use of flexible fiberoptic endoscopy for determination of endotracheal tube position in the pediatric patient. Crit Care Med 1988;16:884–887.

72. Reynolds HY. State of the art: bronchoalveolar lavage. Am Rev Respir Dis 1987; 135:250–263.

73. Wood RE. Flexible bronchoscopy in children. In: Hilman B, ed. Pediatric respiratory disease: diagnosis and treatment. Philadelphia: WB Saunders, 1993:111–122.

74. Perez CR, Wood RE. Update on pediatric flexible bronchoscopy. Pediatr Clin North Am 1994;41:385–400.

75. Kurland G, Blakeslee E, Noyes E, et al. Bronchoalveolar lavage and transbronchial biopsy in children following heart-lung and lung transplantation. Chest 1993;104:1043–1045.

76. Whitehead B, Scott JP, Helms P, et al. Technique and use of transbronchial biopsy in children and adolescents. Pediatr Pulmonol 1992;12:240–246.

77. Wimberley N, Faling JL, Bartlett JG. A fiberoptic bronchoscopy technique to obtain uncontaminated lower airway secretions for bacterial culture. Am Rev Respir Dis 1979; 119:337–343.

78. Wimberley NW, Bass JB, Boyd BW, Kirkpatrick MB, Serio RA, Pollok HM. Use of a bronchoscopic catheter brush for the diagnosis of pulmonary infections. Chest 1982;81:556–562.

79. Timsit JP, Misset B, Francoual S, Goldstein FW, Vary P, Coulet J. Is protected specimen brush a reproducible method to diagnose ICU-acquired pneumonia? Chest 1993;104: 104–108.

80. Meduri GU, Beals DH, Mayub AG, Baselski V. Protected bronchoalveolar lavage: a new bronchoscope technique to retrieve uncontaminated distal airway secretions. Am Rev Respir Dis 1991;143:855–864.

81. Rosenfeld MA, Yoshimura K, Trapnell BC, et al. In vivo transfer of the human cystic fibrosis transmembrane conductance regulator gene to the airway epithelium. Cell 1992; 68:143–155.

82. Crystal RG. Gene therapy strategies for pulmonary diseases. Am J Med 1992; 92(6A):44S–52S.

83. Hubbard RC, Crystal RG. Strategies for aerosol therapy of alpha 1-antitrypsin deficiency by the aerosol route. Lung 1990; 168(suppl):565–578.

84. Prakash UBS. The use of the pediatric fiberoptic bronchoscope in adults. Am Rev Respir Dis 1985;132:715–717.

85. Weiss SM, Hert RC, Gianola FJ, Clark JG, Crawford SW. Complications of fiberoptic bronchoscopy in thrombocytopenic patients. Chest 1993;104:1025–1028.

86. Schnapf BM. Oxygen desaturation during fiberoptic bronchoscopy in pediatric patients. Chest 1991;99:591–594.

87. Krombach F, Fiehl E, Burkhardt D, et al. Short-term and long-term effects of serial bronchoalveolar lavage in a non-human primate model. Am J Respir Crit Care Med 1994;150:153–158.

88. Standifano TJ, Kunkel SL, Strieter RM. Elevated serum levels of tumor necrosis factor-alpha after bronchoscopy and bronchoalveolar lavage. Chest 1991;99: 1529–1530.

89. Wagener JS. Fatality following fiberoptic bronchoscopy in a two-year-old child. Pediatr Pulmonol 1987;3:197–199.

90. Prakash UBS, Stubbs SE. Optimal bronchoscopy. J Bronchol 1994;1:44–62.

24 | The Role of Spiral Computed Tomography in the Evaluation of Lung Cancer

Anwar R. Padhani and Elliot K. Fishman

Over the past 15 years, computed tomography (CT) systems have undergone continuous development in terms of increased spatial resolution, decreased scanning time, and decreased computation time needed for image display. Spiral or helical CT is the latest technical advance in this field.

The concept of spiral CT was introduced at the 1989 Radiological Society of North America meeting and then described by Kalender and colleagues (1) and Vock and colleagues (2). The idea is straightforward: allow for continuous scanning and data acquisition with the patient advanced through a CT gantry at a constant rate. The resultant path described by the x-ray beam is that of a spiral or helix (Figure 24.1). During the acquisition of data, the patient is instructed to breath-hold to eliminate motion artifacts. The resultant data represent a volume of attenuation values. The maximum scan time is a function of both the characteristics of the x-ray tube and the computer storage available. On the Somatom Plus S scanner (Siemens Medical Systems, Iselin, NJ), the maximum imaging time is 32 seconds at 210 mA or 40 seconds at 165 mA. Manufacturers are likely to increase imaging time to 50 to 60 seconds in the near future.

Advantages and Disadvantages

The rapidity with which the CT data can be acquired is the principle advantage of spiral CT. Rapid scanning with intravenous contrast

using spiral CT can consistently be carried out at peak vascular enhancement. Another advantage of spiral CT scanning is reduced contrast media requirements. Costello and associates (3) have shown that contrast volumes can be substantially reduced by at least 30% to 50%. The reduction of contrast dose is particularly beneficial for the elderly, for patients with renal impairment, and for other groups of patients at high risk for nephrotoxicity. Other potential advantages of lower dose scanning include fewer side effects, less contrast artifacts, and greater cost savings.

A major advantage of spiral CT is that images with no respiratory motion are acquired. An essentially gapless volume of data without discontinuities between slices is obtained. This accurate volume of data can be

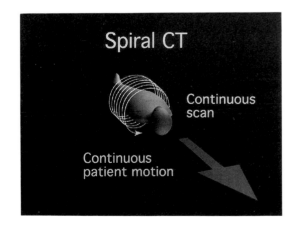

Figure 24.1. Spiral CT scanning. The x-ray tube rotates continuously while the patient moves at a steady rate through the CT gantry, thus describing a helix or spiral.

viewed not only as transaxial images but also as multiplanar reconstructions (e.g., coronal, sagittal, or other user-defined oblique planes). The data so obtained are also ideal for cine display and three-dimensional imaging. The technique may also prove to be useful for the assessment of the airways and to study vascular physiology.

Disadvantages of limitation in the milliamps is mostly seen in the abdomen and are less severe in the chest. This disadvantage is being overcome due to refinements in detector technology and x-ray tubes with larger heat capacities. Longer periods of spiral scanning are possible but the limitations in milliamps limits its widespread applicability due to increasing signal-to-noise ratio with increasing scan time. Other disadvantages include the necessity to allow tube cooling and computer system delays between helical and nonhelical scanning. The ability to acquire images early can result in vascular flow artifacts although these are generally not seen in applications in the chest.

Spiral Applications in the Chest

Evaluation of the Pulmonary Nodule

The introduction of spiral volumetric scanning has added a new dimension to the assessment of pulmonary nodules (4,5). Spiral CT is now the method of choice for the detection and characterization of solitary nodules. Costello and colleagues (5) compared standard and spiral CT in 20 patients with suspected pulmonary nodules less than one cm. Using a spiral CT protocol of 10-mm thickness and a table feed of 10 mm/sec with interpolated data reconstructed at 4-mm intervals, spiral CT detected 4 of 22 nodules that were missed on standard CT due to respiration-induced misregistration.

Spiral CT with smaller interscan spacing is likely to result in increased detection of pulmonary nodules. This is particularly true for small lesions and for nodules at the lung bases.

The ability to retrospectively reconstruct overlapping scans results in better visualization of small lesions without additional radiation exposure and is a chief advantage of spiral CT. This process is currently relatively time consuming, however, with reconstruction times of approximately 8 to 9 seconds per slice. However, upgrades to computer systems on newer scanner models will reduce this to around one second. Equally important, the ability to retrospectively reconstruct the raw data and shift the slice location, together with the high spatial resolution of spiral CT, allow the nodule centers to be accurately assessed by densitometry (2).

Evaluation of the Tracheobronchial Tree, Hila with Multiplanar Reconstructions

The usefulness of multiplanar imaging in patients with lung cancer has been evaluated using magnetic resonance imaging (MRI). Multiplanar imaging has been found useful in the evaluation of superior sulcus tumors, in tumors that abut the diaphragm, in the evaluation of chest wall invasion, and in the assessment of mediastinal invasion (6). MRI, however, has not replaced CT in the primary evaluation of patients with lung cancer. The ability to image in a multiplanar fashion using CT data reinforces CT's dominance in this area.

Traditionally, multiplanar reconstructions (MPRs) using CT data have been poor because the imaging time needed to acquire the large number of cuts often resulted in interscan motion due to uneven respiratory efforts. In addition, the inability to maintain optimal contrast enhancement throughout data acquisition resulted in suboptimal images. These problems can be minimized with a single breath-hold spiral CT data acquisition. Interscan motion can usually be eliminated and fast scanning with properly timed injection of contrast material results in optimal arterial and venous opacification. These data are ideal for MPR and three-dimensional imaging.

Primary Tumor Evaluation with Spiral CT

Tumor Size

Lesion size is one factor that distinguishes a T1 from a T2 lesion. Although maximum dimension has been emphasized, tumor size may not appear accurately in the transaxial dimension and size determined from spiral CT-generated MPRs is more accurate. Volume data sets also provide the ability for accurate tumor volumetrics. Whether this is important in staging remains an unanswered question.

Chest Wall Invasion

Generally the results of CT in predicting chest wall invasion are disappointing, with local pain being as sensitive an indicator of invasion as CT (7). MRI, with a sensitivity of 94% versus 63% for CT, appears to be more sensitive in determining chest wall invasion because of its excellent contrast resolution as well as its multiplanar imaging capability (8). The potential sensitivity of spiral CT-acquired MPRs is undetermined but is likely to be intermediate.

Superior Sulcus Tumors

The MRI is superior to CT in detecting chest wall invasion in cases of superior sulcus or Pancoast tumor, as well as in the evaluation of other structures such as the brachial plexus, blood vessels, and vertebral body and canal. MRI axial images alone have no advantage over axial CT but MRI's multiplanar capability gives it an edge in depicting these structures (6). In addition, signal characteristics are helpful in the evaluation of invasion. However, MRI frequently fails to demonstrate rib destruction and CT-acquired multiplanar images may prove as useful as MRI in the evaluation of these lesions (Figure 24.2). The use of computer workstations for review of multiplanar CT data can be valuable in optimizing the orthogonal planes chosen for image display.

Mediastinal Pleura

Neither CT nor MRI has been valuable in diagnosing mediastinal pleural invasion. Contiguity of tumor with pleura does not necessarily indicate invasion and only with definite evidence of invasion or interdigitation by tumor can invasion be confirmed. Spiral CT-acquired MPRs are unlikely to provide additional information in this regard unless definite invasion is documented.

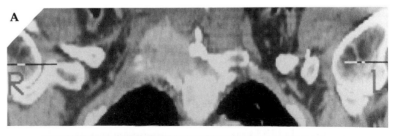

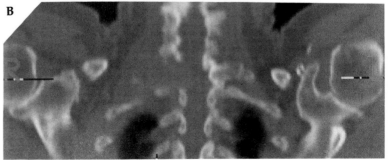

Figure 24.2. *A*, Oblique transaxial (soft tissue window) and (*B*), coronal (bony window) reconstruction in a patient with a right apex mass. The mass is well seen with bony destruction and thecal encroachment. Here the superiority of CT imaging to demonstrate bony pathology together with its multiplanar capability are shown to advantage.

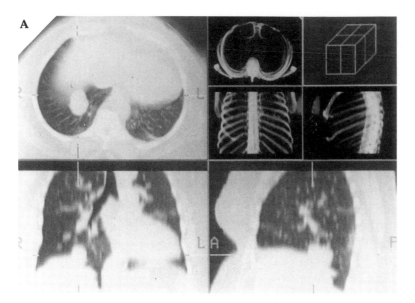

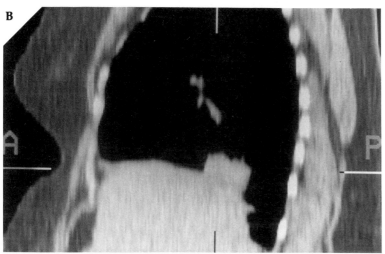

Figure 24.3. *A*, Multiplanar display (lung window) and (*B*), sagittal reconstruction (soft tissue window) show probable tumor invasion of the diaphragm. This was confirmed at lobectomy. The tumor was a metastatic thyroid cancer.

Pericardium and Diaphragm

The continuity of tumor to pericardium and diaphragm also does not necessarily indicate invasion. Lesions that abut the diaphragm are ideally suited for imaging in the coronal or sagittal plane. Spiral-generated multiplanar images are superior to MRI in this regard because the suspended respiratory motion results in sharp delineation of the diaphragm (Figure 24.3).

Tracheobronchial Tree

The relationship of tumor to the tracheo-bronchial tree is important both for staging and for surgical planning. Although trans-axial CT is excellent for the detection of endo-bronchial lesions, its overall accuracy in predicting bronchial involvement is limited. Partial volume averaging can create errors and the transaxial plane of imaging is not ideal. The optimal transaxial technique requires thin sections to evaluate the bronchi, which can be achieved with our protocol. The trachea and the major bronchi, however, are better demonstrated in the coronal plane using spiral-generated MPRs (Figure 24.4). This technique is likely to be more accurate in predicting tracheobronchial invasion but needs further clinical evaluation.

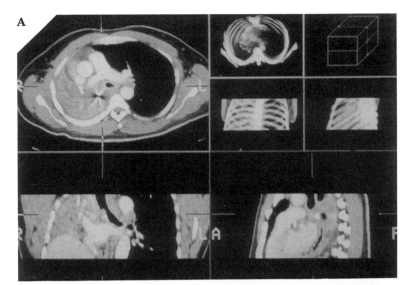

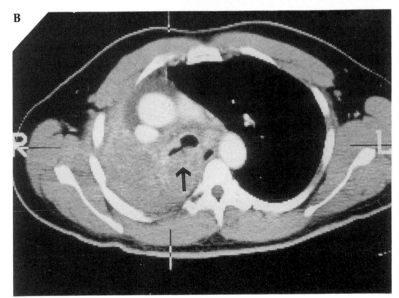

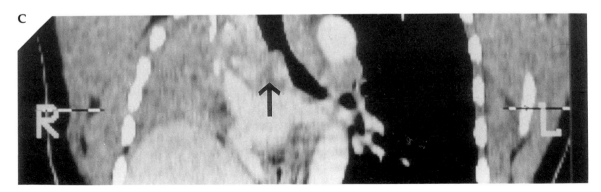

Figure 24.4. Recurrent lung cancer. A non–small–cell lung cancer diagnosed 3 years previously was treated with a right upper lobectomy and postoperative radiation. *A,* Multiplanar display. *B,* Trans-axial image reveals a right hilar and subcarinal recurrence (*arrow*), mediastinal invasion, narrowing of the right lower lobe bronchus and distal atelectasis. *C,* Coronal reconstruction shows tumor involvement of the lower trachea, carina, and both main bronchi with complete occlusion of the right lower lobe bronchus. Bronchoscopy showed tumor involving the lower trachea and carina with almost complete occlusion of the right main bronchus. The left main bronchus was also involved by tumor. The coronal reconstructions were useful in guiding successful laser coagulation.

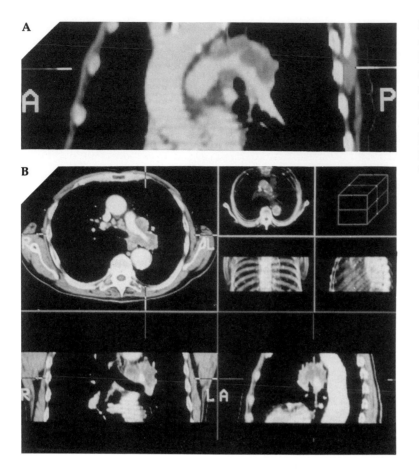

Figure 24.5. A, Multiplanar display demonstrates a left hilar mass with mediastinal adenopathy. B, The oblique sagittal reconstruction shows tumor encasement and narrowing of the left pulmonary artery. Note the prominent pulsation artifacts of the vascular structures.

Invasion of the Mediastinum, Heart, and Great Vessels

Involvement of these structures indicates advanced cancer (T4). Excellent vascular opacification is essential for the diagnosis of vascular invasion. Although this diagnosis using transaxial CT can be made confidently, most investigators believe that MRI is more sensitive than CT. However, the excellent vascular opacification together with thin cuts and the MPR capability of spiral CT should make it more sensitive than conventional CT. In addition, spiral CT should replace the occasional use of angiography in the evaluation of vascular involvement by lung cancer (9) (Figure 24.5).

Lymph Node Evaluation with Spiral CT

A large number of studies have produced an enormous amount of data and with it controversy and confusion regarding the role of CT in staging mediastinal lymph node metastases in patients with lung cancer. The goal of these studies was to determine whether CT can accurately detect the presence of mediastinal metastases in patients with lung cancer. A detailed discussion of this is beyond the scope of this chapter and the reader is directed to many excellent review articles (10,11). Given the variability of CT in the evaluation of lymph nodes in these studies, it is questionable whether CT has much utility in the evaluation of adenopathy. CT and mediastinoscopy should be considered complementary procedures and surgical candidates should be considered for both. Patients without enlarged lymph nodes (less than one cm) should proceed to surgery and, to detect the true pathologic stage of the disease, should have a thorough mediastinal dissection. Metastases to these nodes is uncommon, occurring in approximately 7% of all cases. It seems reasonable to proceed directly to surgery in these patients with an expectation of 90% to 95% that no N2 disease will be found. Furthermore, patients with microscopic metastases noted at time of surgery have improved survival rates if the metastases and the primary tumor are all resected. In patients with enlarged lymph nodes by any criteria, a prethorocotomy staging procedure seems warranted (e.g., mediastinoscopy) due to the higher 20% to 30% false positive rate.

Currently, metastases to peribronchial parenchymal and ipsilateral hilar lymph nodes (N1) have been poorly demonstrated by conventional dynamic incremental CT. This can be attributed to several factors, including poor vascular opacification, older machines with slower scanning times, and the chosen imaging plane. Spiral-generated CT images, because of

their high level of vascular opacification and thin sections, consistently provide excellent depiction of these nodes. The MPRs show hilar nodes well and allow the differentiation of the right hilar pseudotumor from adenopathy (Figure 24.6), a well-known diagnostic pitfall in axial imaging (12). In addition, some lymph node groups are suboptimally evaluated in the transaxial plane, such as those in the anteroposterior window and in the subcarinal areas. Lymph nodes in these stations are well demonstrated with the multiplanar capability of spiral CT. This improved definition is helpful when planning bronchoscopically guided biopsy of mediastinal lymph nodes. The differentiation of malignant and benign lymph nodes, however, by size criteria using any imaging modality is controversial.

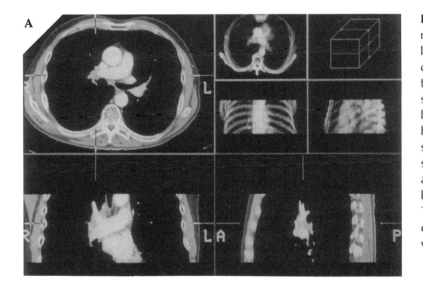

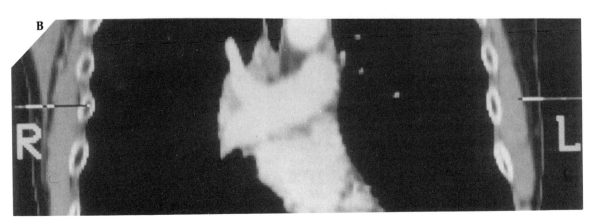

Figure 24.6. A 66-year-old male smoker with a 2.5-cm left upper lobe adenocarcinoma (not shown). The transaxial reconstruction (A), shows a probably enlarged lymph node at the right hilum. The coronal reconstruction (B), shows two small lymph nodes medial and one lateral to the upper lobe pulmonary artery origin. These nodes were anthracotic at surgery and uninvolved by tumor.

Future Roles for Spiral CT

One of the primary goals of imaging in lung cancer is to direct the investigation most likely to lead to a histologic diagnosis (e.g., bronchoscopy, mediastinoscopy, lung biopsy, etc.). Transaxial CT imaging has been shown to correlate well with bronchoscopy (13) in the assessment of solitary lung nodules. The relationship of a lung lesion to an adjacent bronchus is particularly well delineated using spiral CT because of its thin section reconstruction capability. This capability, together with MPR, may prove superior to transaxial imaging alone. In this regard, spiral CT may prove of use in performing needle tip localization for patients undergoing CT-guided lung aspiration/biopsy. We have found the MPRs to be useful in the planning of bronchoscopic sampling of mediastinal lymph nodes, but its value in approaching lung masses has not been studied. We have also found the multiplanar capability a valuable tool in the preplanning of patients for laser coagulation and brachytherapy but have not explored its use in planning radiotherapy.

REFERENCES

1. Kalendar WA, Seissler W, Klotz E, Vock P. Spiral volumetric CT with single-breath-hold technique, continuous transport, and continuous scanner rotation. Radiology 1990; 176:181–183.
2. Vock P, Soucek M, Daepp M, Kalender WA. Lung: spiral volumetric CT with single-breath-hold technique. Radiology 1990;176: 864–867.
3. Costello P, Dupuy DE, Ecker CP, Tello R. Spiral CT of the thorax with reduced volume of contrast material: a comparative study. Radiology 1992;183:663–666.
4. Shaffer K, Pugatch RD. Small pulmonary nodules: dynamic CT with single breath technique. Radiology 1989;173:567–568.
5. Costello P, Anderson W, Blume D. Pulmonary nodule: evaluation with spiral volumetric CT. Radiology 1991;179:875–876.
6. Templeton PA, Caskey CI, Zerhouni EA. Current uses of CT and MR imaging in the staging of lung cancer. Radiol Clin North Am 1990;28:631–646.
7. Glazer HS, Aronberg DJ, Sagel SS, et al. Pleural and chest wall invasion in bronchogenic cancer: CT evaluation. Radiology 1985;157:191–194.
8. Musset D, Grenier P, Carett MF, et al. Primary lung cancer staging: prospective comparative of MR imaging with CT. Radiology 1986;160:607–611.
9. Miyamoto H, Hayakawa K, Hata E, et al. Preoperative evaluation of digital subtraction pulmonary angiography in primary lung cancer. Kokyu To Junkan 1989;37:1209–1214.
10. Aronchick JM. CT of mediastinal lymph nodes in patients with non-small cell lung carcinoma. Radiol Clin North Am 1990; 28:573–581.
11. Libshitz HI. CT of mediastinal lymph nodes in lung cancer: is there a "state of the art"? AJR Am J Roentgenol 1983;141:1081.
12. Ashida C, Zerhouni EA, Fishman EK. CT demonstration of prominent right hilar soft tissue collections. J Comput Assist Tomogr 1987;11:57–59.
13. Naidich DP, Sussman R, Kutcher WL, et al. Solitary pulmonary nodules. CT-bronchoscopic correlation. Chest 1988;93:595–599.

Index